Malnutrition: Impacts on Health and Well-Being

Malnutrition: Impacts on Health and Well-Being

Edited by Logan Bowman

SYRAWOOD
PUBLISHING HOUSE
New York

Published by Syrawood Publishing House,
750 Third Avenue, 9th Floor,
New York, NY 10017, USA
www.syrawoodpublishinghouse.com

Malnutrition: Impacts on Health and Well-Being
Edited by Logan Bowman

International Standard Book Number: 978-1-68286-433-3 (Hardback)

Cataloging-in-publication Data

Malnutrition : impacts on health and well-being / edited by Logan Bowman.
p. cm.
Includes bibliographical references and index.
ISBN 978-1-68286-433-3
1. Malnutrition. 2. Malnutrition in children. 3. Nutrition disorders. 4. Nutrition. 5. Health. I. Bowman, Logan.
RA645.N87 M35 2017
614.593 9--dc23

Printed in China.

TABLE OF CONTENTS

PREFACE

Malnutrition is a vast field of study. It analyzes in detail the impact of diet on human body and effect of no or low nutrients in the diet. This book provides significant information of this discipline to help develop a comprehensive understanding of the subject. It includes some of the vital pieces of work being conducted across the world, on various topics related to malnutrition. Different approaches, evaluations, methodologies and advanced studies on malnutrition have been included in this book. It is a complete source of knowledge on the present status of this important field. This text is an essential guide for both academicians and those who wish to pursue this discipline further.

The information shared in this book is based on empirical researches made by veterans in this field of study. The elaborative information provided in this book will help the readers further their scope of knowledge leading to advancements in this field.

Finally, I would like to thank my fellow researchers who gave constructive feedback and my family members who supported me at every step of my research.

Editor

Follow-Up of Post-Discharge Growth and Mortality after Treatment for Severe Acute Malnutrition (FuSAM Study): A Prospective Cohort Study

Marko Kerac[1,2,3,4*], James Bunn[2,5], George Chagaluka[2], Paluku Bahwere[1,6], Andrew Tomkins[3], Steve Collins[1], Andrew Seal[3]

1 Valid International, Oxford, United Kingdom, **2** Department of Paediatrics and Child Health, College of Medicine, Blantyre, Malawi, **3** Institute for Global Health, University College London, London, United Kingdom, **4** Leonard Cheshire Disability and Inclusive Development Centre, University College London, London, United Kingdom, **5** Liverpool School of Tropical Medicine, Liverpool, United Kingdom, **6** Centre of Research in Epidemiology, Biostatistics and Clinical Research, Free University of Brussels, Brussels, Belgium

Abstract

Background: Management of Severe Acute Malnutrition (SAM) plays a vital role in achieving global child survival targets. Effective treatment programmes are available but little is known about longer term outcomes following programme discharge.

Methods: From July 2006 to March 2007, 1024 children (median age 21.5 months, IQR 15–32) contributed 1187 admission episodes to an inpatient-based SAM treatment centre in Blantyre, Malawi. Long term outcomes, were determined in a longitudinal cohort study, a year or more after initial programme discharge. We found information on 88%(899/1024).

Results: In total, 42%(427/1024) children died during or after treatment. 25%(105/427) of deaths occurred after normal programme discharge, >90 days after admission. Mortality was greatest among HIV seropositive children: 62%(274/445). Other risk factors included age <12 months; severity of malnutrition at admission; and disability. In survivors, weight-for-height and weight-for-age improved but height-for-age remained low, mean −2.97 z-scores (SD 1.3).

Conclusions: Although SAM mortality in this setting was unacceptably high, our findings offer important lessons for future programming, policy and research. First is the need for improved programme evaluation: most routine reporting systems would have missed late deaths and underestimated total mortality due to SAM. Second, a more holistic view of SAM is needed: while treatment will always focus on nutritional interventions, it is vital to also identify and manage underlying clinical conditions such as HIV and disability. Finally early identification and treatment of SAM should be emphasised: our results suggest that this could improve longer term as well as short term outcomes. As international policy and programming becomes increasingly focused on stunting and post-malnutrition chronic disease outcomes, SAM should not be forgotten. Proactive prevention and treatment services are essential, not only to reduce mortality in the short term but also because they have potential to impact on longer term morbidity, growth and development of survivors.

Editor: Philip Bejon, Kenya Medical Research Institute (KEMRI), Kenya

Funding: UNICEF Malawi funded this study. Valid International provided support in the form of salaries for authors MK (from end 2005 to Jan 2008 only - the 'baseline' period of this study) PB, and SC but did not have any additional role in the study design, data collection and analysis, decision to publish, or preparation of the manuscript. The specific roles of these authors are articulated in the 'author contributions' section. MK gratefully acknowledges NIHR for funding his current UCL Academic Clinical Lecturer post.

Competing Interests: Valid International (PB - current; SC - current; MK 2005-2008) provides consultancy services on the rollout of Community-based Management of Acute Malnutrition. All other authors have declared that no competing interests exist. At the time of the study, PB and MK (part time, till 2008 only) were employees of Valid International. SC is the unpaid director of Valid Nutrition. Valid International is the sister company of Valid Nutrition that promotes the development and promotion of RUTF. This does not alter our adherence to all the PLoS ONE policies on sharing data and materials.

* E-mail: marko.kerac@gmail.com

Background

Severe acute malnutrition (SAM) is a major global public health problem [1],[2]. It includes two forms of malnutrition, oedematous malnutrition (kwashiorkor) and severe wasting (low weight-for-height and/or low mid upper arm circumference) [3]. Severe wasting alone affects 18.7 million children (95% CI 14.2 to 23.2 million) aged under 5 years and is responsible for over half a million deaths per year (7.4 to 7.8% of total under-5 child deaths) [4]. Treating SAM thus has an important role to play towards global health initiatives such as Millennium Development Goal 4, decreasing child mortality [5]. For treatment services to improve their effectiveness and impact, it is vital that they are informed by high quality evidence.

Whilst there are no universal performance targets for SAM treatment programmes, there are widely acknowledged minimum standards such as those set by the 'SPHERE' humanitarian charter [6]. The latest version of SPHERE released in 2011 suggests that *overall* therapeutic feeding programme mortality should not exceed 10%, less than 15% should default, and over 75% of discharges should have recovered - defined as "free from medical complications; regained appetite; achieved and maintained appropriate weight gain without nutrition-related oedema, (e.g. for two consecutive weighings)" [6]. Such outcomes are certainly achievable, especially in well run 'Community Management of Acute Malnutrition' (CMAM) programmes which emphasize high population coverage, proactive case-finding, and early treatment [7]. (SPHERE emphasises that the interpretation of outcomes should take into account programme type: programmes which implement outpatient care alone should expect better outcomes than those which include inpatient care, the latter usually having a sicker and more vulnerable patient group). However, even if the SPHERE targets are achieved, it is important for managers, policy makers and funders to appreciate that these are short term outcomes, after a median of some 40 days of treatment. They do not necessarily reflect subsequent child survival and morbidity outcomes. The true public health impact of an intervention is also determined by how the discharged children fare in the longer term.

There is limited data on long term outcomes following discharge from SAM treatment. The few studies that have looked at this are mostly old, pre HIV and even pre current definitions of SAM [8]. This represents an important knowledge gap. Our primary aim in this study was to follow up patients over a year after their treatment for SAM to describe the longer term mortality and growth outcomes. A secondary aim was to identify key risk factors for good/poor long term outcomes, particularly those which might be amenable to change or which would help identify high risk individuals for more targeted future support. By doing this, our goal is to inform improvements in future treatment services.

Methods

Ethics Statement

This follow-up study was approved by the Malawi College of Medicine Research and Ethics Committee (Reference P.03/04/236). Home visits followed the example of a previous study based on MOYO [9] and had an added advantage of potential clinical benefit i.e. if any problems were identified, the carer was advised and where necessary referred.

Study Design

This was a prospective cohort study, arising from an RCT (ISRCTN 19364765) described in detail elsewhere [10]. Briefly, the 'ProNut study' had enrolled malnourished children in a trial examining the efficacy of a prebiotic/probiotic mixture (Synbiotic 2000Forte™) added to ready-to-use therapeutic food during SAM treatment. No significant effects were found.

Study setting

MOYO nutrition ward, Queen Elizabeth Hospital, Malawi. This serves a catchment population of both urban and rural Blantyre district. At the time there were no community programmes for SAM active in the district, so: no community mobilization; no proactive identification of SAM cases; no sub-classification into 'complicated' and 'uncomplicated' SAM [11]. Children diagnosed with SAM (either at local health centres or in the paediatric admissions area of Queen's hospital) were all referred for inpatient care.

Anti-retroviral (ARV) treatment for HIV had been available in Queen's Hospital since 2004, and the process of scaling up and decentralizing was happening at the time of this study. Whilst ARVs were always available, guidance at the time was for children newly diagnosed with HIV to start ARVs if meeting stage 3 or 4 (WHO classification) which included failure to respond to nutritional therapy [12]. As a result many would not have been considered for ARVs until 1–2 months after presenting with SAM, and those with good nutritional recovery not be eligible unless another staging criteria met. From October 2006 we were able to obtain CD4 counts which also informed the decision to start ARVs. Co-trimoxazole prophylaxis was provided from admission, and advised to be continued indefinitely.

Participants

Cohort subjects were children admitted to MOYO nutrition ward for inpatient care from the 12th July 2006 to 9th March 2007. This was the ProNut recruitment period and included both dry (July to November) and rainy seasons (December to March). Whilst not every carer consented to their child's enrolment into ProNUT, almost all answered a detailed baseline questionnaire. Admission criteria to MOYO followed Malawi 2007 national guidelines [13]. These defined SAM as weight-for-height <70% median (NCHS growth references) *and/or* mid upper arm circumference <110 mm *and/or* oedematous malnutrition. Because of the inpatient-only set-up with children self-presenting to care, it is likely that most would have been towards the 'complicated' end of the SAM spectrum [11]. However, since our patient assessment at the time did not include an appetite test, an unknown (but likely small) proportion would have had 'uncomplicated' SAM - which in today's treatment programmes would be treated at home [2].

Children who were successfully cured (defined as two consecutive visits at above 80% weight-for-height, no oedema, clinically stable) in MOYO's combined inpatient/outpatient programme were asked to return for a ward-based review on the 1 year anniversary of their cure date. Non-cures and those failing to return for assessment were followed-up at their home by a mobile team comprising of a study nurse and driver. They used a verbal address obtained from carers during the admission. The mobile team were usually able to determine outcome information at first field visit, and only rarely needed to return if nobody was available to report on what had happened to a child.

Variables

The main study outcome was to describe longer term post-treatment survival. This was defined as the child being seen or reliably reported to be alive at ≥1year after the original discharge date from MOYO. Deaths were subdivided into short term (whilst still an inpatient on MOYO); medium term (within the 1st 90 days of admission but after inpatient care); longer term (defined as death >90 days following programme admission). Ninety days was chosen to be consistent with the upper limits of time normally spent in therapeutic feeding; 3 weeks of inpatient care and 10 weeks in the 'outpatient therapeutic programme' (OTP).

We also assessed long term growth as a secondary outcome. Weight-for-height, weight-for-age, and height-for-age z-scores were all assessed and compared with sibling controls. Sibling controls were identified at home visit and were defined as any child born to the same mother and living in the same household. We measured all siblings present at the time of follow-up visit but due to limited resources were not able to return for a second visit if any live siblings were away from the household at the original visit.

Additional variables were assessed at original admission to MOYO and are available with complete data collection sheets http://discovery.ucl.ac.uk/1306755/1/1306755.pdf [14]. They included clinical history; clinical signs assessed by a doctor or study clinical officer; family and socioeconomic status; HIV status (positive/negative/unknown); HIV clinical staging according to WHO criteria [12].

Data Sources/measurement

During the initial ward admission, weight was measured using on Tanita 1582 digital scales, accurate to 20 g and checked daily. Length was measured to the nearest 1 mm on locally made boards. Baseline measurements were recorded by two independent observers, according to research standard protocols [15]. At follow-up, the same scales were used but with a portable Leicester height board, suitable for field use.

HIV testing was done on an opt-out basis as a routine part of ward protocols. It involved two ELISA rapid tests (Determine HIV-1/2 [Abbott Laboratories, USA] and Uni-Gold HIV [Trinity Biotech PLC, Ireland]), with a third (Hema Strip HIV 1/2 [Chembio Diagnostic System Inc, USA] or SD-Bioline HIV 1/2 [Standard Diagnostics Inc, Korea]) in case of discordant results. PCR for definitive diagnosis in children younger than 18 months of age was unavailable.

Study Size

The RCT in which the cohort was nested determined the sample size [10]. To give an idea of the effect size that could be confidently detected, the original ProNut sample size of 400 per group was large enough, at 95% significance, 80% power, and accommodating 100 losses to follow-up, to detect an inter-group difference of 65% vs. 75% cure. With 1024 patients analysed in FUSAM (more than in ProNUT since not all consented for randomization and some died before the ProNut intervention began) sample size would have been sufficient for most clinically important exposures.

Statistical methods

Data were entered in EpiData 3.1 (EpiData Association, Odense, Denmark, 2003–4). Check files helped ensure high quality data entry, e.g. by checking that variables were in-range and consistent with related variables. Key data (anthropometry, dates, final outcomes, HIV status) were double entered. Unusual results, such as a long time to final outcome, were cross checked against original patient files.

Main analyses were performed using Stata Intercooled 10.0TM (StataCorp LP, USA). Kaplan-Meier time-to-death curves are presented as 'step-up' curves in accordance with suggested best practice [16]. Multivariable analysis was done using Cox regression. Because survival curves for HIV seropositive and seronegative children violated the proportional hazards assumption (confirmed by a formal test using Schoenfeld residuals), complex multivariable analyses in our final results table are presented stratified by HIV. Other key variables (admission oedema, admission age, admission MUAC, admission WAZ) did not violate the assumption. The '*exactp*' option within Stata's '*stcox*' command was specified in all reported regression models.

Chi-square tables and approximate confidence limits for relative risk were used to examine categorical data using StatCalc (CDC, Atlanta, USA, 1993). Where cell numbers are small, Fisher exact results are noted.

Quantitative variables

Z-scores were calculated from weight, height/length, age and sex variables using ENA for SMART software, version October 2007 [17]. Lower (more negative) z-score imply more severe malnutrition. Since children were admitted on the basis of NCHS references, we felt it appropriate to analyse using NCHS references. Given our research-standard measurement protocols using two independent observers, baseline extreme Z-scores were assumed to be real and not excluded [15]. However, with greater potential for error associated with field-based work at the final FuSAM visits, extreme final z-scores were considered more likely to be measurement errors than a child who is truly very small or very large. Following standard criteria [17], individuals with extreme z-scores on follow-up were thus excluded from anthropometry-related analysis: weight-for-height z-scores, WHZ (NCHS) <-4 or $>+6$ or weight-for-age z-score, WAZ (NCHS) <-6 or $>+6$ or height-for-age z-score HAZ (NCHS) <-6 or $>+6$.

For survival analysis and Cox regression, time 0 was the date of admission to MOYO. Time to FuSAM follow-up for other patients was calculated in days by subtracting date of admission from date of final outcome (alive, dead or unknown/other). If patients died within hours of admission, their length of stay was counted as 0.5 days so that they would still contribute to the final model.

Results

Over the eight month study period a total of 1,024 children contributed to 1,187 malnutrition admission episodes. Final outcome information was found on 889/1024(87%). Of the 135(13%) with no 1-year outcome: 45/135(33%) could not be traced at the address given; 42(31%) did not give an address; 31(23%) had missing notes; 7(5%) lived too far away for the outreach team to visit; 10(7%) had an outcome but at less than a year. Outcomes are summarized in **figure 1**.

A total of 462/1024(45%) children were known to be still alive at a year or more after discharge from treatment. Long term survival was greatest amongst those who had been successfully cured following initial treatment. Of 471 discharged from the OTP as nutritionally cured, 365(77%) were still alive at a year or more after their first admission. Of the 427/1024(42%) who died, most did so early on in programme: 238/427(56%) of deaths were during initial inpatient treatment. Most deaths, 274/427(64%), were among children with underlying HIV infection. Differently expressed, 274/445(62%) of known seropositive children died while a total of 77/459(17%) of known seronegative children died.

Kaplan-Meier failure curves in **figures 2 and 3** further illustrate the probability of death during different time periods. These include 1003 children: we could not plot the remaining 21/1024(2.1%) since the date of final outcome was not known. Median time from initial admission to final outcome was 287 days, IQR 11 to 529. The steep initial slope of the curve highlights the fact that most deaths happened soon after admission to programme; median time to death was 10 days, IQR 3 days to 69 days. 278/427(65%) of deaths occurred within 30 days of admission. Failure curves by HIV serostatus (**figure 3**) highlight the significant adverse impact of HIV. For both HIV negative and positive patients, most deaths occurred soon after admission. However, they soon plateau for HIV negative patients but continued to rise for those with HIV. The Log-rank test for the difference between HIV negative and positive children was $p<0.0001$.

Table 1 shows the baseline profile of the cohort according to children's final outcome. Further details are available online [14]. Because admissions at the time were based on NCHS growth references, NCHS z-scores were used for subsequent calculations. To enable future researchers to compare their data against ours we

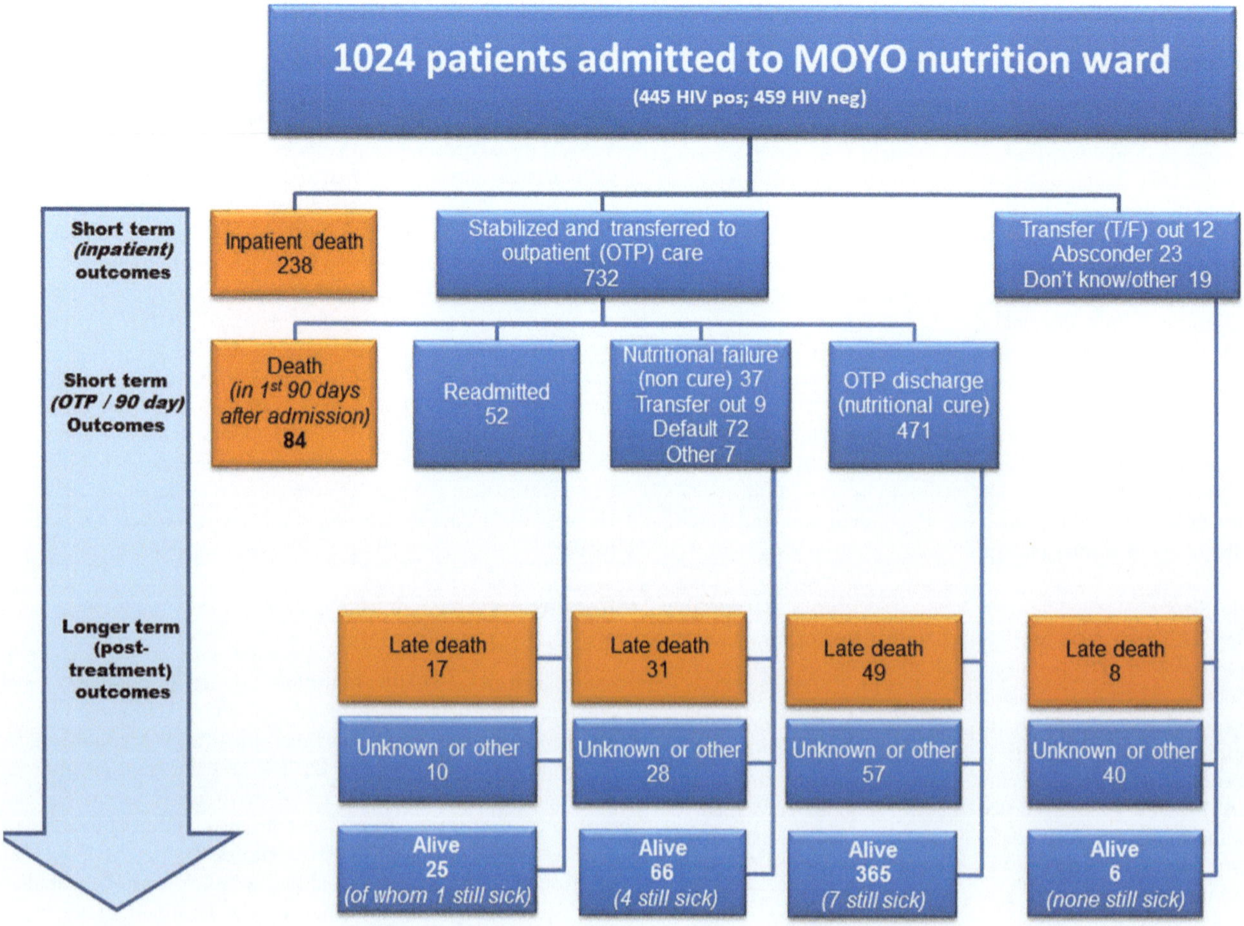

Figure 1. FuSAM study flow chart - all admissions to MOYO. (OTP = 'Outpatient Treatment Programme' – the outpatient part of treatment; T/F = transfer out to different programme). 'Still sick' children were seen or reported to be clinically unwell at follow-up but details were not always known.

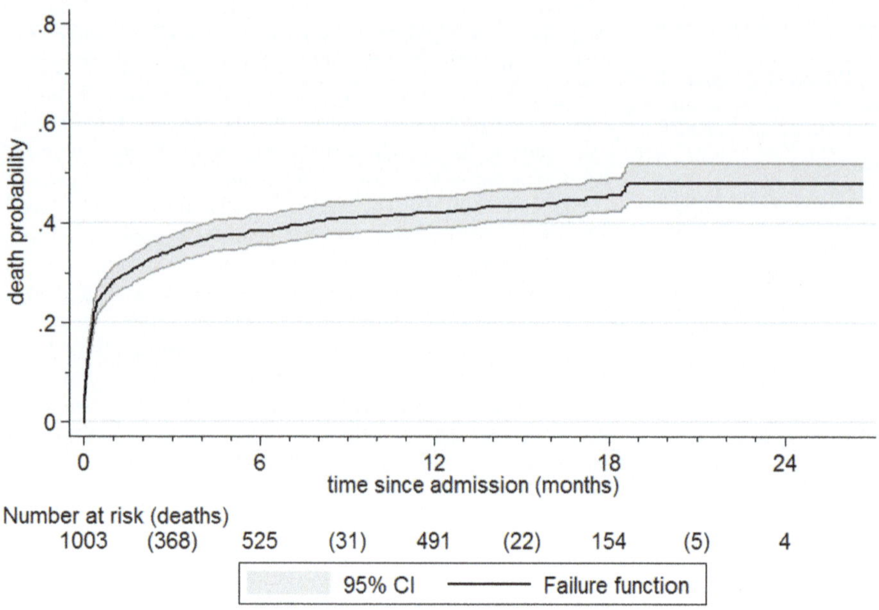

Figure 2. Kaplan Meier failure curve, all patients.

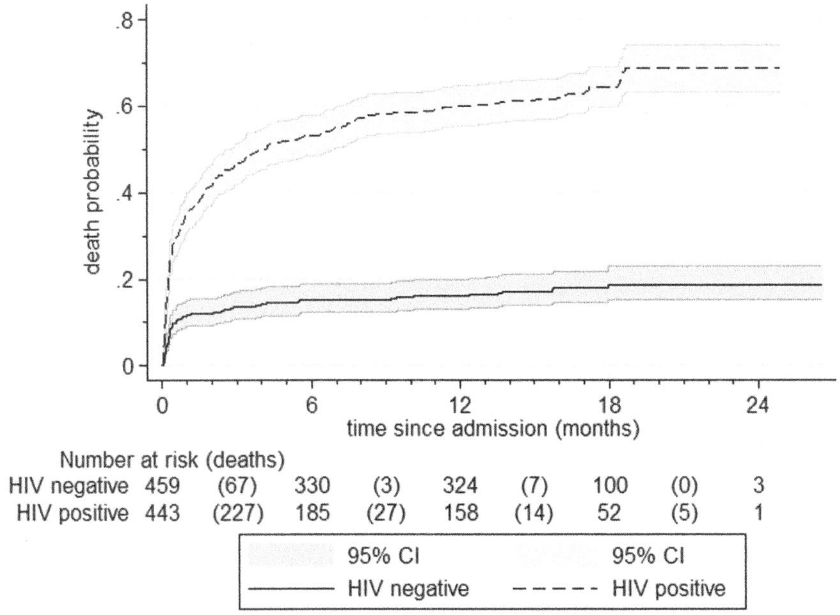

Figure 3. Kaplan Meier failure curves, by HIV serostatus. The tables below figures 2 and 3 show numbers at risk at the beginning of a particular time period. Deaths are in parentheses. Numbers at risk are not simply those previous at-risk minus deaths. Other outcomes also result in children being removed from further analysis (being 'censored'). With this denominator change, the y-axis is mortality *probability* rather than percentage. Whilst our main outcomes focus is on the first year post-discharge, for completeness, data is presented until the last child's follow-up.

also however present admission anthropometry calculated using WHO growth standards [18] (**Table S1**)

Key observations are that: children who died were younger than those still alive at 1 year; kwashiorkor (oedematous malnutrition) was the dominant type of SAM but risk of death was lower than in non-oedematous SAM; children who were more malnourished (lower z-scores); at baseline were more likely to die; HIV was prevalent and HIV-associated mortality was high, especially with advanced disease (as indicated by low CD4 count); disability - mostly neurodisability such as cerebral palsy - was common and deaths among disabled children were high. Another observation was the large number of children who, according to their personal health record (health "passport") or carer, were seen in an outpatient clinic in the six months prior to SAM admission,. In addition, many of these were seen for symptoms potentially

Table 1. Patient profile at baseline (initial admission), by final outcome.

Characteristic	Subcategory	*Death in 1st 90 days (Inpatient or outpatient) (n = 322)*	*Later death (n = 105)*	*Alive at ≥1 year post admission (n = 462)*	*ALL (n = 1024)*
Basic Demographics	**Age in months** (median, IQR)	*19.4 (13 to 30)*	*18.8 (12 to 29)*	*23.3 (17 to 34)*	**21.5 (15 to 32)**
	Boys	*156/322 (48%)*	*66/105 (63%)*	*251/462 (54%)*	**543/1024(53%)**
Type of SAM	**Kwashiorkor†**	*175/322 (54%)*	*45/105 (43%)*	*383/462 (83%)*	**697/1024(68%)**
	Severe wasting	*135/322 (42%)*	*55/105 (52%)*	*69/462 (15%)*	**275/1024 (27%)**
Anthropometry (z-scores)	**Weight-for-height** (WHZ)	*−2.77 (1.2)*	*−2.65 (1.2)*	*−1.92 (1.2)*	***−2.25 (1.3)***
	Weight-for-age (WAZ)	*−4.13 (1.1)*	*−4.30 (1.1)*	*−3.18 (1.2)*	***−3.59 (1.3)***
	Height-for-age (HAZ)	*−3.43 (1.4)*	*−3.88 (1.3)*	*−3.03 (1.4)*	***−3.23 (1.4)***
HIV	**HIV seronegative**	*57 (18%)*	*20 (19%)*	*315 (68%)*	**459 (45%)**
	HIV seropositive	*191 (59%)*	*83 (70%)*	*139 (30%)*	**445 (43%)**
	HIV unknown	*74 (23%)*	*2 (2%)*	*8 (2%)*	**120 (12%)**
Clinical	**Disability** (any)	*24/282 (9%)*	*9/102 (9%)*	**22/453 (5%)**	**60/938 (6%)**
	Outpatient episodes *(last 6 months)*	*233/253 (92%)*	*90/98 (92%)*	*396/440 (90%)*	**797/884 (90%)**
	Outpatient episodes *(last 6 months, symptoms suggestive of malnutrition)*	*60/254 (24%)*	*26/97 (27%)*	*84/437 (19%)*	**187/882 (21%)**

†Numbers with kwashiorkor plus numbers with severe wasting = 972 rather than 1024: the remaining 52 patients had complicated moderate wasting. These children were treated according to exactly the same protocols as those with SAM and hence are included in the follow-up study.

consistent with SAM (e.g. "swelling"; "severely thin" or similar noted in health passport").

Risk factors for mortality were further explored using multivariable Cox Regression in **Table 2**. Adjusting for age, oedema and HIV, low baseline MUAC, WHZ and WAZ are all strongly associated with death. Low HAZ is of borderline significance. Children with oedematous malnutrition were significantly less likely to die than those without. Though the youngest children below 12 months of age were significantly more likely to die, there was no clear age-related risk gradient among older children. HIV stands out as having the greatest adverse impact, an adjusted hazard ratio of 4.03(95% CI 3.08 to 5.25). Deaths among children whose HIV serostatus was unknown were especially high.

Table 3 shows clinical and social factors which might plausibly explain mortality. What is notable here is that after adjusting for baseline anthropometry, very few factors remain as independent predictors of death. Disability stands out as strongly and significantly associated with death in HIV negative patients, and only just outside the $p<0.05$ threshold for HIV positive patients. Severe anaemia (PCV<10) was also associated with increased risk of death, but in HIV positive patients only.

Finally, **Figure 4** shows the final anthropometry of the children who had received treatment on the MOYO ward, compared to sibling controls. Median birth order of the MOYO children was 2nd born. 184 of the ex-MOYO children had one or more siblings measured and with valid anthropometric z-scores: 111 had only one sibling; 54 had two siblings, 18 had three siblings and one had four siblings (total 277 sibling controls). 12 sibling WHZ scores, 65 WAZ scores and 25 HAZ scores were excluded as extreme by our cleaning process. Over 90% of siblings were reported as never having had SAM themselves. Several points are of note. First is the complete catch-up of weight-for-height (WHZ). From an initial programme discharge mean WHZ of −1.96(SD 1.5), there was a 1.92(95% CI 1.76 to 2.08) z-score catch-up, bringing the surviving group to a WHZ of 0.04(1.0), comparable to sibling controls. Weight-for-age also improved by 1.66(95% CI 1.50 to 1.82) z-scores to a 'long-term' final value of −1.77(1.1). This was, however, significantly below that of sibling controls: mean difference in z-scores −0.55(95% CI −0.71 to −0.38, $p<0.01$). Height-for-age also improved, albeit by only 0.37(95% CI 0.21 to 0.53, $p<0.01$) z-scores, to a 'long-term' final value of −2.97(SD1.3). This was again significantly lower than that of the sibling controls: mean difference −1.13(95% CI −1.34 to −0.93, $p<0.01$). Median age of all the siblings who were measured was 61 months and median age of the ex-MOYO children who has a sibling measured was 41 months. Further details of growth outcomes are available online and include sibling-by-sibling comparisons (pages 123–125) and comparisons by HIV and admission oedema (pages 114–118) [14]. **Table S2** in this paper shows main anthropometric changes in the ex-MOYO children over the course of the study.

Discussion

In our SAM treatment programme, overall mortality was high in both the short and medium term, markedly above SPHERE targets of <10% [6]. Long term survivors showed good weight-for-height catch-up growth, some weight-for-age catch-up but minimal height-for-age catch-up, compared to sibling controls. These observations are rare in the SAM literature and therefore offer key lessons for policy makers and programme managers:

First is the need for more information on longer term outcomes so as to assess the true impact of SAM on child mortality. In our setting, routine reporting would have given a falsely optimistic impression of post-SAM mortality. Overall 427/1024(42%)

Table 2. Cox regression exploring main baseline predictors of death.

Risk factor		Number of deaths	Hazard ratio (95% CI)	Adjusted hazard ratio* (95% CI)	P (adj.)
Sex	Girls	202/469 (43%)	Ref.	Ref.	
	Boys	221/530 (42%)	0.92 (0.76 to 1.12)	0.89 (0.73 to 1.08)	0.26
Age group (in months)	>=60	30/88 (34%)	1.11 (0.58 to 2.12)	1.22 (0.63 to 2.36)	0.55
	48–<60	13/42 (31%)	Ref.	Ref.	
	36–<48	25/68 (37%)	1.27 (0.65 to 2.49)	1.66 (0.84 to 3.29)	0.14
	24–<36	85/230 (37%)	1.26 (0.70 to 2.25)	1.38 (0.76 to 2.49)	0.29
	12–<24	176/430 (41%)	1.42 (0.81 to 2.49)	1.57 (0.89 to 2.78)	0.12
	<12	97/145 (67%)	2.89 (1.62 to 5.17)	2.49 (1.38 to 4.51)	0.002
Oedema	No	205/305 (67%)	Ref.	Ref.	
	Yes	220/694 (32%)	0.37 (0.30 to 0.44)	0.58 (0.47 to 0.72)	<0.001
Mid Upper Arm Circumference	Per cm unit increase	418/991 (42%)	0.70 (0.66 to 0.74)	0.80 (0.74 to 0.86)	<0.001
Weight-for-Height	Per 1 unit z-score increase	409/973(42%)	0.65 (0.60 to 0.71)	0.75 (0.68 to 0.83)	<0.001
Weight-for-Age	Per 1 unit z-score increase	425/999 (43%)	0.59 (0.54 to 0.64)	0.73 (0.66 to 0.81)	<0.001
Height-for-age	Per 1 unit z-score increase	417/989 (42%)	0.83 (0.78 to 0.89)	0.92 (0.86 to 0.99)	0.04
HIV	Neg	77/459 (17%)	ref	ref	
	Pos	273/443 (62%)	4.84 (3.75 to 6.24)	4.03 (3.08 to 5.25)	<0.001
	unknown	76/101 (75%)	17.8 (12.8 to 24.8)	16.9 (12.1 to 23.7)	<0.001

* Adjusted for age, oedema, and HIV status.

Table 3. Cox regression exploring clinical and social risk factors for death, by HIV serostatus.

Risk factor (assessed at original admission)		Hazard ratio for all mortality (short and long term)*			
		HIV negative	p	HIV positive	p
CLINICAL RISK FACTORS					
Symptoms in previous 2 weeks	Fever	0.96 (0.58 to 1.58)	0.87	0.85 (0.65 to 1.12)	0.25
	Diarrhoea	1.59 (0.95 to 2.68)	0.08	1.15 (0.88 to 1.51)	0.31
	Vomiting	0.84 (0.52 to 1.37)	0.49	1.23 (0.96 to 1.58)	0.10
	Fast or difficult breathing	1.12 (0.59 to 2.12)	0.72	0.71 (0.51 to 0.99)	0.04*
	Cough	1.06 (0.65 to 1.74)	0.80	1.03 (0.79 to 1.36)	0.80
	Anorexia	0.75 (0.46 to 1.22)	0.25	1.17 (0.91 to 1.51)	0.22
	Flaky paint dermatosis	1.66 (0.93 to 2.96)	0.09	1.14 (0.75 to 1.72)	0.54
Anaemia	Any (PCV<30)	1.08 (0.65 to 1.80)	0.76	1.05 (0.80 to 1.36)	0.73
	Severe (PCV<10)	2.19 (0.66 to 7.23)	0.20	2.62 (1.18 to 5.84)	0.02*
Malaria		0.26 (0.04 to 1.88)	0.18	0.94 to 0.46 to 1.95)	0.88
Ever had TB		2.81 (0.35 to 22.7)	0.33	1.27 (0.77 to 2.09)	0.35
Disability (any)		2.77 (1.43 to 5.34)	0.002*	1.76 (0.94 to 3.28)	0.08
Not breastfed (<2 year olds only)		0.67 (0.36 to 1.26)	0.21	0.98 (0.70 to 1.38)	0.92
Inpatient episodes *(non-SAM, past year)*		1.03 (0.55 to 1.91)	0.94	1.31 (0.99 to 1.75)	0.06
Outpatient episodes	in past 6 months	0.69 (0.34 to 1.40)	0.30	0.69 (0.40 to 1.21)	0.20
past 6 months, symptoms of SAM		1.33 (0.74 to 2.41)	0.34	1.00 (0.74 to 1.36)	1.00
SOCIAL AND ECONOMIC RISK FACTORS					
Orphan	*Mother died*	0.97 (0.35 to 2.70)	0.95	0.72 (0.45 to 1.15)	0.17
	Father died	1.33 (0.52 to 3.42)	0.56	1.35 (0.84 to 2.16)	0.21
	Both died	2.78 (0.92 to 8.34)	0.07	1.07 (0.47 to 2.45)	0.17
Maternal education	*None*	Ref.		Ref.	
	Primary school	1.06 (0.53 to 2.13)	0.87	0.78 (0.51 to 1.20)	0.27
	Secondary school	0.57 (0.21 to 1.54)	0.27	0.97 (0.60 to 1.57)	0.91
Paternal education	*None*	Ref.		Ref.	
	Primary school	2.84 (0.38 to 21.26)	0.31	0.89 (0.39 to 2.04)	0.79
	Secondary school	2.31 (0.30 to 17.53)	0.42	0.80 (0.35 to 1.84)	0.60
Wealth quintile	*Poorest*		Ref.		Ref.
	2nd poorest	1.35 (0.63 to 2.89)	0.43	0.67 (0.41 to 1.09)	0.10
	Middle	1.11 (0.50 to 2.44)	0.80	0.95 (0.61 to 1.47)	0.82
	2nd richest	1.49 (0.69 to 3.26)	0.31	0.93 (0.59 to 1.45)	0.75
	Richest	0.95 (0.38 to 2.42)	0.92	0.91 (0.60 to 1.38)	0.66
Main household water source	*Piped*	Ref.		Ref.	
	Borehole	0.72 (0.42 to 1.23)	0.23	0.90 (0.67 to 1.21)	0.50
	Well or spring	1.09 (0.51 to 2.32)	0.83	0.90 (0.60 to 1.37)	0.63
Rural Residence		0.67 (0.39 to 1.13)	0.13	0.82 (0.62 to 1.10)	0.62

* Adjusted for oedema, age, sex, admission WAZ and admission MUAC.

children died, but 105(25%) of these deaths occurred >90 days after their original admission. They would have been missed by most nutrition programmes which only follow-up patients up to discharge from outpatient care. Other factors which can mislead routine reporting systems but which we were able to describe include: defaulter follow-up so as to ascribe correct survival status; correctly capturing readmissions (of our 52 readmissions, 17(33%) died) – if not done, denominator population is overestimated and % mortality thus underestimated.

The second key lesson is that patient clinical profile needs to be better accounted for, both when managing individual patients and when judging programme performance. Simple targets like those set by SPHERE offer useful 'red flags' for further investigation but cannot alone distinguish between poorly performing programmes and those caring for a clinically complex patient population. Differentiating these will become increasingly important as countries/regions develop and primary SAM due to food insecurity alone becomes less common. A greater proportion of affected children in such areas will have an underlying medical condition either directly causing or significantly contributing to SAM. Whilst our overall mortality was high, sub-analysis by HIV status revealed that HIV infection was associated with much of the excess mortality. We note the even higher mortality among children whose serostatus was unknown. Too sick to be tested

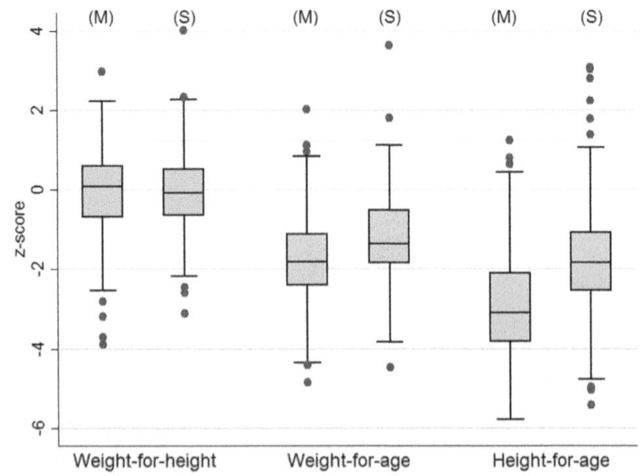

Figure 4. Boxplot showing weight-for-height, weight-for-age and height-for-age of the ex-malnourished surviving child (M) (n = 386) compared to sibling controls (S) (n = 277).

before they died, we believe that most of this group were likely to have been serostatus positive - if so, the known positive results in our paper are a likely under-estimate of the true adverse impact of HIV. Some might argue that children with HIV are therefore better described as dying from 'end-stage HIV disease' (AIDS) rather than from malnutrition with underlying HIV – but to us such distinctions are semantic. What matters is how to better support these children in future programmes: even with more proactive ARV treatment programmes identifying and treating children at an earlier stage, some will end up malnourished and enrolled in feeding programmes such as ours. Therefore, our results, and our message that nutrition programmes need to better care for this especially vulnerable subgroup remains valid. This HIV-associated risk is already well known [19],[20] but other factors are less well described. Notable in FuSAM is the importance of underlying disability. This affected 6% of children and accounted for significant excess mortality - a likely underestimate given that we had no formal screening tool and therefore identified only the most obvious problems. At present, few programmes actively look for disability so this is a key area for future work [21],[22].

The third message relates to the current international emphasis on tackling childhood stunting, championed by the SUN (Scaling up Nutrition) movement [23]. Our results suggest that SUN must take SAM seriously, just as SAM treatment programme should aim to engage more with the SUN. Current treatments for SAM are clearly important and necessary to minimise mortality, but may not be sufficient to address stunting on their own. Whilst it was encouraging to observe good chances of longer term survival following an initial nutritional cure (365/471(77%) of cures being still alive at a year or more after their first admission), limited improvement in survivors' height-for-age was, however, disappointing, as was their significant stunting compared to sibling controls. This is even more notable given the siblings' older median age: population prevalence of stunting increases over the first two years of life so that older cohorts might be expected to be more rather than less stunted [24]. Whilst weight-for-age had improved, it also remained low, significantly below siblings'. The marked improvement of weight-for-height z-scores though in one sense welcome, likely reflects rapid weight gain combined with poor linear growth, a pattern which may be associated with later obesity and chronic disease [25],[26]. This needs further study.

Strengths and consistency with other literature

Our biggest strength is duration of follow-up, at least one year, often longer, after discharge from SAM treatment. Such longer term outcome information is rare. Related to this, our second major strength is a high follow-up rate – 87% is especially good for a developing country setting. This reduces the risk of bias associated with large numbers of 'defaulters', who may be deaths [9].

FuSAM compares favourably to the few other studies looking at longer term SAM outcomes. Most of these other studies however took place pre-HIV [8], FuSAM thus filling a key gap, regarding HIV-era outcomes, especially in sub Saharan Africa where the problem is greatest [27].

In Niger in 1992 [28], of 174 discharged from a TFP, 107(61%) were followed up. At 3–16 months follow-up 17% had died. Though compared to FUSAM this appears better, there is much larger probability of bias due to 39% unknown outcome, a proportion of whom may have been deaths. In Zaire in 1987 [29], 171 SAM children discharged from hospital were followed up and 81.6% found still alive at the end of 5 years. However, kwashiorkor in that study was mainly based on serum albumin and some of the children classified as such might not have met today's oedema, WFH, or MUAC criteria for SAM. In Tanzania in 1987, 87% of 566 children who had been discharged from an NRU were followed over a year [30]. The mortality after discharge was 8% and relapse rate was 13%. In a retrospective cohort study in Guinea Bissau, 1995 [31], 1038 severely malnourished children (defined by weight-for-age <60% NCHS standards) were followed up over 3 years. 354 had received nutritional rehabilitation whereas 684 did not, due to limited programme capacity. Up to 3 years, the relative risk of death in the rehabilitated group was 0.75(0.59 to 0.99). The mortality difference was greatest in the first three months. Weight-for-age z-scores improved from a baseline of −4.52 to −2.76. This is consistent with the weight-for-age improvements we observed in FuSAM.

Weaknesses and generalizability

We acknowledge the limitations of our study so hope that it will inspire more detailed future work to address these:

FuSAM was conducted when CMAM (Community Management of Acute Malnutrition) was not as widespread as it is today. It was not available in Blantyre district where we worked (though it did start shortly after, in mid-2008). This public health orientated approach to SAM treats children mainly as outpatients [2], and emphasises proactive identification through community screening, rather than reactive detection during hospital visits as we had at the time of FuSAM [7]. Even though some risk factors for mortality (e.g. HIV, disability) are likely to be found in both settings, care is needed before generalising our findings to CMAM programmes. However, our results are consistent with CMAM's key principle that earlier treatment is better [7] (i.e. the less severe the malnutrition at baseline, the better the chances of survival). This has recently been confirmed in a follow-up of a CMAM cohort [8], also from Malawi showing much better outcomes than ours. Given this context, our paper is a clear call to any programmes which have not yet switched from inpatient-only SAM care to CMAM, to do so. Whilst in many ways a typical resource poor developing country setting, MOYO ward at the time of FuSAM had inputs and resources (in terms of staff time, clinical expertise, continuity of drug, food and equipment supplies) far above the vast majority of TFPs in Malawi and elsewhere in Sub-Saharan Africa. If our outcomes were poor, they are likely even worse in most other, less well supported settings.

Another limitation related to generalizability is that we examined patients already enrolled in SAM treatment. In-programme risk factors such as we observed are not necessarily the same as those at population-level. Even if a particular risk factor (e.g. HIV infection) is relevant to both general population and within-programme children, the magnitude of effect is likely to be different.

Related to the lack of obvious 'impact' of factors like socioeconomic status (SES), we also acknowledge that we did not model all the possible causal pathways. For instance, low SES could cause/contribute to low admission anthropometry, which did adversely affected outcomes. Hence adjusting for anthropometric status might have concealed the impact of SES. Such pathways need exploration in future work

Resource limitations meant that we were not able to follow-up regularly at fixed time-points after programme discharge, but instead relied on a single long term FuSAM visit. It is possible that some variables such as socioeconomic status or orphaning may have changed over time and hence we may have missed their effects.

Next, is the possibility of systematic reporting or recall bias. We cannot exclude this but do not believe that it is a major problem since death is a very objective outcome, with major findings such as those concerning HIV and disability all highly plausible biologically as well as themselves objective/backed by recorded blood test in case of HIV. We also cannot be sure how missing data from the 13% of children lost to follow-up might have affected results - though as previously stated this is good for a developing country setting so we do not believe it would have significantly altered our key results or affected conclusions. More of a problem is the increased data 'noise' inherent to some of the more subjective, self-reported variables such as socioeconomic status: small but real risks may have been obscured. Another issue is potential selection bias of children seen in the hospital admission departments, before arrival at the MOYO nutrition ward. Very sick patients might die in the admissions area or on the special care ward before transfer to MOYO. Borderline cases might be missed and wrongly sent to the normal paediatric wards instead of to MOYO.

The last potential limitation of our study relates to seasonal variations in the risk of malnutrition. Though recruitment was spread over most of a year and captured both rainy (hungry) season and dry (post-harvest) seasons, there may have been variations in nutritional status depending on when a child was admitted and followed up. Logistic constraints led to variations in time to follow-up. Had a constant time been possible, perhaps different magnitudes of z-score change might have been observed. Again, we doubt that the overall pattern of findings would have been very different. One of the advantages of using sibling controls was that they were measured at the same time as the ex-MOYO child. Where differences were seen they cannot therefore be ascribed solely to seasonal variations.

Conclusions and implications for policy and practice

Although this is an observational study, we believe that our findings have strong policy and practice implications.

The first is the need to be much more aware of longer term as well as short term outcomes of SAM. This long term perspective will also help focus attention on important non-mortality outcomes such as growth, development, co-morbidities and pre-determinants for eventual adult non-communicable disease.

Second is that a more holistic view of SAM management is needed. Treatment is not just about food - this is necessary but not alone sufficient. Programmes should work closer in collaboration with other child health services and form part of a seamless 'continuum of care'. Many SAM treatment programmes already appreciate the need for close links with HIV-related services [32] but the need to improve outcomes for children with disability (and likely other) chronic underlying disease is also clear from our results. Urgent future work is needed to elaborate exactly which interventions are most effective and most cost-effective for these vulnerable individuals.

Finally, our results support calls for on early identification and treatment of SAM. The pioneers of CMAM stressed community engagement and active case finding to identify and treat SAM as early as possible [33],[34]. This emphasis has not always been maintained in subsequent programmes documents [2]. Now is the time for this message to be re-vitalised in all SAM programming [7]. Whilst other confirmatory research is urgently needed, it is very plausible that earlier treatment of SAM would favourably affect stunting and longer term post-SAM chronic disease – both key areas in current international malnutrition policy and programming. Proactive SAM treatment services are essential. They not only have great potential to reduce mortality in the short term but also great potential to impact on longer term morbidity consequences.

Supporting Information

Table S1 Admission Anthropometry by NCHS growth references and WHO growth standards.
(DOCX)

Table S2 Anthropometry over the course of the study (NCHS growth references).
(DOCX)

Acknowledgments

Above all, we thank the children, carers and families who made this study possible. We also thank all the staff of Queen Elizabeth Central Hospital Blantyre, Blantyre, in particular: Agnes Malamula, Hilda Khengere, Christina Mhango, German Chauluka, Elizabeth Molyneux, Tom Heikens, Anne Nesbitt, Hannah Blencowe.

We also thank UNICEF Malawi (Roger Mathisen and Stanley Chitekwe in particular) for their support making the study possible and also colleagues from The Government of Malawi, Office of President and Cabinet and Ministry of Health for their support for MOYO nutrition ward.

Author Contributions

Conceived and designed the experiments: MK JB GC. Performed the experiments: MK JB GC. Analyzed the data: MK JB AS. Wrote the paper: MK JB GC PB SC AT AS. Substantial contribution to interpretation of data: MK JB GC PB SC AT AS. Revised the article critically for important intellectual content: MK JB GC PB SC AT AS. Final approval of the version to be published: MK JB GC PB SC AT AS.

References

1. Collins S (2007) Treating severe acute malnutrition seriously. Arch Dis Child 92: 453–461.
2. WHO/WFP/UNSCN/UNICEF (2007) Community-based management of severe acute malnutrition. A Joint Statement by the World Health Organization, the World Food Programme, the United Nations System Standing Committee on Nutrition and the United Nations Children's Fund. Available: http://www.who.int/nutrition/topics/statement_commbased_malnutrition/en/index.html. Accessed:12 May 2014.

3. WHO child growth standards and the identification of severe acute malnutrition in infants and children. (2009) A joint statement by the World Health Organization and the United Nations Children's Fund. Available: http://www.who.int/nutrition/publications/severemalnutrition/9789241598163/en/index.html. Accessed: 12 May 2014.
4. Black RE, Victora CG, Walker SP, Bhutta ZA, Christian P, et al. (2013) Maternal and child undernutrition and overweight in low-income and middle-income countries. Lancet 382: 427–451.
5. Gillespie SHL (2003) Nutrition and the MDGs: The Relationship Between Nutrition and the Millennium Development Goals: A Strategic Review of the Scope for DfID's Influencing Role. IFPRI Report. International Food Policy Research Institute, Washington.
6. SPHERE (2011) Sphere Project: Humanitarian Charter and Minimum Standards in Disaster Response. Available: http://www.sphereproject.org/. Accessed: 12 May 2014.
7. Collins S, Sadler K, Dent N, Khara T, Guerrero S, et al. (2006) Key issues in the success of community-based management of severe malnutrition. Food Nutr Bull 27: S49–82.
8. Bahwere P, Mtimuni A, Sadler K, Banda T, Collins S (2012) Long term mortality after community and facility based treatment of severe acute malnutrition: Analysis of data from Bangladesh, Kenya, Malawi and Niger. Journal of Public Health and Epidemiology 4: 215–225.
9. Sadler K, Kerac M, Collins S, Khengere H, Nesbitt A (2008) Improving the management of severe acute malnutrition in an area of high HIV prevalence. J Trop Pediatr 54: 364–369.
10. Kerac M, Bunn J, Seal A, Thindwa M, Tomkins A, et al. (2009) Probiotics and prebiotics for severe acute malnutrition (PRONUT study): a double-blind efficacy randomised controlled trial in Malawi. Lancet 374: 136–144.
11. Collins S, Yates R (2003) The need to update the classification of acute malnutrition. Lancet 362: 249.
12. WHO (2006) World Health Organization. WHO Case definitions of HIV for surveillance and revised clinical staging and immunological classification of HIV-related disease in adults and children. Available: http://www.who.int/hiv/pub/guidelines/hivstaging/en/index.html. Accessed: 12 May 2014.
13. Government of Malawi (2007) Interim Guidelines for the Management of Acute Malnutrtion through Community Based Therapeutic Care.
14. Kerac M (2011) Improving the treatment of severe acute malnutrition in childhood: a randomized controlled trial of synbiotic-enhanced therapeutic food with long term follow-up of post-treatment mortality and morbidity. Doctoral Thesis, UCL (University College London). Available: http://discovery.ucl.ac.uk/1306755/1/1306755.pdf. Accessed: 12 May 2014.
15. de Onis M, Onyango AW, Van den Broeck J, Chumlea WC, Martorell R (2004) Measurement and standardization protocols for anthropometry used in the construction of a new international growth reference. Food Nutr Bull 25: S27–36.
16. Pocock SJ, Clayton TC, Altman DG (2002) Survival plots of time-to-event outcomes in clinical trials: good practice and pitfalls. Lancet 359: 1686–1689.
17. Emergency Nutrition Assessment (ENA) software for Standardized Monitoring and Assessment of Relief and Transitions (SMART). Version October 2007. Available: http://www.nutrisurvey.de/ena/ena.html. Accessed: 12 May 2014.
18. de Onis M, Garza C, Onyango AW, Rolland-Cachera MF (2009) WHO growth standards for infants and young children. Arch Pediatr 16: 47–53.
19. Fergusson P, Tomkins A, Kerac M (2009) Improving the management of Severe Acute Malnutrition in HIV prevalent settings. International Health 1: 10–16.
20. Thurstans S, Kerac M, Maleta K, Banda T, Nesbitt A (2008) HIV prevalence in severely malnourished children admitted to nutrition rehabilitation units in Malawi: geographical & seasonal variations a cross-sectional study. BMC Pediatr 8: 22.
21. Groce NE, Kerac M, Farkas A, Schultink W, Bieler RB (2013) Inclusive nutrition for children and adults with disabilities. The Lancet Global Health 1: e180–e181.
22. UNICEF (2013) UNICEF Global Partnership on Children with Disabilities - background note. Available: http://www.unicef.org/disabilities/files/Nutrition_Background_Note-GPcwd(1).pdf. Accessed: 12 May 2014
23. Scaling Up Nutrition (SUN) Available: http://scalingupnutrition.org/about. Accessed: 12 May 2014.
24. Victora CG, de Onis M, Hallal PC, Blossner M, Shrimpton R (2010) Worldwide timing of growth faltering: revisiting implications for interventions. Pediatrics 125: e473–480.
25. Stettler N, Iotova V (2010) Early growth patterns and long-term obesity risk. Curr Opin Clin Nutr Metab Care 13: 294–299.
26. Dulloo AG (2008) Thrifty energy metabolism in catch-up growth trajectories to insulin and leptin resistance. Best practice & research Clinical endocrinology & metabolism 22: 155–171.
27. Fergusson P, Tomkins A (2009) HIV prevalence and mortality among children undergoing treatment for severe acute malnutrition in sub-Saharan Africa: a systematic review and meta-analysis. Trans R Soc Trop Med Hyg 103: 541–548.
28. Pecoul B, Soutif C, Hounkpevi M, Ducos M (1992) Efficacy of a therapeutic feeding centre evaluated during hospitalization and a follow-up period, Tahoua, Niger, 1987–1988. Ann Trop Paediatr 12: 47–54.
29. Hennart P, Beghin D, Bossuyt M (1987) Long-term follow-up of severe protein-energy malnutrition in Eastern Zaire. J Trop Pediatr 33: 10–12.
30. van Roosmalen-Wiebenga MW, Kusin JA, de With C (1987) Nutrition rehabilitation in hospital–a waste of time and money? Evaluation of nutrition rehabilitation in a rural district hospital in South-west Tanzania. II. Long-term results. J Trop Pediatr 33: 24–28.
31. Perra A, Costello AM (1995) Efficacy of outreach nutrition rehabilitation centres in reducing mortality and improving nutritional outcome of severely malnourished children in Guinea Bissau. Eur J Clin Nutr 49: 353–359.
32. Bahwere P, Piwoz E, Joshua MC, Sadler K, Grobler-Tanner CH, et al. (2008) Uptake of HIV testing and outcomes within a Community-based Therapeutic Care (CTC) programme to treat severe acute malnutrition in Malawi: a descriptive study. BMC Infect Dis 8: 106.
33. Collins S (2001) Changing the way we address severe malnutrition during famine. Lancet 358: 498–501.
34. Grobler-Tanner C, Collins S (2004) Community Therapeutic Care (CTC). A new approach to managing acute malnutrition in emergencies and beyond. FANTA (Food and Nutrition Technical Assistance). Technical Report 8. Available: FANTA www.eldis.org/vfile/upload/1/document/0708/DOC17926.pdf. Accessed: 12 May 2014. FANTA (Food and Nutrition Technical Assistance).

2

Starvation Induces Phenotypic Diversification and Convergent Evolution in *Vibrio vulnificus*

Hwajiun Chen[1,2], Chun-Yao Chen[1,2]*

1 Department of Life Science, Tzu-Chi University, Hualien, Taiwan, **2** Institute of Medical Sciences, Tzu-Chi University, Hualien, Taiwan

Abstract

Starvation is a common stress experienced by bacteria living in natural environments and the ability to adapt to and survive intense stress is of paramount importance for any bacterial population. A series of starvation experiments were conducted using *V. vulnificus* 93U204 in phosphate-buffered saline and seawater. The starved population entered the death phase during the first week and approximately 1% of cells survived. After that the population entered a long-term stationary phase, and could survive for years. Starvation-induced diversification (SID) of phenotypes was observed in starved populations and phenotypic variants (PVs) appeared in less than 8 days. The cell density, rather than the population size, had a major effect on the extent of SID. SID was also observed in strain YJ016, where it evolved at a faster pace. PVs appeared to emerge in a fixed order: PV with reduced motility, PV with reduced proteolytic activity, and PV with reduced hemolytic activity. All of the tested PVs had growth advantages in the stationary phase phenotypes and increased fitness compared with 93U204 cells in co-culture competition experiments, which indicates that they had adapted to starvation. We also found that SID occurred in natural seawater with a salinity of 1%–3%, so this mechanism may facilitate bacterial adaptation in natural environments.

Editor: Dongsheng Zhou, State Key Laboratory of Pathogen and Biosecurity, Beijing Institute of Microbiology and Epidemiology, China

Funding: National Science Council grant NSC96-2311-B-320-004, (http://web1.nsc.gov.tw/). Tzu Chi University grant TCIRP96003-01, (http://www.tcu.edu.tw/). The funders had no role in study design, data collection and analysis, decision to publish, or preparation of the manuscript.

Competing Interests: The authors have declared that no competing interests exist.

* E-mail: cychen@mail.tcu.edu.tw

Introduction

Vibrio vulnificus is a notorious human pathogen, which causes clinical manifestations that range from wound infection to primary sepsis, or even death [1]. This species is also a fish pathogen that affects eel and tilapia aquaculture in many Asian and European countries, including Japan [2], Bangladesh [3], Denmark [4], and Spain [5]. It has also been isolated from oysters and shrimps [6,7].

However, *V. vulnificus* is usually found in aquatic environments as free-living bacteria. Environmental *V. vulnificus* isolates are reported to be highly heterogeneous. Arias et al. reported high genetic diversity after ribotyping 132 strains of *V. vulnificus* by random amplified polymorphic DNA PCR [8]. Wong et al. also demonstrated high genetic heterogeneity in environmental isolates from the United States and Taiwan using pulsed-field gel electrophoresis [9]. The mechanism that allows this high genetic diversity to be maintained in marine environments still remains unknown. This high genetic heterogeneity may be derived from a continuous and abundant supply of mutations in natural populations, or it could be the result of relaxed selection in a heterogeneous environment.

In natural environments, bacteria are expected to experience repeated "feast or famine" fluctuations, so the capacities to survive starvation and respond rapidly to transient nutrient bursts are of paramount importance. Gram-negative bacteria react to various types of environmental stress with a general stress response. This response depends on alternative sigma factors such as RpoS, which regulate a suite of genes and redirect resources from supporting growth to self-maintenance (reviewed in [10]). These include genes related to metabolic adaptations to available resources and alterations in the control of motility, cell morphology, stress resistance, and biofilm formation.

Bacteria activate the general stress response early during starvation. They will induce further stringent responses if the nutritional limitation persists and the cells will stop to grow, while there is a switch to a more error-prone DNA polymerase, which may elevate the mutation rate [11]. Stress-directed mutation is considered a universal mechanism of microbial adaptation to environmental stress at the population level during long-term starvation [12]. This mechanism may contribute to adaptive evolution in *Escherichia coli* in laboratory culture [13]. This phenomenon has been described in many microbes in laboratory settings, but its occurrence in natural habitats has not been examined previously.

The population dynamics of *V. vulnificus* in conditions of starvation have been examined in several studies. Biotype 2 strain E22 *V. vulnificus* was reported to survive starvation for 50 days in artificial seawater [14]. In a subsequent study, two- to three-order drops in population size were seen in E22 after 160-day starvation in water with 0.5% or 1.5% salinity at 25°C [15]. Similarly, approximately 1% of biotype 1 strain C7184 cells survived at the end of 35-day starvation in artificial seawater at 22°C [16]. The question is how does starvation affect the physiology of *Vibrio* spp. and does it affect bacterial diversification? Many *Vibrio* spp. can survive long-term starvation, even for several years [15,17]. They enter a viable but non-culturable (VBNC) state when they are starved at a low temperature [18]. The starved cells are known to change their morphology from rod to coccoid cells, as reported in *V. vulnificus* [15], *V. parahaemolyticus* [19], *V. angustum* [20], *V. shilloi*, and *V. tasmaniensis* [21]. Starved *V. parahaemolyticus* cells also exhibit greater cell adherence and hydrophobicity [9]. These results indicate that starvation can lead to dramatic changes in the morphology and physiology of *Vibrio* spp.

Previously, we isolated *V. vulnificus* from diseased tilapia [22]. The epidemics occurred only in fish maintained in a low salinity (<0.5%) environment, which suggests that these tilapia-pathogenic isolates were descendants of low salinity-adapted *V. vulnificus*. Further analysis indicated that these isolates formed several genetic groups (unpublished data), which indicates either that the ability to infect tilapia has evolved more than once, or that horizontal gene transfer is responsible for the emergence of novel pathogenic strains. We hypothesize that if starvation can lead to phenotypic diversification in a natural environment, it may facilitate the generation of virulent bacterial variants by providing a larger pool of diverse progeny for selection. The aim of the present study was to show that starvation can induce the diversification of *V. vulnificus* in laboratory and natural settings, and that this starvation-induced diversification (SID) could promote bacterial adaptation and persistence. We showed that *V. vulnificus* survived for an extended period and exhibited phenotypic diversification. SID was cell density-dependent and a result of adaptive mutation. We provide evidence to demonstrate that SID occurred with various salinity levels and was observed in two different isolates.

Materials and Methods

Bacterial strains, culture media, and growth conditions

All of the bacterial culture experiments were performed at 30°C. Bacteria were grown in tryptic soy broth or agar supplemented with 1.5% NaCl (TSBS and TSAS, respectively). Strain 93U204 is a fish pathogen, which was isolated from moribund tilapia collected from Kaohsiung in Taiwan. This isolate was a kind gift from Dr. Chia-Ben Chao of Kaohsiung Institute of Livestock Disease Control and Prevention, and was identified as *V. vulnificus* by 16S rDNA sequencing (manuscript in preparation). YJ016 was a human clinical strain isolated from Tainan, Taiwan, and its genome has been sequenced [23]. This strain was kind gift from Dr Lien-I Hor of Department of Microbiology and Immunology, National Cheng-Kung University, Taiwan. All bacterial isolates were properly stored by putting 100 μL overnight culture in 1 mL of TSBS supplemented with 50% glycerol, and then kept in −80°C freezer (GV039P/M, Kaltis International, Taipei, Taiwan).

Long-term starvation of bacterial cultures

Bacteria were grown in TSBS with constant 200 rpm horizontal shaking (E450, Deng Yng, New Taipei City, Taiwan). Cells were harvested in the late exponential phase (approximately 1×10^9 CFU/mL), washed twice with phosphate-buffered saline (PBS, 0.1 M phosphate buffer and 0.85% NaCl, pH 7.3), and re-suspended in suitable media. The bacterial cells were diluted in PBS to the desired concentrations if needed.

Most of the starvation experiments were conducted in 30-mL Wheaton glass serum bottles (Z113980, Wheaton, Millville, New Jersey, USA). Experiments conducted in other containers are indicated. The cells were washed twice with PBS, and re-suspended in 10 mL test media. Each serum bottle was capped with a flange red rubber stopper (224100-172, Wheaton) and sealed with an open aluminum cap (224178-01, Wheaton). The cells were incubated at 30°C without shaking and were sampled repeatedly using 1-mL insulin syringes (27-gauge, Terumo, Tokyo, Japan). The viable counts were determined using the drop plate method [24]. The bacterial suspensions were serially diluted in TSBS and five 10 μL drops of each dilution were placed on TSAS plates. The plates were incubated at 30°C for 18 h before they were counted. We chose to use TSBS as diluent to prevent possible loss of viability of these stressed cells on agar plate, which has been documented for *V. vulnificus* [25]. The serial dilution process generally took less than 10 minutes to perform, and in a preliminary test, cells starved in PBS did not increase significantly (n = 6, paired t test, $P>0.05$) after being transferred into TSBS for 20 minutes. Therefore we consider using TSBS as diluent did not invalidate the drop plate results. To compare the bacterial survival in various media, 93U204 cells were re-suspended in PBS, natural seawater with 3% salinity (NSW), half-strength natural seawater diluted with distilled water (HNSW), or TSBS. The salinity of seawater was determined using a hand-held salinity refractometer (MR100ATC, Milwaukee Instruments, Rocky Mount, North Carolina, USA). The starting concentration of 93U204 was approximately 5×10^9 CFU/mL. The survival rate was determined every day for 7 days by plate counts on TSAS after serial dilution. In the long-term starvation experiment, we re-suspended the cells in PBS or TSBS for 214 days using a starting concentration of 1×10^9 CFU/mL. The bacterial viability was measured on days 0, 1, 2, 3, 8, 14, 35, 56, 93, 115, and 214.

Phenotypic characterization

We developed a Motility-Hemolysis-Proteolysis (MHP) grouping system to classify *V. vulnificus* isolates, which was based on three readily identifiable characteristics, namely motility (M), hemolysis (H), and proteolysis (P). The isolates were classified into one of 100 phenotype groups according to their motility (five levels, from M0 to M4), hemolysis (four levels, from H0 to H3), and proteolysis (five levels, from P0 to P4) activity levels. Motility, hemolytic activity and proteolytic activity were measured on motility agar (1% tryptone, 2% NaCl, 0.25% agar), blood agar (LB agar supplemented with 5% sheep blood), and skim milk agar (LB agar supplemented with 2% skim milk). In every test the progenitor 93U204 was inoculated on the same test plate as a control, and the diameters of its colony on motility agar, clear zone on blood agar and clear zone on skim milk agar were recorded. We defined M0 to M4 as having colony size of 0, 0–0.33, 0.33–0.67, 0.67–1.2, or over 1.2 times of that measured in 93U204 control; H0 to H3 as having clear zone on blood agar of 0, 0–0.5, 0.5–1.5, or over 1.5 times of that measured in 93U204 control; and P0 to P4 as having clear zone on skim milk agar of 0, 0–0.33, 0.33–0.67, 0.67–1.2, or over 1.2 times of that measured in 93U204 control. The progenitor 93U204 had the M3H2P3 phenotype, and the human pathogenic strain YJ016 had the M3H1P3 phenotype. Some 93U204 phenotypic variants (PVs) developed opaque or translucent colonies. These PVs included an additional "O" for opaque and "T" for transparent in their MHP label.

To determine the phenotypic composition, colonies from each sample were picked randomly with sterile toothpicks and inoculated into 150 μL LB in a 96-well microtiter plate, followed by overnight incubation at 30°C. We used a stainless steel 96-pin replicator to transfer the bacterial cells onto motility agar, skim milk agar, blood agar, and thiosulfate-citrate-bile salts-sucrose (TCBS) agar. The results for motility, proteolytic activity, hemolytic activity, and growth on TCBS were determined at 6, 20, 48, and 20 h after inoculation at 30°C. Isolates with the same MHP grouping were defined as a PV.

Starvation-induced diversification (SID) experiments

In this study six different SID experiments in PBS were conducted. Each bottle of inoculated PBS was treated as a population. Populations within the same experimental group received the same 93U204 preparation as the inocula. For each population, a sampling series was conducted at the indicated time for each experiment to trace the dynamics of phenotypic change. For each sample, approximately 30 colonies were isolated for phenotypic characterization and the result was used to calculate the relative abundance of each PV. The starting bacterial density was adjusted to approximately 10^9 CFU/mL, and the experiments were conducted in 10 mL of PBS in 30-mL serum bottles, unless indicated otherwise.

The settings for each experiment were as follows. (1) The analysis of temporal change in the PV composition included two sets of experiments, with one population in each set. Both populations received the same inoculum. Samples were taken on days 0, 8, 16, 24, and 32. (2) The analysis of SID in replicate populations comprised two sets of experiments, with five populations in each set. Samples were taken on day 33. (3) The SID and population survival rate analysis comprised 12 sets of experiments, with 1–3 populations in each set and a total of 20. Samples were taken on days 14 or 15. (4) The analysis of the effect of cell density on SID comprised four sets of experiments, with three populations in each set. The bacterial densities in these four sets were adjusted to approximately 10^9, 10^7, 10^5, and 10^3 CFU/mL. Samples were taken on days 14, 28, and 42. (5) The analysis of the effect of population size on SID comprised three sets of experiments, with three populations in each set. The bacterial suspension volumes used in the three sets were 100 mL, 10 mL, and 3 mL, in 125-mL serum bottles (Z114014, Wheaton), 30-mL serum bottles, and 30-mL serum bottles, respectively. Samples were taken on days 14, 28 and 42. (6) Two *V. vulnificus* strains, 93U204 and YJ016, were used to test the effect of salinity on SID. For each strain, the analysis comprised one set of experiments, with three treatments in each set. Samples were taken on days 14, 28, and 42. These sets used natural seawater with 1%, 2%, and 3% salinities. The seawater was sterilized using 0.22 μm filter. The salinity was checked using a refractometer. The desired salinity was achieved by mixing freshly collected seawater with freshwater from the same estuary area.

Competition experiments

Three isolates, each from a separate PBS-starvation survivor population of 93U204, were used in the competition experiments. B33-12 was isolated from the trial B 33-day population; C30-2 was isolated from the trial C 30-day population; and D33-4 was isolated from the trial D 33-day population. All of the strains derived from the starvation cultures were identified as *V. vulnificus* by species-specific *vvp* PCR [26]. Another primer pair of p134/p135 was also used, which targeted *V. vulnificus rpoS* [27]. The *rpoS* primer pair comprised the forward primer p134 (5′-ACATAACgATAATTACCTCAgTgC-3′), which started 264 bp upstream of the YJ016 *rpoS*, and the reverse primer p135 (5′-CgTCAAAAATTgTCTCAACTTg-3′), which ended 276 bp downstream of YJ016 *rpoS* and was located in *mutS*. The expected size of this PCR product was 1530 bp. The PCR protocol comprised a preheating step at 94°C for 6 min, followed by 30 cycles of 94°C for 30 s, 55°C for 30 s, and 72°C for 2 min, with a final extension at 72°C for 7 min. Their *rpoS* DNA sequences were identical to those of the 93U204 progenitor cell according to nucleotide sequencing with an Applied Biosystems 3730xl DNA Analyzer, which was conducted at the VYM Genome Research Center of National Yang-Ming University. The obtained nucleotide sequences were compared with the GenBank DNA database using the BLASTn program.

All of the isolates were stored at −80°C in TSBS with 15% glycerol. The stock was subcultured in 12 mL TSBS in a 125-mL flask and grown to the late exponential phase with 200 rpm horizontal shaking. The culture was then washed twice with PBS by centrifugation (10 min, room temperature, 4500×*g*). The bacterial preparation was re-suspended in PBS to the desired concentration. The progenitor 93U204 was mixed at 1000:1 with each of the isogenic cultures derived from C30-2, D33-4, or B33-12 in PBS at the start of a two-week experiment. Monocultures of the 93U204 progenitor and mutants were included as controls.

The bacterial concentration of each sample was determined using the drop plate method with TSAS plates. The relative abundance of each competing population was determined every 2 days for 14 days. We used phenotypic characterization to identify the relative amount of the two competing phenotypes, because only a small fraction of the cells changed their phenotype up to the late stage of the starvation experiment. In each of these competition experiments, cells with reduced motility and enhanced proteolytic activity were considered to be descendents of C30-2, cells with reduced motility that were unable to grow on TCBS were considered to be descendents of D33-4, and cells with reduced motility and enhanced proteolytic activities were considered to be descendents of B33-12.

Diversity evaluation and statistical analysis

The bacterial diversity was evaluated using the Shannon diversity index, $H' = -\sum p_i \ln p_i$, where p_i is the relative abundance of each phenotype. Each phenotype was defined as having the same motility, hemolysis, and proteolysis activity characteristics. Cluster analysis and linear regression were performed using PAST software (http://folk.uio.no/ohammer/past/) [28].

Electron microscopy

All of the electron microscopy experiments were conducted in the Electron Microscopy Center, Tzu-Chi University. A bacterial suspension from each preparation was centrifuged at 5,000×*g* for 5 min at 4°C to collect bacterial cells. The pellets were re-suspended and fixed with 2.5% glutaldehyde in PBS at 4°C. On the day the observations were made, the bacterial cells were washed twice with 0.1 M phosphate buffer with 5% sucrose, post-fixed with 1% osmium tetraoxide for 1 h, and washed twice with 0.1 M phosphate buffer with 5% sucrose. Next, a 5 μL drop of bacterial suspension was placed on a Formvar/carbon-coated grid for 2 min to allow absorption of bacteria onto the grid. A drop of 2% phosphotungstic acid was placed on the grid to achieve negative staining. The grids were then air-dried and examined using a Hitachi H-7500 transmission electron microscope (Hitachi, Tokyo, Japan) at 80 kV. Digital images were collected using a 2048×2048 Macrofire monochrome CCD camera (Optronics, Goleta, California, USA). Cell diameter and length measurements were made using these images with ImageJ v. 1.46 (http://rsbweb.nih.gov/ij/index.html).

Chemicals and reagents

All of the PCR-related reagents were included in the Taq DNA Polymerase 2X Master Mix Red kit (1.5 mM $MgCl_2$, Ampliqon IIII, Odense, Denmark). The electron microscopy chemicals and reagents were obtained from Electron Microscopy Services (Hatfield, Pennsylvania, USA). The culture media and ingredients were obtained from Becton Dickinson and Company (Sparks, Maryland, USA), while all other chemicals were obtained from Sigma (St Louis, Missouri, USA). All of the primers were purchased from Gene Messenger (Kaohsiung City, Taiwan). Fresh sheep blood was obtained from Creative Media Products Ltd (New Taipei City, Taiwan).

Results

Survival of *V. vulnificus* 93U204 after starvation in various culture media

The repeated appearance of new *V. vulnificus* pathogens in tilapia farms and their high heterogeneity in natural populations (unpublished data) suggests that some environmental biotype 1 strains might repeatedly invade and persist in low-salinity tilapia farms, which later became pathogens. Thus, we aimed to determine whether environmental stresses, such as starvation, could contribute to the emergence of virulence.

First, we examined the survival of *V. vulnificus* 93U204 in nutrient-poor PBS and seawater, or nutrient-rich TSBS. The number of culturable 93U204 in PBS dropped rapidly by two orders from the starting concentration of 5×10^9 CFU/mL during the first week in PBS, NSW and HNSW (Figure 1A). The viable population was even smaller in TSBS, to approximately 8×10^2 CFU/mL on day 1 and below the detection limit (20 CFU/mL) after day 3.

To understand the long-term survival of *V. vulnificus*, we inoculated PBS and TSBS with cells at approximately 1×10^9 CFU/mL, and tracked the viable population dynamics for 7 months (Figure 1B). Three-order and five-order drops were seen after 7 days in the PBS and TSBS groups, respectively. The mortality stabilized after 2 weeks, then the populations entered a slow and gradual declining phase in both groups. In another experiment with a starting cell density of 5×10^8 CFU/mL, approximately 10^3 CFU/mL of *V. vulnificus* survived starvation in PBS at 1215 days after inoculation. We conclude that a starved 93U204 population will typically experience a rapid decrease during the first week, before the mortality stabilizes after the second week. The population then enters a slow period of decline, but can survive for months to years.

We examined the morphology of starved cells by transmission electron microscopy (Figure 1C). The un-stressed log phase cells exhibited the typical vibrioid morphology, whereas the cells starved in PBS for 4 days became more slender. Most of the cells from the 4 day TSBS population were ruptured, which indicated their extremely low viability in this treatment. PBS-starved cells were a similar length to the log-phase cells, but their cell diameters were much smaller (Figure 1D).

Starvation and PBS-induced phenotypic diversification in *V. vulnificus*

The high mortality in starved *V. vulnificus* populations may exert strong selection on survivors. We conducted 2 independent PBS starvation trials of 93U204 and monitored the population for phenotypic change. SID was seen in both trials (Figure 2A). A total of 16 and 13 PVs were found in trial 1 and trial 2, respectively. We designated the progenitor 93U204 M3H2P3 phenotype as the "wild-type (WT)" phenotype. PV was first detected at day 8 in trial 1, and at day 16 in trial 2. The proportion of WT cells decreased with time as the number of detected PVs increased. To confirm that these changes were not transient, we picked five morphologically distinct colonies from each population to assess their phenotypic consistency through subcultures. After at least three subcultures onto TSAS, none reverted back to the WT phenotype, which demonstrated that these changes were not transient and were likely to be genetic.

The PVs in each population were categorized further to detect general trends in the motility, hemolysis, or proteolysis activity (Figure 2B). PVs with reduced motility (mot-R PVs) and with reduced hemolytic activity (hem-R PVs) increased with time, and the mot-R PVs appeared earlier than the hem-R PVs during starvation. PVs with enhanced proteolysis activity (pro-E PVs) appeared transiently on day 24 and disappeared or decreased greatly on day 32 in both trials. We conclude that a reduction in motility, a reduction in hemolytic activity, and an enhancement in proteolytic activity could promote the survival of 93U204 during starvation.

SID was associated with cell survival in populations

If diversification is a bacterial strategy for overcoming environmental stress, there should be a correlation between diversity and population survival. Thus, we collected survival and PV composition data from 20 starved 93U204 populations. All of these populations were started with approximately 10^9 CFU/mL in 10 mL PBS, followed by starvation for 14 or 15 days before sampling. Three of the 20 populations had very low viability at approximately 0.1% of the original population (Figure 2C). SID was seen in all but these three populations, which remained homogeneous and all of the colonies examined (30 for each population) had an unchanged phenotype. This result suggests that SID may be needed for the population to overcome environmental stress.

Source of PVs in starvation survival populations

PVs found in starved population may have been present in low numbers in the original population, or they may have been mutants derived from WT cells during starvation. Thus, we conducted five parallel starvation experiments using the same original population as the inoculum (Figure 3). We hypothesized that if these PVs were original members of the inoculum population and were selected during starvation, the compositions of these five surviving populations should be very similar.

The results showed that each population had a unique phenotypic composition after 33 days of starvation (Figure 3B), which suggested that these PVs were novel mutants that evolved independently in each population. However, similar trends were seen among the populations (Figure 3C). In both trials, mot-R PVs dominated the five populations, which indicates that a reduction in motility may provide more advantages than other mutations during early starvation. In some populations, hem-R PVs also increased in proportion (Figure 3B).

Advantages of starvation survivors compared with wild-type cells

Certain PVs were observed repeatedly in the starvation experiments (Figures 2 and 3), which suggests that these PVs may have been more resistant to starvation-induced death, or that they may have been related to traits that made them more competitive than WT cells during starvation. To demonstrate that PVs performed better than the WT strain during starvation conditions, we selected three isolates, i.e., C30-2, D33-4, and B33-12, from three different survivor populations and performed competition tests with WT cells. C30-2 was isolated from the trial C 30-day population, and had reduced motility and enhanced proteolytic activity (M1H2P4 phenotype). D33-4 was isolated from the trial D 33-day population, and had reduced motility, reduced hemolysis, and increased proteolytic activity, and could not grow on TCBS plates (M1H1P4 phenotype). B33-12 was isolated from

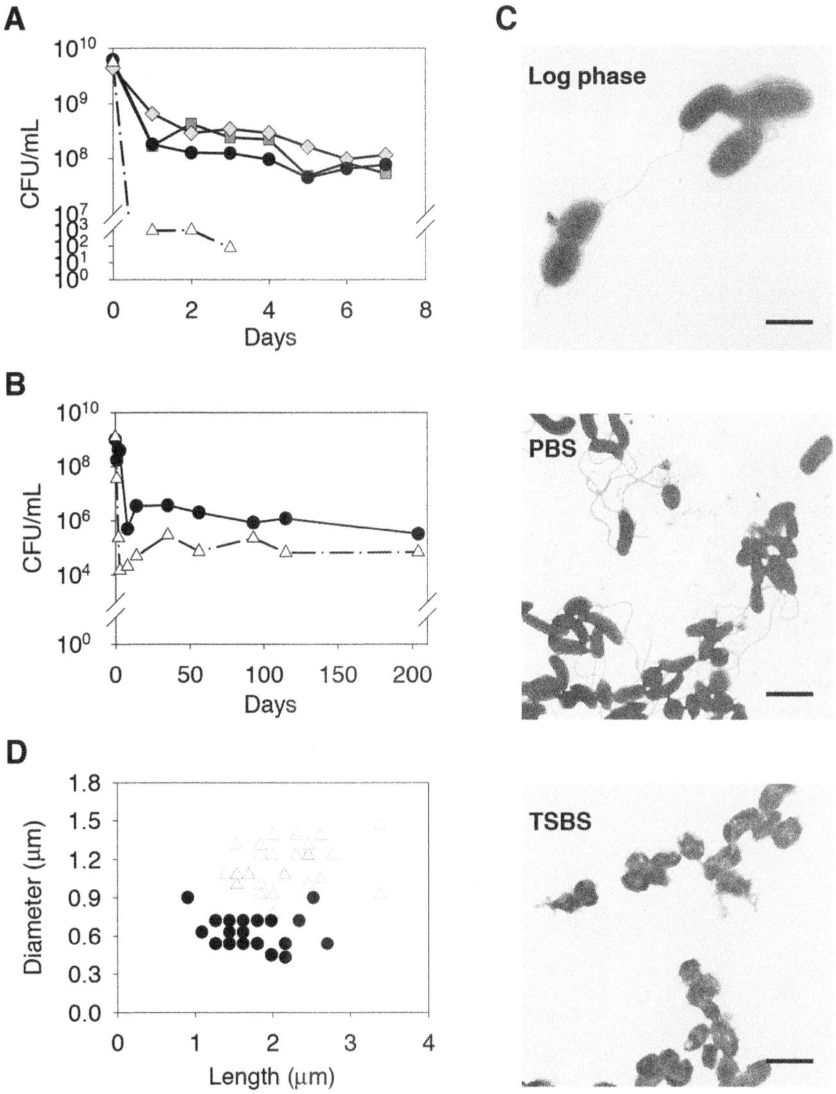

Figure 1. Survival of *V. vulnificus* cultures in various media. (A) Dynamics of *V. vulnificus* populations in phosphate-buffered saline (PBS, ●), natural seawater (NSW, ◇), half-strength natural seawater (HNSW, □), and tryptic soy broth with 1.5% NaCl (TSBS, △) during the first week after inoculation. The results shown were derived from three replicate populations. (B) Dynamics of *V. vulnificus* populations in PBS (●) and TSBS (△) during an extended period of starvation (214 days). Representative results are shown from one experiment. (C) Electron micrographs of *V. vulnificus* cells showing the cellular morphology of a log-phase population (Log phase), a population starved in PBS for 4 days (PBS), and a population starved in TSBS for 4 days (TSBS). Most of the cells starved in TSBS were ruptured. All of the bars represent 2 μm. (D) The diameters and lengths of log-phase cells (△) and cells starved in PBS for 4 days (●).

the trial B 33-day population, and had reduced motility and hemolysis activity levels (M1H1P3 phenotype).

When cultured alone in PBS, the survival rates of all the tested PVs were similar to that of the progenitor control (Figure 4, upper), which indicated that they were not more resistant to starvation-induced death. When inoculated at 0.1% in a mixed culture with progenitor 93U204, the C30-2-like M1H2P4 cells exhibited a slow increase and reached 14% on day 14 (Figure 4A) (95% and 81% in the second and third trials), while D33-4-like M1H2P4 cells reached 56% on day 14 in mixed culture (Figure 4B) (79% and 62% in the second and third trials, respectively). B33-12-like M1H1P3 cells reached 40% on day 2 and continued to increase until they reached 95% on day 14 (Figure 4C) (49% and 79% in the second and third trials, respectively). The relative abundance of each mutant varied among trials, but they dominated from 0.1% in all three trails. In mutant monoculture, no isolates switched back to the WT phenotype. Similarly, only less than 6.5% of mutant-like isolates were detected in the 93U204 progenitor monoculture at the end of the experiments. Therefore, we conclude that all three tested PVs were more competitive than the WT cells at surviving starvation.

Cell density, but not the number of cells, had a major effect on SID

High density can be stressful for bacterial cells and lead to more mutations in the population. Thus, we tested the effect of cell density on the generation of SID. We examined SID at 10^9, 10^7, 10^5, and 10^3 CFU/mL. The PV diversity appeared to increase with density (Figure 5A). The Shannon index correlated positively with log-transformed cell density (linear regression, $r = 0.76684$, $P = 0.0048$). Both percentage of WT cells ($r = -0.81659$,

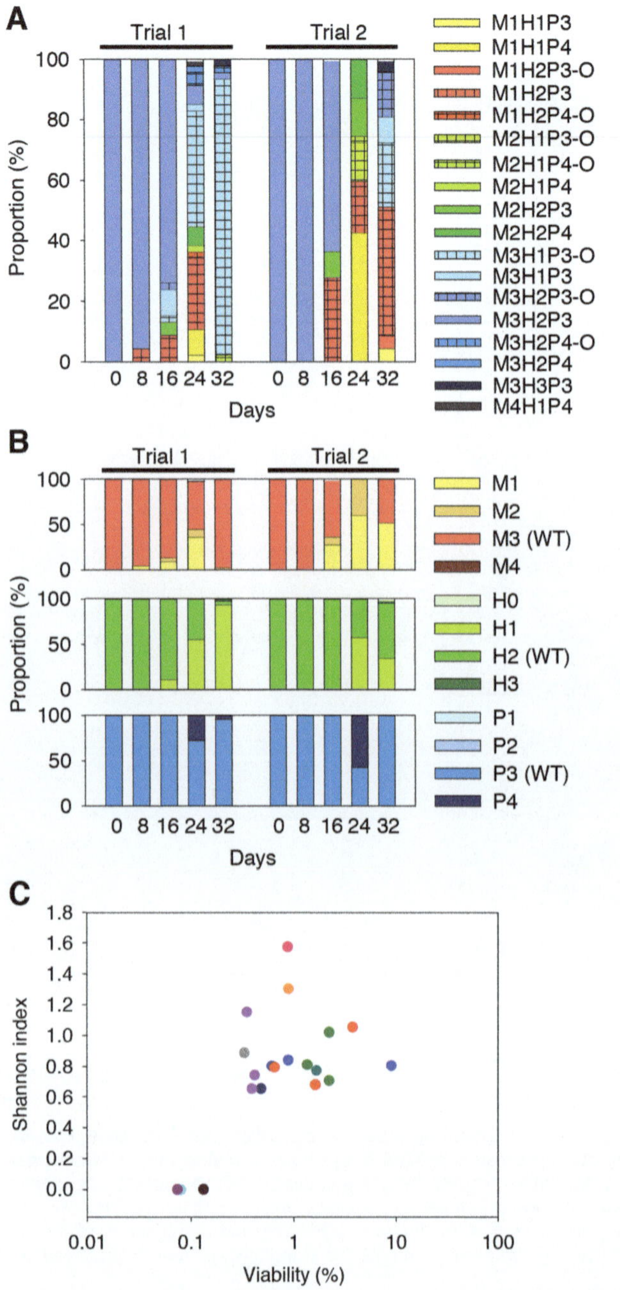

Figure 2. Phenotypic diversification of the *V. vulnificus* 93U204 population during starvation in phosphate-buffered saline. (A) Relative abundance of phenotypic variants in starved populations from two replicate trials. The population gradually diversified from the 93U204 M3H2P3 phenotype. (B) Compositions of populations, which were categorized based on their motility (top panel), hemolytic activity (middle), and proteolytic activity (bottom panel). WT, phenotype of the parental 93U204. (C) Association of diversity with mortality in starved populations. Twenty populations were starved in phosphate-buffered saline, and their survival and diversity were measured on days 14 or 15. The figure shows the distinction between low survival/un-diversified populations (left) and high survival/diversified populations. These 20 populations were derived from 12 separate inoculations (indicated by different colors).

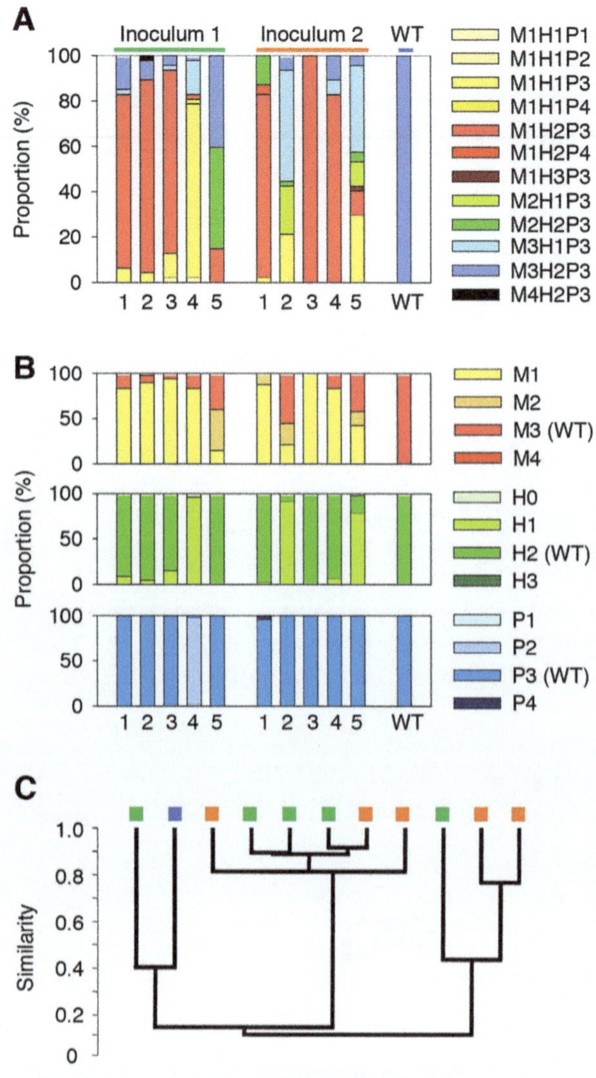

Figure 3. Phenotypic variant (PV) compositions of different sets of starvation populations. (A) The PV compositions of two sets of starvation populations, which started with the same inoculum, were analyzed for 33 days (n = 5). (B) Summaries of the phenotypic composition in terms of the motility (M), hemolysis (H), and proteolysis (P) activity levels are shown in. (C) Cluster analysis of the PV composition of each population. Green rectagulars, populations received inoculum 1; organge, populations received inoculum 2; blue, unstarved control. The analysis was based on the Bray-Curtis similarity and paired group methods.

P = 0.0008) and ratio of final to initial population size (r = − 0.88628, P = 0.0001) correlated negatively with log-transformed cell density. However, this trend was only evident in the day 14 population and was absent on days 28 and 42, which suggests that the density effects were probably masked by saturation because of continuous diversification.

In these experiments, the increase in density was confounded by the increased absolute number of cells in the populations. Larger populations contained more cells so they were more likely to contain more mutants, which meant that there was a higher likelihood of beneficial mutations accumulating in these populations. In the next experiment, we fixed the starting cell density at 10^9 CFU/mL and varied the volume of the medium among 100, 10, or 3 mL, before examining the effect of the population size on SID (Figure 5B). Neither Shannon index nor percentage of WT cell correlated significantly with medium volume. Therefore, we conclude that the cell density has a more important effect than the

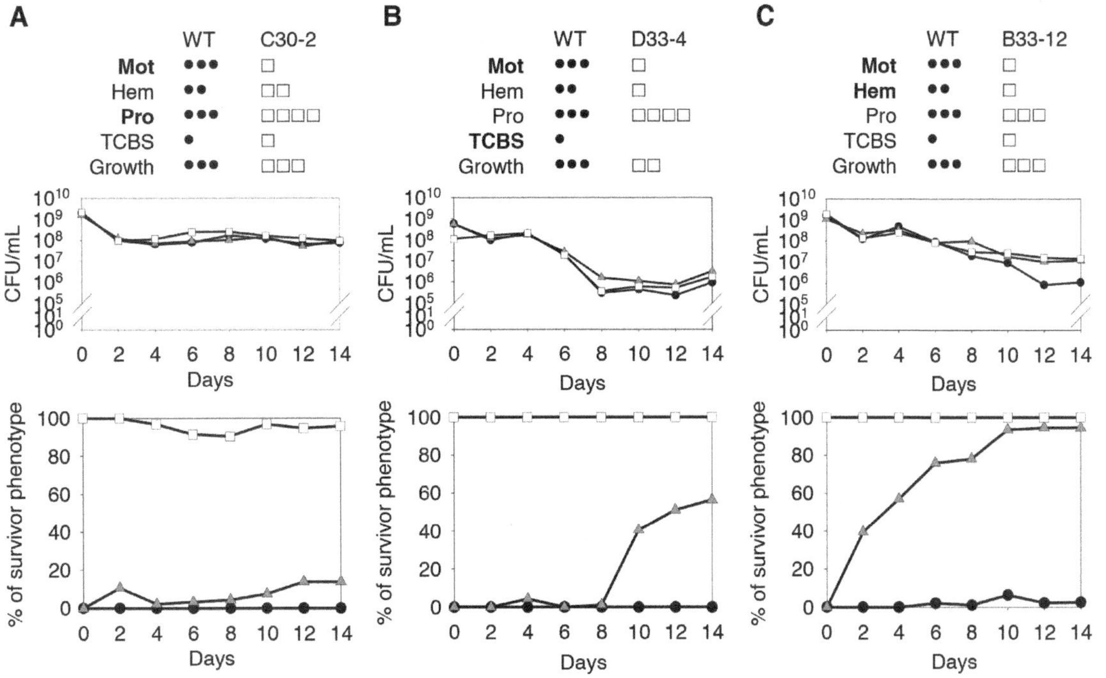

Figure 4. Competition between various phenotypic variants (PVs) derived from different survivor populations during starvation survival. Three PVs, i.e., C30-2 (A), D33-4 (B), and B33-12 (C), were competed with 93U204 cells in starvation conditions. The top panels show the population size and mutant phenotype dynamics. The bottom panels show the results of the competition experiments. For each mutant-wild-type (WT) pair, we measured the survival of the mutant-only (□), WT-only (●), or WT-mixed with 0.1% mutant (△) populations. The relative abundance of cells with the mutant phenotype was determined by examining 94 colonies in each trial. All three of the tested PVs increased their relative abundance after 14 days. Only one representative set of results (trial 1) is shown. The motility (Mot), hemolysis (Hem), proteolytic activity (Pro), growth on TCBS (TCBS), and growth on TSAS (growth) phenotype of each mutant was included in the figure and the characteristics used for differentiate mutant from WT colonies were shown in bold.

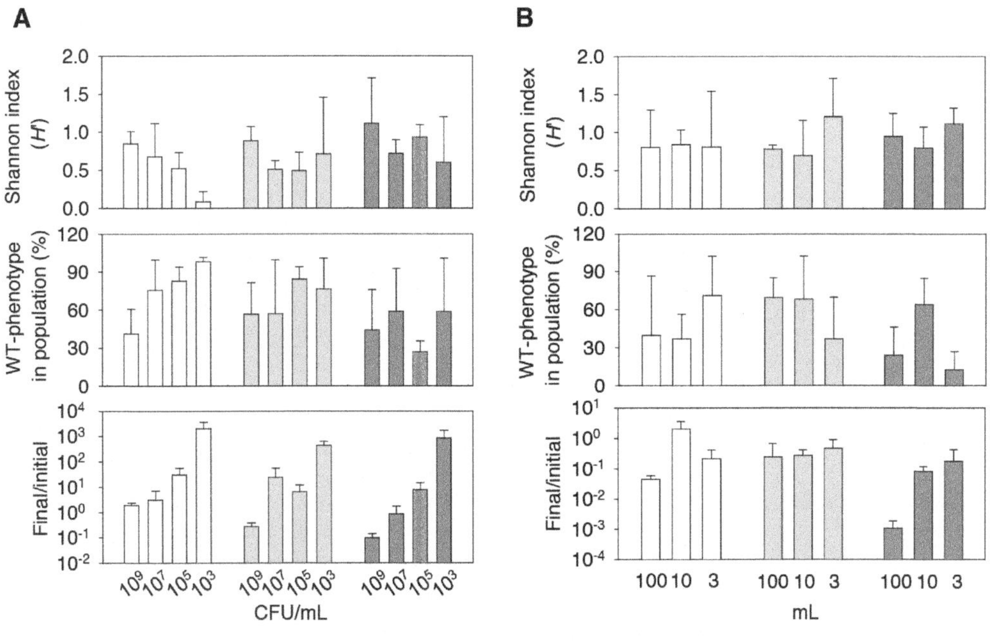

Figure 5. Effects of population density and population size on starvation-induced diversification. 93U204 cells were starved in 10 mL phosphate-buffered saline at densities of 10^9, 10^7, 10^5, and 10^3 CFU/mL (A), or in 100, 10 and 3 mL at a density of 10^9 CFU/mL (B). The Shannon diversity index (top), percentage of cells with the wild-type (WT) phenotype (middle), and survival rate (bottom) of each population on days 14 (white bar), 28 (light grey bar), and 42 (dark grey bar) are shown. At day 14, phenotypic diversity (indicated by Shannon index) correlated positively with cell density, and percentage of WT and ratio of final to initial populations correlated negatively with cell density. After day 14, the trends in Shannon index and WT cell percentage were less apparent. Increased population size did not lead to more beneficial mutations in the population.

population size during phenotypic diversification in conditions of starvation.

SID in seawater

SID was readily observed in a laboratory setting, so we investigated whether this phenomenon also occurs in natural seawater. We starved *V. vulnificus* 93U204 cells in natural seawater samples, which were adjusted to salinities of 1%, 2%, or 3%, and we monitored any phenotypic changes (Figure 6A and B). The SID observed in natural seawater was comparable to that in PBS, which indicates that SID can occur in natural marine environments. For comparison, another *V. vulnificus* isolate YJ016 was also used in this starvation experiment (Figure 6C and D). SID was observed in both 93U204 and YJ016, although YJ016 diversified at a faster rate. The three populations cultured with different salinities had similar SID, which suggests that this phenomenon was not affected by salinity.

Discussion

In this study, we determined the population dynamics of 93U204 during long-term starvation. The survival rates were similar to those reported in previous studies [14–16]. During the first week, there was a dramatic decrease in the viable population. Two weeks after inoculation, the population increased slightly, before the population entered a long and gradual decline (Figure 1). The life cycle of *E. coli* has been classified into lag, log, stationary, death, and long-term stationary phases [29]. *E. coli* cells grow rapidly during the log phase but the growth slows in the stationary phase when the nutrient supply decreases, and finally the cells progress to the death phase. Typically, >99% of the population lose their viability during the death phase, but the remaining cells can survive for several years with few declines in their cell numbers. The survival of *V. vulnificus* followed similar dynamics to those previously reported for *E. coli*, with an apparent death phase (rapid decrease) and a long-term stationary phase (slow decrease). A starved *E. coli* population maintained its size at approximately 10^6 CFU/mL for over 5 years when sterile distilled water was supplied to maintain the volume and osmolarity [29]. In our experiments, *V. vulnificus* remained at approximately 10^6 CFU/mL in PBS and 10^5 CFU/mL in TSBS for 214 days (Figure 1B), while it remained at approximately 10^3 CFU/mL in PBS for 1215 days. Therefore both species have comparable survival in longterm starvation.

After treating the stationary phase *E. coli* population with antibiotics to remove any dividing cells, some non-dividing cells were found to be dividing [30]. These cells were named "persisters" that allowed the population to survive in a harsh environment. Similar persisters may also play a role in the earlier stages during the survival of *V. vulnificus*, but they are not likely to be the major source of survivors because the "revived" persisters had the WT phenotype. The divergence between parallel populations and the fixed phenotype during passages strongly suggests that PVs are mutants derived from the progenitor cells. The cells acquired adaptive mutations during starvation, before subsequent selection, and they survived the stressful conditions.

Vibrios are known to enter the VBNC state under stress. In *V. vulnificus* the VBNC state could be induced through a temperature downshift to 5°C [31] or 4°C [32]. Although the cell viability seen in our starvation experiment may be similar to that in VBNC population, it is unlikely that the loss of viability is due to VBNC. Our experiments were conducted at 30°C, and no VBNC *V. vulnificus* has been reported at this temperature so far. An elevation of temperature to 21°C is sufficient to resuscitate VBNC *V. vulnificus* within 24 h [33]. We compared the property of 93U204 cells kept in PBS at either 30°C or at 4°C. After 9-day starvation treatment, most cells kept at 30°C co-stained with both propidium iodide and SYTO 9 (using LIVE/DEAD *Bac*Light Bacterial Viability Kit, for microscopy & quantitative assays, L7012, Life Technologies, Carlsbad, California, USA)(unpublished data), but co-staining was rarely seen in cells kept at 4°C. Addition of catalase is known to increase the survival of VBNC cells on agar plates [34]. Addition of catalase increased survival of cells kept at 4°C (with vs. without catalase, paired t-test, $P = 0.038$) by 4.6 ±3.2 times, but it had no effect on cells kept at 30°C (paired t-test, $P = 0.4655$). These data suggest that the loss of viability seen in our starvation experiments was not due to the induction of VBNC state.

Most cells that survived the death phase exhibited phenotypic changes (Figure 2). These changes were generally advantageous compared with the progenitor cells and they are referred to collectively as growth advantage in the stationary phase (GASP) phenotypes [29]. Cells that exhibit GASP phenotypes during starvation have been reported in bacteria such as *Campylobacter jejuni* [35], *Pseudomonas* [36,37], *Geobacter* [38], and enterobacteria [39]. A GASP phenotype was also observed in *V. fischeri* [40]. A non-toxigenic *V. cholerae* isolate derived from a starved long-term slab culture was shown to have growth advantages compared with its toxigenic progenitors [41]. Mutations that lead to GASP have been studied in *E. coli* (reviewed in [29]). The loss of a functional *rpoS* may be advantageous in increasing amino acid utilization, while *lrp* and the *ybeJ-gltJKL* cluster encode the leucine-responsive protein and a high-affinity aspartate and glutamate transporter, respectively. In *Vibrio* spp., however, there is still no known genetic basis for GASP phenotypes.

Three types of strategies may facilitate bacterial survival during starvation: persister, scavenger, and replicator strategies. Cells that employ a persister strategy can persist during starvation conditions via physiological adaptation. These cells may have to trade their nutrient acquisition ability (nutritional competence) for self-preservation, according to the SPANC balance hypothesis [42]. Scavengers are cells that can increase their nutrient input, either by acquiring the ability to explore novel resources or by increasing their substrate-binding affinity or substrate-transporting ability. Replicators are cells that reduce their energy expenditure via mutation in functions that are not required for survival so they may have higher rates of replication. Scavengers and replicators may replicate faster than their progenitor cells, so they are more likely to dominate the surviving population.

Several systems have been used to study bacterial responses to nutrient limitation. Lenski's laboratory have conducted a long-term evolution experiment (LTEE) with *E. coli* [43]. In this system, the bacteria are transferred to new broth each day. During the first few hours, replicators may have advantages, but the scavengers are favored over time. Persisters have an advantage only when the population experiences severe nutrient deprivation, which is not likely to happen in the LTEE. Therefore, replicators and scavengers are expected to dominate in this system. The mean fitness increased by approximately 35% in the 2000-generation population [44]. The adaptation led to a decrease in the lag time before growth and an increase in the maximum growth rate, although the death rate and the nutrient concentration required to support half the maximum rate did not change significantly. Therefore, replicators were favored in this system.

Ferenci's laboratory pioneered the use of a chemostat system to study the response and evolution of *E. coli* in a constant low-nutrient environment [45]. The nutrient concentrations were maintained at stable low levels, so the scavengers had an

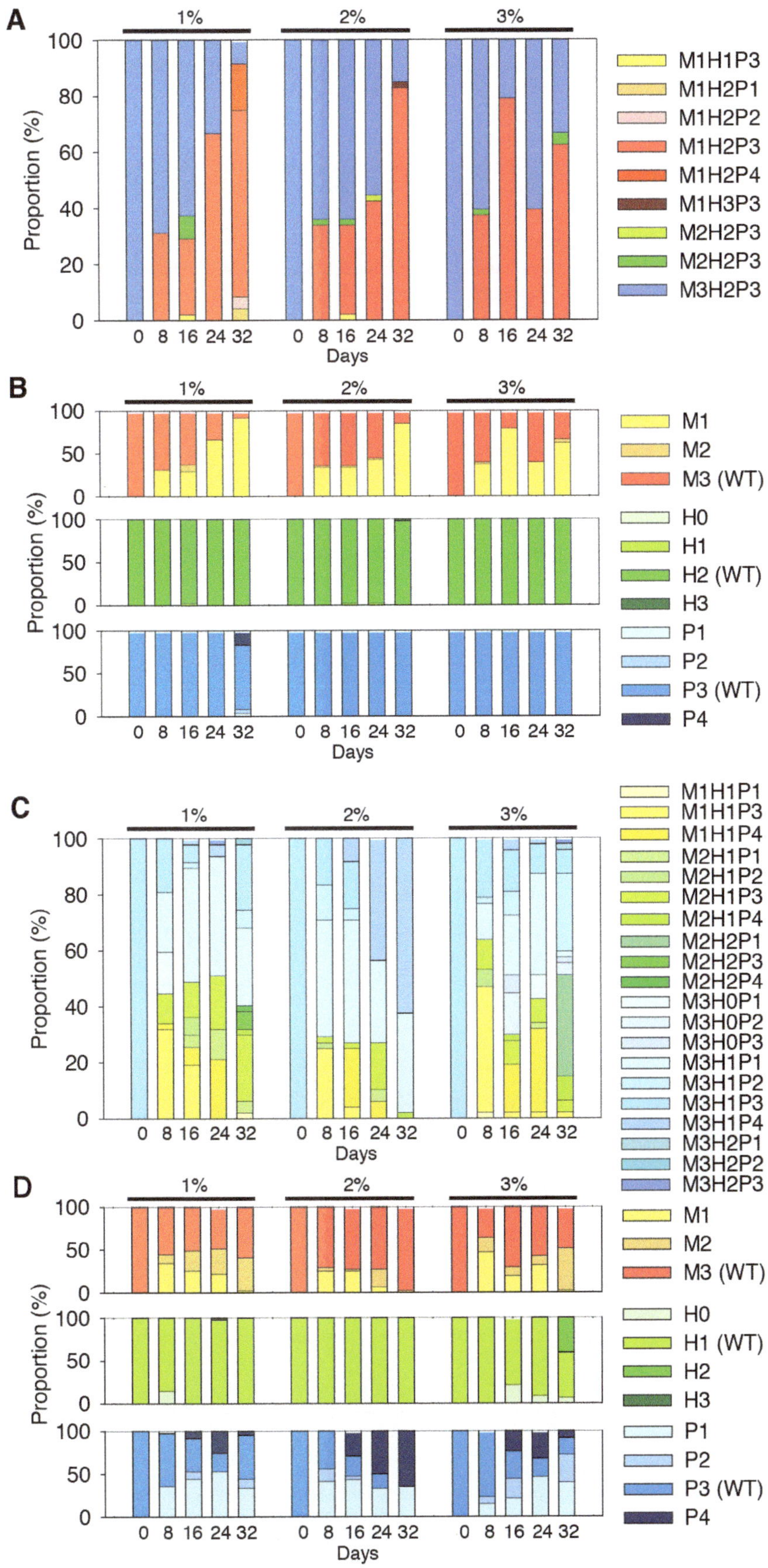
A
1%
2%
3%
Proportion (%)
100
80
60
40
20
0
0 8 16 24 32
0 8 16 24 32
0 8 16 24 32
Days
M1H1P3
M1H2P1
M1H2P2
M1H2P3
M1H2P4
M1H3P3
M2H2P3
M2H2P3
M3H2P3
B
1%
2%
3%
Proportion (%)
100
50
0
Days
M1
M2
M3 (WT)
H0
H1
H2 (WT)
H3
P1
P2
P3 (WT)
P4
C
1%
2%
3%
Proportion (%)
Days
M1H1P1
M1H1P3
M1H1P4
M2H1P1
M2H1P2
M2H1P3
M2H1P4
M2H2P1
M2H2P3
M2H2P4
M3H0P1
M3H0P2
M3H0P3
M3H1P1
M3H1P2
M3H1P3
M3H1P4
M3H2P1
M3H2P2
M3H2P3
D
1%
2%
3%
Proportion (%)
Days
M1
M2
M3 (WT)
H0
H1 (WT)
H2
H3
P1
P2
P3 (WT)
P4

Figure 6. Starvation-induced diversification (SID) of *V. vulnificus* strains 93U204 and YJ016 in seawater. We tested the SID in natural seawater samples with salinities of 1%, 2%, or 3%. The results for 93U204 are shown in (A) and (B), while those for YJ016 are shown in (C) and (D). The starting concentration was 10^9 CFU/mL. The phenotypic variant compositions (A and C) and the summarized population compositions (B and D) for motility (upper), hemolysis (middle), and proteolysis activity (lower) are also shown.

advantage over replicators and persisters. In this system, an *rpoS* mutant rapidly became dominant within the first 3 days [46]. Growth in these conditions is highly *rpoD*-dependent, which supports *rpoS* mutations [47]. Mutations in the *rpoS*, *mlc*, *malT*, and *mgl* have been demonstrated to increase the expression of *ompF*, *lamB*, *mglBAC*, and *ptsG*, which improves high-affinity glucose uptake [48−50]. Thus, the scavengers dominated this system.

In our study, we starved the cells in PBS from the start, so persisters may have possessed advantages compared with other cells during the first few days. Dead cells accumulated rapidly over time and the surviving cells actively utilized the nutrients released from the dead cells, so they gradually increased in number and dominated the population. The first types of PVs that appeared in the starved populations were mot-R PVs (Figures 2 and 6). Reductions or loss of motility after starvation have been reported in diverse bacteria, including *Rhizobium meliloti* [51], *V. angustum* [52], and unidentified marine bacteria [53]. Flagellar motility requires much energy, so a reduction in bacterial motility has the benefit of saving energy, which is consistent with the recently proposed Black Queen hypotheses [54]. However, these PVs did not have an increased growth rate in TSBS. It is likely that these PVs lacked a growth advantage, or they may only possess a growth advantage in low-nutrient conditions. During a stringent response, *E. coli* downregulates the expression of flagellar genes [55], [56]. Recently, it was reported that *V. vulnificus* downregulates its flagellar regulator FlhF in the stationary phase via the quorum sensing master regulator SmcR [57]. This indicates that cells are not motile in the stationary phase so those that lose motility will not be selected against and will tend to be detected. Without appropriate evidence, we were not able to tell whether the rapid appearance of mot-R PVs was a result of a replicator or scavenger strategy. However, based on the presence of large numbers of dead cells, a scavenger strategy was more favored.

In the present study, the average proteolytic activity of the 93U204 survivor populations remained unchanged or increased, but the hemolytic activity decreased with time (Figure 2). These trends may represent a trade-off between using energy to produce the corresponding proteins and acquiring nutrients from dead cells with these proteins. In the set of experiment shown in Figure 6B, the proteolytic activity and hemolytic activity of the survivors remained largely unchanged, although mot-R PVs still dominated. We hypothesize that a reduction in motility is a more reliable strategy for increasing fitness, whereas the advantage of manipulating exoenzyme production is dependent on the environment and the competing bacteria. Similarly, in YJ016, PVs with reduced or enhanced proteolytic activity increased their relative abundance (Figure 6D), so other factors may be more important when surviving starvation.

In the competition experiments, all three PVs dominated the progenitor cells in all three trials. However, there were high variations in their proportions in the final population. The mutants had advantages over the progenitor cells, but newly emerged mutations in the populations could potentially affect the results of the competition, although these new mutations were practically undetectable because we only examined a limited number of phenotypic features. This observation emphasizes the dynamic nature of evolution under starvation conditions, where the exact composition of the starved population will be changing constantly.

In conclusion, the dynamics of *V. vulnificus* population under conditions of starvation were very similar to those of *E. coli*, which may be common in Gammaproteobacteria. In addition, SID was observed in populations cultured in PBS, which also occurred with a wide range of salinities. We suggest that SID is likely to occur in natural settings, which may be the mechanism that maintains the high phenotypic diversity observed in natural populations. Further investigations are required to determine whether this mechanism is linked to the emergence of pathogenic strains from environmental bacteria.

Acknowledgments

The authors acknowledge the staff of the Electron Microscopy Laboratory, Tzu Chi University, Taiwan, for their technical support with electron microscopy, and the High-throughput Genome Analysis Core Facility of National Core Facility Program for Biotechnology, Taiwan (NSC 101-2319-B-010-001), for sequencing. The authors would also like to thank Enago (www.enago.tw) for the English language review.

Author Contributions

Conceived and designed the experiments: HC CYC. Performed the experiments: HC. Analyzed the data: CYC HC. Contributed reagents/materials/analysis tools: CYC. Wrote the paper: CYC HC.

References

1. Jones MK, Oliver JD (2009) *Vibrio vulnificus*: disease and pathogenesis. Infect Immun 77: 1723–1733. doi:10.1128/IAI.01046-08.
2. Tison DL, Nishibuchi M, Greenwood JD, Seidler RJ (1982) *Vibrio vulnificus* biogroup 2: new biogroup pathogenic for eels. Appl Environ Microbiol 44: 640–646.
3. Mahmud ZH, Wright AC, Mandal SC, Dai J, Jones MK, et al. (2010) Genetic characterization of *Vibrio vulnificus* strains from tilapia aquaculture in Bangladesh. Appl Environ Microbiol 76: 4890–4895. doi:10.1128/AEM.00636-10.
4. Dalsgaard I, Høi L, Siebeling RJ, Dalsgaard A (1999) Indole-positive *Vibrio vulnificus* isolated from disease outbreaks on a Danish eel farm. Dis Aquat Org 35: 187–194. doi:10.3354/dao035187.
5. Fouz B, Larsen JL, Amaro C (2006) *Vibrio vulnificus* serovar A: an emerging pathogen in European anguilliculture. J Fish Dis 29: 285–291. doi:10.1111/j.1365-2761.2006.00719.x.
6. Daniels NA (2011) *Vibrio vulnificus* oysters: pearls and perils. Clin Infect Dis 52: 788–792. doi:10.1093/cid/ciq251.
7. Gopal S, Otta SK, Kumar S, Karunasagar I, Nishibuchi M, et al. (2005) The occurrence of *Vibrio* species in tropical shrimp culture environments; implications for food safety. Int J Food Microbiol 102: 151–159. doi:10.1016/j.ijfoodmicro.2004.12.011.
8. Arias CR, Pujalte MJ, Garay E, Aznar R (1998) Genetic relatedness among environmental, clinical, and diseased-eel *Vibrio vulnificus* isolates from different geographic regions by ribotyping and randomly amplified polymorphic DNA PCR. Appl Environ Microbiol 64: 3403–3410.
9. Wong HC, Chang CN (2005) Hydrophobicity, cell adherence, cytotoxicity, and enterotoxigenicity of starved *Vibrio parahaemolyticus*. J Food Prot 68: 154–156.
10. Hengge R (2011) The general stress response in Gram-negative bacteria. In: Storz G, Hengge R, editors. Bacterial Stress Responses. ASM Press. pp. 251–290.
11. Foster PL (2007) Stress-induced mutagenesis in bacteria. Crit Rev Biochem Mol Biol 42: 373–397. doi:10.1080/10409230701648494.
12. Wright BE (2004) Stress-directed adaptive mutations and evolution. Mol Microbiol 52: 643–650. doi:10.1111/j.1365-2958.2004.04012.x.
13. Gonzalez C, Hadany L, Ponder RG, Price M, Hastings PJ, et al. (2008) Mutability and importance of a hypermutable cell subpopulation that produces stress-induced mutants in *Escherichia coli*. PLoS Genet 4: e1000208. doi:10.1371/journal.pgen.1000208.

14. Biosca EG, Amaro C, Marco-Noales E, Oliver JD (1996) Effect of low temperature on starvation-survival of the eel pathogen *Vibrio vulnificus* biotype 2. Appl Environ Microbiol 62: 450–455.
15. Marco-Noales E, Biosca EG, Amaro C (1999) Effects of salinity and temperature on long-term survival of the eel pathogen *Vibrio vulnificus* biotype 2 (serovar E). Appl Environ Microbiol 65: 1117–1126.
16. Hülsmann A, Rosche TM, Kong IS, Hassan HM, Beam DM, et al. (2003) RpoS-dependent stress response and exoenzyme production in *Vibrio vulnificus*. Appl Environ Microbiol 69: 6114–6120.
17. Amel BKN, Amine B, Amina B (2008) Survival of *Vibrio fluvialis* in seawater under starvation conditions. Microbiol Res 163: 323–328. doi:10.1016/j.micres.2006.06.006.
18. González-Escalona N, Fey A, Höfle MG, Espejo RT, A Guzmán C (2006) Quantitative reverse transcription polymerase chain reaction analysis of *Vibrio cholerae* cells entering the viable but non-culturable state and starvation in response to cold shock. Environ Microbiol 8: 658–666. doi:10.1111/j.1462-2920.2005.00943.x.
19. Chen SY, Jane WN, Chen YS, Wong HC (2009) Morphological changes of *Vibrio parahaemolyticus* under cold and starvation stresses. Int J Food Microbiol 129: 157–165. doi:10.1016/j.ijfoodmicro.2008.11.009.
20. Ostling J, Flärdh K, Kjelleberg S (1995) Isolation of a carbon starvation regulatory mutant in a marine *Vibrio* strain. J Bacteriol 177: 6978–6982.
21. Vattakaven T, Bond P, Bradley G, Munn CB (2006) Differential effects of temperature and starvation on induction of the viable-but-nonculturable state in the coral pathogens *Vibrio shiloi* and *Vibrio tasmaniensis*. Appl Environ Microbiol 72: 6508–6513. doi:10.1128/AEM.00798-06.
22. Chen CY, Chao CB, Bowser PR (2006) Infection of tilapia *Oreochromis* sp. by *Vibrio vulnificus* in freshwater and low-salinity environments. Journal of the World Aquaculture Society 37: 82–88. doi:10.1111/j.1749-7345.2006.00010.x.
23. Chen CY, Wu KM, Chang YC, Chang CH, Tsai HC, et al. (2003) Comparative genome analysis of *Vibrio vulnificus*, a marine pathogen. Genome Res 13: 2577–2587. doi:10.1101/gr.1295503.
24. Herigstad B, Hamilton M, Heersink J (2001) How to optimize the drop plate method for enumerating bacteria. J Microbiol Methods 44: 121–129.
25. Park KJ, Kang MJ, Kim SH, Lee HJ, Lim JK, et al. (2004) Isolation and characterization of *rpoS* from a pathogenic bacterium, *Vibrio vulnificus*: role of sigmaS in survival of exponential-phase cells under oxidative stress. J Bacteriol 186: 3304–3312. doi:10.1128/JB.186.11.3304-3312.2004.
26. Hill WE, Keasler SP, Trucksess MW, Feng P, Kaysner CA, et al. (1991) Polymerase chain reaction identification of *Vibrio vulnificus* in artificially contaminated oysters. Appl Environ Microbiol 57: 707–711.
27. Chen C (2005) Regulatory roles of the sigma factors RpoS and RpoN in the pathogenesis of *Vibrio vulnificus* YJ016. [master thesis]. Taiwan: Chung-Shan Medical University.
28. Hammer Ø, Harper DAT, Ryan PD (2001) PAST: Paleontological statistics software: package for education and data Analysis. Palaeontologia Electronica: 1–9.
29. Finkel SE (2006) Long-term survival during stationary phase: evolution and the GASP phenotype. Nat Rev Microbiol 4: 113–120. doi:10.1038/nrmicro1340.
30. Roostalu J, Jõers A, Luidalepp H, Kaldalu N, Tenson T (2008) Cell division in *Escherichia coli* cultures monitored at single cell resolution. BMC Microbiology 8: 68. doi:10.1186/1471-2180-8-68.
31. Oliver JD, Bockian R (1995) In vivo resuscitation, and virulence towards mice, of viable but nonculturable cells of *Vibrio vulnificus*. Appl Environ Microbiol 61: 2620–2623.
32. Smith B, Oliver JD (2006) In situ and in vitro gene expression by *Vibrio vulnificus* during entry into, persistence within, and resuscitation from the viable but nonculturable state. Appl Environ Microbiol 72: 1445–1451. doi:10.1128/AEM.72.2.1445-1451.2006.
33. Oliver JD, Hite F, McDougald D, Andon NL, Simpson LM (1995) Entry into, and resuscitation from, the viable but nonculturable state by *Vibrio vulnificus* in an estuarine environment. Appl Environ Microbiol 61: 2624–2630.
34. Kong IS, Bates TC, Hülsmann A, Hassan H, Smith BE, et al. (2004) Role of catalase and *oxyR* in the viable but nonculturable state of *Vibrio vulnificus*. FEMS Microbiol Ecol 50: 133–142. doi:10.1016/j.femsec.2004.06.004.
35. Martínez-Rodriguez A, Kelly AF, Park SF, Mackey BM (2004) Emergence of variants with altered survival properties in stationary phase cultures of *Campylobacter jejuni*. Int J Food Microbiol 90: 321–329.
36. Silby MW, Giddens SR, Mahanty HK (2005) Mutation of a LysR-type regulator of antifungal activity results in a growth advantage in stationary phase phenotype in *Pseudomonas aureofaciens* PA147-2. Appl Environ Microbiol 71: 569–573. doi:10.1128/AEM.71.1.569-573.2005.
37. Tark M, Tover A, Tarassova K, Tegova R, Kivi G, et al. (2005) A DNA polymerase V homologue encoded by TOL plasmid pWW0 confers evolutionary fitness on *Pseudomonas putida* under conditions of environmental stress. J Bacteriol 187: 5203–5213. doi:10.1128/JB.187.15.5203-5213.2005.
38. Helmus RA, Liermann LJ, Brantley SL, Tien M (2012) Growth advantage in stationary-phase (GASP) phenotype in long-term survival strains of *Geobacter sulfurreducens*. FEMS Microbiol Ecol 79: 218–228. doi:10.1111/j.1574-6941.2011.01211.x.
39. Bacun-Druzina V, Cagalj Z, Gjuracic K (2007) The growth advantage in stationary-phase (GASP) phenomenon in mixed cultures of enterobacteria. FEMS Microbiol Lett 266: 119–127. doi:10.1111/j.1574-6968.2006.00515.x.
40. Petrun B, Lostroh CP (2013) *Vibrio fischeri* exhibit the growth advantage in stationary-phase phenotype. Can J Microbiol 59: 130–135. doi:10.1139/cjm-2012-0439.
41. Paul K, Ghosh A, Sengupta N, Chowdhury R (2004) Competitive growth advantage of nontoxigenic mutants in the stationary phase in archival cultures of pathogenic *Vibrio cholerae* strains. Infect Immun 72: 5478–5482. doi:10.1128/IAI.72.9.5478-5482.2004.
42. Ferenci T, Spira B (2007) Variation in stress responses within a bacterial species and the indirect costs of stress resistance. Annals of the New York Academy of Sciences 1113: 105–113. doi:10.1196/annals.1391.003.
43. Lenski RE, Travisano M (1994) Dynamics of adaptation and diversification: a 10,000-generation experiment with bacterial populations. Proc Natl Acad Sci USA 91: 6808–6814.
44. Vasi F, Travisano M, Lenski RE (1994) Long-term experimental evolution in *Escherichia coli*. II: Changes in life-history traits during adaptative to a seasonal environment. The American naturalist 144: 432–456.
45. Death A, Notley L, Ferenci T (1993) Derepression of LamB protein facilitates outer membrane permeation of carbohydrates into *Escherichia coli* under conditions of nutrient stress. J Bacteriol 175: 1475–1483.
46. Notley-McRobb L, Seeto S, Ferenci T (2003) The influence of cellular physiology on the initiation of mutational pathways in *Escherichia coli* populations. Proc Biol Sci 270: 843–848. doi:10.1098/rspb.2002.2295.
47. Ferenci T (2003) What is driving the acquisition of *mutS* and *rpoS* polymorphisms in *Escherichia coli*? Trends Microbiol 11: 457–461.
48. Notley-McRobb L, Ferenci T (1999) Adaptive *mgl*-regulatory mutations and genetic diversity evolving in glucose-limited *Escherichia coli* populations. Environ Microbiol 1: 33–43.
49. Notley-McRobb L, Ferenci T (1999) The generation of multiple co-existing *mal*-regulatory mutations through polygenic evolution in glucose-limited populations of *Escherichia coli*. Environ Microbiol 1: 45–52.
50. Notley-McRobb L, Ferenci T (2000) Experimental analysis of molecular events during mutational periodic selections in bacterial evolution. Genetics 156: 1493–1501.
51. Wei X, Bauer WD (1998) Starvation-induced changes in motility, chemotaxis, and flagellation of *Rhizobium meliloti*. Appl Environ Microbiol 64: 1708–1714.
52. Stretton S, Danon SJ, Kjelleberg S, Goodman AE (1997) Changes in cell morphology and motility in the marine *Vibrio* sp. strain S14 during conditions of starvation and recovery. FEMS Microbiology Letters 146: 23–29. doi:10.1016/S0378-1097(96)00387-4.
53. Amy PS, Morita RY (1983) Starvation-survival patterns of sixteen freshly isolated open-ocean bacteria. Appl Environ Microbiol 45: 1109–1115.
54. Morris JJ, Lenski RE, Zinser ER (2012) The Black Queen Hypothesis: evolution of dependencies through adaptive gene loss. MBio 3. doi:10.1128/mBio.00036-12.
55. Durfee T, Hansen A-M, Zhi H, Blattner FR, Jin DJ (2008) Transcription profiling of the stringent response in *Escherichia coli*. J Bacteriol 190: 1084–1096. doi:10.1128/JB.01092-07.
56. Lemke JJ, Durfee T, Gourse RL (2009) DksA and ppGpp directly regulate transcription of the *Escherichia coli* flagellar cascade. Mol Microbiol 74: 1368–1379. doi:10.1111/j.1365-2958.2009.06939.x.
57. Kim SM, Lee DH, Choi SH (2012) Evidence that the *Vibrio vulnificus* flagellar regulator FlhF is regulated by a quorum sensing master regulator SmcR. Microbiology (Reading, Engl) 158: 2017–2025. doi:10.1099/mic.0.059071-0.

3

Apolipoprotein E Plays a Key Role against Cryptosporidial Infection in Transgenic Undernourished Mice

Orleâncio G. R. Azevedo[1,3], David T. Bolick[1], James K. Roche[1], Relana F. Pinkerton[1], Aldo A. M. Lima[1,2], Michael P. Vitek[4], Cirle A. Warren[1], Reinaldo B. Oriá[1,3]*, Richard L. Guerrant[1,2]

1 Division of Infectious Diseases and International Medicine, Center for Global Health, School of Medicine, University of Virginia, Charlottesville, Virginia, United States of America, **2** Laboratory of Infectious Diseases, Clinical Research Unit, Institute of the Brazilian Semi-Arid, School of Medicine, Federal University of Ceara, Fortaleza, Ceará, Brazil, **3** Laboratory of the Biology of Tissue Healing, Ontogeny and Nutrition, Institute of the Brazilian Semi-arid, School of Medicine, Federal University of Ceara, Fortaleza, Ceará, Brazil, **4** Duke University Medical Center, Department of Medicine, Durham, North Carolina, United States of America

Abstract

Apolipoliprotein E (apoE), a critical targeting protein in lipid homeostasis, has been found to have immunoinflammatory effects on murine models of infection and malnutrition. The effects of apoE in undernourished and *Cryptosporidium parvum*-infected mice have not been investigated. In order to study the role of apoE in a model of *C. parvum* infection, we used the following C57BL6J mouse genetic strains: APOE-deficient, wild-type controls, and APOE targeted replacement (TR) mice expressing human APOE genes (E3/3; E4/4). Experimental mice were orally infected with 10^7-unexcysted-*C. parvum* oocysts between post-natal days 34–35 followed by malnutrition induced with a low-protein diet. Mice were euthanized seven days after *C. parvum*-challenge to investigate ileal morphology, cytokines, and cationic arginine transporter (CAT-1), arginase 1, Toll-like receptor 9 (TLR9), and inducible nitric oxide synthase (iNOS) expression. In addition, we analyzed stool oocyst shedding by qRT-PCR and serum lipids. APOE4/4-TR mice had better weight gains after infection plus malnutrition compared with APOE3/3-TR and wild-type mice. APOE4/4-TR and APOE knockout mice had lower oocyst shedding, however the latter exhibited with villus blunting and higher ileal pro-inflammatory cytokines and iNOS transcripts. APOE4/4-TR mice had increased ileal CAT-1, arginase-1, and TLR9 transcripts relative to APOE knockout. Although with anti-parasitic effects, APOE deficiency exacerbates intestinal inflammatory responses and mucosal damage in undernourished and *C. parvum*-infected mice. In addition, the human APOE4 gene was found to be protective against the compounded insult of *Cryptosporidium* infection plus malnutrition, thus extending our previous findings of the protection against diarrhea in APOE4 children. Altogether our findings suggest that apoE plays a key role in the intestinal restitution and immunoinflammatory responses with *Cryptosporidium* infection and malnutrition.

Editor: Dipshikha Chakravortty, Indian Institute of Science, India

Funding: This research was supported by NIH Research Grant #5R01HD053131 funded by the Eunice Kennedy Shriver National Institute of Child Health and Human Development (NICHD) and the NIH Office of Dietary Supplements (ODS). WNIH Cooperative Agreement U54 AI57168 for the Mid-Atlantic Regional Center for Excellence (MARCE) funded by the National Institute of Allergy and Infectious Diseases, and by Fogarty International Center grant TW006713-01. Orleancio de Azevedo was supported by the Center Global Infectious Diseases Research Training (GIDRT) program at NIH, grant 5 D43 TW006578-08/GIDRT. The funders had no role in study design, data collection and analysis, decision to publish, or preparation of the manuscript.

Competing Interests: The authors have declared that no competing interests exist.

* E-mail: oria@ufc.br

Introduction

Cryptosporidiosis is a water-borne disease associated with the majority of parasitic protozoan outbreaks recently reported worldwide [1]. Immunocompromised hosts may fail to assemble efficient immune-inflammatory responses against *Cryptosporidium* infections (mainly Th-1-mediated cytokines), leading to intestinal barrier disruption and undernutrition [2].

Malnourished and immune-suppressed children are a particular risk group for *Cryptosporidium* infections, since they are more susceptible to acquiring the infection, more afflicted with a lasting morbidity, and at greater risk of disseminating the infection further, therefore amplifying its spread [3].

A reverberating vicious cycle of infection and malnutrition in young children may cause profound long-term deficits in physical and cognitive development, even without overt diarrhea, which can be irreversible [4]. The predisposition and adverse outcomes from repeated or prolonged exposure to *C. parvum* and other enteric infections may additionally have a strong genetic component in terms of host-parasite and epigenetic interactions [5,6], which could affect the efficacy of nutritional interventions early in life in children at risk in endemic areas [7] and may have long-term consequences. Indeed, we have found that APOE4, the gene associated with increased susceptibility to Alzheimer's disease, is actually protective against early childhood diarrhea and its associated cognitive impairment [8].

Apolipoprotein E (APOE = gene, apoE = protein) is a critical targeting protein in lipid homeostasis where excess cholesterol from somatic cells helps to form apoE-containing lipoprotein particles that are directed to apoE-receptors in the liver, where the particles are internalized and metabolized [9]. The human APOE gene has 3 alleles at its locus on chromosome 19: APOE2, APOE3, the most frequent allele, and APOE4. APOE4 is often associated with late onset Alzheimer's disease [10], poor recovery after neurological injury [11], and associated with increased oxidative stress [12].

ApoE-deficient mice have been shown to have impaired innate immune defenses in models of *Listeria monocytogenes* [13] and *Klebsiella pneumonia* [14] infections. In addition, in a model of maternal-offspring separation, undernourished APOE knockout mice failed to thrive after being re-fed, showing intestinal mucosal atrophy and poor IGF-1 response [15]. Therefore, we examined the effect of the apolipoprotein-E isoforms in a murine model of *C. parvum* infection plus undernutrition, which we have recently validated [16]. The responses of human APOE targeted replacement and APOE knockout mice to *C. parvum* plus undernutrition were measured to determine whether we could confirm and extend our field studies showing the role of apolipoprotein E in the effects of childhood malnutrition and intestinal infection induced by *C. parvum.* This specific infection/undernutrition/APOE genotype mouse model has permitted us to examine whether pro-inflammatory states associated with APOE transgenic mice [12] would be beneficial against cryptosporidial infections.

Materials and Methods

Malnutrition protocol

Thirty-day-old C57BL/6J (APOE$^{-/-}$, APOE$^{+/+}$, APOE3/3 and APOE4/4 targeted replacement male mice) were purchased from Taconic (Albany, New York). Mice were acclimated, body weight matched, and assigned to the experimental groups. Mice assigned to the undernourished groups received an isocaloric diet with 2% of protein (low-protein diet) (Harland Labs, Dublin, VA). Undernourished mice stayed under a low-protein diet for 7 days before *C. parvum* oocyst challenge and continued their diet until the end of the experiment. Nourished control groups received standard chow diet (20% of protein). Weights were monitored daily.

Experimental mice were sacrificed in CO_2 chambers seven days post-infection (mean age of 42 days old). Euthanasia was assured by cervical dislocation. After opening the abdominal cavity, approximately 1 cm-long ileum segment (proximal to the ileocecal valve) was removed and fixed in 4% paraformaldehyde. Another 2 cm-segment, proximal to the first segment, was removed and milked free of stool for quantitative real-time PCR for cryptosporidial DNA analyses (tissues were frozen and stored in −20°C until assay). A final 1-cm ileal segment was harvested and prepared for real time-PCR and cytokine assays, as described below (tissues were frozen immediately in liquid nitrogen and stored in −80°C until further assays). The protocol described herein was approved and is in accordance with the Institutional Animal Care and Use Committee policies of the University of Virginia.

Preparation and administration of inoculum

C. parvum unexcysted oocysts were obtained from experimentally infected calves (Iowa isolate; Waterborne, Inc., New Orleans, Louisiana). *C. parvum* oocysts were stored in phosphate-buffered saline (PBS) at 4°C and used within 8 weeks of their receipt. The tube with oocysts was gently vortexed and incubated at room temperature for 10 min before use. Each infected mouse received 100 μl of PBS plus freshly prepared unexcysted *C. parvum* oocysts in a recently vortexed solution (10^7 oocysts per mouse) by oral gavage directly into the stomach. Control mice received 100 μl of PBS by oral gavage at the same time.

Stool collection and DNA extraction

Stools were collected in pre-weighed tubes daily after gentle abdominal stroking or milked free from the ileum after euthanasia for all groups and stored at −20°C until DNA extraction. The DNA was extracted from the frozen stool samples using Qiagen QIAamp DNA Stool Kit (Qiagen, Inc., Germantown, Maryland) with some modifications. First, 400 μl of ASL buffer was added to each sample, vortexed at 1,500 rpm overnight for complete homogenization. Samples were incubated at 82.5°C for 5 min and then vortexed for 1 min at full speed. The supernatant was pipetted into a new tube containing 30 μl of proteinase K to which 400 μl of AL buffer was added and incubated at 70°C for 10 min with 400 μl of absolute ethanol and mixed, according to manufacturer's instructions. Finally, DNA was eluted in 200 μl Elution Buffer and stored at −20°C.

Morphological analyses

Ileal villus heights and crypt depths (n = 4 for each group) were measured using hematoxylin and eosin-stained slides on a light microscope (BH-2, Olympus, Tokyo, Japan), equipped with a high-resolution digital camera that was connected to a computer with an image capture program. Villus height was measured from the baseline to the villus apex. The crypt depth was measured from the baseline to the crypt bottom. All morphometric measurements were done blindly using NIH Image J 1.44 S (National Institutes of Health, Bethesda, MD) after proper calibration.

C. parvum stool detection by quantitative Polymerase Chain Reaction

Extracted DNA (5 μl) was added to a master mix (20 μl) to give a total reaction volume of 25 μl per sample. The master mix was prepared by mixing 12.5 μl of Bio-Rad iQ SYBR Green Supermix (Bio-Rad Laboratories, Hercules, California), 5.5 μl of DEPC-treated nuclease free sterile water (Fisher Scientific, Pittsburgh, Pennsylvania), and 1.0 μl (6.2 mM) each of both forward and reverse primers (Invitrogen, Carlsbad, California). The primers target the 18 s rRNA gene of the parasite as shown in **Table 1** (GenBank no. AF164102). The reaction was performed in a Bio-Rad iCycler iQ multicolor PCR Detection System using iCycler software (version 3.0). Amplification consisted of 15 min at 95°C followed by 40 cycles of 15 sec at 95°C, 15 sec at 52°C, and 20 sec at 72°C, followed by 0.5-degree increments for 10 sec starting at 75°C and ending with 95°C for the Melt Curve. Fluorescence was measured during the annealing step of each cycle. Ct values of each run were compared to standards with known amounts of *C. parvum* DNA and log transformed into number of organisms per mg of stool sample.

Inflammatory Cytokine Beads Assay (Luminex)

Ileal specimens were stored at −80°C until required for assay. The harvested tissue was homogenized and processed with HEPES buffer (Invitrogen, Carlsbad, CA, USA) (pH = 7.4). Briefly, microtiter plates were coated overnight at 4°C with antibodies against murine TNF-α, IL-1β and IL-10 (2 μg/ml). After blocking the plates, the samples and standards at various dilutions were added in duplicate and incubated at 4°C for 2 h. The plates were washed three times with buffer. After washing the plates, biotinylated sheep polyclonal anti-TNF-α or anti-IL-1β or anti-IL-10 (diluted 1:1000 with assay buffer 1% BSA), was added to the wells. After further incubation at room temperature for 1 h, the plates were washed and 50 μl of avidin-HRP diluted 1:5000 was added. The color reagent phenylenediamine (OPD; 50 μl) was added 15 min later and the plates were incubated in the dark at

Table 1. Primers used in the study.

Primers	Sequence (5′-3′)
Beta-actin	AATTTCTGAATGGCCCAGGT TTTGTGTAAGGTAAGGTGTGC
Arginase -1	TCTGCCAAAGACATCGTGTA GGTAGCTGAAGGTCTCTTCC
CAT - 1	CACTGCTGATCTGTGTACCT GTGGGGACATAAGATGCTCA
RNA 18 s *C. parvum*	CTGCGAATGGCTCATTATAACA AGGCCAATACCCTACCGTCT
iNOS	TCCTGGACATTACGACCCCT AGGCCTCCAATCTCTGCCTA
TLR9	TGGTGTTGAAGGACAGTTCTCTC CACTCGGAGGTTTCCCAGC

37°C for 15–20 min. The enzyme reaction was stopped with 2 N H_2SO_4 and absorbance was measured at 490 nm. Values were expressed as picograms/mililiter (pg/ml).

Serum lipid measurements

The samples were collected at the end of experiment (day 7 after infection). Blood was drawn in anesthetized animals through transcardiac puncture using a 1 ml-syringe. The blood was transferred to a PCR tube and coagulated at room temperature. Tubes were then centrifuged (3.000 rpm) for 10 minutes at 4°C. The serum was stored at −80°C until lipid analyses were performed according to the method of Roeschlau and colleagues [17].

CAT-1 and Arginase 1 qRT-PCR analyses (quantitative reverse transcriptase-polymerase chain reaction)

Total cellular RNA was obtained from each intestinal tissue using the RNeasy kits (Qiagen), and cDNA was synthesized from 1 µ, and cDNA wiScript (Biorad). For quantitative PCR analyses of cytokine mRNA abundance, cDNA was diluted 1:8; 4 µL of this dilution were used for each PCR reaction. Reagents from the BioRad real-time PCR kit containing Sybr Green were used for quantitative PCR reactions. Primer sequences used in the experiment are shown in the **Table 1**.

The PCR conditions were: 95°C 10 min, 95°C 3 min, followed by 40 cycles of 95°C 30 s, 58°C 30 s, and 72°C 30 s, followed by a melt curve analysis. Data were analyzed and are presented based upon the relative expression method [16]. The formula used for calculation was: Relative expression $= 2^{-(\mathbf{S\Delta CT-\ C\Delta CT})}$, where **ΔCT** is the difference in threshold cycle between the gene of interest (i.e., Arginase-1) and the housekeeping gene (β-actin)**S** = *C. parvum* challenged mice and **C** = uninfected mice.

Statistical analysis

Analyses of weight loss/increase were expressed as percent change in baseline body weight. The analyses of stool shedding (number of parasites per mg of stool) were performed using Graph Pad Prism version 5.0 software (Media Cybernetics, CA). Statistical analyses were performed using ANOVA with Bonferroni post-hoc correction or unpaired Student *T* test when appropriate. A *P* value<0.05 was considered significant. Data are presented as mean ± standard error, with the exception of serum lipid levels which are presented as mean ± standard deviation.

Results

APOE 4/4 TR mice lost less weight when challenged by under nutrition and cryptosporidiosis

The inability to reach an expected growth rate has been proposed as a biological marker of under nutrition and/or enteric infections in animal models [15,18]. All experimental groups under the low protein diet showed significant short-term weight loss, as compared with the wild-type nourished controls, however APOE 4/4 targeted replacement mice had less weight loss with under nutrition compared with APOE 3/3 and wild-type undernourished mice. APOE knockout mice showed a slightly better weight adaptation than wild-type controls under the low-protein diet (**Fig. 1A**).

After *Cryptosporidium parvum* infection, undernourished APOE 4/4 TR mice had less weight decrements, at day 2 post-inoculum, when the parasite load was heavier (see below) when compared with undernourished APOE knockout and APOE 3/3 TR. APOE3/3 TR mice had the greatest weight loss on day 2. In addition, undernourished infected APOE knockout mice showed significant weight impairments after the 4th day of *C. parvum* challenge and showed poor growth catch-up after infection (**Fig. 1B**).

APOE 4/4 TR mice have significantly lower fecal C. parvum oocyst shedding

To better evaluate *C. parvum* infection in undernourished experimental mice, we assessed the quantity of *C. parvum* oocyst shedding in stools using quantitative polymerase chain reaction. From day 3 after infection onward, the APOE 4/4 TR mice showed an accelerated pace of oocyst reduction. After one week post-infection, only one (1 out of 14, 7.4%) experimentally infected –APOE 4/4 TR mouse showed *C. parvum* shedding in stool (**Fig. 2**). In addition, the APOE knockout mice had slightly, but significantly lower oocyst shedding per milligram of stool ($p<0.05$) than APOE3/3 TR mice at days 1 and 3 post- infection, when the oocyst burden in stool was higher.

APOE 4/4 TR have improved intestinal villi when challenged by under nutrition and cryptosporidiosis

Undernourished uninfected mice showed ileal villus shortening and crypt derangement, with almost complete absence of mitoses. Cryptosporidial infections were associated with crypt hyperplasia, villus blunting, and inflammation in the lamina propria and submucosa as opposed to nourished controls (data not shown). Infected undernourished APOE knockout mice showed reduced villus height and more scattered villi as compared to wild-type and APOE4/4 TR. APOE 3/3 TR mice presented slightly reduced crypt depth as compared to wild-type mice (**Fig. 3A, B and C**). Furthermore, APOE4/4 TR showed better villus height as compared to APOE 3/3 TR and APOE knockout mice following infection and under nutrition ($p<0.05$) (**Fig. 3A and B**). In addition infected APOE 4/4 TR showed better villus/crypt ratio as opposed to all other challenged groups (**Fig. 3D**).

APOE 4/4 TR mice have lower serum triglyceride levels when challenged by under nutrition and cryptosporidiosis

In order to find whether the host response to infections involves changes in lipid levels, we measured serum lipid fractions. Following *C. parvum* infection in undernourished mice, we found significant increases (8 fold higher) in serum total cholesterol and

A

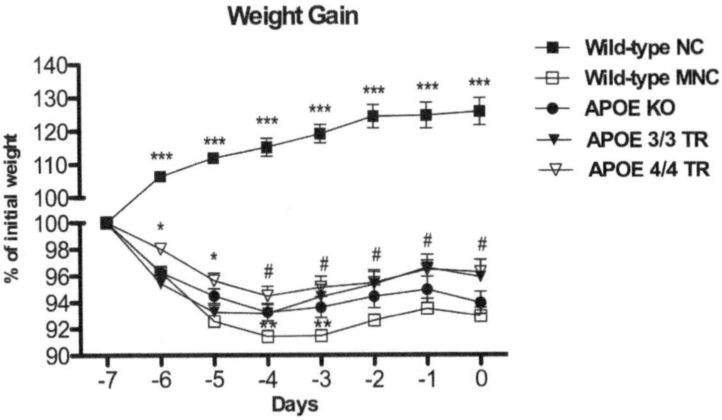

*p<0.05 APOE TR 3/3 vs APOE TR 4/4
**p<0.05 wild-type vs APOE KO
*** p<0.05 vs all
# p<0.05 APOE 4/4 and APOE 3/3 vs wild-type

B

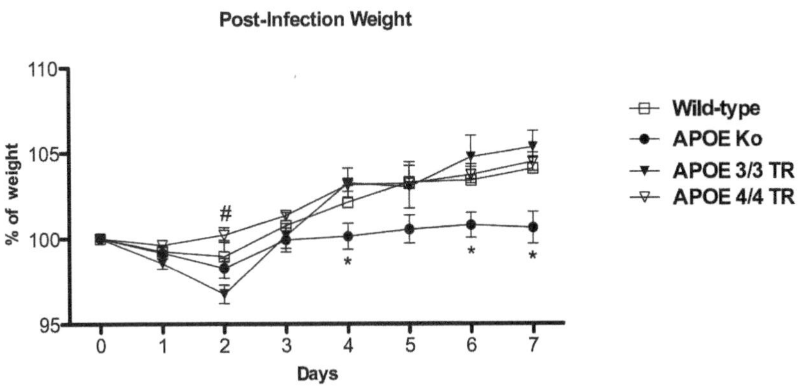

* p<0.05 vs all
# p<0.05 APOE 4/4 TR vs APOE 3/3 TR and APOE Ko

Figure 1. A. Body weight gain (% initial weight) from experimental uninfected and undernourished groups under a low protein diet. APOE 4/4 targeted replacement (APOE 4/4 TR) mice (n = 17) showed 643 a better growth response in comparison with APOE 3/3 targeted replacement (APOE 3/3 TR) mice (n = 8). **B.** Body weight gain (% initial infection weight) from experimental mice challenged by a compounded malnutrition and *Cryptosporidium parvum* insult. Undernourished mice were orally inoculated with 10^7- unexcysted oocysts diluted in 100 µl of PBS. APOE deficient mice show impaired growth following *Cryptosporidium parvum* infection as compared to the other groups. Results are shown as mean ±SEM.

LDL-cholesterol in APOE knockout mice than in C57BL/6J controls.

The APOE 4/4 TR mice had a trend of increased serum HDL cholesterol levels when compared with the other groups. No significant differences were found between APOE 3/3 and APOE 4/4 TR mice. The APOE knockout mice had increased serum triglyceride levels in comparison to APOE 4/4 TR mice. In addition, albeit not significant, APOE 3/3 TR mice showed higher serum triglyceride levels (**Table 2**).

Undernourished APOE knockout mice have increased ileal pro-inflammatory cytokines with cryptosporidial infection

Ileal cytokine analyses revealed significantly higher IL-1β and IFN-γ levels in APOE knockout mice following *C. parvum* infection and undernutrition as compared with respective wild-type controls. In general, there were heavier inflammatory cytokine responses associated with apoE deficiency. Furthermore, both APOE TR undernourished and infected mice showed lower ileal levels of IL-1β than APOE knockout and wild-type challenged mice.

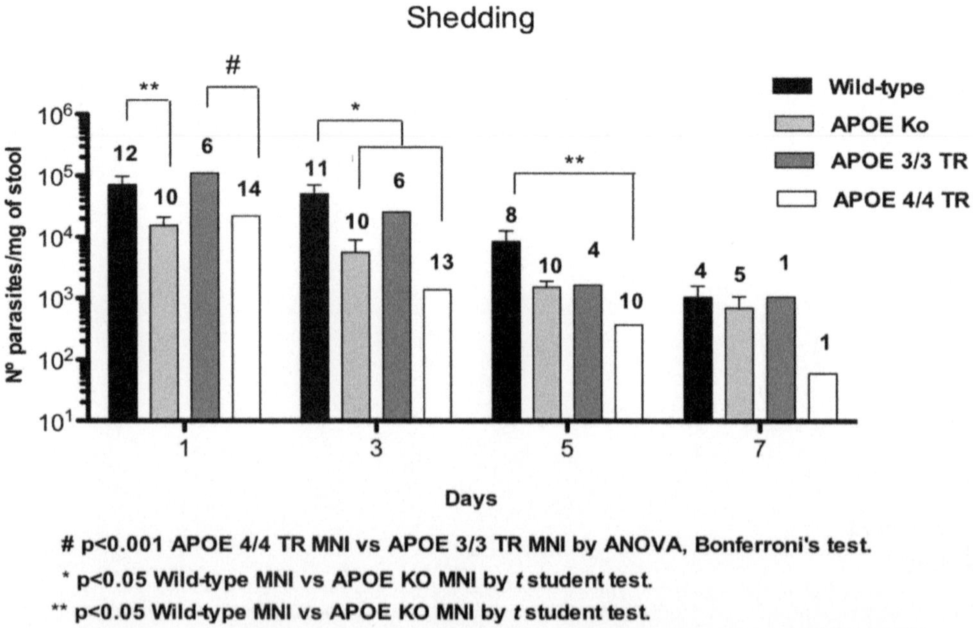

Days	Wild-type	APOE Ko	APOE TR 3/3	APOE TR 4/4
Day 1	12 (100%)	10 (100%)	6 (100%)	14 (100%)
Day 3	11 (91.67%)	10 (100%)	6 (100%)	13 (92.85%)
Day 5	8 (66.67%)	10 (100%)	4 (66.67%)	10 (71.42%)
Day 7	4 (33.33%)	5 (50%)	1 (16.67%)	1 (7.14%)

Figure 2. Fecal shedding of parasites in weaned undernourished C57BL/6 mice orally inoculated with 10^7-unexcysted *Cryptosporidium parvum* oocysts per mouse (given in100 µL of PBS) on day 7 after the onset of the low protein diet. Results are shown in a log scale a mean±SEM. *Cryptosporidium parvum* stool oocyst shedding was determined by qRT PCR. Data were expressed as number of parasites per miligram of stool and percentage and number of infected mice with measurable oocyst shedding per day after *Cryptosporidium parvum* challenge. N above the bars means the number of mice still showing oocyst shedding.

IFN-γ and TNF-α are key cytokines related to *C. parvum* eradication. They were both increased in wild-type undernourished infected mice in comparison with uninfected controls. On the other hand, IL-17 levels were lower in APOE knockout mice after infection and under-nutrition as compared with the APOE knockout uninfected controls and with undernourished infected wild-types. No significant differences were seen between APOE3/3 and APOE4/4 TR mice in all cytokines measured (**Fig. 4**).

APOE 4/4 TR mice showed increased CAT-1, arginase 1, and TLR-9 mRNA when challenged by under nutrition and cryptosporidiosis

In order to assess key mechanisms involved in host-parasite interactions and tissue repair, we addressed the cationic amino acid transporter (CAT-1), arginase-1, and Toll-like receptor 9. We found increased ileal expression of CAT-1 mRNA transcripts in the ileum from undernourished plus infected APOE 4/4 TR mice in comparison to wild-type and APOE-deficient mice on day 7 post-infection. In addition, APOE knockout mice had significantly reduced ileal CAT-1 mRNA expression as compared to wild-type mice ($p<0.05$). Similar changes were also seen with arginase 1, where the highest ileal levels were observed in APOE4/4 TR mice (**Fig. 5 A and B**). In addition we found an increased ileal mRNA levels of TLR9 (Toll-like receptor 9) in APOE 4/4 TR group in comparison to APOE knockout mice ($p<0.05$). Increased ileal levels of inducible nitric oxide synthase (iNOS) mRNA were found in APOE knockout mice in comparison to all groups ($p<0.05$) (**Fig. 5C and D**).

Discussion

Children in developing areas are particularly susceptible to malnutrition associated with *Cryptosporidium parvum* infections, resulting in debilitating diarrhea as well as growth shortfalls [19]. Since nutritional states and the APOE genetic profile may directly affect the host response against infection [20,21] and therefore influence the risk of acquiring and spreading *Cryptosporidia*, we evaluated this infection in different undernourished C57BL6J genetically-engineered mice, including wild-type, APOE-deficient and APOE target-replacement mice.

In this study, we found that APOE-deficient mice had significantly less *C. parvum* oocyst shedding measured by quantitative PCR in stools on the first and third days post-infection, when the infection peaks. In agreement with our findings, greater mucosal immune responses against orally-inoculated pathogens,

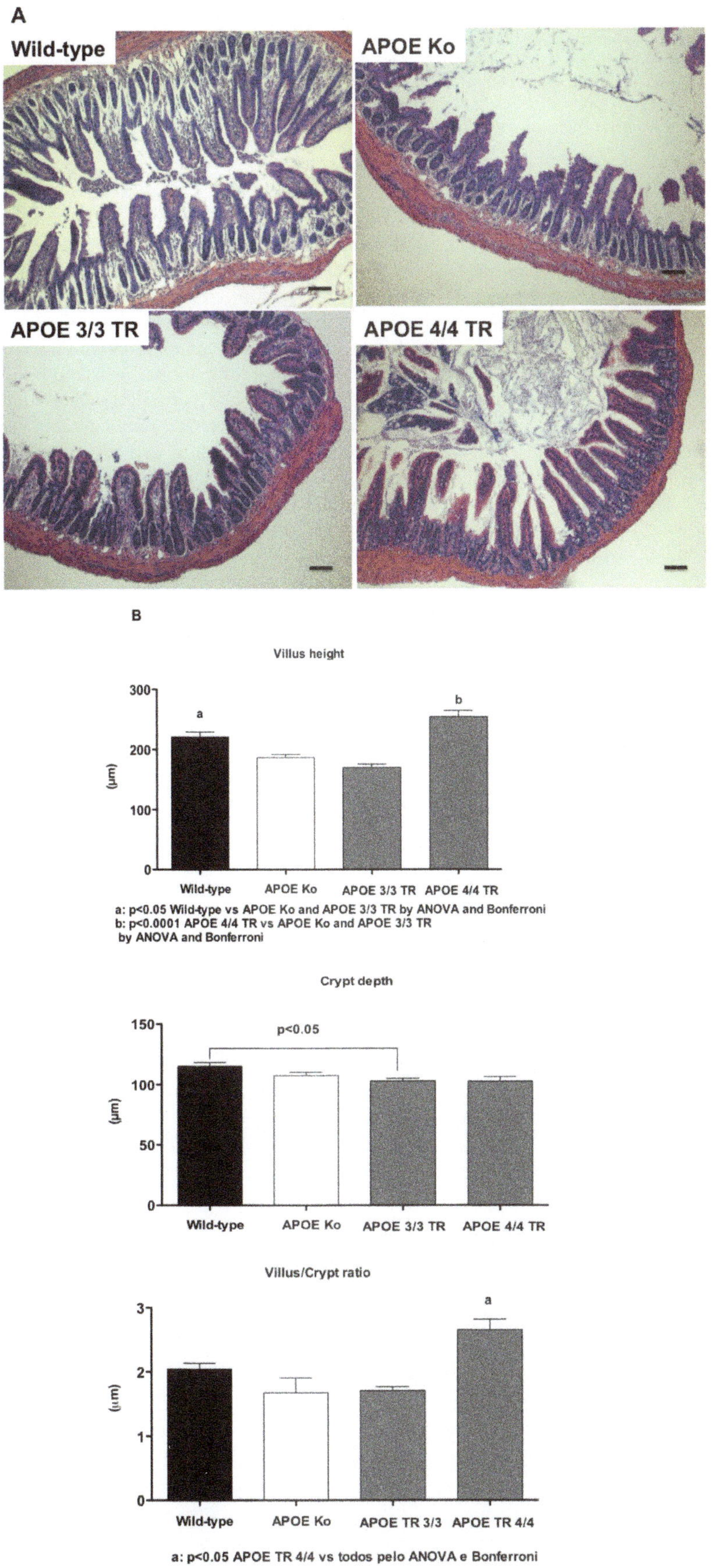
A
Wild-type
APOE Ko
APOE 3/3 TR
APOE 4/4 TR
B
Villus height
(µm)
300
200
100
0
a
b
Wild-type
APOE Ko
APOE 3/3 TR
APOE 4/4 TR
a: p<0.05 Wild-type vs APOE Ko and APOE 3/3 TR by ANOVA and Bonferroni
b: p<0.0001 APOE 4/4 TR vs APOE Ko and APOE 3/3 TR by ANOVA and Bonferroni
Crypt depth
(µm)
150
100
50
0
p<0.05
Wild-type
APOE Ko
APOE 3/3 TR
APOE 4/4 TR
Villus/Crypt ratio
(µm)
3
2
1
0
a
Wild-type
APOE Ko
APOE TR 3/3
APOE TR 4/4
a: p<0.05 APOE TR 4/4 vs todos pelo ANOVA e Bonferroni

Figure 3. A. Representative ileal histology from orally *Cryptosporidium parvum* infected mice. Wild-type, APOE knock-out, and APOE targeted replacement mice (APOE 3/3 TR and APOE 4/4 TR) were fed with a low protein diet during 7 days then infected with 10^7-unexcysted *Cryptosporidium parvum* oocysts and euthanized seven days after infection. H&E ×400. Scale bar 10 μM. **B.** Ileal villus height; **C.** crypt depth, and **D.** villus-crypt ratio from wild-type, APOE knock-out, and APOE targeted replacement mice (APOE 3/3 TR and APOE 4/4 TR). Morphometrics was done from hematoxylin and eosin stained-sections in at least four animals per group at low magnification. Data are presented as mean±SEM. Comparisons were performed by Students unpaired *T* test. Villi and crypts were measured only when their full longitudinal axis was found.

via Th-1 responses, have been shown in APOE knockout mice [22]. In addition, our data suggest that these parasite-killing effects are independent of any increases in IL-17, which was actually found to be low in the ileal tissue of these animals. The Th-17-mediated pathway has been reported to coordinate the immune response against extracellular bacteria [23], suggesting that APOE deficient mice may be poorly adapted against the potential intestinal bacterial translocation due to *C. parvum*-induced intestinal barrier leakage.

Emulsion associated and free-apoE have been shown to bind to LPS (by its exposed hydrophilic domain involving arginine residues) and to redirect LPS from Kupffer cells to liver parenchymal cells, altering lipid metabolism and improving LPS clearance via bile from circulation and reducing LPS-induced lethality [24,25].

Although exhibiting more parasite elimination, undernourished APOE-deficient mice had greater inflammatory cytokine responses and mucosal atrophy in the ileal tissue one week-post inoculum, accompanied by greater weight deficits following 7 days of infection. This can be explained by a constitutive pro-inflammatory state that has been shown with ApoE deficiency in association with hypercholesterolemia [12]. Hypercholesterolemia found in the *C. parvum*-infected APOE knockout mice, even sustained following under nutrition, as shown in our study, may reflect impaired intestinal cholesterol delivery to the liver for metabolism. This effect may be associated with increased bile acid transport in the terminal ileum and diminished fecal bile acid loss, and higher serum and intestinal LDL-cholesterol levels [26].

The transient, slightly better gain weight seen in uninfected APOE knockout mice on the low-protein diet, as compared with wild-type controls, may reflect more available cholesterol, regardless of ApoE/lipoprotein delivery, used as an energy source for growth. Prentice and colleagues have shown that energy-enriched diets are critical for catch-up growth following acute enteric infections [27]. In our earlier studies, we found that neonatal undernourished APOE knockout mice failed to thrive after being re-fed [15]. These seemingly slightly contradictory findings may be explained by the low body-fat mass in the neonatal period that would render these mice with insufficient cholesterol to support rapid growth or the high cholesterol phenotype in APOE knockout mice may occur later after weaning.

Overproduction of TNF-α, IL-1β, and decreased IL-10 ileal levels seen in undernourished and infected ApoE knockout mice could be a consequence of the intestinal barrier disruption and increased luminal LPS-trafficking to the lamina propria. Infections and increased LPS intestinal transit (or cytokines activated by it), even in low amounts, could lead to a hypertriglyceridemic state altering liver lipid metabolism [28]. Endotoxin stimulates arginine transport via TNF-α signaling [29], thus impaired intestinal arginine uptake seen with ApoE deficiency (but improved in APOE4 targeted replacement mice) could contribute to poor bacterial removal and increased mucosal inflammation.

Lipoproteins and lipids present in the serum may contribute to the host innate immunity against pathogens [30]. Studies using APOE deficient mice confirmed the role of APOE in host susceptibility to endotoxemia and *Klebsiella pneumoniae* infection [14], while transgenic mice expressing human APOE3 and APOE4 genes revealed an isoform-specific effect of APOE on the proinflammatory response to lipopolysaccharide [31].

Toll-like receptors are key mediators of the innate immune system against *C. parvum* infections [32]. In our previous study, we have shown that undernourished C57BL6J mice had higher ileal mRNA transcripts for TLR2 and TLR4, but not TLR9, which was diminished by *C. parvum* infection [16]. In the current study, we found that APOE4 mice had increased ileal TLR9 transcripts compared with APOE knockout mice. TLR9-immune mediated responses have been found important to control C. *parvum* infection in a neonatal mouse model [33].

APOE4 may also contribute to elimination of *C. parvum* infection with an inflammatory response that is more regulated compared to the uncontrolled cytokine production noted in ApoE deficient mice. ApoE also enhances microbial lipid antigen presentation (which can be found with increased bacterial intestinal translocation) to antigen-presenting cells via the low-density lipoprotein receptor (LDLR) which could culminate in natural killer T (NKT) cell activation and cytokine secretion [34,35], an effect that could attenuate *C. parvum* infection.

Table 2. Lipid profile of experimental undernourished mice following *Cryposporidium parvum* infection (mice orally infected with 10^7 unexcysted oocysts).

Analytes (mg/dL)	Wild-type (n = 5)	ApoE Ko (n = 5)	ApoE TR 4/4 (n = 5)	ApoE TR 3/3 (n = 4)
Total Cholesterol	60.8±18.5	615.8±69.6*	112±16.9	96.75±14.0
HDL	52±9.3	50±5.7	58±6.2**	47±7.8
LDL	29.80±6.5	576±65.8***	45.8±10.4	38.50±7.0
Triglycerides	53.20±17	59±4.0#	48.6±8.0	68.5±24.0

*p<0.001 ApoE Ko vs all;
** p = 0.05 ApoE TR 4/4 vs ApoE TR 3/3;
*** p<0.001 ApoE Ko vs all;
#p<0.05 ApoE Ko vs ApoE TR 4/4 by Student *t* Test.

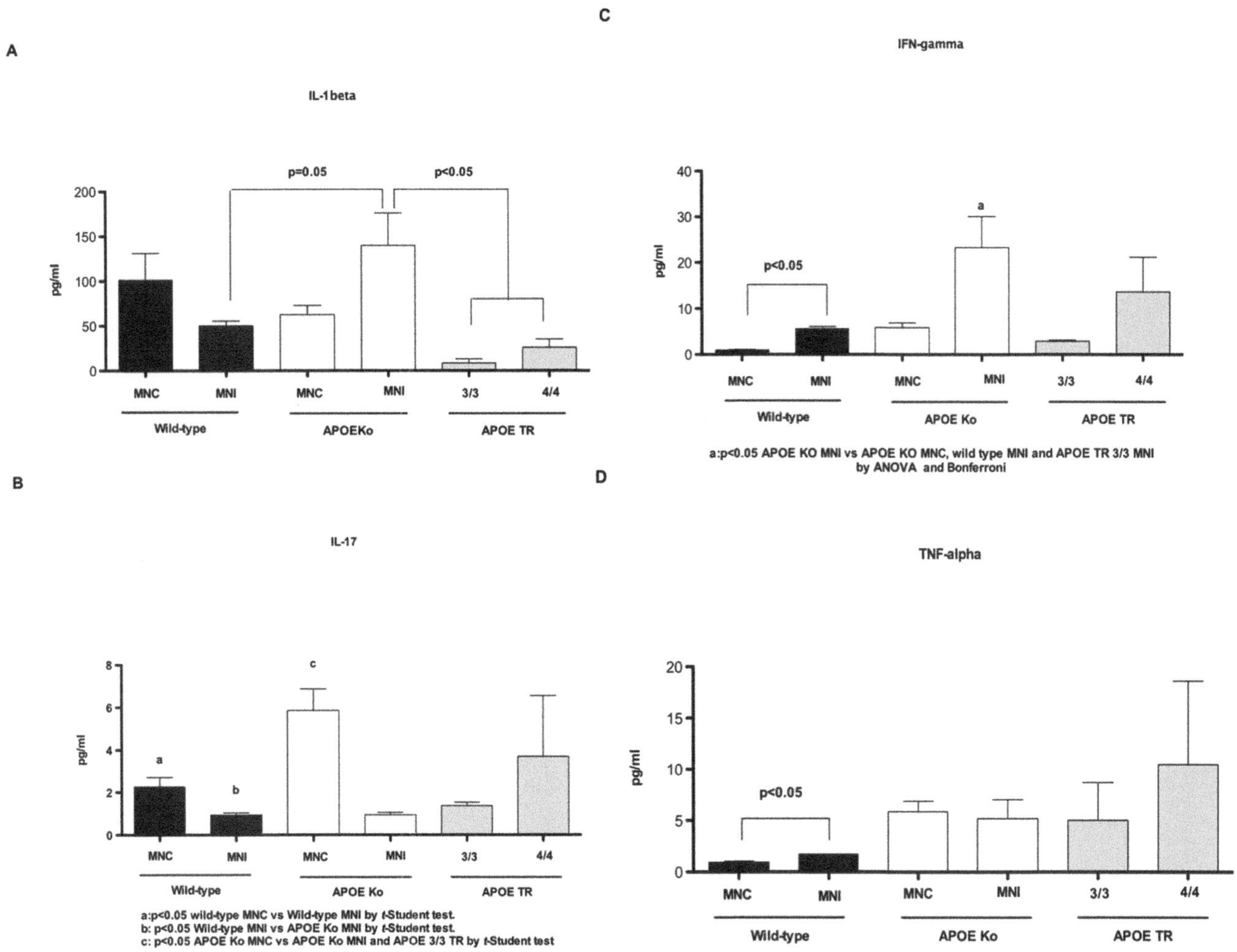

Figure 4. Luminex assays from experimental mice for the following ileal pro-inflammatory cytokines: (A) Interleukin 1-β; (B) Interleukin-17; (C) Interferon-gamma; and (D) Tumor necrosis factor alpha. Experimental mice were challenged by a compounded malnutrition and *Cryptosporidium parvum* insult and samples were harvest on day 7 post-*C. parvum inoculum*. Wild-type, APOE knock-out, and APOE targeted replacement mice (APOE 3/3 TR and APOE 4/4 TR) were orally inoculated with 10^7-unexcysted oocysts diluted in 100 μl of PBS. Groups have at least 4 per groups and the results are shown as mean ±SEM and are expressed in pg/ml. MNC = uninfected undernouorished control group. MNI = undernourished infected group.

Finally, APOE4 has been shown to up-regulate the L-arginine selective cationic protein transporter (CAT-1), part of the amino acid-polyamine-organocation (APC) superfamily, which has been associated with increased L-arginine uptake by neuroglia cells. Our data show that CAT-1 is up-regulated in the ileum of undernourished *C. parvum* infected-APOE4 targeted replacement mice compared to APOE3 controls. Increased uptake of L-arginine preferentially by enterocytes may enhance the intestinal barrier function, mucosal blood flow, and the immune system in addition to mucosal repair (cell proliferation and migration) following injury, by increasing polyamine synthesis and constitutive nitric oxide synthase (cNOS) activity [36]. Indeed, we have observed that arginine can enhance the killing of cryptosporidial parasites in our murine model, via both iNOS and arginase pathways [37]. In addition, protozoa could utilize arginine and therefore reducing the NO production by the host and weakening the innate immune defenses against infection [37].

Arginase-1 is an enzyme that catalyzes arginine's conversion into ornithine, which may then enter into the polyamine pathway [38]. Taken with our previous findings and those Colton et al. see below and reference [46], these findings with ApoE 4/4 targeted replacement transgenic mice suggest that increased uptake of arginine through CAT-1 activity and the arginine shift to the arginase pathway for improving mucosal restitution following *C.parvum*-induced mucosa injury in undernourished mice.

Recently, we have demonstrated that L-arginine supplementation improved mucosal recovery following *C. parvum* infection plus undernutrition and that ileal arginase 1 was a marker of infection severity [37]. In contrast with that finding, APOE4 targeted replacement mice up-regulated arginase 1 which may indicate that mucosal recovery is still underway. More studies are warranted to evaluate the role of arginase 1 during *C. parvum* infection and mucosal recovery.

APOE4 targeted gene replacement and APOE knockout mice have been found with increased pro-inflammatory states [39], an effect that is potentially undesirable for neurodegenerative diseases, but beneficial during exposure to gut-infectious pathogens early in life [40]. The beneficial effect of apoE4 in boosting host innate immunity against infectious agents is a potential explanation for the prevalence of the APOE4 in our genetic pool

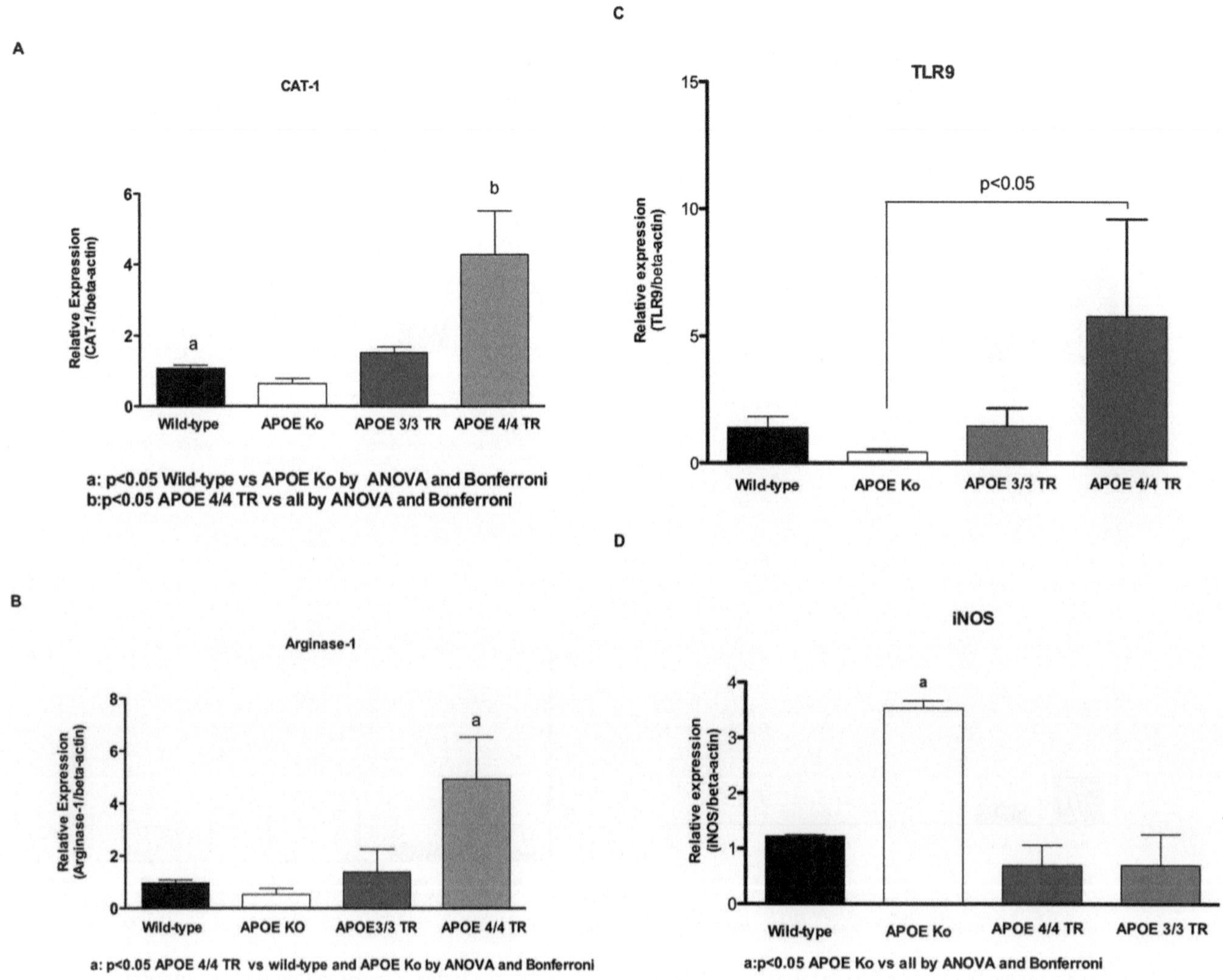

Figure 5. Quantitative real-time PCR assays from experimental mice for the following ileal mRNA transcripts: (A) cationic amino acid transporter (CAT-1); (B) arginase 1; (C) Toll-like receptor 9 (TLR9); and (D) Inducible nitric oxide synthase (iNOS). Experimental mice were challenged by a compounded malnutrition and *Cryptosporidium parvum* insult and samples were harvested on day 7 post-*C. parvum inoculum*. Wild-type, APOE knockout, and APOE targeted replacement mice (APOE 3/3 TR and APOE 4/4 TR) were orally inoculated with 10^7-unexcysted oocysts diluted in 100 μl of PBS. Groups have at least 4 per groups and the results are shown as mean ±SEM and expressed after β-actin normalization.

[41], and recognized as a thrifty allele [42]. This gene is considered important to enhance energy usage and storage and to foster host defenses at times of food scarcity and when repeated bouts of infection outbreaks occur and energy usage for catch-up growth and fit immunity are critical requirements for immediate survival [43].

Interestingly, data from the Tsiname population in lowland Bolivia (an indigenous forager-farmer population, with high infectious morbidity and shortened life expectancy) when bearing APOE4 show lower C-reactive protein levels, suggesting low rates of environmental-related infections [44]. In our study, targeted transgenic mice expressing human apoE4 protein have an advantage in eliminating *C. parvum* oocysts after being exposed to a high load of parasitic inoculum supporting the concept of antagonistic pleiotropy for the APOE4 gene [45].

Altogether, our findings support that APOE4 is protective during *C. parvum* infections early in life, improving parasite elimination with enhanced intestinal mucosal recovery. These effects may be caused by boosting innate immunity but without the overt inflammation seen with apoE deficiency and improving arginine uptake and arginase 1-driven mucosal restitution.

The APOE4 allele has been associated with increased nitric oxide production in platelet cells and in macrophages also is associated with increase expression of CAT-1 (cationic amino acid transporter), and with increased arginine uptake in brain microglia [46].

Our mouse model data support the beneficial effect of the APOE4 allele seen in cohort shantytown children afflicted with malnutrition and enteric infections who harbor this allele [20]. Although the orchestrated epithelial restitution and immune-inflammatory responses against malnutrition and enteric infections constitute a multi-factorial gene-to-gene interplay, the APOE gene appears to enable better intestinal adaptation against *Cryptosporidium parvum*.

One limitation of this study is the lack of the undernourished uninfected controls for comparisons of baseline levels for the APOE TR 4/4 and TR3/3 mice. In addition, we cannot rule out that the level of *Cryptostoridium* excystation after oral inoculation may have varied in the different genetic mouse strains used, however, after 6 h of *C. parvum* challenge in a model of human HCT-8 epithelial monolayers a considerable excystation of the oocysts is already seen [47].

In summary, our overall findings suggest that ApoE is one of the key players modulating the intestinal architecture and immune and inflammatory responses following malnutrition and *C. parvum* infection.

Acknowledgments

The authors would like to thank Gina Calabrese and Mary Stout for technical assistance and Glynis Kolling, Ph.D., for helpful comments to improve this manuscript.

Author Contributions

Conceived and designed the experiments: RG RO JR. Performed the experiments: OA DB. Analyzed the data: RP. Contributed reagents/materials/analysis tools: RG RO JR. Wrote the paper: RG RO JR OA DB. Approved the final version of the manuscript: AL MV CW RO.

References

1. Karanis P, Kourenti C, Smith H (2007) Waterborne transmission of protozoan parasites: a worldwide review of outbreaks and lessons learnt. J Water Health 5: 1–38.
2. Marcos LA, Gotuzzo E (2013) Intestinal protozoan infections in the immunocompromised host. Curr Opin Infect Dis 26: 295–301. doi: 10.1097/QCO.0b013e3283630be3.
3. Dillingham RA, Lima AA, Guerrant RL (2002) Cryptosporidiosis: epidemiology and impact. Microbes Infect 4: 1059–1066. doi: 10.1016/S1286-4579(02)01630-1.
4. Guerrant RL, Oria RB, Moore SR, Oria MO, Lima AA (2008) Malnutrition as an enteric infectious disease with long-term effects on child development. Nutr Rev 66: 487–505. doi: 10.1111/j.1753-4887.2008.00082.x.
5. Turan N, Ghalwash MF, Katari S, Coutifaris C, Obradovic Z., et al.(2012) DNA methylation differences at growth related genes correlate with birth weight: a molecular signature linked to developmental origins of adult disease? BMC Med Genomics 5: 10. doi: 10.1186/1755-8794-5-10.
6. Pinkerton RC, Oria RB, Kent JW, Jr., Kohli A, Abreu C., et al. (2011) Evidence for genetic susceptibility to developing early childhood diarrhea among shantytown children living in northeastern Brazil. Am J Trop Med Hyg 85: 893–896. doi: 10.4269/ajtmh.2011.11-0159.
7. Mitter SS, Oria RB, Kvalsund MP, Pamplona P, Joventino ES, et al.(2012) Apolipoprotein E4 influences growth and cognitive responses to micronutrient supplementation in shantytown children from northeast Brazil. Clinics (Sao Paulo) 67: 11–18. doi: 10.6061/clinics/2012(01)03.
8. Oria RB, Patrick PD, Blackman JA, Lima AA, Guerrant RL (2007) Role of apolipoprotein E4 in protecting children against early childhood diarrhea outcomes and implications for later development. Med Hypotheses 68: 1099–1107. doi: 10.1016/j.mehy.2006.09.036.
9. Mahley RW, Rall SC, Jr. (2000) Apolipoprotein E: far more than a lipid transport protein. Annu Rev Genomics Hum Genet 1: 507–537. doi: 10.1146/annurev.genom.1.1.507.
10. Strittmatter WJ, Bova HC (2002) Molecular biology of apolipoprotein E. Curr Opin Lipidol 13: 119–123.
11. Chapman J, Vinokurov S, Achiron A, Karussis DM, Mitosek-Szewczyk K, et al. (2001) APOE genotype is a major predictor of long-term progression of disability in MS. Neurology 56: 312–316.
12. Jofre-Monseny L, Minihane AM, Rimbach G (2008) Impact of apoE genotype on oxidative stress, inflammation and disease risk. Mol Nutr Food Res 52: 131–145. doi: 10.1002/mnfr.200700322.
13. Roselaar SE, Daugherty A (1998) Apolipoprotein E-deficient mice have impaired innate immune responses to Listeria monocytogenes in vivo. J Lipid Res 39: 1740–1743.
14. De BN, Netea MG, Demacker PN, Kullberg BJ, van der Meer JW, et al. (2000) Apolipoprotein E-deficient mice have an impaired immune response to Klebsiella pneumoniae. Eur J Clin Invest 30: 818–822. eci715 [pii].
15. Oria RB, Vieira CMG, Pinkerton RC, De Castro-Costa CM, Lopes MB, et al. (2007) Apolipoprotein E knockout mice have accentuated malnutrition with mucosal disruption and blunted insulin-like growth factor responses to refeeding. Nutrition Research 26: 427–435. doi: 10.1016/j.nutres.2006.06.020.
16. Costa LB, JohnBull EA, Reeves JT, Sevilleja JE, Freire RS, et al. (2011) Cryptosporidium-malnutrition interactions: mucosal disruption, cytokines, and TLR signaling in a weaned murine model. J Parasitol 97: 1113–1120. doi: 10.1645/GE-2848.1.
17. Roeschlau P, Bernt E, Gruber W (1974) Enzymatic determination of total cholesterol in serum. Z Klin Chem Klin Biochem 12: 226.
18. Coutinho BP, Oria RB, Vieira CM, Sevilleja JE, Warren CA, et al. (2008) Cryptosporidium infection causes undernutrition and, conversely, weanling undernutrition intensifies infection. J Parasitol 94: 1225–1232. doi: 10.1645/GE-1411.1.
19. Checkley W, Epstein LD, Gilman RH, Black RE, Cabrera L, et al. (1998) Effects of Cryptosporidium parvum infection in Peruvian children: growth faltering and subsequent catch-up growth. Am J Epidemiol 148: 497–506.
20. Oria RB, Patrick PD, Zhang H, Lorntz B, de Castro Costa CM, et al. (2005) APOE4 protects the cognitive development in children with heavy diarrhea burdens in Northeast Brazil. Pediatr Res 57: 310–316. doi: 10.1203/01.PDR.0000148719.82468.CA.
21. Vasunilashorn S, Finch CE, Crimmins EM, Vikman SA, Stieglitz J, et al. (2011) Inflammatory gene variants in the Tsimane, an indigenous Bolivian population with a high infectious load. Biodemography Soc Biol 57: 33–52.
22. De BN, Netea MG, Demacker PN, Verschueren I, Kullberg BJ, et al. (1999) Apolipoprotein E knock-out mice are highly susceptible to endotoxemia and Klebsiella pneumoniae infection. J Lipid Res 40: 680–685.
23. Serrano HA (2009) [Helper (TH1, TH2, TH17) and regulatory cells (Treg, TH3, NKT) in rheumatoid arthritis]. Reumatol Clin 5S1: 1–5. doi: 10.1016/j.reuma.2008.11.012.
24. Rensen PC, Oosten M, Bilt E, Eck M, Kuiper J, et al. (1997) Human recombinant apolipoprotein E redirects lipopolysaccharide from Kupffer cells to liver parenchymal cells in rats In vivo. J Clin Invest 99: 2438–2445. doi: 10.1172/JCI119427.
25. Van OM, Rensen PC, Van Amersfoort ES, Van EM, Van Dam AM, et al. (2001) Apolipoprotein E protects against bacterial lipopolysaccharide-induced lethality. A new therapeutic approach to treat gram-negative sepsis. J Biol Chem 276: 8820–8824. doi: 10.1074/jbc.M009915200.
26. Bhat BG, Rapp SR, Beaudry JA, Napawan N, Butteiger DN, et al. (2003) Inhibition of ileal bile acid transport and reduced atherosclerosis in apoE−/− mice by SC-435. J Lipid Res 44: 1614–1621. doi: 10.1194/jlr.M200469-JLR200.
27. Hoare S, Poppitt SD, Prentice AM, Weaver LT (1996) Dietary supplementation and rapid catch-up growth after acute diarrhoea in childhood. Br J Nutr 76: 479–490.
28. Feingold KR, Staprans I, Memon RA, Moser AH, Shigenaga JK, et al. (1992) Endotoxin rapidly induces changes in lipid metabolism that produce hypertriglyceridemia: low doses stimulate hepatic triglyceride production while high doses inhibit clearance. J Lipid Res 33: 1765–1776.
29. Pan M, Choudry HA, Epler MJ, Meng Q, Karinch A, et al. (2004) Arginine transport in catabolic disease states. J Nutr 134: 2826S–2829S.
30. Barcia AM, Harris HW (2005) Triglyceride-rich lipoproteins as agents of innate immunity. Clin Infect Dis 41 Suppl 7: S498–S503. 10.1086/432005 [doi].
31. Zhang H, Wu LM, Wu J (2011) Cross-talk between apolipoprotein E and cytokines. Mediators Inflamm 2011: 949072. doi: 10.1155/2011/949072.
32. McDonald V, Korbel DS, Barakat FM, Choudhry N, et al. (2013) Innate immune responses against Cryptosporidium parvum infection. Parasite Immunol 35: 55–64. doi: 10.1111/pim.12020.
33. Barrier M, Lacroix-Lamande S, Mancassola R, Auray G, Bernardet N, et al. (2006) Oral and intraperitoneal administration of phosphorothioate oligodeoxynucleotides leads to control of Cryptosporidium parvum infection in neonatal mice. J Infect Dis 193: 1400–1407. doi: 10.1086/503748.
34. Chuang K, Elford EL, Tseng J, Leung B, Harris HW (2010) An expanding role for apolipoprotein E in sepsis and inflammation. Am J Surg 200: 391–397. doi: 10.1016/j.amjsurg.2009.10.017.
35. van den Elzen P, Garg S, Leon L, Brigl M, Leadbetter EA, et al. (2005) Apolipoprotein-mediated pathways of lipid antigen presentation. Nature 437: 906–910. doi: 10.1038/nature04001.
36. Li P, Yin YL, Li D, Kim SW, Wu G (2007) Amino acids and immune function. Br J Nutr 98: 237–252.
37. Castro IC, Oliveira BB, Slowikowski JJ, Coutinho BP, Siqueira FJ, et al. (2012) Arginine decreases Cryptosporidium parvum infection in undernourished suckling mice involving nitric oxide synthase and arginase. Nutrition 28: 678–85. doi: 10.1016/j.nut.2011.09.011.
38. Wu G, Morris SM, Jr. (1998) Arginine metabolism: nitric oxide and beyond. Biochem J 336 (Pt 1): 1–17.
39. Vitek MP, Brown CM, Colton CA (2009) APOE genotype-specific differences in the innate immune response. Neurobiol Aging 30: 1350–1360. doi: 10.1016/j.neurobiolaging.2007.11.014.
40. Finch CE, Morgan TE (2007) Systemic inflammation, infection, ApoE alleles, and Alzheimer disease: a position paper. Curr Alzheimer Res 4: 185–189. doi: 10.2174/156720507780362254.
41. Oria RB, Patrick PD, Oria MO, Lorntz B, Thompson MR, et al. (2010) ApoE polymorphisms and diarrheal outcomes in Brazilian shanty town children. Braz J Med Biol Res 43: 249–256. doi: 10.1590/S0100-879X2010007500003.
42. Corbo RM, Scacchi R (1999) Apolipoprotein E (APOE) allele distribution in the world. Is APOE*4 a 'thrifty' allele? Ann Hum Genet 63: 301–310.

43. Hoare S, Poppitt SD, Prentice AM, Weaver LT (1996) Dietary supplementation and rapid catch-up growth after acute diarrhoea in childhood. Br J Nutr 76: 479–490.
44. Vasunilashorn S, Crimmins EM, Kim JK, Winking J, Gurven M, et al. (2010) Blood lipids, infection, and inflammatory markers in the Tsimane of Bolivia. Am J Hum Biol 22: 731–740. doi: 10.1002/ajhb.21074.
45. Moreau PH, Bott JB, Zerbinatti C, Renger JJ, Kelche C, et al. (2013) ApoE4 confers better spatial memory than apoE3 in young adult hAPP-Yac/apoE-TR mice. Behav Brain Res 243: 1–5. doi: 10.1016/j.bbr.2012.12.043.
46. Colton CA, Brown CM, Czapiga M, Vitek MP (2002) Apolipoprotein-E allele-specific regulation of nitric oxide production. Ann N Y Acad Sci 962: 212–225.
47. Costa LB, Noronha FJ, Roche JK, Sevilleja JE, Warren CA, et al. (2012) Novel in vitro and in vivo models and potential new therapeutics to break the vicious cycle of cryptosporidium infection and malnutrition. J Infect Dis 205: 1464–1471. doi: 10.1093/infdis/jis216.

4

Quantifying and Exploiting the Age Dependence in the Effect of Supplementary Food for Child Undernutrition

Milinda Lakkam[1], Stefan Wager[2], Paul H. Wise[3], Lawrence M. Wein[4]*

1 Institute for Computational and Mathematical Engineering, Stanford University, Stanford, California, United States of America, **2** Statistics Department, Stanford University, Stanford, California, United States of America, **3** School of Medicine, Stanford University, Stanford California, United States of America, **4** Graduate School of Business, Stanford University, Stanford, California, United States of America

Abstract

Motivated by the lack of randomized controlled trials with an intervention-free control arm in the area of child undernutrition, we fit a trivariate model of weight-for-age z score (WAZ), height-for-age z score (HAZ) and diarrhea status to data from an observational study of supplementary feeding (100 kCal/day for children with WAZ < -2.5) in 17 Guatemalan communities. Incorporating time lags, intention to treat (i.e., to give supplementary food), seasonality and age interactions, we estimate how the effect of supplementary food on WAZ, HAZ and diarrhea status varies with a child's age. We find that the effect of supplementary food on all 3 metrics decreases linearly with age from 6 to 20 mo and has little effect after 20 mo. We derive 2 food allocation policies that myopically (i.e., looking ahead 2 mo) minimize either the underweight or stunting severity – i.e., the sum of squared WAZ or HAZ scores for all children with WAZ or HAZ <0. A simulation study based on the statistical model predicts that the 2 derived policies reduce the underweight severity (averaged over all ages) by 13.6–14.1% and reduce the stunting severity at age 60 mo by 7.1–8.0% relative to the policy currently in use, where all policies have a budget that feeds $\approx$4% of children. While these findings need to be confirmed on additional data sets, it appears that in a low-dose (100 kCal/day) supplementary feeding setting in Guatemala, allocating food primarily to 6–12 mo infants can reduce the severity of underweight and stunting.

Editor: C. Mary Schooling, CUNY, United States of America

Funding: Graduate School of Business, Stanford University and a B.C. and E.J. Eaves Stanford Graduate Fellowship. The funders had no role in study design, data collection and analysis, decision to publish, or preparation of the manuscript.

Competing Interests: The authors have declared that no competing interests exist.

* Email: lwein@stanford.edu

Introduction

With over 3 M deaths per year of children under 5 years attributable to undernutrition [1] and the level of food aid far less than required [2,3], it is vital to optimally allocate food to the appropriate children in the appropriate amounts. To address this problem in a rigorous manner requires knowledge about three key aspects [4]: (i) the evolution of weight and height (and perhaps disease) of children under 5 years in the absence of food aid; (ii) the impact that weight and height (and perhaps other factors such as age, sex and disease) have on morbidity and mortality, and (iii) the impact of supplementary or therapeutic food on weight and height (and perhaps other factors such as disease).

A bivariate statistical model of weight and height can be constructed from a longitudinal data set [4] to address (i), and logistic regression [4,5] or proportional hazards [6] models can estimate the impact of anthropometric measurements on mortality to address (ii). The ideal approach to (iii) would use longitudinal measurements of weight and height from a large randomized control trial with a control arm that does not receive any food. There appears to be only one study that possesses these characteristics for therapeutic food [7] and no studies involving supplementary feeding [8]. As a result, very little is known about how the impact of food on weight and height is influenced by a child's age, sex and pre-intervention weight, height and presence of disease, and the amount of therapeutic or supplementary food consumed. Furthermore, the ethical issues inherent in using a control group that does not receive food suggests that there may not be any large randomized control trials with intervention-free arms performed in the future.

Consequently, the most promising approach to making headway on aspect (iii) is to jointly estimate aspects (i) and (iii) – i.e., fit a statistical model of weight and height in the presence of nonrandom food aid – using observational or dose-response studies of nutrition programs that do not include intervention-free control arms. In this study, we make a first step in this direction and analyze data from a nutrition program in Guatemala, where every child under 5 years in 17 villages has his weight, height and diarrhea status (the number of days in the previous week with diarrhea) measured every 2 mo, and children with weight-for-age z score (WAZ) less than -2.5 receive supplementary food of ≈ 100 kCal/day. We use the WAZ $= -2.5$ threshold to cast the nutrition program as a natural experiment – where children with WAZ just above -2.5 (who do not receive treatment) act as a control group for the children with WAZ just below -2.5 (who do receive treatment) – and analyze it via a regression discontinuity design [9], which is a design where the assignment of an intervention is based on the value of an observed covariate lying below (or above) a fixed threshold. By comparing observations that are just above and just below WAZ $= -2.5$, the regression discontinuity design allows us to estimate the average treatment effect. In econometrics, statistics and related fields, regression discontinuity designs have become the preferred approach for evaluating the effects of intervention in a setting such as ours, where randomization is not possible [9]. More specifically, a generalized additive model (GAM) [10] is used to predict future (i.e., 2 mo hence) WAZ, height-for-age z score (HAZ) and diarrhea status (because deaths from wasting do not occur in this setting, we focus on WAZ and HAZ instead of weight-for-height z score, WHZ) in terms of current and past values of (WAZ,HAZ,diarrhea) along with seasonal and age-interaction terms. This statistical model allows us to isolate how age influences the impact that supplementary food has on WAZ, HAZ and diarrhea status. We use these statistical results to derive 2 allocation policies that minimize the underweight (or stunting) severity, i.e., the sum of squared expected WAZ (or HAZ) scores among children with WAZ <0(or HAZ <0), 2 mo into the future. We build a simulation model based on our GAM that compares the derived allocation policies to the allocation policy that is currently used in the nutrition program in Guatemala, and to the counterfactual of no supplementary food.

Materials and Methods

Data

Our data set tracks 2125 children (1047 boys, 1078 girls) from 17 communities participating in a nutrition program in Guatemala from November 2009 to April 2012. Every 2 months, children from birth to age 60 mo had their WAZ, HAZ – both measured according to World Health Organization (WHO) child growth standards [11] – and the number of days with diarrhea in the previous week recorded. The nutrition program provided supplementary food to all children with WAZ <-2.5. Children over 12 mo received ≈ 100 kCal/day of Incaparina (a supplement made from maize and soy flours) and sugar, and children between 6–12 mo received half this amount and – for children with inadequate or no breastfeeding despite promoter efforts to support breastfeeding until at least 1 year of age –2 400-gm cans of powdered infant formula (Nestle NAN Pro 1 or 2, made of whey and casein milk proteins) per mo. The Stanford Institutional Review Board, which includes members with medical and social science expertise, and the Review Committee of the Hospital Obras Sociales de Monsignor Gregorio Schaffer, San Lucas Toliman reviewed and approved this study prior to study initiation. Informed consent in Spanish and/or the local indigenous language was obtained from a parent/guardian for all children at enrollment. All patient information was anonymized and de-identified prior to analysis.

Generalized Additive Model

For boys and girls, we build separate GAMs for the evolution of (W_t,H_t,D_t) for age t varying from 1 to 60 mo, which are the WAZ, HAZ and the number of days with diarrhea in the previous week for a child of age t mo (see Table 1 for a description of most of the variables). Define the Intention To Treat (ITT) indicator variable $I_t=1$ if $W_t<-2.5$ and $I_t=0$ otherwise, and let M_t be the month of the year when a child is of age t. Let $\hat{t}=(t-31.76)/15.74$ be the standardized age, where 31.76 mo and 15.74 mo are the mean and standard deviation of the ages among all entries in the data set.

An analysis of GAM results with varying amounts of history suggests that we need to maintain 4 mo of history; i.e., if we are trying to estimate a child's $(W_{t+2},H_{t+2},D_{t+2})$ then we need to use (W_t,H_t,D_t) and $(W_{t-2},H_{t-2},D_{t-2})$. To ease the interpretation of our GAM coefficients, we let the response variables be

Table 1. The estimated parameters for boys from the GAM.

Variable	Description	Estimating $W_{t+2}-W_t$			Estimating $H_{t+2}-H_t$			Estimating D_{t+2}		
		Est.	S.E.	*p*	Est.	S.E.	*p*	Est.	S.E.	*p*
	Intercept	−0.230	0.018	0.000	−0.907	0.025	0.000	−0.751	0.081	0.000
W_t	WAZ	−0.095	0.007	0.000	0.124	0.009	0.000	−0.184	0.039	0.000
$W_t\hat{t}$	WAZ × age	0.014	0.006	0.026	−0.068	0.009	0.000	−0.056	0.036	0.115
W_t-W_{t-2}	WAZ increment	−0.256	0.011	0.000	−0.000	0.016	0.981	0.183	0.066	0.006
$(W_t-W_{t-2})\hat{t}$	WAZ incr. × age	−0.090	0.010	0.000	0.021	0.013	0.116	0.084	0.055	0.122
H_t	HAZ	0.038	0.006	0.000	−0.177	0.008	0.000	−0.007	0.033	0.835
$H_t\hat{t}$	HAZ × age	0.006	0.005	0.280	0.092	0.007	0.000	0.068	0.030	0.024
H_t-H_{t-2}	HAZ increment	−0.020	0.009	0.030	−0.205	0.013	0.000	0.063	0.053	0.236
$(H_t-H_{t-2})\hat{t}$	HAZ incr. × age	−0.007	0.008	0.375	−0.022	0.011	0.036	−0.041	0.042	0.337
D_t	Diarrhea	0.003	0.003	0.387	−0.003	0.004	0.429	0.102	0.014	0.000
$D_t\hat{t}$	Diarrhea × age	0.014	0.003	0.000	0.007	0.004	0.091	−0.021	0.013	0.100

For each variable, we give the estimated coefficient (Est.), the standard error (S.E.) and the p-value.

$(W_{t+2}-W_t,H_{t+2}-H_t,D_{t+2})$. We fit $W_{t+2}-W_t$ and $H_{t+2}-H_t$ by least squares and model D_t by a Poisson random variable. We let the link functions be the identity function for $W_{t+2}-W_t$ and $H_{t+2}-H_t$ and the natural logarithm for D_{t+2}. The predictor variables include the current values (W_t,H_t,D_t) and their age-interaction terms $(W_t\hat{t},H_t\hat{t},D_t\hat{t})$, the most recent increments $((W_t-W_{t-2}),(H_t-H_{t-2}))$ and their age interaction terms $((W_t-W_{t-2})\hat{t},(H_t-H_{t-2})\hat{t})$, as well as seasonal functions $(f_M^W(M_t),f_M^H(M_t),f_M^D(M_t))$ for the month of the year, age functions $(g^W(t),g^H(t),g^D(t))$ in the absence of supplementary food, and age functions $(g_I^W(t)I_t,g_I^H(t)I_t,g_I^D(t)I_t)$ due to the ITT. The seasonal functions are modeled as periodic cubic splines and the age functions are modeled as cubic smoothing splines. We denote the sample covariance matrix calculated from the residuals of the GAM by Σ. The 3 GAM equations are stated with their resulting coefficients in §1 of File S1.

To make the most use of the available data without imputing any missing data, we include every set of 3 consecutive measurements by assuming they occur at ages t −2, t and t +2 for some t. We also discard as outliers any z scores outside the range of $[-5,5]$.

Proposed Allocation Policies

Because of the difficulty of solving a dynamic program with a system state that is the joint population-wide probability density function (PDF) of (W_t,H_t,D_t), we derive 2 derived policies – referred to as the derived WAZ policy and the derived HAZ policy – that estimate every child's $(W_{t+2},H_{t+2},D_{t+2})$ given all the information known at age t, and minimizes the sum of $E[W_{t+2}]^2$ (or $E[H_{t+2}]^2$) over all children with $W_t<0$(or $H_t<0$), subject to a constraint on the amount of supplementary food allocated. As in [12], this objective captures moderate and mild forms of undernutrition and also incorporates the fact that more severe undernutrition leads to more severe consequences; however, we use $E[W_{t+2}]^2$ rather than $E[W_{t+2}^2]$ so that the proposed policy is relatively simple.

Let $c_t=0.5$ if $t\in[6,12]$ and $c_t=1$ if $t>12$, which represents the normalized amount of supplementary food consumed by a child at age t. The allocation policy that solves this constrained optimization problem prioritizes all children with $W_t<0$ by $(E[W_{t+2}|I_t=1)]^2-E[W_{t+2}|I_t=0]^2)/c_t$ (with smaller values getting higher priority), and allocates the food until it is gone (§2 of File S1).

Simulation Model

The simulation model tracks 1 M children of each sex from age 6 to 60 mo. A child's initial (W_t,H_t,D_t) at 6 mo is randomly sampled with replacement from all children of the same sex in the data set when they were 6 mo. At each 2-mo time step, the values of $(W_{t+2},H_{t+2},D_{t+2})$ are calculated using the GAM and then adding an additive trivariate noise term that is normally distributed with mean zero and covariance matrix Σ (and rounding the value of D_{t+2} to the nearest integer).

We consider the 5 policies described in Table 2. All policies except the no food policy allocate the same amount of food, which is dictated by the amount of food allocated under the current policy (i.e., $W_t<-2.5$). This food budget is 1.2 (0.7) units of food per boy (girl) over a child's 27 feeding opportunities, which corresponds to 4.7% of children being fed at any given time. We do a 1-dimensional search for thresholds (for the quantities being prioritized in Table 2) for the simple WAZ policy and the 2 derived policies so that the amount of food allocated by these policies is equal to this food budget. The thresholds for the simple WAZ policy are −1.8 for boys (i.e., a boy under 2 yr receives food if $W_t<-1.8$) and −1.7 for girls, the thresholds for the derived WAZ policy are −0.082 for boys (i.e., a boy receives food if $(E[W_{t+2}|I_t=1)]^2-E[W_{t+2}|I_t=0]^2)/c_t<-0.082$) and −0.138 for girls, and the thresholds for the derived HAZ policy are −0.44 for boys and −0.56 for girls.

For each policy and various values of θ, we report $P(H_t<\theta)$ and $P(W_t<\theta)$ for all $t\in[6,60]$ mo. We also compute 2 variants of the severity index considered in [12], the average of $\sum_{t=6}^{60} W_t^2 I_{\{W_t<0\}}/28$ over all children and the average of $H_{60}^2 I_{\{H_{60}<0\}}$, where $I_{\{x\}}$ is the indicator function of the event x. These quantities are the average squared shortfalls below the reference median (i.e., zero) for WAZ averaged over all ages and for HAZ at age 60 mo. We refer to these measures as the underweight severity and the stunting severity, respectively.

Results

GAM Results

The GAM parameters are very similar for boys (Table 1) and girls (Table 1 of File S1), and the statistically significant parameters have the following interpretations. WAZ exhibits global mean reversion (i.e., heavier children tend to lose weight and lighter children tend to gain weight), which is more pronounced in younger children, and local mean reversion (i.e., children who have recently lost weight tend to gain it back and vice versa), which is more pronounced in older children. Taller children tend to gain weight although children who recently grew taller are less likely to gain weight. Current diarrhea status has no impact on weight gain overall, although older boys are more likely to gain weight after a diarrhea episode while younger boys are more apt to lose weight (this effect is not observed in girls). HAZ also exhibits global mean reversion that is more prominent in younger children and local mean reversion that is more prominent in older children, and the magnitude of global mean reversion for HAZ is larger than it is for WAZ. Heavier children are more apt to grow taller, an effect that is more evident in younger children. Current diarrhea status and recent weight gain are not associated with height gain. Diarrhea is reinforcing; i.e., current diarrhea tends to lead to future diarrhea. Lighter children and children who recently gained weight both tend to get more diarrhea, and the former effect is more pronounced in older girls than younger girls. Current height of boys has no overall impact on getting diarrhea, although taller girls are more likely to get diarrhea than shorter girls. Older tall children are more likely to get diarrhea than younger tall children.

Turning to the spline functions, which are also very similar for boys (Fig. 1) and girls (Fig. 1 of File S1), we see that low WAZ and high diarrhea prevalence are on very similar annual cycles (with November - April being the most severe months), while HAZ has a more rapid increase and lags slightly behind WAZ, peaking during August - November (Figs. 1a–c). In the absence of intervention, faltering in WAZ and HAZ occurs during the first 2 yr, at which point WAZ stabilizes and HAZ increases for boys (Figs. 1d–e); for girls, WAZ does not stabilize until ≈40 mo and HAZ begins to increase at 30 mo. The prevalence of diarrhea decreases with age (Fig. 1f). The effect of ITT (i.e., supplementary food) has a similar pattern for all 3 variables: the impact is beneficial (i.e., higher WAZ and HAZ, lower diarrhea) and linearly decreasing between 6 and 20 months, and thereafter has little or no effect (with the exception that ITT leads to an increase in diarrhea for older girls). ITT's effect on HAZ is twice as large as its effect on WAZ.

Table 2. Food allocation policies.

Name of Policy	Children Receiving Food	Severity Index	
		Underweight	Stunting
No Food	None	1.87	5.44
Current	$W_t < -2.5$	1.84	5.50
Simple WAZ	Under 2 yr and prioritized by W_t	1.77	5.35
Derived WAZ	Prioritized by $(E[W_{t+2}\|I_t=1)]^2 - E[W_{t+2}\|I_t=0]^2)/c_t$	1.59	5.11
Derived HAZ	Prioritized by $(E[H_{t+2}\|I_t=1)]^2 - E[H_{t+2}\|I_t=0]^2)/c_t$	1.58	5.06

A description of the food allocation policies and their severity indices for boys, which measure the average of squared shortfalls below the reference median (i.e., zero) for WAZ averaged over all 28 measured ages (underweight) and for HAZ at age 60 mo (stunting).

The covariance parameters are very similar for boys and girls (§1 of File S1), where weight gain and height gain are positively correlated, weight gain and diarrhea are negatively correlated, and height gain and diarrhea are the least correlated. The adjusted R^2 for $(W_{t+2} - W_t, H_{t+2} - H_t, D_t)$ are 0.151, 0.259 and 0.041 for boys, and 0.226, 0.309 and 0.052 for girls.

Food Allocation Results

The results for boys (Figs. 2–5) and girls (Figs. 2–5 of File S1) are very similar, aside from the fact that girls are less underweight than boys, and hence have a smaller food budget. Given the strong influence of age on the effect of intervention (Figs. 1g–i), it is not surprising that the two derived policies allocate much of the food to children <12 mo (Fig. 2). Consequently, the two derived policies reduce the far left tail of the HAZ and WAZ distributions between 6–12 mo (Figs. 3–4). Although some of this gain is dissipated through the next 4 years, these 2 policies still dominate the other policies throughout the first 5 years. The current policy incurs a significant increase in extreme underweight (WAZ <-3) during 12–30 mo because it fails to feed enough children <12 mo who are in danger of faltering. A similar outcome – but at WAZ <-2.5– is incurred by the simple WAZ policy for children during 20–24 mo.

The severity indices (Table 2 for boys, Table 2 of File S1 for girls) reveal that the derived HAZ policy achieves slightly smaller underweight and stunting severity indices than the derived WAZ policy, although both policies perform well on both measures relative to the other policies, and achieve a 13.6–14.1% reduction in WAZ severity and a 7.1–8.0% reduction in HAZ severity relative to the current policy. The performance gap between the 2 derived policies and the simple WAZ policy is 2–3 times larger than the gap between the simple WAZ policy and the no food policy. In our simulations, the current policy increases the HAZ severity index by 1.1% relative to the no food policy for boys, and increases it by 0.1% for girls. An examination of the stunting PDFs for the 5 policies (Fig. 5) reveals that the current policy reduces the number of children with $H_{60} \in [-3.5, -1]$, but increases the number of children with $H_{60} < -4$. This increase in the extreme tail occurs because there is a small group of children with WAZ values that are consistently <-2.5 and with very low HAZ levels, and ITT further lowers their HAZ levels during months 18–36 and 46–60 (although even at the lowest points in Fig. 1 h of -0.08 at 25 mo and -0.1 at 60 mo, children continue to grow taller under ITT). In contrast, the 2 derived policies reduce the number of children with $H_{60} < -2$ and move them to the $H_{60} > -2$ region.

Sensitivity Analysis

We perform a sensitivity analysis for boys to assess the robustness of our main result that the 2 derived policies outperform the current policy. We perform the following procedure 10^3 times: take a random sample with replacement of 1047 boys (which is the original sample size in the data set) from our data set, re-estimate the statistical model (i.e., get new values for the parameters in Table 1 and the functions in Fig. 1), use the statistical model to simulate 10^4 boys under the current policy and the derived WAZ policy (for all runs, the derived WAZ policy is based on the results in Table 1 and Fig. 1, not on the re-estimated model), and compute the percentage reduction in the two severity indices that the derived WAZ policy achieves relative to the current policy. The PDFs of the 10^3 percentage reductions (Figs. 6a–b) show that the derived WAZ policy achieves a mean percentage reduction of 14.7% for underweight severity and 7.6% for stunting severity relative to the current policy, and the percentage of times that the current policy performs better than the derived WAZ policy is 4.7% for underweight severity and 0.2% for stunting severity.

We perform an identical sensitivity analysis to assess whether the current policy reduces the underweight and stunting severities relative to the no food policy. We find that the current policy reduces underweight severity by 1.4% on average and reduces it 79.7% of the time, whereas the current policy increases stunting severity by 1.2% on average and increases it 90.6% of the time (Figs. 6c–d).

Discussion

Statistical Results

The similarity between some of our statistical results and the existing literature is reassuring, and provides some confidence in the remaining statistical results that have no counterpart in the literature. The patterns of growth faltering in Figs. 1d-e are similar to the patterns seen elsewhere [13], as are the decrease in diarrhea prevalence with age (Fig. 1f and [14]). Similarly, the seasonal patterns in Figs. 1a-c are not unlike those found in Malawi [15], and – as is typical in Latin America [16] – stunting is much more prevalent than underweight. Rearranging equations (13)-(16) in the Supporting Material of [4] shows that the model there, which is based on data from Bwamanda in the Democratic Republic of Congo [17], also exhibits global and local mean reversion; global mean reversion in HAZ data is also observed in [15].

Turning to the cross terms, we find that high weight leads to a future increase in HAZ, but that recent weight gain does not; the latter finding agrees with correlations derived in [15]. An analysis

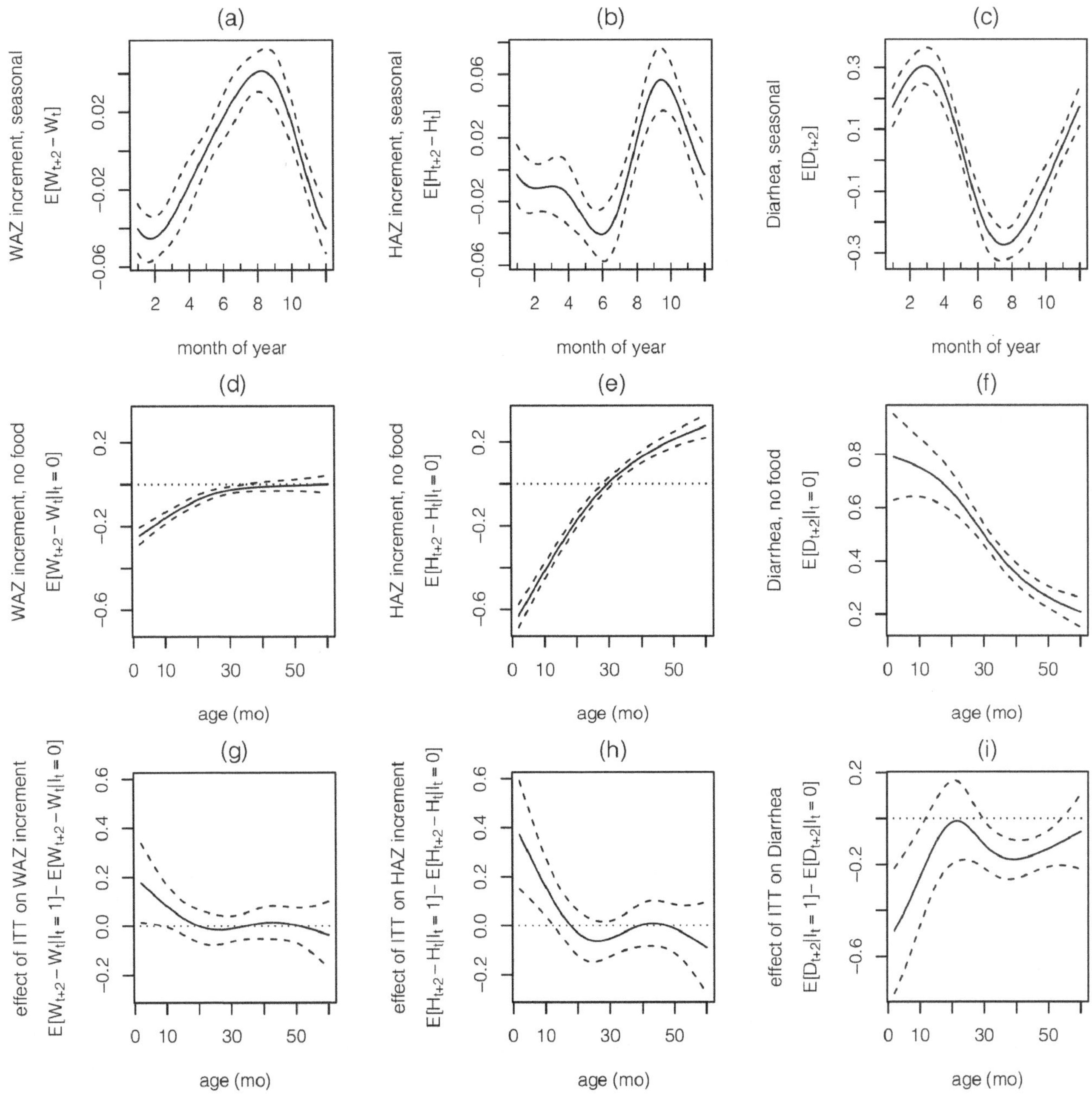

Figure 1. The estimated spline functions (and 95% confidence intervals) for boys from the GAM. The seasonal functions (**a**) $f_M^W(M_t)$, (**b**) $f_M^H(M_t)$ and (**c**) $f_M^D(M_t)$ for WAZ and HAZ increments and diarrhea. The age functions in the absence of supplementary food (**d**) $g^W(t)$, (**e**) $g^H(t)$ and (**f**) $g^D(t)$ for WAZ and HAZ increments and diarrhea. The age functions due to ITT (**g**) $g_I^W(t)$, (**h**) $g_I^H(t)$ and (**i**) $g_I^D(t)$for WAZ and HAZ increments and diarrhea.

of WHZ (rather than WAZ) and HAZ find that both low WHZ and a recent drop in WHZ lead to future reductions in HAZ [18].

Our statistical results provide limited evidence to support the fact that diarrhea can reduce nutritional status. The lack of significance of the D_t coefficient in predicting future WAZ or HAZ gain may be because most of the catch-up growth occurs before the next visit. In addition, the coefficient of $D_t\hat{t}$ in the WAZ equation for boys is consistent with the observation that infants take longer to catch up in weight than older children [19]. Although our model predicts that underweight children are more apt to get diarrhea, which is consistent with earlier results [20,21], the same is not true of stunted children (in fact, taller girls are more likely to get diarrhea than shorter girls in our model); some of the anticipated effect (i.e., stunted children are more likely to get diarrhea) may be partially masked by the age dependence (i.e., the value of the $H_t\hat{t}$ coefficient) and the 2-mo follow-up period. In any case, diarrhea is very difficult to predict and the only factors that play a strong role are seasonality, being underweight, and currently having diarrhea, which collectively suggest environmental and microbiome causes.

Our most intriguing statistical result is the strong dependence of age on the impact of intervention (Figs. 1g–i). Considerable

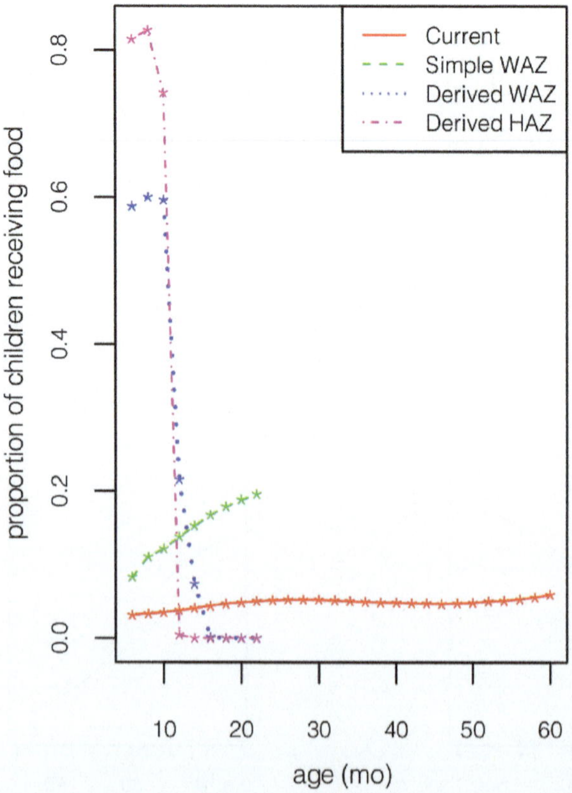

Figure 2. The proportion of boys by age who receive food under the various allocation policies.

evidence has been amassed about the importance of nutrition in the first 1000 days (from conception to 24 mo) [1,22], and Figs. 1g-i can be viewed as a refinement of this principle. Our age-dependent results are similar to those in an earlier study in Guatemala [23], which found that – after controlling for diarrhea, previous height and weight, sex, home diet and socioeconomic status – height gain and weight gain due to supplemental food decreased throughout the first 3 years of life and had little effect after age 3. A meta-analysis in Web Appendix 4 of [24] suggests that linear growth during 6–12 mo is larger than during 12–18 mo in populations with average per capita income >\$1/day, but is smaller for incomes <\$1/day. Fig. 1 h is not inconsistent with this observation because the income in Guatemala is >\$1/day.

The magnitude of the seasonality in Figs. 1a-b and of the global and local mean reversion (Table 1) implies that approaches that ignore these factors can lead to misleading estimates – and systematic overestimates in the case of global mean reversion – of the increase in weight and height that is due to supplementary feeding.

Food Allocation Results

The 2 derived policies anticipate growth faltering and exploit the age dependence in the impact of intervention by front-loading much of the intervention on infants (Fig. 2), who gain a substantial head start relative to the current policy (Figs. 3–4). Although some of the gap disappears by the time children reach age 5 years (perhaps partly due to global mean reversion), much of the improvement remains intact at age 5. The derived policies are fairly simple to implement, although they do require knowledge of a child's height and weight from his previous visit.

Due to the very limited amount of food distributed by the current policy (≈4% of children receive food at any point in time) and the fact that many more children are stunted than underweight, the improvements achieved by the 2 derived policies are modest when measured by stunting (HAZ <-2), but are more pronounced for severe stunting (HAZ <-3) and in the extreme left tail of the HAZ distribution (Fig. 4).

Because of the reinforcing cross terms – i.e., large HAZ leads to future increases in WAZ and large WAZ leads to future increases in HAZ – and the similar age dependence in how intervention increases WAZ and HAZ, the 2 derived policies have very similar performance with respect to reducing the severity of underweight and stunting.

There has been increasing focus on the lifetime effects of stunting [25], and in Latin America, where severe wasting is rare and stunting is prevalent, reducing stunting is one of the primary goals of supplementary feeding programs. To this end, we note that our model predicts that the current policy – because it allows some underweight, stunted children to become very severely

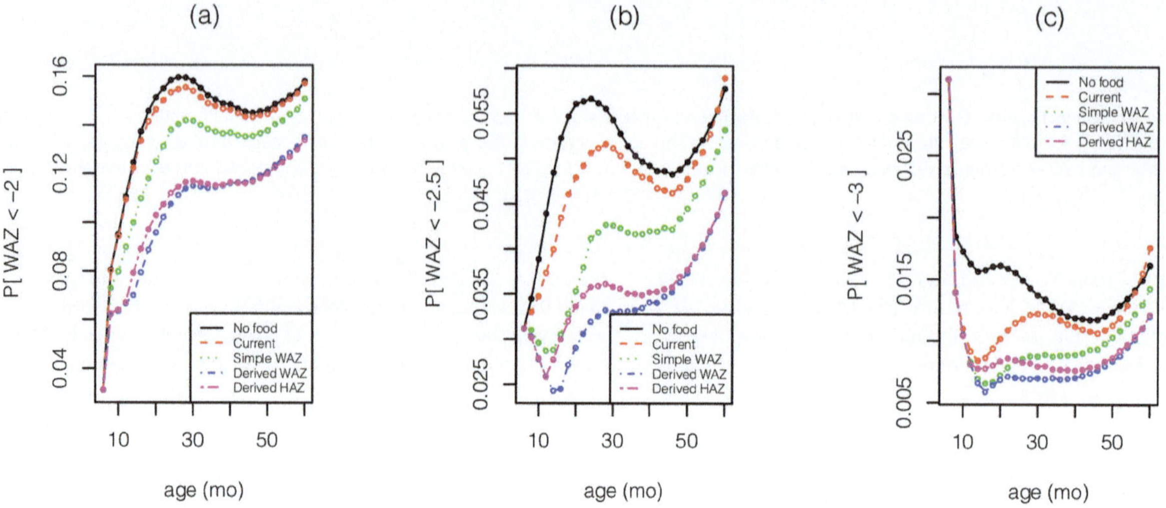

Figure 3. For boys, the left tails, P(WAZ $<\theta$) for θ equals (a) −2, (b) −2.5, (c) −3 vs. age under the various policies.

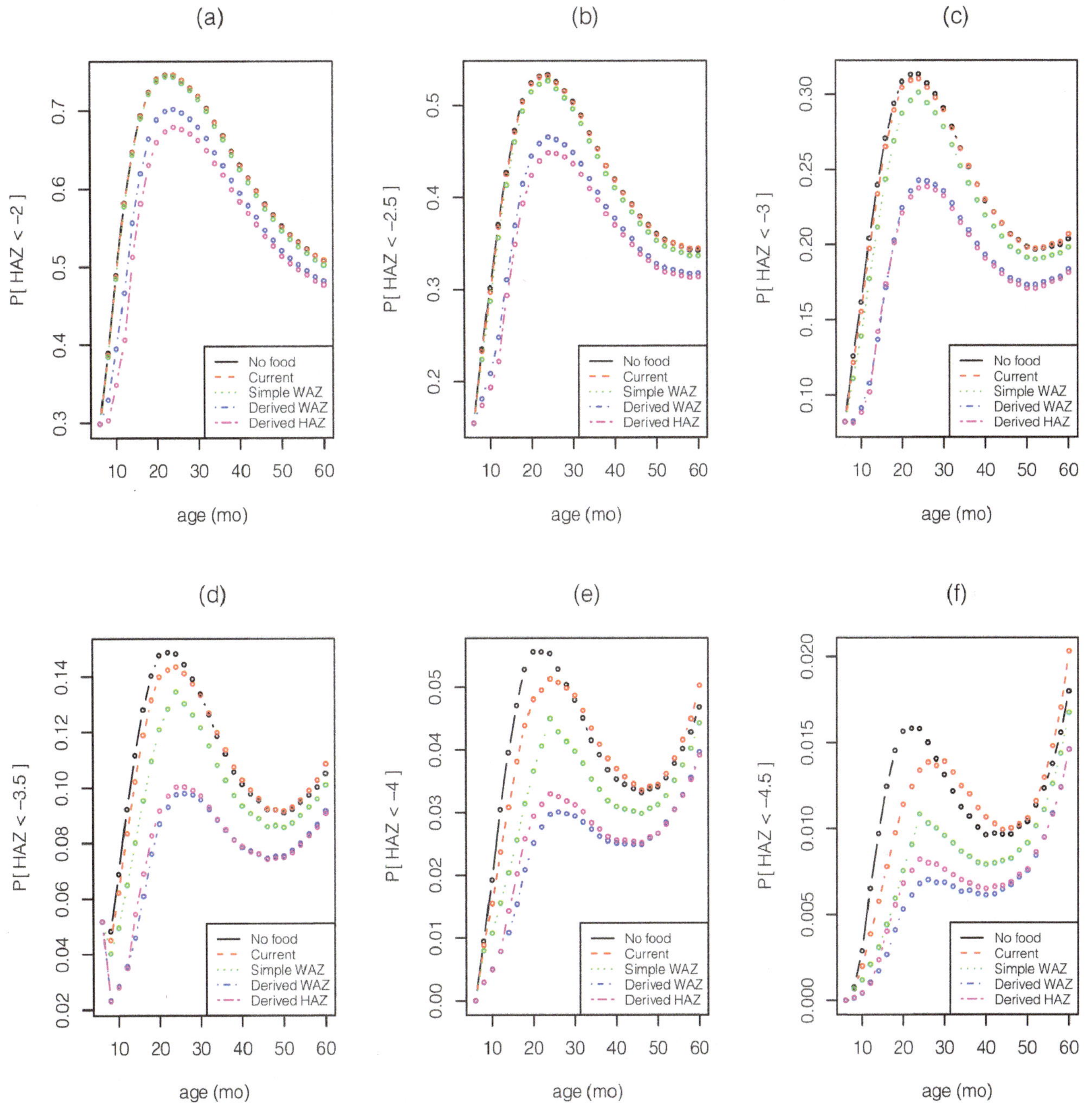

Figure 4. For boys, the left tails, P(HAZ <θ) for θ equals (a) −2, (b) −2.5, (c) −3, (d) −3.5, (e) −4, (f) −4.5 vs. age under the various policies.

stunted (Fig. 5b) – has a slightly higher severity of stunting than the no food policy (Fig. 6d). This result is driven by the fact that ITT leads to a slight decrease in HAZ in our model during months 18–36 and 46–60 (Fig. 1h); it is not clear whether this effect is real (albeit small), or is caused by overshooting of the cubic spline in Fig. 1h. In contrast, despite the wide confidence intervals in Figs. 1g–i, our sensitivity analysis (Figs. 6a–b) suggests that our main result – i.e., that the 2 derived policies outperform the current policy – is somewhat robust.

There has also been concern about the long-term cardiovascular risks associated with catch-up growth in early childhood [26]. While this remains an important issue, particularly for rapid weight gain among infants born at low birth weight, the immediate mortality and developmental risks associated with serious childhood malnutrition would seem to warrant monitored nutritional supplementation.

Limitations of Analysis

Aside from the obvious shortcoming that our analysis is based on data from a non-randomized study, there are 2 major limitations in our data set. The first is that health promoters in the Guatemala nutrition program had discretion to feed sick children, and hence ITT did not exactly coincide with the actual receipt of food. We use ITT so as not to be biased by the behavior

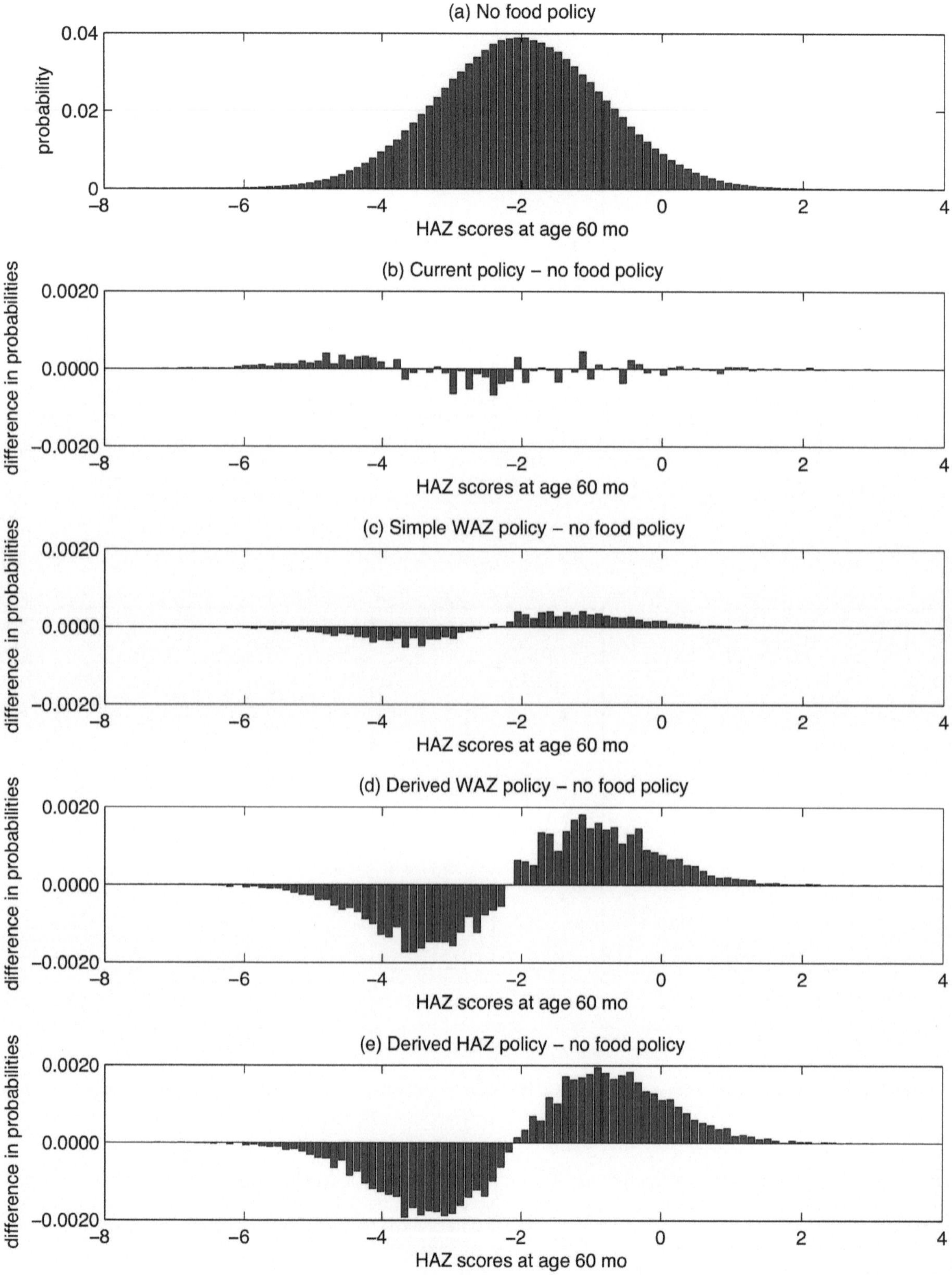

Figure 5. For boys, (a) the PDF for HAZ at age 60 mo, and (b)-(e) the difference in PDFs for HAZ at age 60 mo between 2 policies.

of health promoters. Note that if the health promoters were not given discretion to feed sick children, there may have been an incentive to alter WAZ data (e.g., change −2.3 to −2.6 so as to feed a sick child). The second limitation in our data set is the amount of missing data. While children were supposed to see a health promoter every 2 mo, the actual time between consecutive visits in the data set was 1 mo, 2 mo, 3 mo, 4 mo and >4mo with probabilities 0.094, 0.638, 0.122, 0.121 and 0.024, respectively.

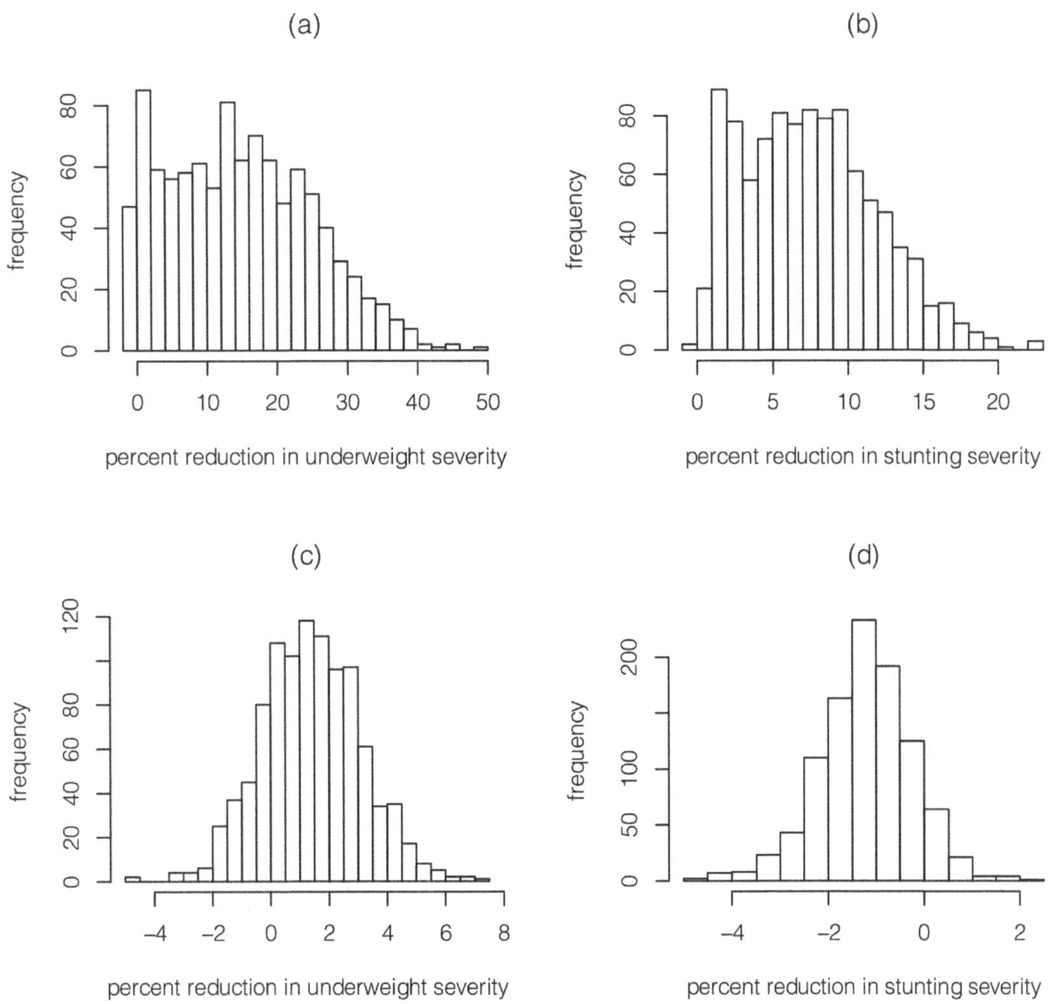

Figure 6. For boys, the PDFs of the percent reduction of the severity indices of (a)-(b) the derived WAZ policy relative to the current policy, and (c)-(d) the current policy relative to the no food policy.

With respect to estimating the impact of ITT and its age interaction, the primary concern with our assumption that consecutive visits are exactly 2 mo is if ITT causes children to visit more or less frequently relative to no ITT. To assess this issue, we re-ran the GAM with the same predictor variables as before but now with the time until the next visit as the response variable. The overall mean effect of ITT was very close to zero (see Fig. 6 of File S1, which is the analogue to Figs. 1g-i in the main text) and the 3 p-values for the cubic spline were 0.91, 0.88 an 0.96.

There are other aspects that could be investigated: estimating the variance of ITT, the interaction of diarrhea and z scores (e.g., a $D_t W_t$ interaction term could address whether diarrhea lowers future weight gain only when current WAZ is low [19]), and whether ITT is a function of D_t [19]. However, we note that our qualitative conclusions would not change even if diarrhea was omitted from the model. Also, the data used here are not well suited to estimate the influence that pre-intervention (WAZ,HAZ) levels have on the impact of intervention because of the lack of intervention-free children with low WAZ and because of the presence of global mean reversion, which may have a similar effect (Fig. 2 in [27]).

The age dependence in the impact of treatment should not be extrapolated to other settings, other doses or other undernutrition thresholds without performing similar statistical analyses of other longitudinal data sets. It should be noted that the community health system within which the nutritional surveillance and supplementation program is embedded also provides basic preventive and therapeutic health services, including routine antihelminthic medication for children greater than 2 years of age and when needed, referral to local and regional, clinical facilities. In addition, identification of malnutrition and the provision of supplementation may elevate the nutritional needs of the child in question and result indirectly in a relative reallocation of some family resources to the child. This in turn could modify the impact of supplementation on growth in different cultural or resource settings. It may be the case that 100 kCal/day is an insufficient dose – particularly after taking into account the possibility of food sharing within families – to improve the nutritional status of children over 2 years old, but that larger doses are sufficient. Similarly, even at the current dose, our findings should not be extrapolated to thresholds other than WAZ $= -2.5$. It is possible that age-specific treatment effects differ by level of undernutrition. In particular, children >20 mo may respond more to supplementary feeding when their initial undernutrition levels are more severe, because of the developmental delays associated with undernutrition. If so, regression discontinuity around a more extreme threshold might have yielded flatter estimated age functions in Figs. 1g–i.

Conclusion

Fitting a trivariate statistical model of WAZ, HAZ and diarrhea to a longitudinal data set from a nutritional program in Guatemala generates results that reinforce and quantify relationships that are already known, and identify new relationships, including a strong age dependence in the impact of supplementary food on WAZ, HAZ and diarrhea, with the benefits decreasing from 6 mo to 20 mo old and staying at a small level between 20 and 60 mo old. Our statistical results highlight the danger of ignoring seasonality and global and local mean reversion when estimating the impact of supplementary food. The food allocation policies derived here perform better than the current policy: by allocating much of the food to infants, the derived policies reduce the underweight severity by 13.6–14.1% and the stunting severity by 7.1–8.0% relative to the current policy, despite using a budget that allocates food to only 4.7% of the children at any time under the current policy. This result should not be extrapolated to other geographical regions, to doses other than 100 kCal/day, or to undernutrition thresholds other than $WAZ = -2.5$. To confirm this result, the derived policies should be compared to the current policy or the simple WAZ policy in a randomized study. More generally, given the paucity of randomized controlled trials with intervention-free control groups, our statistical approach has the potential to uncover new knowledge from observational studies pertaining to therapeutic and supplementary food for children, and our optimization approach allows this knowledge to be leveraged to improve nutritional status in a budget-constrained setting.

Supporting Information

File S1 Supporting Material. Gives the regression model equations, the derivation of the proposed food allocation policies, and the results for girls.
(PDF)

Acknowledgments

We thank Mike Baiocchi and Jeremy Goldhaber-Fiebert for helpful conversations. We also wish to thank Dr. Rafael Tun, Jos Vicente Macario Cosigu, and Dominga Pic Salazar for coordination of the community health worker and nutrition program.

Author Contributions

Conceived and designed the experiments: SW LMW. Performed the experiments: ML SW. Analyzed the data: ML SW LMW. Contributed reagents/materials/analysis tools: PHW. Wrote the paper: LMW.

References

1. Black RE, Victora CG, Walker SP, Bhutta ZA, Christian P, et al. (2013) Maternal and child undernutrition and overweight in low-income and middle-income countries. Lancet 382: 427–451.
2. Horton S, Shekar M, McDonald C, Mahal A, Krystene Brooks J (2010) Scaling up nutrition: What will it cost? Washington, DC: World Bank.
3. Shoham J, Dolan C, Gostelow L (2013) The management of acute malnutrition at scale: a review of donor and government financing arrangements. Technical report, Humanitarian Practice Network, Overseas Development Institute.
4. Yang Y, Van den Broeck J, Wein LM (2013) Ready-to-use food-allocation policy to reduce the effects of childhood undernutrition in developing countries. PNAS 110: 4545–4550.
5. Garenne M, Maire B, Fontaine O, Briend A (2006) Distributions of mortality risk attributable to low nutritional status in niakhar, senegal. J Nutrition 136: 2893–2900.
6. McDonald CM, Olofin I, Flaxman S, Fawzi WW, Spiegelman D, et al. (2013) The effect of multiple anthropometric deficits on child mortality: Meta-analysis of individual data in 10 prospective studies from developing countries. Am J Clinical Nutrition 97: 896–901.
7. Isanaka S, Nombela N, Djibo A, Poupard M, Van Beckhoven D, et al. (2009) Effective of preventive supplementation with ready-to-use therapeutic food on the nutritional status, mortality and morbidity of children aged 6 to 60 months in niger. JAMA 301: 277–285.
8. Dewey KG, Yang Z, Boy E (2009) Systematic review and meta-analysis of home fortification of complementary foods. Maternal Child Nutrition 5: 283–321.
9. Imbens GW, Lemieux T (2008) Regression discontinuity designs: A guide to practice. J Econometrics 142: 615–635.
10. Hastie TJ, Tibshirani RJ (1990) Generalized additive models, volume 43. CRC Press.
11. De Onis M, Garza C, Onyango AW, Borghi E (2007) Comparison of the who child growth standards and the cdc-2000 growth charts. J Nutrition 137: 144–148.
12. Bhagowalia P, Chen SE, Masters WA (2011) Effects and determinants of mild underweight among preschool children across countries and over time. Economics Human Biology 9: 66–77.
13. Victora CG, de Onis M, Hallal PC, Blössner M, Shrimpton R (2010) Worldwide timing of growth faltering: revisiting implications for interventions. Pediatrics 125: e473–e480.
14. Walker CLF, Rudan I, Liu L, Nair H, Theodoratou E, et al. (2013) Global burden of childhood pneumonia and diarrhoea. Lancet 381: 1405–1416.
15. Maleta K, Virtanen SM, Espo M, Kulmala T, Ashorn P (2003) Seasonality of growth and the relationship between weight and height gain in children under three years of age in rural malawi. Acta Paediatrics 92: 491–497.
16. Victora CG (1992) The association between wasting and stunting: An international perspective. J Nutrition 122: 1105–1110.
17. Van den Broeck JV, Eeckels R, Vuylsteke J (1993) Influence of nutritional status on child mortality in rural zaire. Lancet 341: 1491–1495.
18. Richard SA, Black RE, Gilman RH, Guerrant RL, Kang G, et al. (2012) Childhood infection malnutrition network: Wasting is associated with stunting in early childhood. J Nutrition 142: 1291–1296.
19. Dewey KG, Mayers DR (2011) Early child growth: How do nutrition and infection interact. Maternal Child Nutrition 7: 129–142.
20. Yoon PW, Black RE, Moulton LH, Becker S (1997) The effect of malnutrition on the risk of diarrheal and respiratory mortality in children less than 2 y of age in cebu, phillipines. Am J Clinical Nutrition 65: 1070–1077.
21. Caulfield LE, de Onis M, Blossner M, Black RE (2004) Undernutrition as an underlying cause of child deaths associated with diarrhea, pneumonia, malaria, and measles. Am J Clinical Nutrition 80: 193–198.
22. Adair LS, Fall CHD, Osmond C et al (2013) Associations of linear growth and relative weight gain during early life with adult health and human capital in countries of low and middle income: Findings from five birth cohort studies. Lancet 382: 525–534.
23. Schroeder DG, Martorell R, Rivera JA, Ruel MT, Habicht JP (1995) Age differences in the impact of nutritional supplementation on growth. The Journal of nutrition 125: 1051S–1059S.
24. Bhutta ZA, Ahmed T, Black RE, Cousens S, Dewey K, et al. (2008) What works? interventions for maternal and child undernutrition and survival. Lancet 371: 417–440.
25. Victora CG, Adair C L Fall, Hallal PC, Martorell R, Richter L, et al. (2008) Maternal and child undernutrition: Consequences for adult health and human capital. Lancet 371: 340–357.
26. Singhal A, Lucas A (2004) Early origins of cardiovascular disease: Is there a unifying hypothesis? Lancet 363: 1642–1645.
27. Singh AS, Kang G, Ramachandran A, Sarkar R, Peter P, et al. (2010) Locally made ready-to-use therapeutic food for treatment of malnutrition: A randomized control trial. Indian Pediatrics 47: 679–686.

5

Differential Activity of *Striga hermonthica* Seed Germination Stimulants and *Gigaspora rosea* Hyphal Branching Factors in Rice and Their Contribution to Underground Communication

Catarina Cardoso[1], Tatsiana Charnikhova[1], Muhammad Jamil[1¤a], Pierre-Marc Delaux[2,3¤b], Francel Verstappen[1,4], Maryam Amini[1¤c], Dominique Lauressergues[2,3], Carolien Ruyter-Spira[1,5], Harro Bouwmeester[1,4]*

1 Laboratory of Plant Physiology, Wageningen University, Wageningen, the Netherlands, **2** Laboratoire de Recherche en Sciences Végétales, Unité Mixte de Recherche (UMR) 5546, Université de Toulouse, Castanet-Tolosan, France, **3** Laboratoire de Recherche en Sciences Végétales, Unité Mixte de Recherche (UMR) 5546, Centre National de la Recherche Scientifique (CNRS), Castanet-Tolosan, France, **4** Centre for Biosystems Genomics, Wageningen, the Netherlands, **5** Bioscience, Plant Research International, Wageningen, the Netherlands

Abstract

Strigolactones (SLs) trigger germination of parasitic plant seeds and hyphal branching of symbiotic arbuscular mycorrhizal (AM) fungi. There is extensive structural variation in SLs and plants usually produce blends of different SLs. The structural variation among natural SLs has been shown to impact their biological activity as hyphal branching and parasitic plant seed germination stimulants. In this study, rice root exudates were fractioned by HPLC. The resulting fractions were analyzed by MRM-LC-MS to investigate the presence of SLs and tested using bioassays to assess their *Striga hermonthica* seed germination and *Gigaspora rosea* hyphal branching stimulatory activities. A substantial number of active fractions were revealed often with very different effect on seed germination and hyphal branching. Fractions containing (−)−orobanchol and *ent*-2′-*epi*-5-deoxystrigol contributed little to the induction of *S. hermonthica* seed germination but strongly stimulated AM fungal hyphal branching. Three SLs in one fraction, putative methoxy-5-deoxystrigol isomers, had moderate seed germination and hyphal branching inducing activity. Two fractions contained strong germination stimulants but displayed only modest hyphal branching activity. We provide evidence that these stimulants are likely SLs although no SL-representative masses could be detected using MRM-LC-MS. Our results show that seed germination and hyphal branching are induced to very different extents by the various SLs (or other stimulants) present in rice root exudates. We propose that the development of rice varieties with different SL composition is a promising strategy to reduce parasitic plant infestation while maintaining symbiosis with AM fungi.

Editor: Maarja Öpik, University of Tartu, Estonia

Funding: This work was financed by The Netherlands Organization for Scientific Research with VICI grant nr 865.06.002 and Equipment grant nr 834.08.001, attributed to HB, and co-financed by the Centre for Biosystems Genomics, a part of the Netherlands Genomics Initiative/Netherlands Organization for Scientific Research, attributed to HB. The funders had no role in study design, data collection and analysis, decision to publish, or preparation of the manuscript.

Competing Interests: The authors have declared that no competing interests exist.

* Email: harro.bouwmeester@wur.nl

¤a Current address: Department of Biosciences, COMSATS Institute of Information Technology, Islamabad, Pakistan
¤b Current address: Department of Agronomy, University of Wisconsin – Madison, Madison, Wisconsin, United States of America
¤c Current address: Syngenta Seeds B.V., Enkhuizen, the Netherlands

Introduction

Parasitic plants of the genus *Striga* are economically important species that parasitize the dicotyledonous cowpea, and cereal crops such as rice sorghum and maize [1]. In the most affected areas, parasitic plants constitute a major constraint to food production and efficient control methods are scant. *Striga* seeds will only germinate after exposure to host derived molecules, called germination stimulants that the parasite uses to detect host presence. The first phases of root parasitism occur underground and the presence of the parasite is difficult to diagnose until the emergence of its shoots. However, crop yield is already compromised at that stage making timely control of this pest even more difficult [2,3]. It is therefore important to develop control strategies that act before infection is initiated, for example by avoiding or reducing germination of the parasites' seeds. Strigolactones (SLs) are the best described class of germination stimulants and a reduction in the production of these compounds indeed resulted in reduced *Striga* infection [4–6]. However, SLs are also signaling compounds for the establishment of symbiosis with arbuscular mycorrhizal (AM) fungi and are plant hormones that modulate plant architecture [7–12] and therefore, non-discriminate reduction of their production would likely have negative side effects. The symbiotic AM fungi perceive SLs and respond with extensive pre-symbiotic hyphal branching, thus increasing the efficiency of root colonization. In this symbiotic interaction, the fungus takes up nutrients (especially phosphate and nitrogen) and water from the soil and supplies them to the plant in exchange for carbon assimilates [13]. Plants under phosphate starvation increase production and release of SLs into the rhizosphere to promote the symbiosis [14–16]. In soils contaminated with seeds of the parasitic plants, low phosphate availability results in increased levels of infestation by parasitic plants [4].

Adaptation responses to low phosphate such as reduced shoot branching and root system expansion are mediated by SLs [11,17,18]. SL biosynthetic mutants suffer, to some extent, from reduced symbiosis with AM fungi and exhibit altered plant shoot and root architecture which may negatively affect crop yields [9–11,19,20].

SLs are derived from all-*trans*-β-carotene that is isomerized into 9-*cis*-β-carotene by β-carotene isomerase D27 (DWARF27) followed by two consecutive cleavage steps by CAROTENOID CLEAVAGE DIOXYGENASE 7 (CCD7; HIGH TILLERING DWARF1 - HTD1/DWARF17 – 17 in rice) and CAROTENOID CLEAVAGE DIOXYGENASE 8 (CCD8; DWARF10 – D10 in rice) resulting in the production of carlactone [21]. The biosynthetic steps that convert carlactone to SL are not yet elucidated. SLs are a reasonably large class of natural compounds consisting of over 15 structural variants, most of which differ only by having one instead of two methyl groups on the cyclohexenyl A-ring or by having various combinations of hydroxyl or acetoxyl substituents on the A- and B-rings [22]. SLs occur in two distinct stereochemical configurations and the stereochemistry of some SLs was recently revised [23]. SLs from the orobanchol-like family have an *ent* oriented C-ring (Figure 1, structures **1–5** and **8c**). In the strigol-like family the C-ring has the opposite chirality of the orobanchol-like family (Figure 1, structures **6**;**7** and **8a**) [23]. Plants produce a mixture of SLs that differs between and sometimes even within species [16,24,25]. So far, only orobanchol-like SLs have been identified in rice: (−)−orobanchol (**1**), *ent*-2'-*epi*-5-deoxystrigol (**2**), orobanchyl acetate (**3**), 7-oxoorobanchyl acetate (**4**) [10,23]. In addition, three putative methoxy-5-deoxystrigol isomers (**5**) have been reported with unknown structure and stereochemistry [4].

Parasitic plant seeds and AM fungi have different sensitivities to different SL variants [26,27]. Interestingly, it was reported that orobanchol-like SLs (of the same type as found in rice exudates) are considerably less active at inducing *Striga hermonthica* seed germination [27]. Here, we extensively survey the chemical composition (SL content) and biological activity of rice root exudates to understand the relevance of the different SLs, and possible other signalling molecules, in the establishment of mycorrhizal symbiosis with the AM fungus, *Gigaspora rosea*, and infection by the parasitic plant, *Striga hermonthica*.

Materials and Methods

Strigolactone standards

The synthetic SL GR24 (**9a–d**) and (±)-strigol (**8a,d**, $R^1 = CH_3$; $R^2 = OH$) were kindly provided by Prof. Binne Zwanenburg (Radboud University Nijmegen, Netherlands); (−)−orobanchol (**1**) and (+)-*ent*-2'-*epi*-orobanchol (**6**), solanacol, orobanchyl acetate (**3**), 7-oxoorobanchyl acetate (**4**), 7-oxoorobanchol, and sorgomol (**7**) were provided by Prof. Koichi Yoneyama (Utsunomiya University, Japan); (±)-2'-*epi*-strigol (**8b,c**, $R^1 = CH_3$; $R^2 = OH$), (±)-2'-*epi*-5-deoxystrigol (**8b,c**, $R^1 = CH_3$; $R^2 = H$) and (±)-5-deoxystrigol (**8a,d**, $R^1 = CH_3$; $R^2 = H$) were a gift from Prof. Tadao Asami (University of Tokyo, Japan) (Structures **1** to **8a–d** represented in Figure 1).

Plant growth and root exudate collection

The exudates were collected from rice seedlings of the variety Nipponbare and the SL biosynthetic mutant line *d10-2* with Nipponbare background, kindly provided by Prof. Junko Kyozuka (University of Tokyo, Japan) [10]. The seeds were sown in pots of 14 cm diameter filled with quartz sand. The experiment was conducted with three pots per treatment. One pot containing 25 plants represents one replicate. Plants were watered every three days during the first week and every two days during the remaining weeks to full substrate saturation with half-strength modified Hoagland nutrient solution containing NH_4NO_3 (5.6 mM), K_2HPO_4 (0.4 mM), $MgSO_4$ (0.8 mM), $FeSO_4$ (0.18 mM), $CaCl_2$ (1.6 mM), K_2SO_4 (0.8 mM), $MnCl_2$ (0.0045 mM), $CuSO_4$ (0.0003 mM), $ZnCl_2$ (0.0015 mM), Na_2MoO_4 (0.0001 mM). After 3 weeks, phosphate starvation and phosphate starvation in combination with 0.01 μM fluridone – an inhibitor of carotenoid and therefore SL biosynthesis – were applied. Control plants were watered with the half-strength modified Hoagland nutrient solution described above. For the phosphate starvation treatment, KNO_3 (0.8 mM) was substituted for K_2HPO_4 to maintain the same the K^+ concentration. Residual phosphate was removed from the pots by applying 1 L of the concentration nutrient solution and draining the pots. Six days after the start of the treatments the treatment was repeated. Root exudates were collected 24 hours later by applying 1 L of the corresponding nutrient solution and collecting the flow through.

Sample preparation

The root exudates were concentrated using an SPE cartridge (GracePure™ SPE C18 – Max 500 mg) and eluted in 4 mL of 100% acetone. For HPLC, 250 μL of water was added to 1 mL of this acetone eluent after which the acetone was evaporated under a flow of N_2. The remaining 250 μL sample was injected into the HPLC and 1 min fractions (corresponding to 1 mL) were collected. The fractions were evaporated to dryness and dissolved in 200 μL water for further analysis. For MRM-LC-MS analysis, 50 μL of the C18 acetone eluent was diluted 3-fold in water and HPLC fractions were diluted 2-fold in water. For seed germination bioassays, C18 acetone eluents (crude exudates) were diluted 32-fold in water and HPLC fractions 5-fold. For the AM fungal hyphal branching bioassay the HPLC fractions of each replicate were pooled and tested in the same concentration as in the seed germination bioassay.

Fractionation of root exudates

Root exudates were fractioned by HPLC. The samples were injected into a XBridgeTM C18 column (4,6*150 mm from 5 μm, Waters) using a U6K injector (Waters). For the gradient model 510 pumps (Waters) were used. The mobile phase was water and the following gradient to acetonitrile used: 1 min 100% water, 2 min 27% acetonitrile, 15 min 45% acetonitrile, 24 min 80% acetonitrile and 24.2 min 100% acetonitrile which was maintained for 4 minutes to clean the column. The flow rate was 1 mL min^{-1} and the column temperature 25°C. Fractions of one minute were collected using a Biofrac fraction collector (Biorad).

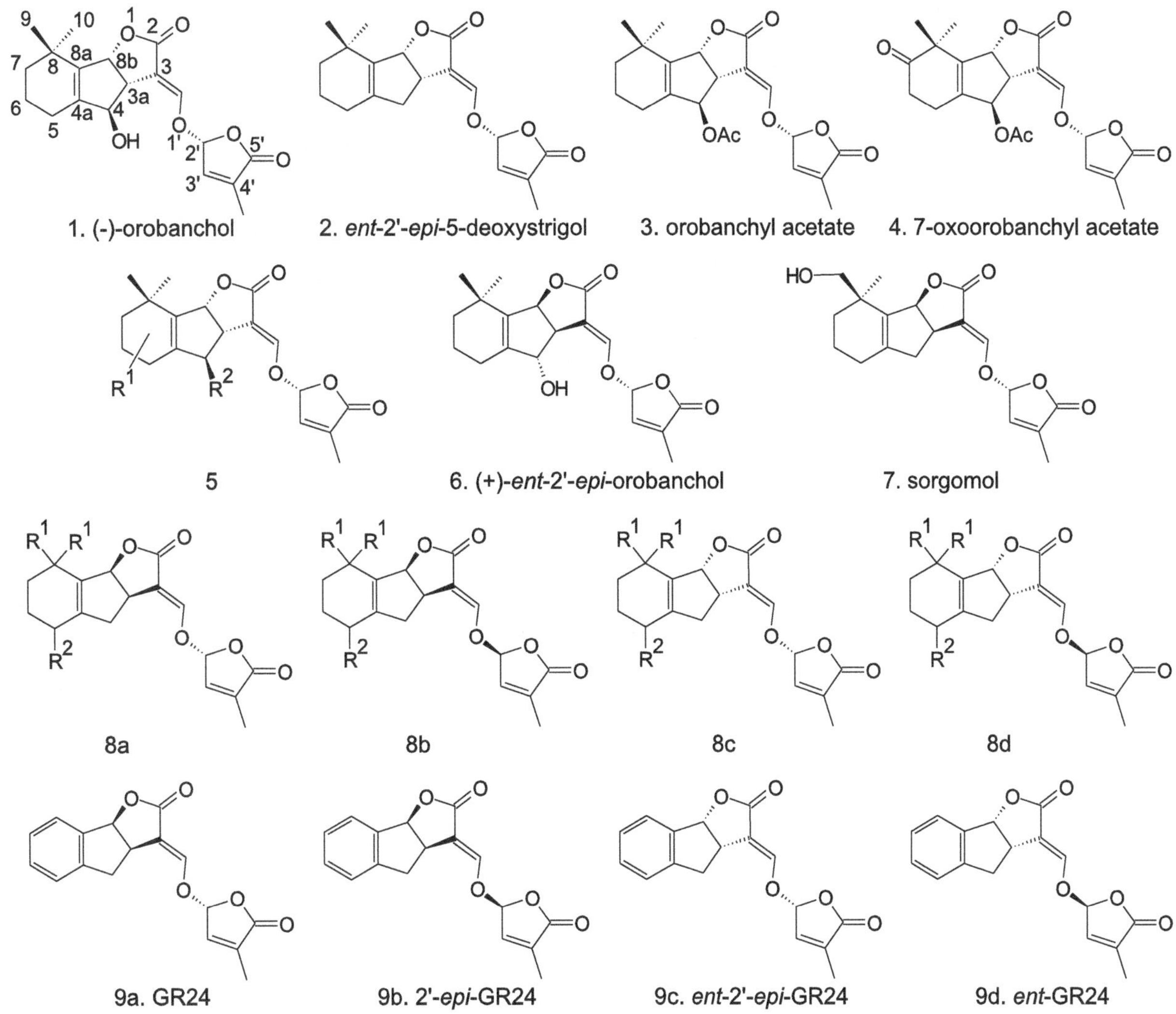

Figure 1. SL structures present in rice root exudates or tested in a seed germination or hyphal branching bioassay. (**1**) (−)-orobanchol; (**2**) *ent*-2′-*epi*-5-deoxystrigol; (**3**) orobanchyl acetate and (**4**) proposed structure of 7-oxoorobanchyl acetate [23]; (**5**) proposed structure of methoxy-5-deoxystrigol isomers (R^1 = OMe; R^2 = H) or the methyl ether of orobanchol (R^1 = H; R^2 = OMe); (**6**) (+)-*ent*-2′-*epi*-orobanchol; (**7**) sorgomol; (**8a–d**) stereoisomers of strigol ($R^1 = CH_3$; R^2 = OH); 5-deoxystrigol ($R^1 = CH_3$; R^2 = H), stereochemical configurations **8a** and **8c** are natural (strigol-type and orobanchol-type, respectively) while configurations **8b** and **8d** are not naturally occurring; (**9a–d**) stereoisomers of SL analogue GR24.

MRM-LC-MS analysis

For LC-MS analysis, samples were filtered through mini syringe filters (Minisart SRP4). The retention times, mass transitions and MS/MS spectra of available SL standards such as (+)-*ent*-2'-*epi*-orobanchol (**6**), (−)-orobanchol (**1**), (±)-5-deoxystrigol (**8a,d**, $R^1 = CH_3$; R^2 = H), (±)-2'-*epi*-5-deoxystrigol (**8b,c**, $R^1 = CH_3$; R^2 = H), (±)-sorgolactone, (±)-strigol (**8a,d**, $R^1 = CH_3$; R^2 = OH), solanacol, orobanchyl acetate (**3**), (±)-7-oxoorobanchol and (±)-7-oxoorobanchyl acetate (**4**) were compared with each sample to quantify SLs using ultra performance liquid chromatography coupled to tandem mass spectrometry (UPLC-MS/MS). Analyses were performed using a Waters Xevo tandem quadrupole (TQ) mass spectrometer equipped with an ESI source. Chromatographic separation was achieved on an Acquity UPLC BEH C18 column (150 × 2.1 mm, 1.7 µm) (Waters) by applying a water/acetonitrile gradient to the column, starting from 5% (v/v) acetonitrile for 2.0 min and rising to 50% (v/v) acetonitrile at 8.0 min, followed by a 1.0 min gradient to 90% (v/v) acetonitrile, which was maintained for 0.1 min before going back to 5% (v/v) acetonitrile using a 0.2 min gradient, prior to the next run. Finally, the column was equilibrated for 2.8 min, using this solvent composition. Operation temperature and flow-rate of the column were 50°C and 0.4 mL min^{-1}, respectively. Sample injection volume was 15 µL. The mass spectrometer was operated in positive electrospray ionization (ESI) mode. Cone and desolvation gas flows were set to 50 and 1000 L h^{-1}, respectively. The capillary voltage was set at 3.0 kV, the source temperature at 150°C and the desolvation temperature at 650°C. The cone voltage was optimized for each SL standard using the IntelliStart MS Console. Argon was used for fragmentation by MS/MS spectra in the collision cell.

The identification of SLs in rice root exudates and extracts was done using Multiple Reaction Monitoring (MRM) and by comparing retention times and MRM mass transitions with those of the available SL standards mentioned above. MRM transitions were optimized for each standard using the IntelliStart MS Console. The MRM transitions for putative 4-methoxy-5-deoxystrigol isomers were initially set based on the theoretically predicted fragmentation (see Results and Discussion section). MRM-transitions for the predicted putative SLs were incorporated in the MRM-method. The structures of all detected SLs were confirmed by MS/MS fragmentation spectra. Data acquisition and analysis were performed using MassLynx 4.1 software (Waters). Full mass scan and precursor ion scan for $m/z = 97$ were performed to search for unknown SLs in biologically active HPLC-fractions 15 to 19. The LC-MS results of the measurements of (−)-orobanchol (**1**) and *ent*-2'-*epi*-5-deoxystrigol (**2**) (of 3 biological replicates) were compared using ANOVA followed by pair wise comparisons with t-test (LSD values) in Genstat (Genstat for Windows 12th Edition; VSN International).

S. hermonthica seed germination bioassay

Seeds of *Striga hermonthica* used for the bioassay were kindly provided by Bob Vasey and originating from a sorghum field in Sudan, collected in 1995. The bioassays were performed as described [28]. The samples were tested in three technical replicates (three discs) and 3 biological replicates were tested, one independent bioassay per biological replicate. Given the binomial distribution nature of the measurements the mean values of the seed germination scores (3 replicates per treatment per fraction) were compared using a Chi-square test in Genstat (Genstat for Windows 12th Edition; VSN International).

AM fungal hyphal branching bioassay

For the AM branching bioassay spores of *Gigaspora rosea* (DAOM 194757) were used. The spores were routinely produced in pots containing leek and collected by wet sieving. They were washed in water/0.05% Tween 20 (v/v), soaked with 2% (w/v) Chloramine T (Sigma) for 10 min, washed again three times in sterile water for 30 s per wash, and stored in an antibiotic solution containing 100 mg L^{-1} gentamycin and 200 mg L^{-1} streptomycin. After 2 days at 4 °C, a second treatment with Chloramine T was carried out under the same conditions. They were then stored in the antibiotic solution at 4°C before use. Branching bioassays were carried out according to Buee *et al.* [29]. Four spores of *Gi. rosea* were germinated (in 2% CO_2 at 30 °C in dark) on M medium (Becard & Fortin, 1988) supplemented with 10 µM quercetin (Sigma) and solidified with 0.6% Phytagel (Sigma). Seven days after inoculation, each spore produced a single germ tube growing upwards. Two small wells on each half of the Petri dish, near the hyphal tip, were made in the gel with a Pasteur pipette tip and 5 µL of the test solution (SL analogue GR24 or purified fraction) or 10% acetonitrile (control) was injected in each well. After 24 h, hyphal branching was recorded by counting newly formed hyphal tips. Twenty to thirty spores were used for each treatment. Values of each tested fraction were compared with the corresponding control using the Student's t-test in Genstat (Genstat for Windows 12th Edition; VSN International).

Results

Rice root exudates were profiled to find compounds responsible for *S. hermonthica* seed germination and AM fungi hyphal branching. Plants were submitted to phosphate starvation with and without the application of 0.01 µM fluridone, an inhibitor of carotenoid and hence SL biosynthesis [28]. A reduction in seed germination stimulatory activity of root exudate fractions by fluridone treatment would suggest that the compound(s) responsible for the biological activity in that fraction is a (are) SL(s). The root exudates were fractioned by HPLC and the biological activity of the resulting fractions as well as the crude exudates (not fractioned) was assessed. Each of the three biological replicates was tested in independent seed germination bioassays of which one is shown in Figure 2 A, and the remaining are shown in Figure S1. Preliminary results showed that fractions eluting before 14 min (fractions 1 to 14) do not exhibit seed germination stimulatory activity (data not shown). Fractioned and crude exudates of control plants with sufficient phosphate showed almost no activity across all fractions. The seed germination stimulatory activity was significantly increased by phosphate starvation in crude exudates and in fractions 15–21, 23–25 and 28 ($P<0.05$ using X^2 test). This was observed consistently in all replicates (Figure 2 A and Figure S1). Fluridone treatment significantly reduced the activity of crude exudates and of fractions 15 to 19 and 24) with 99.9% confidence ($P<0.001$ using X^2 test) in all biological replicates. In fractions 20, 21, and 25 fluridone treatment also reduced the activity but the effect was not consistently significant; in two replicates these fractions showed significance at $P<0.001$ using the X^2 test, but not in the third replicate, likely because the germination stimulatory activity in these fractions was sometimes low. Also in fraction 28 that induces low germination activity the fluridone treatment did not significantly reduce seed germination. The effect of crude and fractioned root exudates on AM fungal hyphal branching was also assessed using *Gi. rosea* spores (Figure 2 B and C). Just as for *S. hermonthica* seed germination, phosphate starvation significantly increased branching stimulatory activity of crude exudates and most fractions (16–20, 24–25 and 27–28, at $P<0.005$, using Student t-test). Crude and fractioned exudates of control, non-phosphate starved plants did not show a significant difference in branching activity compared with the negative control, 10% acetonitrile. All the active fractions (of phosphate starvation treated rice) induced hyphal branching to a similar level. Interestingly, however, fraction 18 - the most active in the *S. hermonthica* seed germination bioassay - induced less AM fungal hyphal branching than the other active fractions (Figure 2 C).

To gain insight into the identity of the compounds responsible for the biological activity, MRM-LC-MS analysis was performed. The MRM chromatograms of crude exudates revealed an intense peak in the channels *m/z* 347>233, 347>205 and 347>97 at retention time 8.05 min, which matches with an authentic standard of (−)-orobanchol (**1**) (Figure 3 A and B). In the channels *m/z* 331>234 and 331>97 there was a peak at 12.51 min, which matches with *ent*-2'-*epi*-5-deoxystrigol (**2**) (Figure 3 C and B). MS/MS fragmentation spectra, and the addition of authentic orobanchol and (±)-2'-*epi*-5-deoxystrigol (**8b,c**, $R^1 = CH_3$; $R^2 = H$) to the samples, confirmed that the compounds detected were indeed orobanchol and *ent*-2'-*epi*-5-deoxystrigol. The same two SLs were barely detectable in exudates of control plants supplied with full nutrient solution, were most abundant in the phosphate starvation treatment and were both significantly reduced by fluridone treatment ($P<0.001$) (Figure 4 A). In addition to (−)−orobanchol (**1**) and *ent*–2'–*epi*–5–deoxystrigol (**2**) three unknown peaks were detected using the channels for 7-oxoorobanchol (*m/z* 361>247 and 361>97) at the retention times 9.9, 10.3 and 10.9 min (Figure 3 E and F), which is substantially later than 7-oxoorobanchol, which elutes at 3.7 min. The three unknown compounds (from here on referred to as methoxy-5-deoxystrigol isomers; see Discussion) were most abundant in the phosphate starvation treatment and were reduced by fluridone treatment (Figure 4 B - D) suggesting they are SL-like compounds.

MRM-LC-MS analysis was also performed on the HPLC fractions to try to correlate the presence of SLs with the seed germination and hyphal branching activity. (−)−orobanchol (**1**) was detected in fractions 19 to 21 with highest abundance in fraction 20 and *ent*-2'-*epi*-5-deoxystrigol (**2**) in fractions 27 and 28 with highest signal in fraction 28 (data not shown). The three

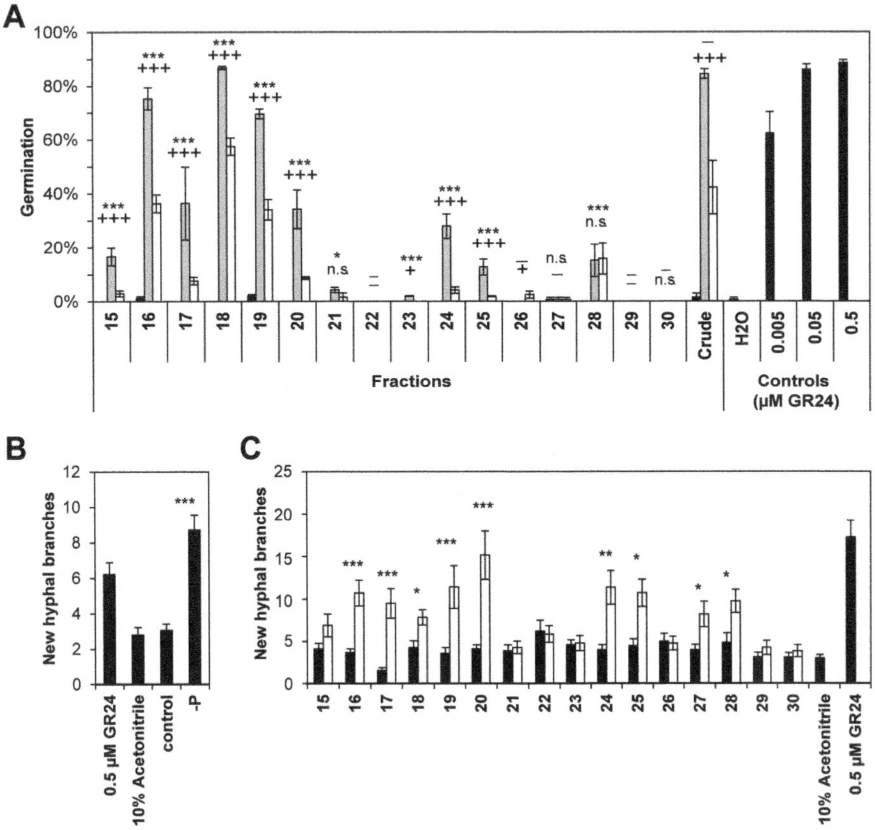

Figure 2. Activity profiles of rice root exudates. Germination of *S. hermonthica* (one biological replicate; the other two are shown in Figure S1) obtained with crude exudates and exudate fractions from rice plants (**A**) treated with full nutrition (black bars); phosphate starvation (grey bars) and phosphate starvation plus 0.01 μM fluridone (white bars). Water and SL analogue GR24 (0.005, 0.05 and 0.5 μM) were used as controls. The error bars represent the standard error of 3 technical replicates. Significance levels between treatments as determined using a X^2 test are indicated: */+ = $P<0.05$; **/++ = $P<0.01$; ***/+++ = $P<0.001$; n.s. = $P>0.05$; * = control vs. phosphate starvation treatment; + = phosphate starvation vs. phosphate starvation plus fluridone treatment. When germination values are close to zero the statistical test cannot be performed, which is indicated with "−". AM fungal hyphal branching induced by crude exudates (**B**) and exudate fractions (**C**) of rice treated with full nutrition (black bars) and phosphate starvation (white bars) in germinating *Gi. rosea* spores. The assay was performed with pooled samples of three biological replicates. GR24 (0.005, 0.05 and 0.5 μM) and 10% acetonitrile in water were used as controls. The bars represent the mean of the total number of new branches, the error bar the standard error of the mean (n = 20). Significance values comparing means between control treatments and phosphate starvation treatment are indicated above the bars. (* = $P<0.05$, ** = $P<0.01$, *** = $P<0.001$).

methoxy-5-deoxystrigol isomers detected in the channel for 7-oxoorobanchol (m/z 361> 247 and 361>97) at the retention times 9.95, 10.3 and 10.9 min eluted in fractions 23-25 with highest abundance in fraction 24 and are likely responsible for the seed germination stimulant/hyphal branching activity peak in fractions 24-25. The activity of the three compounds could not be evaluated individually as they did not separate on HPLC due to their highly similar retention time.

The fractions with highest seed germination inducing activity (16 and 18) were also analyzed using known MRM transitions typical for SLs as well as full mass scan and precursor ion scan for $m/z = 97$. However, we could not detect any masses that could be indicative for SLs and displayed an expected abundance pattern across the treatments similar as the known SLs: low in control, high in P starvation, low upon fluridone treatment.

To further investigate the nature of the active compounds in fractions 16, 18, 24 and 25, exudates of the SL biosynthetic mutant *d10-2* were studied [10]. HPLC fractions 16–25 collected from *d10-2* and its background Nipponbare were tested using the seed germination bioassay. All active fractions in the wild type had reduced activity in the mutant (Figure 5 A) supporting the SL (CCD8-dependent) nature of the compounds responsible for the biological activity of these fractions.

The MRM-LC-MS spectra of *d10-2* mutant root exudates confirmed that (−)-orobanchol (**1**) and *ent*-2'-*epi*-5-deoxystrigol (**2**) as well as the three methoxy-5-deoxystrigol isomers detected at 9.9, 10.35 and 10.95 were strongly decreased in *d10-2* mutant root exudates (Figure 5 B,C), further indicating that the latter three are SLs/require CCD8. Fractions 16 and 18 of *d10-2* exudates were also analyzed by LC-MS and compared with those from wild type plants using full-scan mass spectrometry, but no differential masses were found that could explain the seed germination activity in the wild type and give a hint on the identity of the seed germination stimulant(s) in these fractions.

The activity profiles obtained with the exudate fractions, when tested with the seed germination and hyphal branching are different. Some fractions that stimulate high seed germination percentages induce low fungal response and the contrary is also observed. To further investigate the differences in activity observed in our bioassays, we performed a seed germination bioassay using pure or racemic mixtures of SLs (Table 1). We observed that sorgomol (**7**) is the most active of the tested SLs

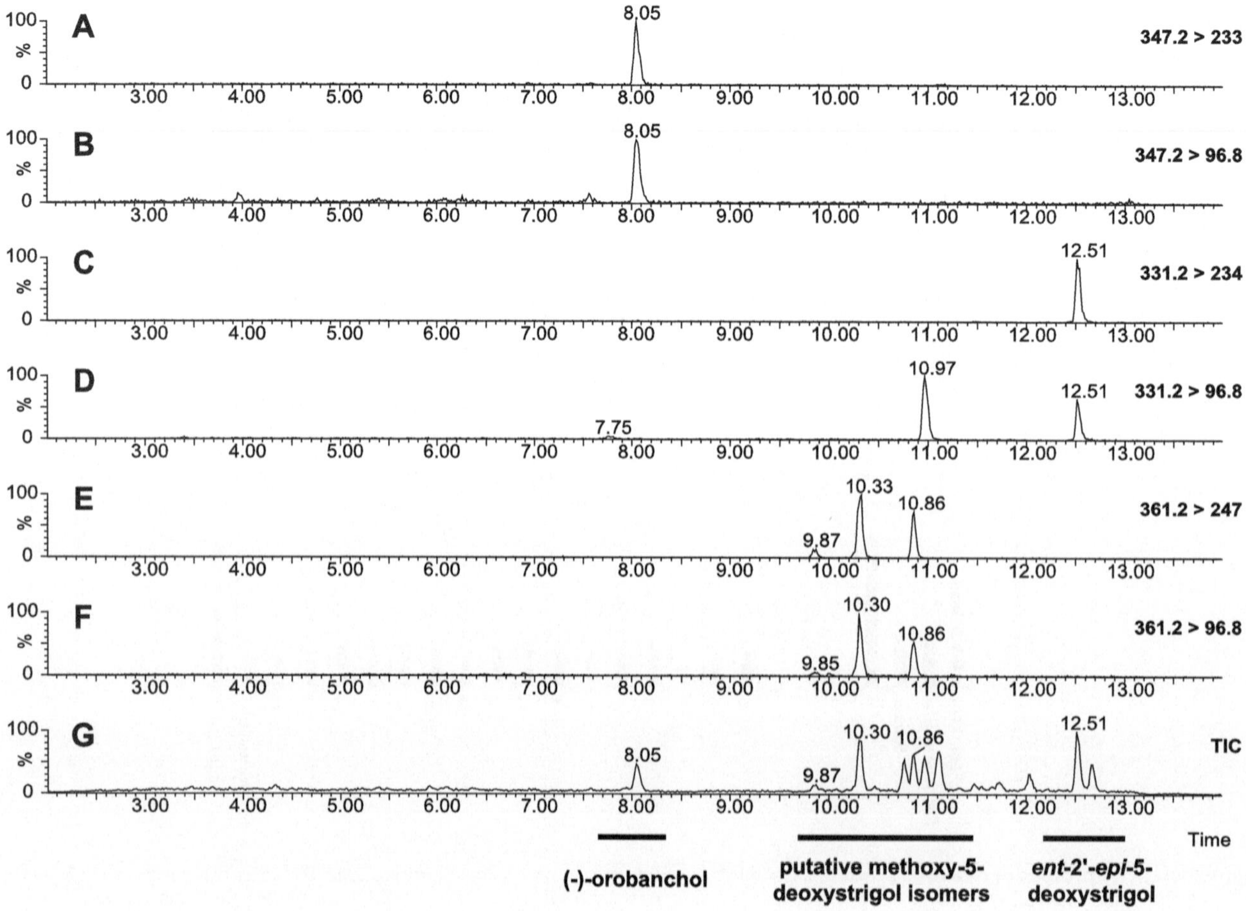

Figure 3. SL analysis of rice root exudates. Root exudates from rice plants grown under phosphate starvation were analyzed with liquid chromatography coupled with tandem mass spectrometry (LC-MS/MS) using multiple reaction monitoring (MRM). Chromatograms of (**A**) transitions 347.2 > 233 and (**B**) 347.2>96.8 for orobanchol; (**C**) transitions 331.2> 234 and (**D**) 331.2>96.8 for 2'-*epi*-5-deoxystrigol; (**E**) transitions 361.2>247 and (**F**) 361.2>96.8 for three putative methoxy-5-deoxystrigol isomers; (**G**) the total ion count (TIC) showing of all measured transitions and where orobanchol (8.05 min), *ent*-2'-*epi*-5-deoxystrigol (12.51 min) and the three putative methoxy-5-deoxystrigol isomers (9.87; 10.33; 10.86 min) are visible.

inducing 36% seed germination at 200 nM and 26% seed germination at 20 nM followed by (+)-*ent*-2'-epi-orobanchol (**6**, 34% seed germination at 200 nM and 8.7% at 20 nM). The racemates of (±)-strigol (**8a,d**, $R^1=CH_3$; $R^2=OH$); (±)-5-deoxystrigol (**8a,d**, $R^1=CH_3$; $R^2=H$) and the racemic mixture of all 4 stereoisomers of GR24 (**9a–d**) have intermediate activity inducing 9.3%, 6.0% and 2.0% seed germination at 20 nM and inducing 19%, 26% and 25% seed germination at 200 nM, respectively. The racemate of (±)-2'-*epi*-5-deoxystrigol (**8b,c**, $R^1=CH_3$; $R^2=H$) induced less seed germination (11 % at 200 nM) and was not active at 20 nM. The least active SLs were (−)-orobanchol (**1**) and the racemate of (±)-2'-*epi*-strigol (**8b,c**, $R^1=CH_3$; $R^2=OH$) that induced less than 1% seed germination in both concentrations. Table 1 also summarises data from a study by Akiyama et al. that analysed the *Gigaspora margarita* hyphal branching activity of a range of different SLs [26]. In contrast to what is observed with *S. hermonthica*, both orobanchol (**1**) and *ent*-2'-*epi*-5-deoxystrigol (**2**) are highly active at inducing hyphal branching and their activity is similar to their natural stereoisomers. Strigol (**8a**, $R^1=CH_3$; $R^2=OH$), sorgomol (**7**), GR24 (**9a**) and (±)-2'-*epi*-strigol (**8b,c**, $R^1=CH_3$; $R^2=OH$) were considerable less active (100 fold) than orobanchol (**1**), and the remaining GR24 stereoisomers (**9b–d**) were 10000- to 1000-fold less active than GR24 (**9a**).

Discussion

Rice root exudates were fractioned to evaluate the contribution of SLs and potentially other signalling molecules to the *S. hermonthica* seed germination stimulant and AMF hyphal branching activity of rice root exudate. MRM–LC–MS analysis of these HPLC fractioned rice root exudates showed the presence of (−)−orobanchol (**1**) in fractions 19, 20 and 21 and *ent*-2'-*epi*-5-deoxystrigol (**2**) in fraction 28 suggesting that these SLs are responsible for the seed germination and hyphal branching stimulatory activities of these fractions. These results confirm the presence of SLs found previously in root exudates of the rice variety Nipponbare except for orobanchyl acetate (**3**) that was not detected in the present study but is reported by others [23]. A fourth SL -7-oxoorobanchyl acetate (**4**) – was also reported to be produced in Nipponbare between days 10 to 17 after germination [23]. In the present study the exudates were collected at a later stage and this SL was not detected.

The relative abundance of (−)−orobanchol (**1**) and *ent*-2'-*epi*-5-deoxystrigol (**2**), measured by MRM-LC-MS across the different

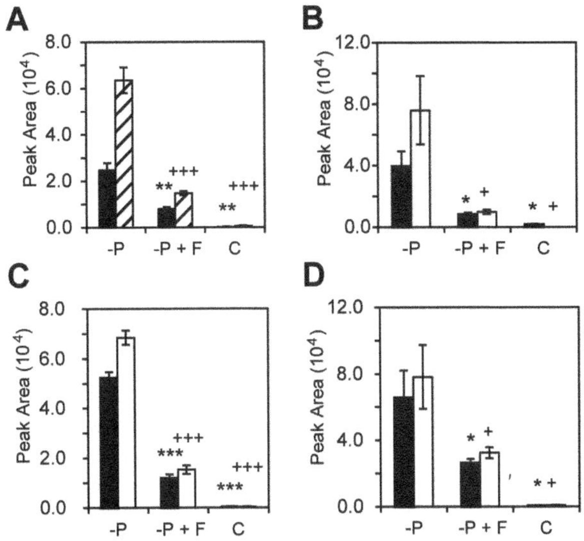

Figure 4. Abundance of (−)−orobanchol, *ent*-2'-*epi*-5-deoxystrigol and putative SL-like compounds in phosphate starvation and fluridone treatments. Peak areas obtained with liquid chromatography coupled with tandem mass spectrometry (LC-MS/MS) analysis using multiple reaction monitoring (MRM) of root exudates of rice. **(A)** (−)−orobanchol (MRM transition 347.2 >96.8; black bars) and *ent*-2'-*epi*-5-deoxystrigol (MRM transition 331.2>234; hatched bars); **(B–D)** three putative SL-like compounds measured in crude exudates with the retention times: rt = 9.87 **(B)**; rt = 10.3 and **(C)** rt = 10.9 **(D)** and the MRM transitions 361>96.8 (black bars) and 361>247 (white bars). All measurements taken from crude exudates of plants grown in different treatments: phosphate starvation (−P); phosphate starvation combined with fluridone (−P+F) and control treatment with full nutrient supply (C). The error bars represent the standard error of 3 biological replicates. Significance values are indicated with * (for *ent*-2'-*epi*-orobanchol and for 361>96.8 transition) and + (for 2'-*epi*-5-deoxystrigol and for 331.2>234 transition) and compare phosphate starvation (-P) treatment vs. phosphate starvation with fluridone (-P+F) and -P vs. full nutrition (C) (*/+ = $P<0.05$, **/++ = $P<0.01$, ***/+++ = $P<0.001$).

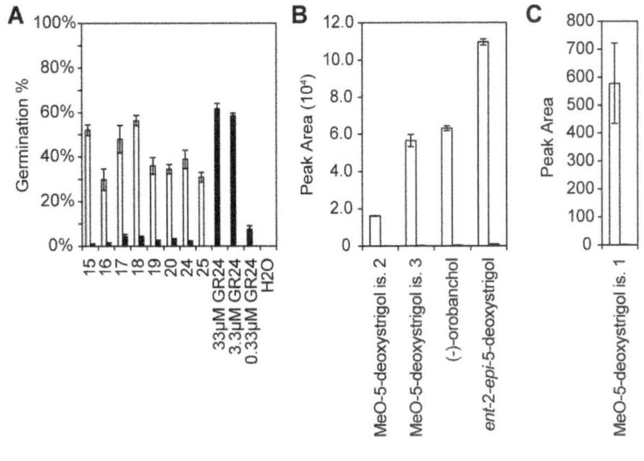

Figure 5. Characterization of rice mutant *d10* exudate. Germination assay with *S. hermonthica* seeds on exudate fractions of full nutrition (black bars) and phosphate starvation (white bars) treated plants **(A)**. Water and GR24 (0.33, 3.3 and 33 µM) were used as controls. Peak areas of *ent*-2'-*epi*-5-deoxystrigol, (−)−orobanchol and putative methoxy-5-deoxystrigol isomers 2 and 3 **(B)** and putative methoxy-5-deoxystrigol isomer 1 **(C)** obtained with liquid chromatography coupled with tandem mass spectrometry (LC-MS/MS) analysis using multiple reaction monitoring (MRM) of root exudates of *d10-2* (black bars) and WT (white bars) under phosphate starvation treatment.

treatments matches the seed germination stimulatory activity of the fractions where these SLs elute (19–20 and 28 respectively). Phosphate starvation induced the highest production of (−)−orobanchol (**1**) and *ent*-2'-*epi*-5-deoxystrigol (**2**) which resulted in the highest germination of *Striga* seeds. Fluridone application inhibited the biosynthesis of these SLs which resulted in a lower biological activity of the fractions and crude exudates, confirming the inhibitory effect of fluridone on SL production that was previously described [28]. MRM-LC-MS analysis of fractions 24–25 revealed the presence of three compounds with the same mass *m/z* 361 showing up in the 361.2>247 and 361.2>96.8 MRM channels. These metabolites were most abundant in exudates of phosphate starved plants and were reduced by fluridone application. The seed germination activity obtained with fractions 24 and 25 correlates with the abundance of the detected masses. MS/MS analysis of the compounds eluting in fractions 24 and 25 shows fragmentation patterns typical for SLs [30]: loss of the D-ring and H_2O yields fragment ions $[M+H - \text{D-ring} - H_2O]^+$ with m/z = 247 and the fragment ion of the D-ring itself $C_5H_5O_2$ with m/z = 97 (Figure 6). The loss of methanol $[M+H - MeOH]^+$, yielding the fragment ion m/z = 329, is not typical for the fragmentation of known SLs and could indicate the presence of a methoxy-group in the molecule (Figure 6). This feature could explain the late retention time of these putative SLs compared with orobanchol (Figure 3 G) and other known SLs given that methyl ethers are less polar than alcohols (Figure 3 E and G). The MS/MS fragmentation spectra of all three compounds are very similar (Figure 6). Based on these data we suggest that the compounds eluting at 9.5, 10.3 and 10.9 are methoxy-5-deoxystrigol isomers (**5**). Isolation followed by NMR or chemical synthesis should give the final proof of the structure of these three isomers. As we do not have this proof as yet, we will refer to these new compounds under the combined name methoxy-5-deoxystrigol isomers [4]. The absence of the putative methoxy-5-deoxystrigol isomers in *d10-2* exudate further supports that these compounds are produced from the SL pathway (Figure 5 B and C).

Fractions 16 and 18 induced the highest level of *S. hermonthica* germination (Figure 2 and Figure S1) and do not contain any of the SLs discussed above. As mentioned above, two other SLs, orobanchyl acetate (**3**) and 7-oxoorobanchyl acetate (**4**), were recently reported in rice [23]. Orobanchyl acetate (**3**) elutes after (−)-orobanchol (**1**) and is unlikely to be responsible for the activity in fractions 16 and 18. 7-Oxoorobanchyl acetate (**4**) elutes before (−)−orobanchol (**1**) and could be present in fraction 16 to 18. This SL was previously detected in exudates collected 10 to 17 days after germination [23]. In the present study, exudates were collected in later stages and this SL was not detected in crude exudates nor in any of the fractions. We could also not detect any other known SLs in fractions 16 to 18; however the seed germination bioassays showed that the activity of fractions 16 and 18 followed the same trend across the treatments as the activity of SL containing fractions. They were increased by phosphate starvation and reduced by fluridone application (Figure 2 A). The seed germination stimulatory activity of these fractions in *d10-2* root exudate was also clearly reduced (Figure 5 A). All this strongly suggests that the activity in these fractions is caused by compounds derived from the SL pathway after carlactone (as CCD8 is required for their production). Considering their high activity in the induction of *S. hermonthica* germination it is of great interest to identify these compounds.

Overall, the activity profiles for *S. hermonthica* seed germination and AM fungal hyphal branching are similar but not the same (Figure 2). All active fractions in the seed germination bioassay

Table 1. *Striga hermonthica* germination and *Gigaspora margarita* hyphal branching in the presence of SL standards.

	S. hermonthica **germination (%)**		*Gi. margarita* **hyphal branching**[1]
	200 nM	**20 nM**	**MEC**[2] **in pg per disc**
(±)-2′-*epi*-strigol	0.00 ± 0.00	0.00 ± 0.00	100
(−)−orobanchol[3]	0.67 ± 0.67	0.00 ± 0.00	1
ent-2′-*epi*-5-deoxystrigol	–	–	3
2′-*epi*-5-deoxystrigol	–	–	30
(±)-2′-*epi*-5-deoxystrigol	11.33 ± 1.76	0.00 ± 0.00	–
GR24	–	–	100
ent-GR24	–	–	10000
2′-epi-GR24	–	–	1000
ent-2′-epi-GR24	–	–	1000
GR24 (4 stereoisomers)	25.33 ± 1.76	2.00 ± 1.15	
ent-5-deoxystrigol	–	–	30
5-deoxystrigol	–	–	3
(±)-5-deoxystrigol	26.00 ± 9.87	6.00 ± 3.05	–
(±)-strigol	19.33 ± 8.82	9.33 ± 4.67	100
Ent-2′-*epi*-orobanchol[4]	34.00 ± 1.15	8.67 ± 2.40	1
sorgomol	36.00 ± 3.05	26.00 ± 5.03	100

[1]Results extracted from Akiyama et al. [26]; [2] MEC = minimum effective concentration; [3] in Akiyama et al. [26] these compounds are named (+)−orobanchol and (+)-2′-*epi*-orobanchol respectively, before revision of stereochemical structure whereas the present table indicates the revised stereochemistry [23].

exhibited hyphal branching stimulatory activity albeit to a different extent. Fraction 20 [(−)−orobanchol (**1**)] induced high AM fungal hyphal branching but stimulated little germination of *S. hermonthica* seeds compared with other fractions. Also, *ent*-2'-*epi*-5-deoxystrigol (**2**, fraction 28; low seed germination), the methoxy-5-deoxystrigol isomers (fractions 24–25; low seed germination) and fraction 16 and 18 (high seed germination) have very different activity with regard to the induction of seed germination whereas being quite similar in the induction of hyphal branching. Fraction 27 did not display seed germination stimulatory activity, but it did induce hyphal branching. This is probably due to the presence of *ent*-2'-*epi*-5-deoxystrigol (**2**) that is still detected in this fraction but at lower concentration than in fraction 28. Hence the concentration of *ent*-2'-*epi*-5-deoxystrigol (**2**) in fraction 27 may not be sufficient to induce *S. hermonthica* seed germination but is apparently high enough to induce AM fungal hyphal branching.

The separation on HPLC is not good enough to separate all the active compounds. This results in tailing peaks for example for (−)−orobanchol (**1**), present in fractions 19 to 21 and with highest abundance in fraction 20. Fraction 19 induces response of both *S. hermonthica* seeds and AM fungi to an extent that is intermediate to fractions 18 and 20. The activity in fraction 19 is probably a result from the cumulative effect of (−)−orobanchol (**1**) and the tail of the unknown active compound eluting mostly in fraction 18. Similarly, the activity observed in fraction 17 might also be due to fronting of fraction 18 and tailing of fraction 16. However, we cannot exclude the presence of other active compounds in fractions 17 and 19.

The two activity profiles show that some of the most active mycorrhizal hyphal branching stimulants present in rice root exudates play only a minor role in the induction of *S. hermonthica* germination. The seed germination stimulatory activity of known concentrations of SLs was assessed and compared with results of a study relating structural differences in SLs to AM fungal hyphal branching stimulatory activity [26] (Table 1). The structure of (−)−orobanchol (**1**) and (+)-*ent*-2'-*epi*-orobanchol (**6**) have been revised after the study by Akiyama et al. [26] hence, these compounds were originally labeled (+)−orobanchol and (+)-2'-*epi*-orobanchol respectively [23,26,31]. As previously shown by Nomura et al. [27] sensitivity of *S. hermonthica* seeds is highly dependent on the orientation of the C-ring, and is more sensitive to the strigol–type configuration. In our bioassays this preference is confirmed, the highest seed germination was obtained with sorgomol (**7**) and (+)-*ent*-2'-epi-orobanchol (**6**) while (−)−orobanchol (**1**) hardly induced any seed germination (Table 1).

AM fungi also have different sensitivity to different SL structures [26]. The strigol–type configuration is sometimes more active, as was observed for GR24 (**9a**) but not always [26]. For instance, all strigol stereoisomers (**8a–d**, $R^1 = CH_3$; $R^2 = OH$) have equal activity just as (−)−orobanchol (**1**) and (+)-*ent*-2'-epi-orobanchol (**6**) (Table 1) [26]. Also the two natural stereoisomers of 5-deoxystrigol (**8a** and **8c**, $R^1 = CH_3$; $R^2 = H$) have each the same activity at inducing hyphal branching (Table 1) [26]. Indeed, the activity of SLs to stimulate hyphal branching seems to be more influenced by modifications in rings A and B than by stereochemical variation [26,32]. In our hyphal branching assay with a different AM species, *Gi. margarita*, we obtained a similar response to the different SLs as reported for *Gi. rosea* [26]. Fraction 20, where (−)−orobanchol (**1**) elutes, displays high activity in the branching bioassay whereas there is no clear activity peak in the seed germination bioassay (Figure 2). Similarly, *ent*-2'-*epi*-5-deoxystrigol (**2**) detected in fractions 27 and 28 induced hyphal branching and only fraction 28 with highest amounts of this SL induced low seed germination (Figure 2). SL activity is also affected by different chemical and structural properties that influence diffusion and stability [26,33]. However compared to other SLs, (−)−orobanchol (**1**) and *ent*-2'-*epi*-5-deoxystrigol (**2**) are highly active at stimulating hyphal branching. Therefore, the low activity of (−)−orobanchol (**1**) and *ent*-2'-*epi*-5-deoxystrigol (**2**) at inducing seed germination does not seem to be a result of

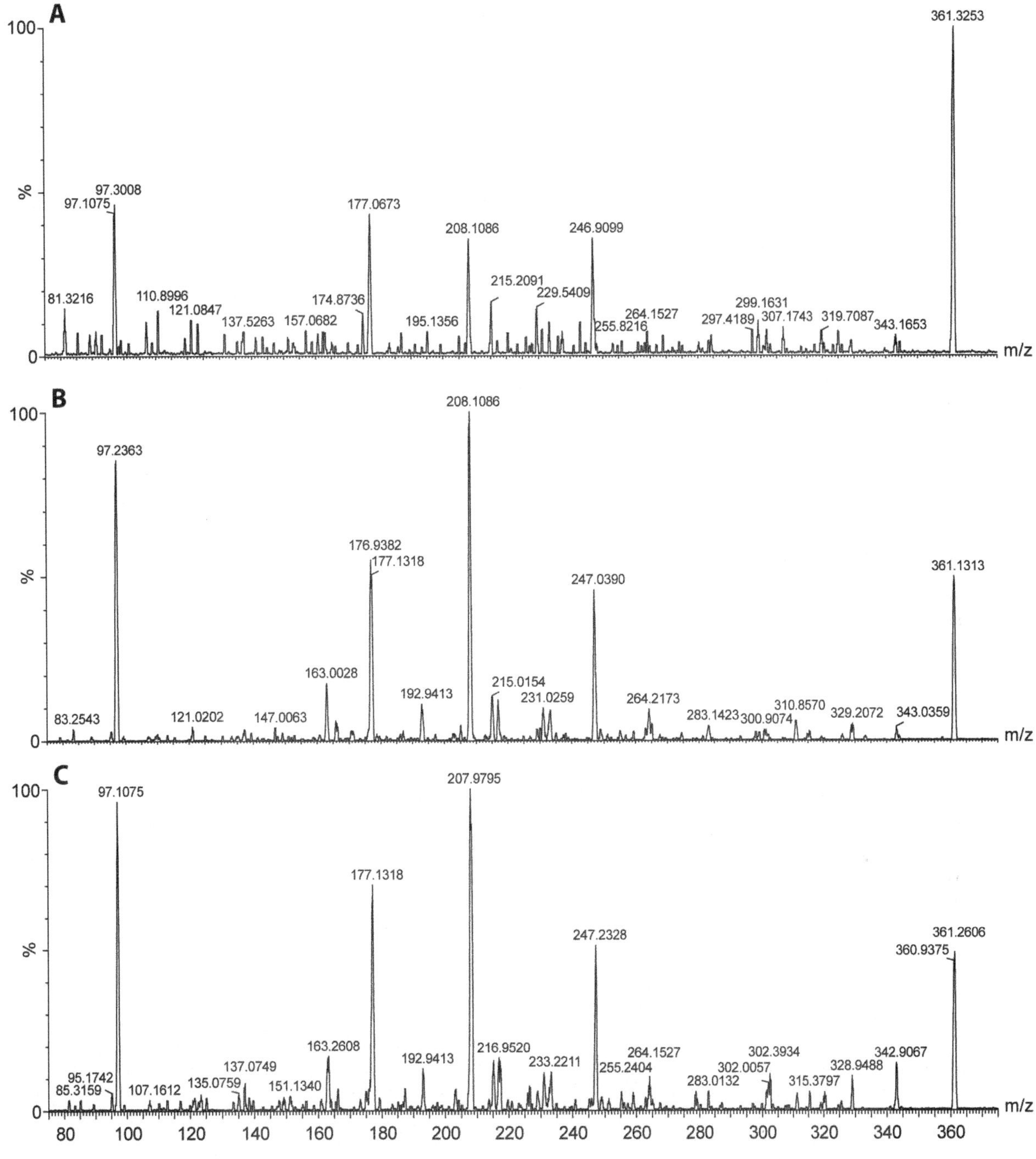

Figure 6. MS/MS spectra of putative SL-like compounds. The spectra were measured at the retention time of each isomer: 9.87 min (**A**), 10.35 min (**B**) and 10.95 min (**C**).

instability or poor diffusion of these two SLs but rather a result of lower sensitivity of the seeds to these compounds.

Our bioassays suggest that strong hyphal branching stimulators make little contribution to the overall stimulation of parasitic seed germination. Moreover, the fractions showing the largest effect on seed germination (fractions 16 and 18) contain stimulants of unknown structure. The reduction of activity in these fractions by fluridone and by mutation in *D10 (CCD8)* suggests that they are SL-like. The strong differences in activity across the exudate fractions suggest that *S. hermonthica* infection and potentially also the infection by other parasitic plant species could be reduced by altering the qualitative composition of SLs rather than just quantitatively reducing their production. New varieties with such altered SL composition could maintain their ability to establish symbiosis with AM fungi while at the same time they induce less *Striga* seed germination. In a recent study, 20 rice cultivars were screened for the abundance of SLs in their root exudates [6]. The authors observed that the relative amounts of (−)−orobanchol (**1**) and *ent*-2'-*epi*-5-deoxystrigol (**2**) differ across cultivars, suggesting that selection for different SL composition is possible.

ent-2'-*epi*-5-Deoxystrigol (**2**) and 5-deoxystrigol (**8a**, $R^1 = CH_3$; $R^2 = H$) have the most simple structure of all SLs so far identified in plants. They have been suggested to be produced from carlactone through the action of MAX1 [and possibly additional enzyme(s)] [21,34] which would imply that the orientation of the C-ring, a structural feature of major importance for the induction of seed germination as well as hyphal branching, is determined by MAX1. We propose that *ent*-2'-*epi*-5-deoxystrigol (**2**) is the precursor for the remaining rice SLs. Further supporting this hypothesis, it has been recently shown that a sorghum enzyme(s) - likely a cytochrome P450 - converts *ent*-2'-*epi*-5-deoxystrigol (**1**) and 5-deoxystrigol (**8a**, $R^1 = CH_3$; $R^2 = H$) into *ent*-2'-*epi*-sorgomol and sorgomol respectively [35]. Breeding for a different SL composition would be greatly aided by the characterization of these later steps in SL biosynthesis, that is the decoration of the SLs' core-structure.

As a word of caution, the sensitivity to specific SLs may vary between *Striga* species and/or races [36]. Therefore, assessment of the seed germination and hyphal branching requirements for the host/parasite and host/AM combination present in a certain region would be necessary in order to direct the development of new, locally adapted, cultivars that are less affected by *Striga* parasitism but still efficient in AM symbiosis establishment. A study performed in sorghum has shown that host plants are especially vulnerable to plant parasitism in the early stages of their life cycle [37]. Since SL composition in rice exudates changes according to the age of the plants [23] efforts to produce new rice varieties should take into consideration SL variation throughout the life cycle.

Finally, we can only speculate about the driving forces for the diversification in SL structures that we see in rice. Unlike for the gibberellins, it seems that there are not just one or two active molecules accompanied by inactive precursors and degradation products. In their role as rhizosphere signaling molecules the different SLs all display activity, albeit admittedly with different efficiency. With regard to their endogenous function, as plant hormones regulating a suit of developmental processes, we only just begin to understand the structure-activity relationships [38]. As a result of all these different functions the consequences of evolutionary and human (breeding) selection pressures are complex – which is reflected in the large structural diversification - and the resulting structural diversification so far difficult to explain.

Supporting Information

Figure S1 Activity profiles of rice root exudates tested with *S. hermonthica* seed germination assay. Two biological replicates are shown here and the third replicate is shown in Figure 2 A. Crude exudates and exudate fractions from rice plants treated with full nutrition (black bars); phosphate starvation (grey bars) and phosphate starvation plus 0.01 μM fluridone (white bars). Water and SL analogue GR24 (0.005, 0.05 and 0.5 μM) were used as controls. The error bars represent the standard error of 3 technical replicates. Significance levels between treatments as determined using a X^2 test are indicated: */+ = $P<$ 0.05; **/++ = $P<0.01$; ***/+++ = $P<0.001$; n.s. = $P>0.05$; * = control vs. phosphate starvation treatment; + = phosphate starvation vs. phosphate starvation plus fluridone treatment. When germination values are close to zero the statistical test cannot be performed, which is indicated with "–".
(TIF)

Acknowledgments

We would like to thank, Bob Vasey for providing *S. hermonthica* seeds, Prof. Binne Zwanenburg, Prof. Koichi Yoneyama, Prof. Tadao Asami and Prof. Guillaume Bécard for providing SL standards. We also thank Jacques Withagen for helping with the statistical analysis.

Author Contributions

Conceived and designed the experiments: CC TC PMD CRS HB. Performed the experiments: CC TC MJ FV MA PMD DL. Analyzed the data: CC TC MJ PMD CRS HB. Contributed reagents/materials/analysis tools: CC TC FV PMD DL. Contributed to the writing of the manuscript: CC TC CRS HB.

References

1. Parker C (2009) Observations on the current status of *Orobanche* and *Striga* problems worldwide. Pest Manag Sci 65: 453–459. doi:10.1002/ps.1713
2. Cardoso C, Ruyter-Spira C, Bouwmeester HJ (2011) Strigolactones and root infestation by plant-parasitic *Striga*, *Orobanche* and *Phelipanche* spp. Plant Science 180: 414–420. doi:10.1016/j.plantsci.2010.11.007
3. Scholes JD, Press MC (2008) Striga infestation of cereal crops – an unsolved problem in resource limited agriculture. Current Opinion in Plant Biology 11: 180–186. doi:10.1016/j.pbi.2008.02.004
4. Jamil M, Charnikhova T, Cardoso C, Jamil T, Ueno K, et al. (2011) Quantification of the relationship between strigolactones and *Striga hermonthica* infection in rice under varying levels of nitrogen and phosphorus. Weed Research 51: 373–385. doi:10.1111/j.1365-3180.2011.00847.x
5. Jamil M, Rodenburg J, Charnikhova T, Bouwmeester HJ (2011) Pre-attachment *Striga hermonthica* resistance of new rice for Africa (NERICA) cultivars based on low strigolactone production. New Phytol 192: 964–975. doi:10.1111/j.1469-8137.2011.03850.x
6. Jamil M, Charnikhova T, Houshyani B, Ast A, Bouwmeester HJ (2012) Genetic variation in strigolactone production and tillering in rice and its effect on *Striga hermonthica* infection. Planta 235: 473–484. doi:10.1007/s00425-011-1520-y
7. Akiyama K, Matsuzaki K, Hayashi H (2005) Plant sesquiterpenes induce hyphal branching in arbuscular mycorrhizal fungi. Nature 435: 824–827. doi:10.1038/nature03608
8. Besserer A, Puech-Pagès V, Kiefer P, Gomez-Roldan V, Jauneau A, et al. (2006) Strigolactones stimulate arbuscular mycorrhizal fungi by activating mitochondria. PLoS Biology 4: e226. doi:10.1371/journal.pbio.0040226
9. Gomez-Roldan V, Fermas S, Brewer PB, Puech-Pagès V, Dun EA, et al. (2008) Strigolactone inhibition of shoot branching. Nature 455: 189–194. doi:10.1038/nature07271
10. Umehara M, Hanada A, Yoshida S, Akiyama K, Arite T, et al. (2008) Inhibition of shoot branching by new terpenoid plant hormones. Nature 455: 195–200. doi:10.1038/nature07272
11. Ruyter-Spira C, Kohlen W, Charnikhova T, van Zeijl A, van Bezouwen L, et al. (2011) Physiological effects of the synthetic strigolactone analog GR24 on root system architecture in *Arabidopsis*: another belowground role for strigolactones?Plant Physiology155721734 . doi:10.1104/pp.110.166645
12. Kapulnik Y, Delaux P-M, Resnick N, Mayzlish-Gati E, Wininger S, et al. (2011) Strigolactones affect lateral root formation and root-hair elongation in *Arabidopsis*. Planta 233: 209–216. doi:10.1007/s00425-010-1310-y
13. Nadal M, Paszkowski U (2013) Polyphony in the rhizosphere: presymbiotic communication in arbuscular mycorrhizal symbiosis. Current Opinion in Plant Biology 16: 473–479. doi:10.1016/j.pbi.2013.06.005
14. Yoneyama K, Xie X, Kusumoto D, Sekimoto H, Sugimoto Y, et al. (2007) Nitrogen deficiency as well as phosphorus deficiency in sorghum promotes the production and exudation of 5-deoxystrigol, the host recognition signal for arbuscular mycorrhizal fungi and root parasites. Planta 227: 125–132. doi:10.1007/s00425-007-0600-5
15. Yoneyama K, Yoneyama K, Takeuchi Y, Sekimoto H (2007) Phosphorus deficiency in red clover promotes exudation of orobanchol, the signal for mycorrhizal symbionts and germination stimulant for root parasites. Planta 225: 1031–1038. doi:10.1007/s00425-006-0410-1
16. López-Ráez JA, Charnikhova T, Gómez-Roldán V, Matusova R, Kohlen W, et al. (2008) Tomato strigolactones are derived from carotenoids and their biosynthesis is promoted by phosphate starvation. New Phytol 178: 863–874. doi:10.1111/j.1469-8137.2008.02406.x
17. Umehara M, Hanada A, Magome H, Takeda-Kamiya N, Yamaguchi S (2010) Contribution of strigolactones to the inhibition of tiller bud outgrowth under phosphate deficiency in rice. Plant and Cell Physiology 51: 1118–1126. doi:10.1093/pcp/pcq084
18. Kohlen W, Charnikhova T, Liu Q, Bours R, Domagalska MA, et al. (2011) Strigolactones are transported through the xylem and play a key role in shoot architectural response to phosphate deficiency in nonarbuscular mycorrhizal host *Arabidopsis*. Plant Physiology 155: 974–987. doi:10.1104/pp.110.164640

19. Kohlen W, Charnikhova T, Lammers M, Pollina T, Tóth P, et al. (2012) The tomato CAROTENOID CLEAVAGE DIOXYGENASE8 (SlCCD8) regulates rhizosphere signaling, plant architecture and affects reproductive development through strigolactone biosynthesis. New Phytologist 196: 535–547. doi:10.1111/j.1469-8137.2012.04265.x
20. Koltai H (2011) Strigolactones are regulators of root development. New Phytol 190: 545–549. doi:10.1111/j.1469-8137.2011.03678.x
21. Alder A, Jamil M, Marzorati M, Bruno M, Vermathen M, et al. (2012) The path from β-carotene to carlactone, a strigolactone-like plant hormone. Science 335: 1348–1351. doi:10.1126/science.1218094
22. Yoneyama K, Xie X, Yoneyama K, Takeuchi Y (2009) Strigolactones: structures and biological activities. Pest Management Science 65: 467–470. doi:10.1002/ps.1726
23. Xie X, Yoneyama K, Kisugi T, Uchida K, Ito S, et al. (2013) Confirming stereochemical structures of strigolactones produced by rice and tobacco. Mol Plant 6: 153–163. doi:10.1093/mp/sss139
24. Awad AA, Sato D, Kusumoto D, Kamioka H, Takeuchi Y, et al. (2006) Characterization of strigolactones, germination stimulants for the root parasitic plants *Striga* and *Orobanche*, produced by maize, millet and sorghum. Plant Growth Regul 48: 221–227. doi:10.1007/s10725-006-0009-3
25. Xie X, Kusumoto D, Takeuchi Y, Yoneyama K, Yamada Y, et al. (2007) 2′-*epi*-Orobanchol and solanacol, two unique strigolactones, germination stimulants for root parasitic weeds, produced by tobacco. J Agric Food Chem 55: 8067–8072. doi:10.1021/jf0715121
26. Akiyama K, Ogasawara S, Ito S, Hayashi H (2010) Structural requirements of strigolactones for hyphal branching in AM fungi. Plant Cell Physiol 51: 1104–1117. doi:10.1093/pcp/pcq058
27. Nomura S, Nakashima H, Mizutani M, Takikawa H, Sugimoto Y (2013) Structural requirements of strigolactones for germination induction and inhibition of *Striga gesnerioides* seeds. Plant Cell Rep 32: 829–838. doi:10.1007/s00299-013-1429-y
28. Matusova R, Rani K, Verstappen FWA, Franssen MCR, Beale MH, et al. (2005) The strigolactone germination stimulants of the plant-parasitic *Striga* and *Orobanche* spp. are derived from the carotenoid pathway. Plant Physiology 139: 920–934. doi:10.1104/pp.105.061382
29. Buee M, Rossignol M, Jauneau A, Ranjeva R, Bécard G (2000) The pre-symbiotic growth of arbuscular mycorrhizal fungi is induced by a branching factor partially purified from plant root exudates. Mol Plant Microbe Interact 13: 693–698. doi:10.1094/MPMI.2000.13.6.693
30. Sato D, Awad AA, Chae SH, Yokota T, Sugimoto Y, et al. (2003) Analysis of strigolactones, germination stimulants for *Striga* and *Orobanche*, by high-performance liquid chromatography/tandem mass spectrometry. J Agric Food Chem 51: 1162–1168. doi:10.1021/jf025997z.
31. Ueno K, Nomura S, Muranaka S, Mizutani M, Takikawa H, et al. (2011) *Ent*-2′-*epi*-orobanchol and its acetate, as germination stimulants for *Striga gesnerioides* seeds isolated from cowpea and red clover. J Agric Food Chem 59: 10485–10490. doi:10.1021/jf2024193
32. Zwanenburg B, Pospíšil T (2013) Structure and activity of strigolactones: new plant hormones with a rich future. Mol Plant 6: 38–62. doi:10.1093/mp/sss141
33. Zwanenburg B, Mwakaboko AS, Reizelman A, Anilkumar G, Sethumadhavan D (2009) Structure and function of natural and synthetic signalling molecules in parasitic weed germination. Pest Manag Sci 65: 478–491. doi:10.1002/ps.1706
34. Seto Y, Sado A, Asami K, Hanada A, Umehara M, et al. (2014) Carlactone is an endogenous biosynthetic precursor for strigolactones. PNAS: 201314805. doi:10.1073/pnas.1314805111
35. Motonami N, Ueno K, Nakashima H, Nomura S, Mizutani M, et al. (2013) The bioconversion of 5-deoxystrigol to sorgomol by the sorghum, *Sorghum bicolor* (L.) Moench. Phytochemistry 93: 41–48. doi:10.1016/j.phytochem.2013.02.017
36. Matusova R, Bouwmeester HJ (2006) The effect of host-root-derived chemical signals on the germination of parasitic plants. Frontis 16: 39–54.
37. Gurney AL, Press MC, Scholes JD (1999) Infection time and density influence the response of sorghum to the parasitic angiosperm *Striga hermonthica*. New Phytologist 143: 573–580. doi:10.1046/j.1469-8137.1999.00467.x
38. Boyer F-D, Germain A de S, Pillot J-P, Pouvreau J-B, Chen VX, et al. (2012) Structure-activity relationship studies of strigolactone-related molecules for branching inhibition in garden pea: molecule design for shoot branching. Plant Physiol 159: 1524–1544. doi:10.1104/pp.112.195826.

6

Motor, Psychiatric and Fatigue Features Associated with Nutritional Status and Its Effects on Quality of Life in Parkinson's Disease Patients

Seyed-Mohammad Fereshtehnejad[1,2]*, Ladan Ghazi[3], Mahdiyeh Shafieesabet[4], Gholam Ali Shahidi[5], Ahmad Delbari[1,6], Johan Lökk[1,7]

1 Division of Clinical Geriatrics, Department of Neurobiology, Care Sciences, and Society (NVS), Karolinska Institutet, Stockholm, Sweden, **2** Firoozgar Clinical Research Development Center (FCRDC), Firoozgar Hospital, Iran University of Medical Sciences, Tehran, Iran, **3** Department of Biosciences and Nutrition, Karolinska Institutet, Stockholm, Sweden, **4** Medical Students Research Committee (MSRC), Faculty of Medicine, Iran University of Medical Sciences, Tehran, Iran, **5** Movement Disorders Clinic, Department of Neurology, Faculty of Medicine, Iran University of Medical Sciences, Tehran, Iran, **6** Aging Research Center, Sabzevar University of Medical Sciences, Sabzevar, Khorasan, Iran, **7** Department of Geriatric Medicine, Karolinska University Hospital, Stockholm, Sweden

Abstract

Objectives: Parkinson's disease (PD) patients are more likely to develop impaired nutritional status because of the symptoms, medications and complications of the disease. However, little is known about the determinants and consequences of malnutrition in PD. This study aimed to investigate the association of motor, psychiatric and fatigue features with nutritional status as well as the effects of malnutrition on different aspects of quality of life (QoL) in PD patients.

Methods: One hundred and fifty patients with idiopathic PD (IPD) were recruited in this study. A demographic checklist, the Unified Parkinson's Disease Rating Scale (UPDRS), the Hospital Anxiety and Depression Scale (HADS) and the Fatigue Severity Scale (FSS) were completed through face-to-face interviews and clinical examinations. The health-related QoL (HRQoL) was also evaluated by means of the Parkinson's Disease Questionnaire (PDQ-39). For evaluation of nutritional status, the Mini Nutritional Assessment (MNA) questionnaire was applied together with anthropometric measurements.

Results: Thirty seven (25.3%) patients were at risk of malnutrition and another 3 (2.1%) were malnourished. The total score of the UPDRS scale ($r = -0.613$, $P<0.001$) and PD duration ($r = -0.284$, $P = 0.002$) had a significant inverse correlation with the total MNA score. The median score of the Hoehn and Yahr stage was significantly higher in PD patients with abnormal nutritional status [2.5 vs. 2.0; $P<0.001$]. More severe anxiety [8.8 vs. 5.9; $P = 0.002$], depression [9.0 vs. 3.6; $P<0.001$] and fatigue [5.4 vs. 4.2; $P<0.001$] were observed in PD patients with abnormal nutritional status. Except for stigma, all other domains of the PDQ-39 were significantly correlated with the total score of the MNA.

Conclusion: Our study demonstrates that disease duration, severity of motor and psychiatric symptoms (depression, anxiety) and fatigue are associated with nutritional status in PD. Different aspects of the HRQoL were affected by patients' nutritional status especially the emotional well-being and mobility domains.

Editor: John Duda, Philadelphia VA Medical Center, United States of America

Funding: These authors have no support or funding to report.

Competing Interests: The authors have declared that no competing interests exist.

* E-mail: sm.fereshtehnejad@ki.se

Introduction

Nutritional status is an important contributor to quality of life (QoL) and general condition of daily living in the elderly [1,2]. In theory, Parkinson's disease (PD) patients are susceptible to impaired nutritional status because of different motor and non-motor symptoms, including psychiatric features and fatigue [3]. Moreover, pharmacological treatment administered in PD can influence nutritional status through the drugs themselves and their side effects such as nausea, vomiting and weight loss [4].

Malnutrition can influence immune system, functional status [5,6], some complications of the disease such as constipation [7] and potentially increases the likelihood of falling [8]. On the other hand, dysphagia increases the risk of malnutrition [9] in PD patients. Despite its important role, nutritional status does not receive the necessary attention in the management of PD and most of the time it is ignored.

So far, there have been a number of studies that have evaluated weight change and/or body mass index (BMI) in PD. However, only a few of them have focused on general nutritional status using validated tools such as the Subjective Global Assessment (SGA) [4,10] and the mini nutritional assessment (MNA) [11,12,13]. Although a few reports used the MNA in PD population, there are still not enough reports to broadly evaluate the relationship between different features of the disease and nutritional status, as well as its effects on the health-related QoL in PD patients. Therefore, our study aimed to investigate the association of motor, psychiatric and fatigue features with nutritional status in PD using the MNA as a comprehensive instrument. In addition, we also evaluated the effects of abnormal nutritional status on different domains of QoL in a population of PD patients.

Subjects and Methods

One hundred and fifty consecutive patients with idiopathic Parkinson's disease (IPD) from a single referral Movement Disorders Clinic in Tehran, Iran, were recruited between October 2011 and December 2012. This was a collaborative project between the Iran University of Medical Sciences (Tehran, Iran) and the Karolinska Institutet (Stockholm, Sweden).

Ethics Statement

The ethics committee of the Firoozgar Clinical Research Development Center (FCRDC) (affiliated with Iran University of Medical Sciences) approved the study protocol. All of the collected data were stored and treated according to the ethical guidelines of medical research. Prior to the launch of the study, all patients were informed about the aims and procedures. All participants provided their verbal informed consent to participate in this study. As the project was designed as an observational research, the verbal form of consent was approved by the aforementioned ethics committee. If any patient did not agree to enroll into the study, no extra evaluation was performed in addition to his/her routine work-up in the clinic and the research checklist was left blank in the documentation procedure. Moreover, participation in this study was voluntary and the patients were free to withdraw from the project whenever they wanted. Furthermore, the identity of research participants was protected, since the data files were anonymous and all of the names were omitted.

Patient Recruitment

Recruited patients fulfilled the United Kingdom Brain Bank criteria for the diagnosis of IPD [14], which was assessed by the same neurologist who had specialized in movement disorders for all of them. All of the IPD patients who were eligible for this study were required to be 30 years or older with motor disability in the mild to moderate severity range according to the Hoehn and Yahr staging criteria [15]. Patients with moderate to severe dementia [mini-mental state examination (MMSE)$<$24] [16] were excluded from the study, as were those who were following special diets or suffering from other diseases considerably influencing nutritional state. Also, any patient with atypical Parkinsonism, including multiple system atrophy (MSA), progressive supranuclear palsy (PSP), and vascular or drug-induced Parkinsonism were not eligible.

Assessments

Data collection was performed through face-to-face interviews with the patients and, whenever possible, their caregivers, along with clinical examinations by means of a checklist and questionnaires. The demographic checklist consisted of baseline variables (age and sex), educational status, co-morbidities, duration of PD (time passed from diagnosis) and history of levodopa administration. These data were collected based on both participants' self-reports and their medical records at the referral centre. Clinical characteristics of PD were assessed using the Unified Parkinson's Disease Rating Scale (UPDRS) [17], Hoehn and Yahr stage [15] and Schwab and England activity of daily living (ADL) scale [18]. The Hospital Anxiety and Depression Scale (HADS) [19] questionnaire was used to focus on aspects of anxiety and depression and the Fatigue Severity Scale (FSS) [20] was used for fatigue measurement. Moreover, the health-related quality of life (HRQoL) was also evaluated by means of the Parkinson's disease quality of life questionnaire (PDQ-39) [21]. In order to assess the nutritional status, the MNA questionnaire was applied together with anthropometric measurements.

All of the assessments were done when the patients were in the "On" state. A movement disorder specialist performed all of the physical examinations and a team of interviewers consisting of trained medical students and general physicians completed the interviews to complete the questionnaires.

Scales and Questionnaires

Unified Parkinson's Disease Rating Scale (UPDRS). UPDRS is the most commonly used scale in the clinical study of PD [22], and is used to assess the severity of PD in different aspects including non-motor symptoms (part I), activities of daily living (ADL) (part II), motor examination (part III) and drug complications (part IV). The UPDRS is scored from a total of 147 points where higher scores reflect worsening disability [17].

Hoehn and Yahr Stage. The Hoehn and Yahr stage is a widely used clinical rating scale, supplanted by the UPDRS, which defines broad categories of motor function in PD. It evaluates the severity of PD based on functional disability and clinical findings. It contains five stages, where 0 indicates no visible symptoms of PD, and 5 shows symptoms on both sides of the body, identifying those PD patients who are unable to walk. Therefore, a higher stage shows greater levels of functional disability [15].

Schwab and England Activities of Daily Living (ADL) scale. The Schwab and England ADL scale is a global scale that is used for assessing a PD patient's ability to perform daily activities in terms of speed and independence through a percentage figure, where 100% indicates total independence, and 0% indicates a state of complete dependence, which is seen in bed-ridden individuals. Therefore, higher scores show greater level of independence [18].

39-item PD questionnaire (PDQ-39). The PDQ-39 is the most commonly used instrument for measuring health-related quality of life in PD patients. It has been developed to assess treatments and interventions that may benefit PD patients. In its long format, it contains 39 items assessing eight aspects of QoL in PD patients: mobility, ADL, emotional well-being, stigma, social support, cognitions, communication and bodily discomfort. All questions on the PDQ-39 are coded in a Likert-scale from 0–4, where 0 = never, 1 = occasionally, 2 = sometimes, 3 = often and 4 = always. The maximum score of 100 on the PDQ-39 scale represents the worst condition, with a score of zero representing the best level of QoL in PD patients [21]. In this study, we used the Persian-translated version of the PDQ39 questionnaire, which has been previously shown to have a high reliability with a Cronbach's alpha coefficient of 0.93 for the total summary index [23].

Hospital Anxiety and Depression Score (HADS). The HADS is a screening tool that was designed to assess the levels of anxiety and depression in a non-psychiatric population attending medical clinics. It is comprised of 14 questions divided into two sections; seven questions are related to anxiety and the other seven focus on depression. Each questionnaire is worth 0–21 points, providing separate scores for either the anxiety or depression sub-scales. Responses are determined or calculated by adding up the sum of 0–3 scores for each question, where 0 = not at all, and 3 = very often indeed [19]. The Cronbach's alpha coefficient has been reported as 0.78 for anxiety and 0.86 for the depression sub-scale of the Persian-version of the HADS questionnaire [24] used in our study.

Fatigue Severity Scale (FSS). The FSS is an instrument that assesses the physical aspects of fatigue and their impact on the patient's daily function in a variety of medical and neurologic disorders. It evaluates the impact of fatigue on motivation, exercise, physical functioning, and carrying out duties and responsibilities, as well as interfering with work, family, or social life. It contains nine questions, with a maximum score of 36 points. We asked each patient to rate the level of fatigue during the past week with scores from 1 to 7 for each statement. Lower values indicate strong disagreement with the statement, whereas higher values indicate strong agreement [20]. A total score is obtained as the average of all of the item-specific scores where higher scores correspond with more severe fatigue. The FSS questionnaire was previously translated into the Persian language and showed acceptable validity and reliability [25]. In this project, we used this Persian-translated version of the FSS questionnaire in our sample of IPD patients.

Mini Nutritional Assessment (MNA). The MNA is a rapid nutrition-assessment tool that can be used for the elderly in order to identify the risk of malnutrition. Moreover, its usefulness extends as a comprehensive geriatric assessment tool that can help in identifying patients who may benefit from early intervention [26]. It has also been seen as a combined screening and assessment tool [27]. The MNA questionnaire consists of brief questions and simple measurements that can be completed in about 10–15 minutes [26]. The full format of the MNA includes 18 items grouped into two sub-sections: six screening questions in the first section and 12 assessment questions in the second section. The MNA scale includes body mass index (BMI), weight loss, arm and calf circumference, appetite, medication, general and cognitive health, dietary matters, autonomy of feeding, and self-perception of health and nutrition, as well as a subjective judgment of malnutrition. The maximum score in the MNA questionnaire is 30 points, where 16 points are obtained by screening questions and 14 points are gained through assessment questions. A total score of less than 17 points indicates "*malnutrition*", scores of 17–23.5 points signify cases that are "*at risk for malnutrition*", while scores equal to or more than 24 points represent "*normal nutritional status*" [28]. In this study, we have used the full format of the Persian-translated MNA provided by the *Nestlé* Nutrition Institutet [29] and the total score is reported. Moreover, according to the small sample size in subgroup comparisons, all of the patients with a total MNA score of <24 are mentioned as "*abnormal nutritional status*", including both malnourished and at-risk patients.

Anthropometric Measurements. As a part of the MNA questionnaire, each participant underwent anthropometric measurements including mid arm circumference (MAC), calf circumference (CC), weight and height. Body weight was recorded in a standardised manner using calibrated floor scales while the subjects wore light clothing with no shoes or coats. For all patients, the weight measurement was performed between 3 p.m. and 5 p.m. when they were supposed to have left at least 2 hours since their lunch and had not yet had their dinner. The standing height was measured using a stadiometer at head level, with the subject's bare feet close together, standing erect and looking straight ahead. Of note, there was no case of considerable stooped posture for any height adjustment. Body mass index was calculated as body weight (*kg*) divided by the square value of height (m^2). For the MAC, the examiner marked the mid-point between the acromial surface of the scapula (bony protrusion surface of upper shoulder) and the olecranon process of the elbow (bony point of the elbow) on the back of the arm, while the subject was asked to hold the forearm in a horizontal position with their palm up. Thereafter, the MAC was measured with a flexible inextensible tape that was applied snugly around the maximum girth of the proximal part of forearm while the subject's arm was hanging down freely along their trunk at their sides. For the CC, the maximal circumference between the ankle and the knee was measured with a flexible tape that was applied horizontally around the maximum girth of the calf, while the subject was standing with their weight evenly distributed on both feet [30]. In order to accurately measure the MAC and CC, we asked the participants to roll up their trouser leg or sleeve to uncover their calf or arm, respectively.

Statistical Analysis

All of the data obtained from the checklists and questionnaires were entered into SPSS software version 20 (IBM; Chicago, IL, USA). Numerical variables are described using the mean and standard deviation (SD), whereas, the discrete values of the Hoehn and Yahr stage are presented as the median and interquartile range (IQR). The relative frequency percentage is also used to describe the nominal or categorical variables. The Kolmogorov-Smirnov (K-S) test was used to check the normality of the distribution of the total MNA score, which was shown to be skewed and non-normal (K-S test $P = 0.003$). The univariate relationship between the total MNA score and those obtained from other scales and questionnaires was assessed by means of the Spearman correlation test. In subgroup analysis, the independent samples *T* test was performed to compare the mean scores of different questionnaires between the IPD patients with normal versus abnormal nutritional status. Moreover, the Mann-Whitney *U* test was used to compare the mean of the total MNA score between female and male patients. It must be noted that according to the rather small sample size in subgroup comparisons, the two subgroups of patients with "*malnutrition*" and "at *risk of malnutrition*" were merged together in one group called "*abnormal nutritional status*".

Further multivariate analysis was performed using a stepwise linear regression model in order to evaluate the factors independently related to the total score of the MNA questionnaire among IPD patients. In addition, binary logistic regression analysis was performed using a forward conditional model to identify the factors that could independently discriminate the IPD patients with abnormal nutritional status. In both regression models, age at the time of diagnosis, sex, weight-adjusted daily levodopa dosage, the score of each part of the UPDRS scale, total UPDRS score, Hoehn and Yahr stage, Schwab and England ADL score, anxiety, depression and fatigue scores were defined as the predictor list. A two-tailed *P*-value of less than 0.05 was considered to show a statistically significant difference or correlation in all analytical procedures.

Results

Baseline and Anthropometric Characteristics

In total, 150 PD patients were recruited into this study consisting of 103 (68.7%) males and 47 (31.3%) females with a mean age of 60.8 (SD = 10.8) *yrs*, ranging between 32 and 84 years, and a mean disease duration of 6.8 (SD = 5.3) *yrs*. Table 1 summarises information on the baseline, anthropometric and clinical characteristics of the recruited PD patients. The mean of the total UPDRS score was 31.7 (SD = 17.2) ranging from 6 to 88. The median score of Hoehn and Yahr staging was 2.0 (IQR = 1.5) and the mean percentage of the Schwab and England ADL scale was 81.7% (SD = 16.7).

Table 1. Baseline, anthropometric and clinical characteristics of the recruited Parkinson's disease patients (n = 150).

Characteristics	Value
Age *(yr)*-Mean (SD)	60.8 (10.8)
Gender *NO.(%)*	
Female	47 (31.3)
Male	103 (68.7)
Level of Education *NO.(%)*	
Illiterate	15 (10.1)
Primary and/or Secondary	36 (24.3)
High School/Diploma	41 (27.8)
College and/or University	56 (37.8)
Duration of Disease *(yr)*-Mean (SD)	6.8 (5.3)
Co-morbidities *NO.(%)*	
Depression	36 (24.5)
Hypertension	24 (16.2)
Cardiovascular Disease	23 (15.8)
Osteoarthritis	19 (13.0)
Diabetes	18 (12.3)
UPDRS Score-Mean (SD)	
Part I-*mental*	2.1 (2.3)
Part II-*ADL*	11.2 (6.9)
Part III-*motor*	15.3 (8.8)
Part IV-*complications*	3.5 (2.8)
Total	31.7 (17.2)
Hoehn & Yahr Stage-Median (IQR)	2.0 (1.5)
Schwab and England Activities of Daily Living Score *(%)*-Mean (SD)	81.7 (16.7)
Daily levodopa dose-Mean (SD)	
Crude *(mg)*	812 (490)
Weight-adjusted *(mg/kg)*	11.75 (7.72)
Anthropometric Measurements-Mean (SD)	
Weight *(kg)*	71.8 (13.6)
Height *(cm)*	166.7 (8.8)
Body Mass Index (BMI) *(kg/m^2)*	25.8 (4.2)
Mid-Arm Circumference (MAC) *(cm)*	28.2 (4.9)
Calf Circumference (CC) *(cm)*	34.9 (3.8)

Table 2 shows the descriptive results for nutritional status (MNA), disease-related quality of life (PDQ-39), and severity of anxiety, depression (HADS) and fatigue (FSS) in PD patients. The highest scores (worst conditions) of PDQ-39 were observed in emotional well-being [27.7 (SD = 22.7)] and mobility [26.8 (SD = 25.1)] domains. The mean of the total MNA score was 25.1 (SD = 3.3) and regarding the cut-off points, 37 (25.3%) PD patients were at risk of malnutrition and another 3 (2.1%) cases were already malnourished.

Univariate Correlations with the MNA Score

Table 3 summarises the univariate correlation coefficients between the scores of different motor, psychiatric, fatigue and quality of life (PDQ-39) scales and nutritional status (MNA). Except for stigma, all other domains of PDQ-39 were significantly and inversely correlated with the total score of the MNA questionnaire (all $P<0.05$). The mobility domain of the disease-related QoL had the largest inverse correlation with the total MNA score (Spearman $r = -0.590$, $P<0.001$), and the emotional well-being domain was the second most important related factor to the total MNA score (Spearman $r = -0.461$, $P<0.001$) in the population of recruited PD patients.

As listed in Table 3, all sections of the UPDRS scale of disease severity had a significant inverse correlation with the total score of the MNA including the mental (Spearman $r = -0.503$, $P<0.001$), ADL (Spearman $r = -0.518$, $P<0.001$), motor (Spearman $r = -0.473$, $P<0.001$) and complication (Spearman $r = -0.336$, $P<0.001$) parts as well as the total UPDRS score (Spearman $r = -0.613$, $P<0.001$). Also, the more severe motor symptoms (Hoehn and Yahr: Spearman $r = -0.414$, $P<0.001$) and morbidity (Schwab and England: Spearman $r = 0.492$, $P<0.001$) observed, the lower the total MNA scores recorded among the recruited PD patients. All of the evaluated non-motor symptoms were significantly correlated with the MNA scores (all $P<0.01$). However, the

Table 2. Descriptive characteristics of nutritional status (MNA), disease-related quality of life (PDQ-39), anxiety, depression (HADS) and fatigue (FSS) in Parkinson's disease (PD) patients.

Questionnaire/Domain	Mean (SD)	Range
MNA (Total)	25.1 (3.3)	6–30
PDQ-39 *domains*		
Mobility	26.8 (25.1)	0–100
Activities of daily living (ADL)	23.4 (22.9)	0–100
Emotional well-being	27.7 (22.7)	0–100
Stigma	21.6 (25.1)	0–100
Social support	7.1 (13.3)	0–75
Cognitive impairment (Cognition)	16.6 (18.3)	0–81
Communication	14.2 (17.9)	0–83
Bodily discomfort	20.9 (20.8)	0–75
HADS *domains*		
Anxiety	6.8 (5.1)	0–20
Depression	5.1 (4.5)	0–17
FSS	4.5 (1.9)	1–7

HADS score of depression was the strongest one associated with the total score of the MNA questionnaire (Spearman r = −0.577, *P*<0.001). Moreover, both anxiety (Spearman r = −0.369, *P*< 0.001) and fatigue (Spearman r = −0.413, *P*<0.001) scores were inversely correlated with the total MNA score. The probable associations of two other continuous variables, age and disease duration, with the MNA score were also assessed. Interestingly, total MNA score was significantly inversely correlated with disease duration (Spearman r = −0.284, *P*= 0.001) in the absence of such an association with patients' age (*P*= 0.271). In addition, while no correlation was found between the cumulative daily dosage of levodopa and total MNA score (Spearman r = −0.085, *P*= 0.310), the weight-adjusted levodopa dose was inversely correlated with total MNA score (Spearman r = −0.218, *P*= 0.009). The result of the Mann-Whitney *U* test demonstrated that the mean of the total MNA score was significantly lower among the female PD patients compared to the male cases [23.7 (SD = 4.3) vs. 25.8 (SD = 2.6); *P*= 0.002].

Univariate Comparisons between Patients with Normal versus Abnormal Nutritional Status

As shown in Table 4, the patients with abnormal nutritional status had a significantly longer history of PD compared to those with normal nutritional status [8.2 (SD = 6.9) *yrs* vs. 6.2 (SD = 4.6) *yrs*; t-value = −2.02, *P*= 0.045]. The results of the independent samples *T* test confirmed that except for stigma, the mean score of other domains of the PDQ-39 questionnaire was significantly different between PD patients with different nutritional status (all *P*<0.05). In addition to each part of the UPDRS scale, the mean of the total UPDRS score was significantly higher among the PD patients with abnormal nutritional status [45.9 (SD = 18.0) vs. 26.4 (SD = 13.6); t-value = −6.50, *P*<0.001]. Accordingly, the median score of the Hoehn and Yahr staging was significantly higher in PD patients at risk of malnutrition compared to those with normal nutritional status [2.5 (IQR = 1.0) vs. 2.0 (IQR = 1.5); t-value = − 4.55, *P*<0.001]. Based on the Schwab and England ADL score, the PD patients with abnormal nutritional status were also more disabled compared to the subgroup with normal nutrition [71.2 (SD = 19.6) vs. 85.7 (SD = 13.9); t-value = 4.29, *P*<0.001]. In addition, more severe anxiety [8.8 (SD = 5.2) vs. 5.9 (SD = 4.9); t-value = −3.08, *P*= 0.002], depression [9.0 (SD = 4.2) vs. 3.6 (SD = 3.5); t-value = −7.77, *P*<0.001] and fatigue [5.4 (SD = 1.5) vs. 4.2 (SD = 2.0); t-value = −4.00, *P*<0.001] were found in PD patients with abnormal nutritional status.

Multivariate Analysis

The continuous score of the whole MNA scale was assigned as the outcome of interest in a forward (stepwise) multivariate linear model where the entire regression was statistically significant (R^2 = 0.539, *P*<0.001, Table 5- model 1). Of interest, with regard to independent variables that remained significant in the regression model, depression (regression coefficient = −0.352, *P*<0.001), total score of the UPDRS scale (regression coefficient = −0.313, *P*<0.001), weight-adjusted daily levodopa dosage (regression coefficient = −0.190, *P*= 0.006) and patients' sex (regression coefficient = −0.196, *P*= 0.003) were found to be significantly associated with the total MNA score.

The logistic regression model was also statistically significant (R^2 = 0.496, *P*<0.001, Table 5- model 2). The forward conditional model revealed that the Hoehn and Yahr stage [OR = 2.4 (95% CI: 1.3–4.5); *P*= 0.007] and depression score [OR = 1.4 (95% CI: 1.2–1.6); *P*<0.001] independently discriminated the PD patients suffering from malnutrition.

Discussion

In this study, we used MNA to assess nutritional status in a group of PD patients with the mean age of 61 (SD = 10) *yrs*, which is close to the age range of the previous report by Wang et al. [65 (SD = 9) *yr*] who used MNA in the PD population [11]. Although the age distribution of our participants was skewed through the inclusion of elderly individuals, it ranged between 32 and 84 *yr*. As an assessment tool, MNA has shown reliable and valid results to screen those elderly patients at risk of malnutrition [31]; however, there are some reports that reveal reproducible results of using MNA in younger adults aged >18 years [32] or in those with a mean age of around 41 *yrs* [33], though both studies were conducted in patients with chronic kidney disease. Specifically in

Table 3. Pearson correlation between the scores of different motor, psychiatric, fatigue and quality of life (PDQ-39) scales and nutritional status (MNA) in Parkinson's disease (PD) patients.

Scale	Domains	Correlation Index	MNA (Total)
PDQ39	**Mobility**	*Spearman R*	−.590**
		P-value	<.001
	Activities of daily living (ADL)	*Spearman R*	−.450**
		P-value	<.001
	Emotional well-being	*Spearman R*	−.461**
		P-value	<.001
	Stigma	*Spearman R*	−.027
		P-value	.744
	Social support	*Spearman R*	−.246**
		P-value	.005
	Cognitive impairment (Cognition)	*Spearman R*	−.320**
		P-value	<.001
	Communication	*Spearman R*	−.414**
		P-value	<.001
	Bodily discomfort	*Spearman R*	−.451**
		P-value	<.001
Disease Severity	**UPDRS** Part I-*mental*	*Spearman R*	−.503**
		P-value	<.001
	UPDRS Part II-ADL	*Spearman R*	−.518**
		P-value	<.001
	UPDRS Part III-motor	*Spearman R*	−.473**
		P-value	<.001
	UPDRS Part IV-complications	*Spearman R*	−.336**
		P-value	<.001
	UPDRS Total	*Spearman R*	−.613**
		P-value	<.001
	Hoehn & Yahr stage	*Spearman R*	−.414**
		P-value	<.001
	Schwab & England stage	*Spearman R*	.492**
		P-value	<.001
HADS	**Anxiety**	*Spearman R*	−.369**
		P-value	<.001
	Depression	*Spearman R*	−.577**
		P-value	<.001
FSS	**Fatigue**	*Spearman R*	−.413**
		P-value	<.001

**Correlation is significant at the 0.01 level (2-tailed).
*Correlation is significant at the 0.05 level (2-tailed).

the case of the PD population, Sheard et al. showed the superior validity of the short form of the MNA compared to other screening tools such as BMI and weight changes. Nevertheless, the Patient-Generated Subjective Global Assessment (PG-SGA) demonstrated better results compared to the full MNA questionnaire for nutritional assessment in a group of PD patients who are aged between 35 and 92 *yrs* [34].

In our study population, malnutrition was found in 2% of the PD patients, while almost a quarter of them were at risk of malnutrition. This figure is close to the reports from the studies by Wang et al. [11] and Barichella et al. [12], illustrating 20% and 22.9% of the risk of malnutrition in Chinese and Italian PD populations, respectively. The rate of malnutrition was also estimated to be as low as 1.7% by Wang et al., which was contributed to race, age, Hoehn and Yahr stage, source of participants' recruitment (from outpatient clinics) and disease duration [11]. On the other hand, there are some other reports showing more prevalent malnutrition in PD populations to as high as 15.6% [35], 19.5% [36] and 23.6% [37] using BMI measures.

Our findings demonstrate that many motor, psychiatric and fatigue symptoms are significantly associated with nutritional status in PD patients. PD patients with abnormal nutritional status

Table 4. Comparison of the mean [standard deviation (SD)] scores of different motor, psychiatric, fatigue and quality of life (PDQ-39) scales between subgroups of Parkinson's disease (PD) patients regarding nutritional status (MNA).

Scale	Domain	Abnormal nutritional status (*n* = 40)	Normal nutritional status (*n* = 106)	*t*-value	*P*-value
Baseline	**Age** *(yr)*	61.3 (12.3)	61.3 (9.8)	−0.02	.982
	Disease duration *(yr)*	8.2 (6.9)	6.2 (4.6)	−2.02	.045*
	Body mass index (BMI) *(kg/m²)*	23.9 (3.8)	26.6 (4.3)	3.57	.001*
	Daily levodopa dose				
	Crude *(mg)*	817 (450)	841 (490)	0.27	.789
	Weight-adjusted *(mg/kg)*	13.55 (8.92)	11.50 (6.94)	−1.46	.146
PDQ39	**Mobility**	45.6 (26.6)	19.4 (20.7)	−5.61	<.001*
	Activities of daily living (ADL)	38.4 (28.9)	18.0 (17.9)	−3.97	<.001*
	Emotional well-being	41.3 (22.4)	22.1 (20.8)	−4.90	<.001*
	Stigma	22.0 (24.4)	21.5 (25.4)	−0.11	.913
	Social support	13.0 (17.2)	5.1 (10.9)	−2.51	.016*
	Cognitive impairment	25.5 (20.5)	13.5 (16.6)	−3.64	<.001*
	Communication	24.6 (23.9)	10.3 (13.6)	−3.56	.001*
	Bodily discomfort	32.5 (20.3)	16.4 (19.6)	−4.30	<.001*
Disease Severity	**UPDRS:** Part I-*mental*	3.8 (3.2)	1.3 (1.4)	−4.69	<.001*
	UPDRS: Part II-*ADL*	15.9 (7.8)	9.4 (5.8)	−5.17	<.001*
	UPDRS: Part III-*motor*	20.6 (10.1)	13.3 (7.4)	−4.18	<.001*
	UPDRS: Part IV-*complications*	5.1 (3.4)	2.9 (2.2)	−3.80	<.001*
	a. Dyskinesia	1.7 (2.5)	.8 (1.4)	−2.08	.042*
	b. Wearing off	2.3 (1.4)	1.5 (1.2)	−3.06	.003*
	UPDRS: Total	45.9 (18.0)	26.4 (13.6)	−6.50	<.001*
	Hoehn & Yahr stage #	2.5 (1.0)	2.0 (1.5)	−4.55	<.001*
	Schwab & England stage *(%)*	71.2 (19.6)	85.7 (13.9)	4.29	<.001*
HADS	**Anxiety**	8.8 (5.2)	5.9 (4.9)	−3.08	.002*
	Depression	9.0 (4.2)	3.6 (3.5)	−7.77	<.001*
FSS	**Fatigue**	5.4 (1.5)	4.2 (2.0)	−4.00	<.001*

(including malnourished and at risk of malnutrition) had more severe symptoms in all parts of the UPDRS scale including motor, non-motor, ADL and complications. Both dyskinesia and the wearing-off phenomenon were more common among PD patients with abnormal nutritional status in whom the Hoehn and Yahr stage and the Schwab and England ADL scores also showed more severe disease. Among the evaluated psychiatric features, more severe depression, anxiety and fatigue were reported in PD patients with nutritional problems. Besides PD symptoms, health-related QoL was also affected by nutritional status. As our findings show, except for stigma, in all other domains of the PDQ-39, the PD patients with abnormal nutritional status showed worse QoL-scores. In other words, poor nutritional status was accompanied with poor QoL in a group of patients with chronic conditions such as PD. It is noteworthy that different domains of QoL such as disability-related features, cognition, communication, and emotional and social aspects were all correlated with the MNA score in the PD population. To our knowledge, this study is one of the few that directly assess the relationship between nutritional status and HRQoL by means of MNA and PDQ-39 tools in the PD population. However, using MNA in another elderly population, malnourished subjects or those at risk of malnutrition have been shown to have poorer QoL and function in rehabilitation centres [2].

Based on multivariate regression analysis, female gender, higher weight-adjusted daily levodopa dosage, more severe disability (higher UPDRS score, more advanced Hoehn and Yahr stage) and more severe depression predicted a lower MNA score or a higher risk of nutritional deficiency in the PD population, when univariate-independent relationships were adjusted for other covariates. These factors represent the role of demographic (sex), disease severity (UPDRS, Hoehn and Yahr stage), psychiatric (depression) and pharmaceutical (weight-adjusted daily levodopa dosage) features of PD in association with nutritional status. We found significantly lower MNA scores among the female PD population, which is in line with the previously published reports indicating female gender as a risk factor for malnutrition in the elderly based on the total MNA score [38]. With regard to the Hoehn and Yahr stage as a measure of PD severity, the current literature is controversial. Two previous reports have shown no significant difference in the Hoehn and Yahr stage when comparing poor nutritional status with the well-nourished PD patients [11,39]. In contrast to these previous reports and similar to our current study, Markus et al. [37], Beyer et al. [40], Uc et al. [35] and Sheard et al. [41] reported a statistically significant correlation between Hoehn and Yahr stage and either BMI, the amount of weight change or nutritional status in a PD population.

Table 5. Multivariate regression models to determine the motor and non-motor factors independently related to total score of the MNA questionnaire (model 1) and having abnormal versus normal nutritional status (model 2) in recruited Parkinson's disease (PD) patients.

Model 1: Linear regression *(Dependent variable: total MNA score)*

Significant Variables	Unstandardized Coefficients		Standardized Coefficients	*t*	*P-value*
	B	*SEM*	*Beta*		
Depression score	−.292	.064	−.352	−4.547	<.001
Total score of UPDRS	−.064	.016	−.313	−3.903	<.001
Gender	−1.525	.503	−.196	−3.032	.003
Weight-adjusted levodopa dosage	−.085	.030	−.190	−2.815	.006
Constant	30.153	.504	-	59.868	<.001

Model 2: Binary Logistic regression *(Dependent variable: abnormal vs. normal nutritional status)*

Significant Variables	*B*	*SEM*	*OR (95% CI)*	*Wald*	*P-value*
Hoehn & Yahr stage	.865	.322	2.38 (1.26–4.46)	7.232	.007
Depression score	.354	.072	1.42 (1.24–1.64)	24.262	<.001
Constant	−4.984	.971	-	26.330	<.001

In both regression models, age at the time of diagnosis, sex, weight-adjusted levodopa dosage, the score of the each part of the UPDRS scale, total UPDRS score, Hoehn & Yahr stage, Schwab & England ADL score, anxiety, depression and fatigue scores were entered as the predictor list.

Regarding psychiatric symptoms and fatigue, there are few similar studies to directly evaluate the relationship between these symptoms and nutritional status in PD. Our findings are in line with previous reports, which show that neuropsychiatric symptoms such as depression, anxiety, dementia, confusion, and apathy contribute to decreased food intake and subsequent weight loss in an elderly PD population [35,42,43]. In line with the results of our study, both Wang et al. [11] and Sheard et al. [41] reported depression as a significant predictor of nutritional status in PD patients. Wang et al. [11] considered many non-motor symptoms in their study and showed that both depression and anxiety were associated with a risk of malnutrition in PD. More recently, a higher depression score was shown in malnourished PD patients by using the Beck's depression inventory (BDI) [41]. Our study uniquely considered fatigue as another factor that might interact with the negative association of depression and anxiety with nutritional status in PD patients. We showed that in addition to previously evaluated psychiatric symptoms, fatigue significantly correlated with malnutrition in PD. Having assessed nutritional status by MNA in another elderly population, Bollwein et al. underlined the close association between frailty syndrome (including exhaustion, low physical activity and slow walking speed) and nutritional status [44]. However, fatigue and exhaustion seem to be both the cause and consequence of malnutrition in the elderly. Emotional well-being, depression and fatigue are important determinants in health status as they are directly associated with the general condition in PD. Additionally, PD can lead to a reduction in mobility, hindering older persons from performing daily activities, such as shopping or food preparation [45].

Our study confirms that more severe motor symptoms and more common dyskinesia are found among PD patients with abnormal nutritional status, which is in line with a similar study performed by Sheard et al. [41]. Although using another scale (SGA) to evaluate nutritional status in a PD population, they also observed higher UPDRS scores among the malnourished participants [41]. The association between malnutrition and disease severity may be due to eating and digesting difficulties occurring in PD [46]. Hypothetically, people with better nutritional status, as indicated by a higher MNA score, may demonstrate a more nutritious dietary pattern when younger, having maintained their healthy diet into late-adulthood. This would increase their odds of being in the groups with higher MNA scores. However, it is not possible to determine the temporality between nutritional status and PD severity by a cross-sectional designed study.

In the present study, BMI was also closely correlated with the nutritional status assessed by MNA. An average of a three-unit lower BMI was observed in PD patients at risk of malnutrition in our study. This finding is in line with a previous report that shows an even lower BMI among the moderately malnourished PD cases compared to the well-nourished patients (20.0 kg/m^2 vs. 25.9 kg/m^2) [10]. In parallel, it has been previously shown that different doses of levodopa administered as the main PD treatment may affect BMI levels [46]. In contrast, no association was detected by Nozaki et al. between PD treatment and weight loss [47]. This can be seen in other studies where no correlation was found between levodopa dose, duration, and weight changes [48]. Similarly, we did not find any relationship between the daily dosage of levodopa and nutritional status, and Sheard et al. also reported this lack of association [41]. However, they found a relationship between the weight-adjusted dose of levodopa (*mg* per *kg* body weight) and MNA score [41]. Of interest, we also observed an inverse correlation between the weight-adjusted daily dosage of levodopa and total MNA score, which demonstrates a higher adjusted dose in PD patients with worse nutritional status (lower MNA score). This finding is consistent with the report by Barichella et al. who recently confirmed that nutritional risk depends on weight-adjusted levodopa dose in PD outpatients [49]. These findings highlight an intrinsic association between nutritional status and both the course of disease and levodopa-related complication in PD patients [49,50,51].

Most interestingly, an inverse relationship was also found between MNA score and disease duration. While a lower MNA score was accompanied by longer disease duration in PD patients, no association was found between the MNA score and patient's age. Previously published evidence shows conflicting results on this issue. While no difference in nutritional status, assessed by MNA, was found regarding PD duration in one study [11], Barichella et al. demonstrated a linear correlation between the MNA score and the duration of PD, even though no correlation was observed between MNA and the chronological age of the patients [12]. These patterns are quite consistent with our findings in the Iranian PD population, which showed an independent association between MNA and PD duration.

Our study suffers from some limitations, which must be taken into account when generalising its findings. One issue refers to the fact that no serum measurement was performed to quantify blood indicators of nutrition. Similar to most previous reports on this issue, the primary focus is on BMI and weight loss, whereas other indicators of nutritional condition such as food intake, fat and muscle status are not considered in our study. However, as an innovative clinical evaluation instrument, the MNA questionnaire provides several questions and four anthropometric measurements without any need for blood sampling or other clinical measurements. MNA is an acceptable tool to assess nutritional status especially among those elderly who are aged >65 *yrs*; therefore, our findings regarding younger patients might not be as valid as those of older ones. Nevertheless, this is the real-life condition of PD population in referral movement disorder centres, and other reports with rather similar ranges of age also used this tool and showed its validity in PD [11,34]. Our study has primarily been designed as a cross-sectional study, which did not allow for the determination of directionality of the association or the so-called causality between malnutrition and PD-related factors. Similar to previous studies, it is not clear whether poor nutritional status is "the chicken or the egg", i.e. the cause or the effect [52]. In a cross-sectional study, such as ours, the relationship between PD symptoms and nutritional status can be reciprocal. While poor symptom control can increase the risk of poor nutritional status, malnutrition can also result in poor symptom control. Moreover, the recruited patients in our study were PD outpatients who attended a referral movement disorder clinic. This selection bias has restricted our samples to the group of mild-to-moderate stage non-hospitalised PD patients. The more severe or end-stage cases, which are potentially at a higher risk of malnutrition, were not able to participate in this study. In order to have more valid data, patients with moderate to severe dementia were also excluded. However, as dementia is a known risk factor of poor nutritional status, this exclusion criterion can also further restrict the generalisability of our findings. As a result, our findings are better to be generalised into an outpatient PD population with mild-to-moderate stages of the disease who are not suffering from severe dementia. Finally, as has been observed in other clinical recordings, some parts of the information were self-reported and based on interviews with the patients and/or their caregivers, hence liable to inaccuracies. Recall bias may have also occurred, causing over- or under-estimated reports for some of the answers. Besides the limitations, our study is the first investigation to contribute to a better understanding of the nutritional status among Iranian PD patients. This study benefits from a large sample size, leading to an acceptable statistical power, as well as a comprehensive list of motor and psychiatric symptoms and the HRQoL, which makes the findings reliable and precise. In addition, we used the MNA questionnaire as an accepted tool to assess nutritional status, while many of the previous studies commonly used BMI and/or body weight instead.

In conclusion, evaluation of nutritional status using the MNA questionnaire in this population of PD patients has demonstrated that there is a significant correlation between PD duration and nutritional status. This significant correlation without considering chronological age, reduces the possibility that the worse MNA scores in patients with longer PD duration were due only to increasing age. In addition, we indicated that PD-related factors are associated with malnutrition in these patients. Many non-motor psychological aspects of PD were related to nutritional status as well as disease severity and level of morbidity. Different aspects of the HRQoL were also closely associated with patients' nutritional status. These cross-sectional data raise further questions and hypotheses regarding whether the individuals with insufficient nutrient intake in the past are more likely to experience malnutrition and a more severe course of PD, or if the presence of PD symptoms can hinder the capability or willingness to engage in appropriate nutritious meal preparation.

The significant correlations between the non-motor and motor symptoms of PD with malnutrition and its association with QoL bring to light the idea of using a tool to assess nutritional status in the routine evaluation of PD as the disease progresses. MNA appears to be a practical, user-friendly and cheap assessment tool for this purpose. Although the role of nutrition in the progression of neurodegenerative disorders still needs more clarification, theoretically, a vicious circle can be created if nutritional features of PD are ignored that can themselves worsen their QoL. Nevertheless, conducting follow-up longitudinal assessments and further studies involving PD patients with more severe stages of the disease may help in providing a more comprehensive picture of the nutritional status and the inter-relationships with motor and psychiatric symptoms and fatigue in PD patients.

Overall, nutritional screening using instruments such as MNA is an easy and quick way to identify patients with PD who may be at risk of malnutrition. They can then be assessed to determine if they are malnourished and to determine appropriate interventions. Based on our findings, PD patients with more depressive symptoms, severe fatigue and more severe disability who are under higher weight-adjusted levodopa dose are more likely to suffer from poor nutritional status and may benefit more from nutritional screening and follow-up assessment. Regardless of the direction of this relationship, including dietary education in the care approaches used for PD patients seems to improve their QoL.

Acknowledgments

The authors are grateful to their colleagues who contributed to the data collection from the movement disorder clinic: Hasti Hadizadeh, Farzaneh Farhadi, Nader Naderi, Arash Rahmani, Dena Khaefpanah and Ms Mahmoudi. The authors also thank all patients and caregivers for their collaboration in the collection of the data.

Author Contributions

Conceived and designed the experiments: SMF LG MS AD JL. Performed the experiments: SMF MS GAS. Analyzed the data: SMF. Contributed reagents/materials/analysis tools: SMF LG MS GAS. Wrote the paper: SMF LG MS GAS AD JL. Critically revised the final version of the manuscript for submission: SMF LG MS GAS AD JL.

References

1. Crogan NL, Pasvogel A (2003) The influence of protein-calorie malnutrition on quality of life in nursing homes. J Gerontol A Biol Sci Med Sci 58: 159–164.
2. Neumann SA, Miller MD, Daniels L, Crotty M (2005) Nutritional status and clinical outcomes of older patients in rehabilitation. J Hum Nutr Diet 18: 129–136.
3. Amaral TF, Matos LC, Teixeira MA, Tavares MM, Alvares L, et al. (2010) Undernutrition and associated factors among hospitalized patients. Clin Nutr 29: 580–585.
4. Sheard JM, Ash S, Silburn PA, Kerr GK (2013) Nutritional status in Parkinson's disease patients undergoing deep brain stimulation surgery: a pilot study. J Nutr Health Aging 17: 148–151.
5. Ahmed T, Haboubi N (2010) Assessment and management of nutrition in older people and its importance to health. Clin Interv Aging 5: 207–216.
6. Chapman IM (2006) Nutritional disorders in the elderly. Med Clin North Am 90: 887–907.
7. Kaye J, Gage H, Kimber A, Storey L, Trend P (2006) Excess burden of constipation in Parkinson's disease: a pilot study. Mov Disord 21: 1270–1273.
8. Visvanathan R, Macintosh C, Callary M, Penhall R, Horowitz M, et al. (2003) The nutritional status of 250 older Australian recipients of domiciliary care services and its association with outcomes at 12 months. J Am Geriatr Soc 51: 1007–1011.
9. Miller N, Allcock L, Hildreth AJ, Jones D, Noble E, et al. (2009) Swallowing problems in Parkinson disease: frequency and clinical correlates. J Neurol Neurosurg Psychiatry 80: 1047–1049.
10. Sheard JM, Ash S, Mellick GD, Silburn PA, Kerr GK (2013) Malnutrition in a sample of community-dwelling people with Parkinson's disease. PLoS One 8: e53290.
11. Wang G, Wan Y, Cheng Q, Xiao Q, Wang Y, et al. (2010) Malnutrition and associated factors in Chinese patients with Parkinson's disease: Results from a pilot investigation. Parkinsonism Relat Disord 16: 119–123.
12. Barichella M, Villa MC, Massarotto A, Cordara SE, Marczewska A, et al. (2008) Mini Nutritional Assessment in patients with Parkinson's disease: correlation between worsening of the malnutrition and increasing number of disease-years. Nutr Neurosci 11: 128–134.
13. Jaafar AF, Gray WK, Porter B, Turnbull EJ, Walker RW (2010) A cross-sectional study of the nutritional status of community-dwelling people with idiopathic Parkinson's disease. BMC Neurol 10: 124.
14. Hughes AJ, Daniel SE, Kilford L, Lees AJ (1992) Accuracy of clinical diagnosis of idiopathic Parkinson's disease: a clinico-pathological study of 100 cases. J Neurol Neurosurg Psychiatry 55: 181–184.
15. Hoehn MM, Yahr MD (1967) Parkinsonism: onset, progression and mortality. Neurology 17: 427–442.
16. Folstein MF, Folstein SE, McHugh PR (1975) "Mini-mental state". A practical method for grading the cognitive state of patients for the clinician. J Psychiatr Res 12: 189–198.
17. Disease MDSTFoRSfPs (2003) The Unified Parkinson's Disease Rating Scale (UPDRS): status and recommendations. Mov Disord 18: 738–750.
18. Schwab RS, EA (1969) Projection techniques for evaluating surgery in Parkinson's disease.
19. Zigmond AS, Snaith RP (1983) The hospital anxiety and depression scale. Acta Psychiatr Scand 67: 361–370.
20. Krupp LB, LaRocca NG, Muir-Nash J, Steinberg AD (1989) The fatigue severity scale. Application to patients with multiple sclerosis and systemic lupus erythematosus. Arch Neurol 46: 1121–1123.
21. Peto V, Jenkinson C, Fitzpatrick R (1998) PDQ-39: a review of the development, validation and application of a Parkinson's disease quality of life questionnaire and its associated measures. J Neurol 245 Suppl 1: S10–14.
22. Ramaker C, Marinus J, Stiggelbout AM, Van Hilten BJ (2002) Systematic evaluation of rating scales for impairment and disability in Parkinson's disease. Mov Disord 17: 867–876.
23. Nojomi M, Mostafavian Z, Shahidi GA, Jenkinson C (2010) Quality of life in patients with Parkinson's disease: Translation and psychometric evaluation of the Iranian version of PDQ-39. J Res Med Sci 15: 63–69.
24. Montazeri A, Vahdaninia M, Ebrahimi M, Jarvandi S (2003) The Hospital Anxiety and Depression Scale (HADS): translation and validation study of the Iranian version. Health Qual Life Outcomes 1: 14.
25. Azimian M, Shahvarughi Farahani A, Dadkhah A, Fallahpour M, Karimlu M (2009) Fatigue Severity Scale: The Psychometric Properties of the Persian-Version in Patients with Multiple Sclerosis. Research Journal of Biological Sciences 4: 974–977.
26. Guigoz Y, Vellas B, Garry PJ (1996) Assessing the nutritional status of the elderly: The Mini Nutritional Assessment as part of the geriatric evaluation. Nutr Rev 54: S59–65.
27. Bauer JM, Volkert D, Wirth R, Vellas B, Thomas D, et al. (2006) [Diagnosing malnutrition in the elderly]. Dtsch Med Wochenschr 131: 223–227.
28. Persson MD, Brismar KE, Katzarski KS, Nordenstrom J, Cederholm TE (2002) Nutritional status using mini nutritional assessment and subjective global assessment predict mortality in geriatric patients. J Am Geriatr Soc 50: 1996–2002.
29. Amirkalali B, Sharifi F, Fakhrzadeh H, Mirarefin M, Ghaderpanahi M, et al. (2010) Evaluation of the Mini Nutritional Assessment in the elderly, Tehran, Iran. Public Health Nutr 13: 1373–1379.
30. Lefton J, Malone A (2009) Anthropometric Assessment. In Charney P, Malone A, eds. ADA Pocket Guide to Nutrition Assessment, 2nd edition. Chicago, IL: American Dietetic Association: 160–161.
31. Guigoz Y, Vellas B, Garry PJ (1994) The Mini Nutritional Assessment (MNA): a practical assessment tool for grading the nutritional stade of elderly patients. Facts Res Gerontol 4: 15–59.
32. Tsai AC, Chang MZ (2011) Long-form but not short-form Mini-Nutritional Assessment is appropriate for grading nutritional risk of patients on hemodialysis-a cross-sectional study. Int J Nurs Stud 48: 1429–1435.
33. Afsar B, Sezer S, Arat Z, Tutal E, Ozdemir FN, et al. (2006) Reliability of mini nutritional assessment in hemodialysis compared with subjective global assessment. J Ren Nutr 16: 277–282.
34. Sheard JM, Ash S, Mellick GD, Silburn PA, Kerr GK (2013) Nutrition screening and assessment in Parkinson's disease: A comparison of methods. e-SPEN Journal 8: e187–e192.
35. Uc EY, Struck LK, Rodnitzky RL, Zimmerman B, Dobson J, et al. (2006) Predictors of weight loss in Parkinson's disease. Mov Disord 21: 930–936.
36. Jaafar A, Porter B, Gray WK, Turnbull EJ, Walker RW (2010) A study of the nutritional status of people with idiopathic Parkinson's disease: comparison of urban and rural community dwellers. In: Abstracts of the 14th International Congress of Parkinson's Disease and Movement Disorders. Mov Disord (Suppl 2): S424.
37. Markus HS, Tomkins AM, Stern GM (1993) Increased prevalence of undernutrition in Parkinson's disease and its relationship to clinical disease parameters. J Neural Transm Park Dis Dement Sect 5: 117–125.
38. Serrano-Urrea R, Garcia-Meseguer MJ (2013) Malnutrition in an Elderly Population without Cognitive Impairment Living in Nursing Homes in Spain: Study of Prevalence Using the Mini Nutritional Assessment Test. Gerontology 59: 490–498.
39. Yapa RSS, Playfer JR, Lye M (1989) Anthropometric and nutritional assessment of elderly patients with Parkinson's disease. J Clin Exp Gerontol. 11: 155–164.
40. Beyer PL, Palarino MY, Michalek D, Busenbark K, Koller WC (1995) Weight change and body composition in patients with Parkinson's disease. J Am Diet Assoc 95: 979–983.
41. Sheard JM, Ash S, Mellick GD, Silburn PA, Kerr GK (2013) Markers of disease severity are associated with malnutrition in Parkinson's disease. PLoS One 8: e57986.
42. Sheard JM, Ash S, Silburn PA, Kerr GK (2011) Prevalence of malnutrition in Parkinson's disease: a systematic review. Nutr Rev 69: 520–532.
43. Lorefalt B, Ganowiak W, Palhagen S, Toss G, Unosson M, et al. (2004) Factors of importance for weight loss in elderly patients with Parkinson's disease. Acta Neurol Scand 110: 180–187.
44. Bollwein J, Volkert D, Diekmann R, Kaiser MJ, Uter W, et al. (2013) Nutritional status according to the mini nutritional assessment (MNA(R)) and frailty in community dwelling older persons: a close relationship. J Nutr Health Aging 17: 351–356.
45. Andersson I, Sidenvall B (2001) Case studies of food shopping, cooking and eating habits in older women with Parkinson's disease. J Adv Nurs 35: 69–78.
46. Barichella M, Marczewska A, Vairo A, Canesi M, Pezzoli G (2003) Is underweightness still a major problem in Parkinson's disease patients? Eur J Clin Nutr 57: 543–547.
47. Nozaki S, Saito T, Matsumura T, Miyai I, Kang J (1999) [Relationship between weight loss and dysphagia in patients with Parkinson's disease]. Rinsho Shinkeigaku 39: 1010–1014.
48. Durrieu G LM, Rascol O, Senard JM, Rascol A, Montastruc JL (1992) Parkinson's disease and weight loss: a study with anthropometric and nutritional assessment. Clin Auton Res 2(3): 153–157.
49. Barichella M, Cereda E, Madio C, Iorio L, Pusani C, et al. (2013) Nutritional risk and gastrointestinal dysautonomia symptoms in Parkinson's disease outpatients hospitalised on a scheduled basis. Br J Nutr 110: 347–353.
50. Barichella M, Cereda E, Pezzoli G (2009) Major nutritional issues in the management of Parkinson's disease. Mov Disord 24: 1881–1892.
51. Cereda E, Pezzoli G, Barichella M (2010) Role of an electronic armband in motor function monitoring in patients with Parkinson's disease. Nutrition 26: 240–242.
52. Teasdale N, Hue O, Simoneau M, Tremblay A, Marceau P, et al. (2007) Predictors of weight loss in Parkinson's disease: is weight loss the chicken or the egg? Mov Disord 22: 436–437.

Differential Pathways to Adult Metabolic Dysfunction following Poor Nutrition at Two Critical Developmental Periods in Sheep

Kirsten R. Poore*, Lisa J. Hollis, Robert J. S. Murray, Anna Warlow, Andrew Brewin, Laurence Fulford, Jane K. Cleal, Karen A. Lillycrop, Graham C. Burdge, Mark A. Hanson, Lucy R. Green

Academic Unit of Human Development and Health, Faculty of Medicine, University of Southampton, Southampton, United Kingdom

Abstract

Epidemiological and experimental studies suggest early nutrition has long-term effects on susceptibility to obesity, cardiovascular and metabolic diseases. Small and large animal models confirm the influence of different windows of sensitivity, from fetal to early postnatal life, on offspring phenotype. We showed previously that undernutrition in sheep either during the first month of gestation or immediately after weaning induces differential, sex-specific changes in adult metabolic and cardiovascular systems. The current study aims to determine metabolic and molecular changes that underlie differences in lipid and glucose metabolism induced by undernutrition during specific developmental periods in male and female sheep. Ewes received 100% (C) or 50% nutritional requirements (U) from 1–31 days gestation, and 100% thereafter. From weaning (12 weeks) to 25 weeks, offspring were then fed either *ad libitum* (CC, UC) or were undernourished (CU, UU) to reduce body weight to 85% of their individual target. From 25 weeks, all offspring were fed *ad libitum*. A cohort of late gestation fetuses were studied after receiving either 40% nutritional requirements (1–31 days gestation) or 50% nutritional requirements (104–127 days gestation). Post-weaning undernutrition increased *in vivo* insulin sensitivity, insulin receptor and glucose transporter 4 expression in muscle, and lowered hepatic methylation at the delta-like homolog 1/maternally expressed gene 3 imprinted cluster in adult females, but not males. Early gestational undernutrition induced lower hepatic expression of gluconeogenic factors in fetuses and reduced *in vivo* adipose tissue insulin sensitivity in adulthood. In males, undernutrition in early gestation increased adipose tissue lipid handling mechanisms (lipoprotein lipase, glucocorticoid receptor expression) and hepatic methylation within the imprinted control region of insulin-like growth factor 2 receptor in adulthood. Therefore, undernutrition during development induces changes in mechanisms of lipid and glucose metabolism which differ between tissues and sexes dependent on the period of nutritional restriction. Such changes may increase later life obesity and dyslipidaemia risk.

Editor: Nick Ashton, The University of Manchester, United Kingdom

Funding: This work was supported by a Wessex Medical Research Innovation Fund (M13) (www.wesmed.org.uk), a Biotechnology and Biosciences project grant (D17858) (http://www.bbsrc.ac.uk) and a Gerald Kerkut Trust PhD Studentship (http://www.southampton.ac.uk/~gktrust/). Professor Mark Hanson is funded by British Heart Foundation (http://www.bhf.org.uk). The funders had no role in study design, data collection and analysis, decision to publish, or preparation of the manuscript.

Competing Interests: The authors have declared that no competing interests exist.

* E-mail: kpoore@soton.ac.uk

Introduction

The worldwide incidence of obesity nearly doubled between 1980 and 2008, affecting both developed countries and developing societies that are undergoing socio-economic transition [1]. Strategies to reduce obesity by promoting healthy eating and an active lifestyle are producing disappointing results [2] and lifestyle factors do not appear to have the same impact on obesity in all individuals. Epidemiological and animal studies demonstrate that early life nutrition can exert a major influence on susceptibility to obesity, cardiovascular and metabolic diseases in adulthood [3,4]. Thus, knowledge of an individual's nutritional pathway during development may be beneficial in devising effective strategies to reduce the risk of obesity and its consequences.

The timing of nutritional challenges during development dictates the type, direction and magnitude of changes in the offspring's metabolic and cardiovascular phenotype. Mid- and late-gestation exposure to the Dutch Famine reduced birth weight and glucose tolerance in adulthood, which worsened with obesity [5] while early gestation famine exposure did not affect birth weight, but increased coronary heart disease prevalence and atherogenic risk factors [6,7]. Postnatally, nutrition and growth patterns also influence later metabolic health, with reduced birth size, persistent thinness in infancy but accelerated childhood growth and later obesity conferring increased risk of insulin resistance and dyslipidaemia [8–11]. Malnutrition in the first year also reduces glucose tolerance and insulin sensitivity in young men, independent of birth weight [12]. As well as investigating low birth weight and thinness at birth [13,14] it is now clear that a range of possible developmental pathways to poor health in adulthood should be considered. These include the periconceptional and fetal periods and/or early postnatal infant life and beyond.

Animal models have confirmed the influence of different windows of sensitivity on offspring phenotype and work towards elucidating mechanisms in different tissues [15–20]. In sheep, undernutrition either during the first month of gestation or immediately after weaning (before puberty/adolescence) induces differential, sex-specific changes in metabolic and cardiovascular systems in adulthood. In males, cardiovascular abnormalities such as left ventricular hypertrophy were observed following exposure to undernutrition in early gestation (with no effect on birth weight) which was ameliorated if postnatal nutrition was relatively 'matched' to that prenatally [21]. In contrast, post-weaning undernutrition improved glucose tolerance and insulin sensitivity in both young and mature females, regardless of early gestation undernutrition [22]. Small for gestational age human infants also show increased sensitivity to insulin [23]. In females particularly, this may help return body weight towards a threshold necessary for successful reproductive function [23]. No such adaptation was observed in male sheep undernourished post-weaning [22], suggesting they must employ different strategies to regain body weight. Although an increase in fat was observed in young but not mature adult females exposed to both early gestation and post-weaning undernutrition [22], metabolic abnormalities may become apparent before overt obesity [24]. We suggest that enhanced insulin sensitivity in postnatally undernourished females may facilitate body weight recovery but increase their susceptibility to later obesity so long as nutrient supply is abundant. Indeed alterations in glucose metabolism and liver function in aged sheep exposed to maternal undernutrition have been observed only following a later period of unlimited feeding [25].

Epigenetic regulation by DNA methylation provides a mechanism linking suboptimal nutrition with long-lasting changes in specific gene expression and later phenotype [26,27,28]; for example epigenetic markers in neonatal blood and cord tissue have been linked with later adiposity and cardiometabolic risk factors [29,30]. Furthermore, hepatic epigenetic modifications are detectable in early postnatal life following maternal undernutrition, before the phenotypic changes appear within the liver or other metabolic tissues, suggesting an interaction between the later environment and these modifications [24,31]. The influence of early postnatal diet on epigenetic mechanisms remains little studied [32].

To develop biomarkers of risk and suggest preventative measures for obesity requires a detailed molecular phenotype in metabolically active tissues and understanding of lipid metabolism that may predispose to inappropriate adipose deposition. Large animal models allow links between specific molecular and epigenetic alterations in a range of tissues and whole animal phenotype. The aim of this study was therefore to determine underlying differences in lipid metabolism in male and female sheep following early gestation and/or post-weaning undernutrition, both *in vivo* and at the molecular level. We have measured circulating non-esterified fatty acid (NEFA) and triacylglycerol (TAG) during a glucose tolerance test (GTT) and mRNA levels of peroxisome proliferator-activated receptor γ (PPARγ; regulation of adipocyte differentiation), lipoprotein lipase (LPL; hydrolyses triglycerides and regulates their movement into adipocytes) and glucocorticoid receptor (GR; mediates glucocorticoid effects on adipose lipid accumulation and mobilisation) in metabolically active tissues. The mechanistic basis of the persistent, sex-specific effect of post-weaning undernutrition on metabolic homeostasis was also examined in tissues that regulate glucose and lipid uptake by measuring insulin receptor (IR), glucose transporter 4 (GLUT4), GR, phosphoenolpyruvate carboxykinase (PEPCK) and glucose-6-phosphatase (G6Pase). We have also investigated epigenetic modifications of hepatic genes regulating metabolic homeostasis and body composition by measuring methylation of imprinting control regions (ICRs) of the insulin-like growth factor (IGF) 2/H19 and insulin-like growth factor-2 receptor (IGF2R) imprinted clusters and of the delta-like homolog 1 (DLK1)/ maternally expressed gene 3 (MEG3) imprinted cluster, which are involved in fetal and early postnatal growth and in adipocyte development, respectively, and have been linked with metabolic abnormalities and changes in adiposity [33–35]. We proposed that for females undernutrition prior to puberty will have a greater impact on mechanisms that control lipid and glucose metabolism, given the importance of maintaining adequate body condition for future reproductive success. In males, we proposed early gestation undernutrition will have a greater impact on mechanisms regulating adiposity, due to the relatively greater need for nutrients to drive their faster growth rate during gestation. We found that exposure to both gestational and post-weaning undernutrition induces sex- and tissue-specific effects on lipid and glucose handling mechanisms that may increase obesity and dyslipidaemia risk in later life.

Materials and Methods

Study of Adult Offspring Exposed to Early Life Undernutrition

Animals. All procedures were carried out in accordance with the regulations of the UK Home Office Animals (Scientific Procedures) Act, 1986 (PPL 30/1858). The data in this study comes from the same cohort of sheep previously studied by us and for which other data have been published elsewhere [21,22,36]. Fifty-nine Welsh Mountain ewes in their second or third parity (2–3 years old), carrying singleton and twin pregnancies, and of uniform good body condition score (BCS; ~3 on a scale of 1–5 [37]) were used in this study. Full details about ewe mating, ewe and lamb housing and diets are presented elsewhere [22]. All manipulations of ewes and of lambs until 1.5 years of age took place at the Royal Veterinary College, North Mymms. A flow diagram showing the allocation of ewes and their offspring to the different dietary regimes is presented in Figure S1.

Before conception, ewes were randomly assigned to a control or a dietary restricted group. Control ewes (early gestation control, C; $n = 29$; 12 singleton (s), 17 twin (t)) received 100% nutritional requirements before and throughout gestation. From 1–31 days gestation (dGA; term = 147 days), ewes in the dietary restricted group (early gestation undernutrition, U; $n = 31$; 15 s, 15 t) received 50% nutritional requirements and then 100% requirements for the remainder of gestation. From −7 dGA, ewes were weighed weekly. The starting pelleted diet ration for each ewe was calculated using RUMNUT software (Ruminant Nutrition) version 5 for sheep (AT Chamberlain, Hampshire) based on initial body weight. This ration was adjusted weekly according to their weight measurement. The RUMNUT software was based on AFRC Guidelines for pregnant sheep [38] and incorporated adjustments for weight gain according to gestational age. Water was provided *ad libitum*. Ewes were individually penned from −7 to 37 dGA and group housed thereafter with animals at a similar gestational age. Ewes delivered and suckled lambs naturally while receiving 100% nutritional requirements, with further feed ration adjustments according to lactational needs [38].

A total of 77 male and female, singleton and twin, lambs were included in the study (Figure S1). Lambs were weaned at 12 weeks, after gradual introduction of the post-weaning diet [22]. Lambs from C and U ewes were grouped with approximately 10 others of similar body weight and post-weaning treatment group in open barns. For each lamb, an individual linear weight trajectory was calculated for the period 12–25 weeks that was based on weights taken at birth, 4, 8 and 12 weeks. Lambs were assigned to either a post-weaning control diet (yielding early gestation control/post-weaning control, CC; early gestation undernutrition/post-weaning control, UC) or post-weaning undernutrition diet (early gestation control/post-weaning undernutrition, CU; early gestation undernutrition/post-weaning undernutrition, UU). Post-weaning control lambs were fed 100% nutritional requirements to follow their individual trajectory from 12–25 weeks and post-weaning undernutrition lambs were fed a restricted pelleted diet such that body weight was reduced to 85% of their individual target weight from 12–25 weeks. Lambs had free access to hay throughout. To keep body weight on the desired trajectory, lambs were monitored individually by weekly weighing and feed ration adjustment. If necessary, lambs were temporarily removed to individual pens to maintain body weight at the desired level. For twin lambs, one twin was assigned to the post-weaning control diet and the other to the post-weaning undernutrition diet, except for twin pairs from 14 ewes in which only one offspring of the pair was used (Figure S1). The number, sex and proportion of singleton to twin lambs in each group are as follows; males: CC, $n = 13$ (5 s, 8 t), CU, $n = 8$ (3 s, 5 t), UC, $n = 8$ (4 s, 4 t), UU, $n = 11$ (5 s, 6 t); females: CC, $n = 9$ (2 s, 7 t), CU, $n = 7$ (2 s, 5 t), UC, $n = 10$ (2 s, 8 t), UU, $n = 11$ (4 s, 7 t).

From 25 week onwards, all lambs were returned to larger group housing and received 100% nutritional requirements. All lambs were weighed at 35 weeks and just prior to experiments (see below) at 16.5±0.1 months (1.5 years) and 29.6±0.2 months (2.5 years) of age. At each experimental age, body condition score was assessed manually and fat and muscle depths were measured by ultrasound in the third lumbar region by a small number of experienced animal technicians, as described previously [22].

For technical reasons e.g catheter loss prior to *in vivo* experiments or difficulty with laboratory procedures, data from the full number of animals in each group were not always achieved. The number of observations for each data set is indicated in the legend of each table or figure or within the text of the results section.

Surgical techniques. As described previously [22], surgery at 9.9 months (to create carotid artery loops for repeated arterial access and to vasectomise male lambs) and experiments at 1.5 years of age were performed at the Royal Veterinary College and experiments at 2.5 years were performed at the University of Southampton. Prior to each set of experiments, sheep were moved into individual cages and acclimatised for 4–6 days, with no change in their feeding regime. Indwelling carotid artery and jugular vein catheters were inserted under general anaesthesia (at 1.5 years: 2–4% halothane in O_2 by face mask; at 2.5 years: induced by thiopentone sodium (10 mg.kg^{-1}, *i.v.*) and maintained by 2–4% halothane in O_2 by endotracheal tube). Antibiotic treatment (15 mg.kg^{-1}, *i.m.*; Betamox) was administered to all sheep. At 1.5 years, catheters were maintained for 3 days then removed prior to sheep returning to group housing. At 2.5 years, catheters were maintained for up to 17 days during a series of experiments and subsequent *post mortem* that are described elsewhere [21,22,39].

Experimental protocol. At 1.5 and 2.5 years of age, a glucose tolerance test (GTT) was performed following an overnight fast (16.00 h–09.00 h). Glucose (0.5 g.kg body weight^{-1}) was administered as an intravenous bolus over 3 minutes and arterial blood samples (3 ml into chilled EDTA tubes) were collected immediately before (0 min) and at 10, 20, 30, 60, and 120 min after the start of the glucose administration (time 0). All blood samples were centrifuged immediately (10 min at 4°C) and plasma was stored at –20°C for later laboratory analysis.

Study of Fetuses Exposed to Gestational Undernutrition

Animals. A separate cohort of 23 Welsh Mountain primiparous ewes, carrying singleton fetuses, of uniform body condition score were used for collection of late gestation fetal tissues. As described previously [40], ewes were randomly assigned to a control or one of two dietary restricted groups, housed individually on straw and from −16 dGA (adjusted to gestational age) were fed a complete pelleted diet (89.2% dry matter as fed, providing 10.7 MJ.(kg dry matter)$^{-1}$ (metabolisable energy) and 14.8% protein) with water available *ad libitum*. Control ewes (C, $n = 8$; 4 male and 4 female fetuses) were fed 100% nutritional requirements throughout gestation. Early gestation nutrient-restricted ewes (E, $n = 9$; 5 male and 4 female fetuses) were fed 40% of nutrient requirements from 1−31 dGA and late gestation nutrient-restricted ewes (L, $n = 6$; 4 male and 2 female fetuses) were fed 50% of nutrient requirements from 104−127 dGA (term ~147 dGA). At all other times, ewes received 100% nutrient requirements. Full details about ewe mating, surgical and experimental procedures in these fetuses that are not presented in the current study are described elsewhere [40,41].

Post Mortem Procedures

At the completion of all experimental protocols, *i.v.* pentobarbitone sodium overdose (200 mg.ml^{-1} Pentoject, Animalcare Ltd, UK) was used to kill adult sheep (2.5 years) or pregnant ewes and their fetuses (at 127 dGA). Samples of left and right lobes of the liver were removed from both adults and fetuses and skeletal (flexor digitorum longus) muscle and perirenal adipose tissue was removed from adults. All tissues were snap frozen in liquid nitrogen and stored at −80°C.

Laboratory Analysis

mRNA expression analysis. Total RNA was extracted from adult muscle, adult adipose tissue and fetal and adult left and right liver lobe using the TRIzol method and reverse transcribed into cDNA. Real-time RT PCR (ABL Prism 7700 and 7500 Sequence Detection System, Applied Biosystems Step One Plus) was used to measure mRNA expression for IR in all adult and fetal tissues, GLUT4 in adult muscle and adipose tissue, GR in adult adipose tissue and adult and fetal liver, LPL and PPAR-γ in adult adipose tissue, PEPCK and G6Pase in adult and fetal liver, IGFII and IGF2R in the left lobe of adult liver. Primers and probes (Table S1) were designed using Primer Express Software (Applied Biosystems, USA). GR in adult adipose tissue, IGFII and IGF2R gene expression and expression of housekeeping genes were measured using SYBR Green (JumpStart Taq ReadyMix, Sigma Aldrich S4438). Gene expression in adult muscle and adipose tissues was normalised to the geometric mean of β-actin and glyceraldehyde 3-phosphate dehydrogenase (GAPDH) mRNA expression, as determined using a GeNorm normalising kit (Primer Design, Southampton, UK) validated for use in the sheep. In adult and fetal liver, gene expression was normalised to the geometric mean of glyceraldehyde 3-phosphate dehydrogenase (GAPDH), ribosomal protein 19 large subunit (RPL-19) and β-actin mRNA expression, as determined using the GeNorm normalising kit. GR gene expression in adult adipose tissue was performed before the GeNorm kit became available so these data were normalised to 18S mRNA expression. Coefficients of variation ranged from 6% to 10%.

PCR-based methylation analysis. PCR was used to amplify regions within the imprinting control regions (ICRs) of the DLK1/MEG3, IGF2R and IGF2/H19 imprinted clusters (Table S1) then DNA methylation levels were analysed by pyrosequencing using a PyroMark Q96 (Biotage/Qiagen), as described previously [42]. In brief, genomic DNA from adult left liver lobe was bisulfite converted using the EZ DNA Methylation-Gold Kit (Zymo Research), following manufacturer's guidelines. The expression of the DLK1/MEG3 imprinted cluster is regulated, like the IGF2/H19 cluster, by binding of CTCF within the ICR region, which is itself influenced by the presence or absence of DNA methylation at CTCF binding sites. We identified a potential CTCF site within the MEG3 ICR, based upon reported CTCF consensus sequences [43–45] that contained CpG dinucleotides 2, 3, and 4, and was directly adjacent to CpG1 within the pyrosequencing assay. Methylation at the H19 loci was examined across CTCF binding site IV, which has previously been shown to regulate H19 expression [44,46]. Methylation within the ICR of IGF2R, a 2.3 Kb CpG island regulates IGF2R expression in sheep [46,47].

Determination of DNA methylation within the GR promoter region was undertaken prior to the availability of the above methodology, therefore for this data set methylation-sensitive PCR was used. PCR was used to amplify DNA extracted from adult left and right liver lobes and treated with methylation-sensitive restriction enzymes (AciI and HpaII). GR primers were designed to amplify two regions within the CpG island within the GR promoter region, based on a partial ovine sequence determined by express sequence tag mapping to the bovine sequence (Table S1).

Plasma lipid analysis. Plasma NEFA and TAG concentrations during GTT at 1.5 and 2.5 years were measured to assess insulin-induced inhibition of lipolysis in adipose tissue. A randomly chosen subset of animals was included for these measurements. Plasma NEFA concentrations were measured by a spectrophotometric two-stage enzymatic assay kit (Wako NEFA HR2, ACS-ACOD method; Alpha Laboratories, Eastleigh, UK) on a Konelab 20 autoanalyser (Thermo Fisher Scientific, Hemel Hempstead, UK). This method was not sensitive enough to measure TAG concentrations. Therefore, gas chromatography (HP 6890 Series GC System equipped with a flame ionisation detector and 7683B Series Injector) was used, following separation of lipid classes by solid phase extraction, to measure plasma TAG concentrations (extracted from 0.4 g plasma, made up to 0.8 ml) or adipose total lipid content (extracted from 20 mg adipose tissue), as described previously [48].

Data Analysis

For NEFA and TAG analysis during GTT in adult sheep, summary measures (baseline, slope, maximum fall from baseline and area under curve relative to baseline (AUC)) were calculated. For all adult data except liver, the effects of four main factors were tested (early gestation diet, post-weaning diet, sex and offspring number (i.e. singleton or twin)) using multifactorial analyses of variance (4-way ANOVA). For adult liver, the same factors were examined using multifactorial analyses of variance for repeated measures (RM ANOVA), with liver lobe as the repeated measure. For fetal liver, the main factors of maternal dietary group and fetal sex were used in a RM ANOVA, with liver lobe as the repeated measure. Where significant effects of a main factor or interactions between the main factors were found, further analyses were performed within subsets of the data. Linear regression analysis was used to examine relationships between two factors: this was done within each sex, across all nutritional groups. Statistical analyses were performed using GraphPad Prism version 5 and SPSS version 11. Data are expressed as mean ± S.E.M. and significance was accepted at $p<0.05$, with a trend noted when $0.05<p<0.1$.

Results

Lipid Metabolism during Glucose Tolerance Test

Diminished insulin-induced inhibition of lipolysis in adult males and females undernourished in early gestation. Plasma NEFA and TAG concentrations during a glucose tolerance test (GTT), performed in both young (1.5 years) and mature (2.5 years) adulthood [22] were determined as a surrogate measure of insulin-induced adipose tissue lipid metabolism. The insulin-induced fall in NEFA output during GTT was reduced ($p<0.05$) at 2.5 years in sheep exposed to early gestation undernutrition, regardless of post-weaning nutrition (Fig. 1B). There was no effect of sex on this response. The slope from 10–30 min during the GTT tended to be shallower in UC and UU groups (-9.4 ± 0.9 *vs.* -7.2 ± 1.4 μmol.l.min^{-1}, $p<0.1$). Basal NEFA and TAG concentrations at 2.5 years were not influenced by early life nutrition (Table 1). There was no effect of early gestation undernutrition on plasma NEFA and TAG concentrations during the GTT at 1.5 years. Faster relative growth during the first 12 postnatal week was associated with reduced NEFA AUC at 2.5 years ($r^2=0.20$, $p<0.05$). Low birth weight was associated with increased NEFA AUC at 2.5 years ($r^2=0.16$, $p<0.005$).

Increased insulin sensitivity in mature adult females undernourished post-weaning. At 1.5 years, there were no overall effects of post-weaning nutrition or sex on plasma NEFA or TAG concentrations before (Table 1) or during GTT (data not shown). Basal NEFA and TAG concentrations in 1.5 year-old males and females combined were positively related to current fatness (back fat depth corrected for body weight; $r^2=0.16$ and 0.19, respectively; $p<0.01$). At 2.5 years, in females only, the maximum fall in plasma TAG concentrations during GTT was greater (indicating increased insulin sensitivity) in animals undernourished only in the post-weaning period (CU, 11.5 ± 5.5 μg.ml^{-1}) compared to controls (CC, 8.7 ± 1.4 μg.ml^{-1}). Adipose tissue lipid content was also reduced ($p<0.05$) in CU compared to CC females at 2.5 years (Table 2).

Tissue Expression of Factors Involved in Lipid Metabolism

Increased adipose tissue lipid handling factors in adult males undernourished in early gestation. In males, but not females, both LPL and GR mRNA levels in adipose tissue at 2.5 years were significantly higher in sheep exposed to early gestation undernutrition (Fig. 2). This was not associated with an effect on adipose tissue lipid content (Table 2). PPARγ (Table 2), LPL (Fig. 2) and GR mRNA (1.49 ± 0.05 *vs.* 0.97 ± 0.05 arbitrary units) levels in adipose tissue at 2.5 years were significantly ($p<0.001$) higher in males than females. Faster relative growth during the first 12 postnatal weeks was associated with higher GR mRNA levels in adipose tissue ($r^2=0.11$, $p<0.05$).

Adipose tissue factors are unaffected by post-weaning undernutrition. There were no significant effects of post-weaning nutrient restriction on mRNA levels of PPARγ, LPL or GR in adipose tissue of either male or female sheep at 2.5 years (Fig. 2, Table 2).

Tissue Expression of Factors Involved in Glucose Metabolism

Hepatic gluconeogenic gene expression during fetal but not adult life is reduced by early and late gestation undernutrition. In a cohort of late gestation (127 days) singleton fetuses exposed to a 40% nutrient restriction in early gestation (compared to 50% in the adult cohort), PEPCK mRNA levels were reduced ($p<0.05$) in both hepatic lobes (Fig. 3). Levels

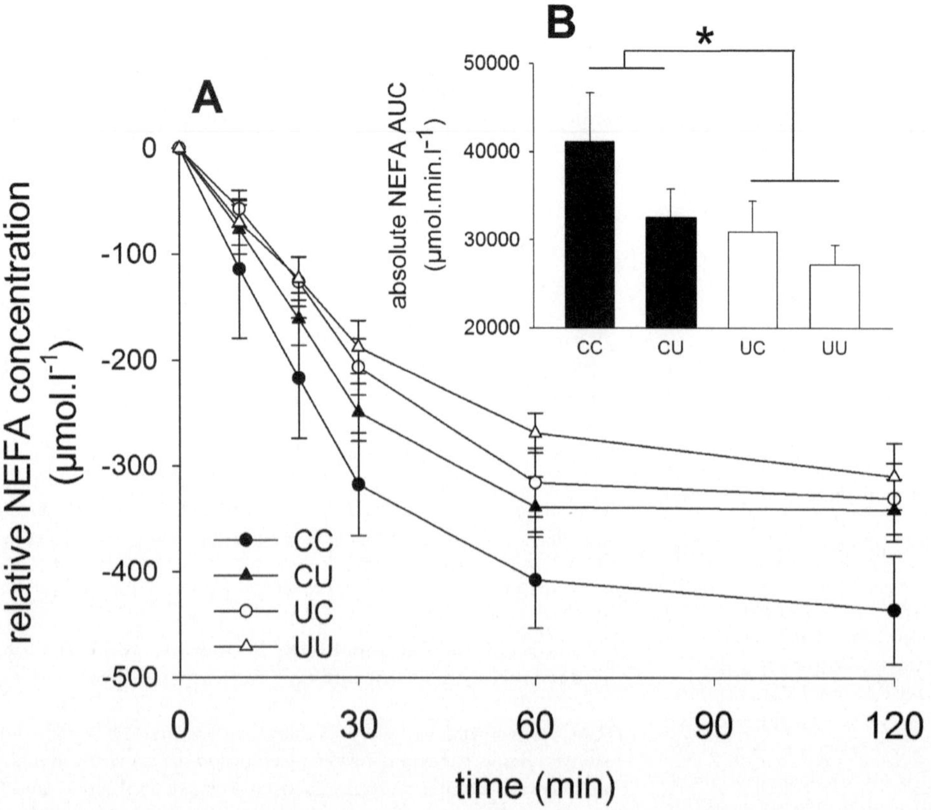

Figure 1. ***In vivo*** **lipid handling in 2.5 year-old sheep.** (A) Plasma non-esterified fatty acid (NEFA) concentrations relative to baseline in male and female sheep combined during a glucose tolerance test at 2.5 years. Glucose (0.5 g.kg^{-1}) was given at time 0. (B) Absolute area under the NEFA response curve (AUC); *p<0.05, early gestation undernutrition groups less than early gestation control groups. CC: *n* = 13; CU: *n* = 14; UC: *n* = 15; UU: *n* = 13). Values are mean ± S.E.M.

of GR ($p<0.01$) and G6Pase ($p<0.05$) mRNA in fetal liver were also reduced by early gestation undernutrition, but in a lobe-specific manner. PEPCK, GR and G6Pase mRNA levels were similarly reduced in fetuses exposed during late gestation (104–127 days) (Fig. 3).

In adult tissues, early gestation undernutrition had no effect on IR mRNA levels in muscle (Fig. 4), adipose tissue or liver (Table 2), or on hepatic GR, PEPCK or G6Pase mRNA levels (Fig. 2, Table 2). While being a twin had no bearing on adult glucose tolerance in this model, GLUT4 mRNA levels in muscle were elevated in adult female twins undernourished in early gestation (UC and UU combined ($n = 11$), 1.28±0.08 *vs.* CC and CU combined ($n = 12$), 0.90±0.08 arbitrary units; $p<0.005$). Early gestation undernutrition increased PEPCK mRNA levels ($p<0.05$) in the adult right liver lobe compared to controls, but only in singleton males (0.31±0.04 *vs.* 0.18±0.04 arbitrary units).

Gluconeogenic genes in liver differs between the lobes. There was differential expression of gluconeogenic genes between the fetal liver lobes, with G6Pase ($p<0.01$) and GR ($p = 0.065$) expression overall greater in the left (29.09±5.93 and 8.85±0.66, respectively) compared to the right (20.34±4.15 and 7.18±0.73 arbitrary units, respectively) liver lobe. Regardless of early gestation or post-weaning undernutrition, in adult liver GR mRNA levels overall were greatest ($p<0.001$) in the right lobe compared to left lobe in males and females (males: 7.14±0.53 *vs.* 3.24±0.23; females: 3.56±0.25 *vs.* 2.30±0.16 arbitrary units) and PEPCK mRNA levels were greatest ($p<0.05$) in the left lobe compared to right lobe in males (0.27±0.02 *vs.* 0.22±0.02 arbitrary units). Both GR and PEPCK mRNA levels overall were higher ($p<0.001$) in adult male than female liver, regardless of lobe (5.19±0.22 *vs.* 2.93±0.26 and 0.24±0.02 *vs.* 0.14±0.02 arbitrary units, respectively) and in female twins compared to singletons (3.89±0.26 *vs.* 3.24±0.43 arbitrary units (right liver lobe) and 0.21±0.02 *vs.* 0.10±0.03 (left liver lobe), respectively, see also Table 2). DNA methylation within the GR promoter region in adult liver was not affected by lobe, nutrition, sex or offspring number (Table 2).

Increased insulin signalling factors in muscle in adult females undernourished post-weaning. Post-weaning undernutrition in adult female, but not male sheep, regardless of early gestation undernutrition, significantly ($p<0.05$) increased mRNA levels of IR and GLUT4 in skeletal muscle but not in perirenal adipose tissue (Fig. 4, Table 2). Reduced growth rate during the period of post-weaning undernutrition from 12–25 weeks was also directly associated with increased IR and GLUT4 mRNA levels in muscle from females ($r^2 = 0.17$, $p<0.05$ and $r^2 = 0.22$, $p<0.01$, respectively). The effect of post-weaning undernutrition on GLUT4 mRNA levels was strongest in singleton sheep, as revealed by investigation of a significant ($p<0.05$) interaction between post-weaning undernutrition and offspring number: CU and UU singletons combined, 1.25±0.10 ($n = 4$) *vs.* CC and UC singletons combined, 0.74±0.12 ($n = 4$) arbitrary units. Post-weaning nutrition restriction had no effect in the liver on IR, GR, PEPCK or G6Pase mRNA levels (Table 2), except in the right liver lobe where PEPCK mRNA levels in singleton male sheep were reduced by post-weaning undernutrition (CU and UU combined,

Table 1. Basal plasma NEFA and TAG concentrations in young (1.5 years) and mature (2.5 years) adult male and female sheep.

	Males				Females			
	CC	CU	UC	UU	CC	UC	CU	UU
1.5 Years:								
NEFA (μmol.l^{-1})	792±70$^{(5)}$	647±53$^{(5)}$	747±104$^{(5)}$	748±132$^{(5)}$	828±93$^{(6)}$	914±72$^{(5)}$	907±52$^{(5)}$	815±90$^{(5)}$
TAG (μmol.l^{-1})	36.4±4.0$^{(6)}$	27.1±6.5$^{(4)}$	5.3±5.3$^{(6)}$	34.9±11.6$^{(6)}$	38.2±11.4$^{(5)}$	38.6±4.9$^{(5)}$	33.9±4.0$^{(5)}$	41.5±12.0$^{(5)}$
2.5 Years:								
NEFA (μmol.l^{-1})	482±65$^{(7)}$	410±35$^{(8)}$	375±52$^{(8)}$	384±46$^{(8)}$	544±83$^{(6)}$	448±49$^{(6)}$	443±52$^{(7)}$	399±50$^{(6)}$
TAG (μmol.l^{-1})	22.8±3.2$^{(9)}$	30.8±6.7$^{(6)}$	19.0±1.8$^{(6)}$	27.3±5.0$^{(7)}$	25.0±2.3$^{(6)}$	29.9±7.5$^{(5)}$	17.4±3.2$^{(7)}$	21.3±1.6$^{(6)}$

Data are mean ± S.E.M. Values in brackets represent number of observations.

0.16±0.02 (n = 8) *vs.* CC and UC combined, 0.31±0.06 (n = 10) arbitrary units).

Hepatic Methylation Pattern of Factors Regulating Metabolic Homeostasis and Body Composition

Increased methylation of imprinted genes regulating growth in adult males undernourished in early gestation. There was a significant ($p<0.05$) increase in methylation within the ICR of IGF2R at CpG 11, 13 and 15 in left liver lobe from 2.5 year-old males undernourished in early gestation but not from females (Fig. 5). Early gestation undernutrition had no effect on methylation at the IGF2/H19 or DLK/MEG3 loci in adult liver in either sex (Fig. 5). There were no effects of early gestation undernutrition on IGFII or IGF2R mRNA levels in adult liver (Table 2).

Decreased methylation of adipocyte development factor DLK/MEG3 in adult females undernourished post-weaning. In female but not male sheep, post-weaning undernutrition significantly reduced hepatic DLK/MEG3 methylation at CpG dinucleotides 1, 2, 3, and 4 (Fig. 5), an effect that could reduce expression of DLK1. There was no significant effect of post-weaning undernutrition on IGF2R or IGF2/H19 imprinted clusters (Fig. 5). Poor growth in females between 12 and 25 weeks was associated with decreased DLK/MEG3 methylation at CpG 2, 3 and 4 (r^2 = 0.24, 0.29 and 0.18, respectively, $p<0.005$). There was a positive relationship in 2.5 year-old males between DLK/MEG3 methylation at CpG 4 in left liver lobe and muscle depth (r^2 = 0.13, $p<0.05$).

Discussion

This large animal study is unique in its comparison of the effects of a postnatal nutrient restriction challenge in the context of a previous prenatal nutritional challenge. We have shown that exposure to both early gestation and post-weaning undernutrition have sex- and tissue-specific effects on mechanisms of lipid and glucose metabolism, effects that may increase the risk of obesity and dyslipidaemia in later life. The presence of sex differences in the current study confirms differential effects on metabolic and cardiovascular parameters previously reported in sheep [21,22], and goes further to suggest that males and females adopt different strategies in the face of reduced nutrition at critical windows of development.

We showed previously that female sheep undernourished in the post-weaning period make metabolic adaptations, improving their glucose handling, that persist from young through to mature adulthood [22]. In the current study, we show that this effect is likely brought about by enhanced insulin-induced glucose uptake specifically into muscle, via increased insulin receptor and glucose transporter 4 mRNA levels. Factors which are known to be involved in hepatic insulin sensitivity, in the regulation of gluconeogenesis and in adipose tissue differentiation and lipid hydrolysis, were unaffected by post-weaning undernutrition in this study. The effect in muscle is consistent with studies of improved insulin signalling capacity in intra-uterine growth restricted fetal sheep [49] and in rat offspring exposed to maternal low protein diet [19], and provides a mechanism whereby post-weaning undernutrition in females induces adaptations in muscle that enhance nutrient uptake and storage. If this effect was initiated shortly after the post-weaning challenge, prior to puberty, it may provide a strategy to facilitate the return to control body weight observed by 1.5 years (young adulthood) [22], which could be critical to ensure reproductive success. However with ageing and/or an over-abundant nutrient environment, these mechanisms

Table 2. Genes of interest in liver and adipose tissue of mature (2.5 years) adult male and female sheep.

	Males				Females			
	CC	CU	UC	UU	CC	CU	UC	UU
	n=13	*n*=7	*n*=8	*n*=11	*n*=9	*n*=7	*n*=9	*n*=11
Liver – left lobe:								
GR mRNA[x, z]	3.41±0.49	2.85±0.40	3.41±0.40	3.35±0.49	2.73±0.37	2.20±0.29	2.32±0.14	2.37±0.24
IR mRNA	0.187±0.023	0.222±0.066	0.304±0.081	0.282±0.056	0.268±0.030	0.203±0.025	0.276±0.041	0.228±0.041
PEPCK mRNA[y,z]	0.258±0.049	0.190±0.021	0.313±0.033	0.294±0.055	0.166±0.036	0.194±0.038	0.224±0.041	0.140±0.027
G6Pase mRNA	0.485±0.051	0.521±0.116	0.463±0.059	0.522±0.100	0.536±0.084	0.486±0.078	0.471±0.078	0.455±0.060
GR methylation	0.013±0.004	0.021±0.012	0.010±0.002	0.018±0.004	0.013±0.004	0.011±0.005	0.049±0.043	0.013±0.004
IGFII mRNA	0.512±0.076	0.523±0.097	0.552±0.136	0.513±0.056	0.380±0.059	0.405±0.041	0.378±0.067	0.426±0.041
IGF2R mRNA	0.015±0.006	0.006±0.002	0.023±0.011	0.017±0.006	0.062±0.056	0.011±0.003	0.017±0.001	0.040±0.023
Liver – right lobe:								
GR mRNA[x]	7.18±0.67	7.57±0.66	6.68±0.94	7.42±1.44	3.67±0.56	3.51±0.30	3.75±0.60	3.77±0.47
IR mRNA	0.234±0.041	0.302±0.050	0.238±0.064	0.266±0.039	0.203±0.017	0.217±0.024	0.250±0.051	0.242±0.019
PEPCK mRNA	0.198±0.029	0.219±0.046	0.307±0.072	0.182±0.027	0.106±0.008	0.150±0.025	0.126±0.017	0.141±0.021
G6Pase mRNA	0.512±0.076	0.523±0.097	0.552±0.136	0.513±0.056	0.380±0.059	0.405±0.041	0.378±0.067	0.426±0.041
GR DNA methylation	0.015±0.006	0.006±0.002	0.023±0.011	0.017±0.006	0.062±0.056	0.011±0.003	0.017±0.001	0.040±0.023
Adipose tissue:								
IR mRNA	1.63±0.15	1.75±0.25	1.56±0.17	1.29±0.10	1.55±0.24	1.37±0.19	1.54±0.19	1.35±0.18
GLUT4 mRNA	1.55±0.16	1.66±0.12	1.38±0.18	1.51±0.13	1.06±0.18	1.28±0.18	1.42±0.15	1.49±0.32
PPARγ mRNA	1.85±0.17	1.83±0.24	1.82±0.15	1.68±0.15	0.97±0.16	0.88±0.11	0.96±0.09	0.97±0.14
Lipid content (mmol. mg^{-1})	507±27	500±34	514±15	491±37	567±14[a]	500±34[b]	535±14	551±14

Data are mean ± S.E.M.
[a, b]significant difference (p<0.05) between CU and CC groups in females;
[x]significant difference (p<0.001) between left and right liver lobes;
[y]significant difference (p<0.05) between left and right liver lobes in males;
[z]significant difference (p<0.001) between males and females: see text for more details. Values given have arbitrary units and are normalised to geometric means of β-actin, GAPDH and RPL-19 (liver) or β actin and GAPDH (adipose tissue).

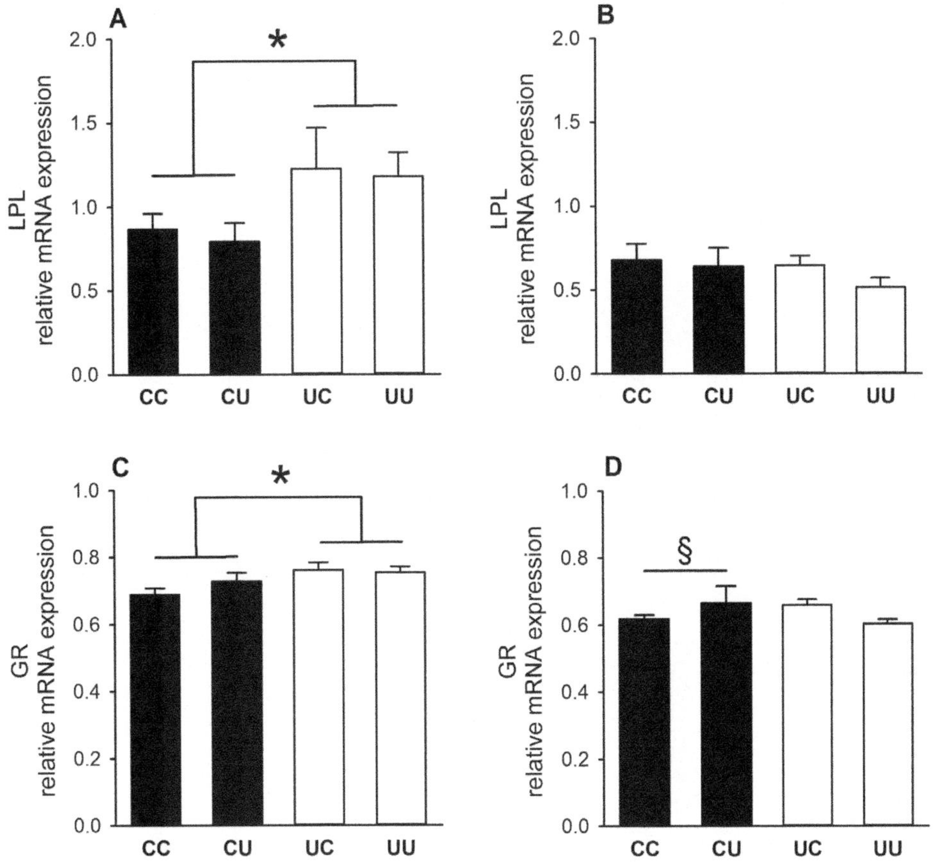

Figure 2. Factors involved in lipid handling in adipose tissue of 2.5 year-old sheep. Messenger RNA levels of lipoprotein lipase (LPL, normalised to geometric mean of β actin and GAPDH) and glucocorticoid receptor (GR, normalised to 18S) from male (A, C) and female (B, D) sheep (CC: male, $n=13$, female, $n=9$; CU: male, $n=9$; CU: male, $n=7$, female $n=7$; UC: male, $n=8$, female, $n=9$; UU: male, $n=11$, female, $n=11$). Values are mean ± S.E.M. *$p<0.05$, early gestation undernutrition groups greater than early gestation control groups. § $p=0.08$, CU greater than CC.

may lead to inappropriate effects on body composition or fatness and metabolic homeostasis [25]. Indeed in human infants, a transition from enhanced insulin sensitivity during rapid early weight gain to insulin resistance has been observed, in association with a propensity for central fat accumulation [23].

We show for the first time in sheep, epigenetic modifications of the DLK1/MEG imprinted cluster in mature adult liver of females exposed to post-weaning undernutrition. Genetic ablation of DLK1 in the myogenic lineage impairs muscle development and DLK1 knock-out increases adiposity [34,35]. In addition, an endocrine role of hepatic DLK1 has been suggested since specific manipulation of hepatic DLK1 expression can influence adipose tissue mass [50]. Although hepatic DLK1 expression was too low to measure in this study, it may be possible that the reduction in hepatic genes regulated by the DLK1/MEG3 imprinted cluster expression in females undernourished post-weaning is associated with reduced muscle mass and altered adipocyte development. Persistence of these effects in females may also negatively impact on metabolic homeostasis in the longer term.

These effects of post-weaning undernutrition on glucose metabolism were similar in females with or without prior exposure to early gestation undernutrition. However, in mature adult females exposed to post-weaning undernutrition without gestational undernutrition (CU group), adipose tissue and/or liver triglyceride handling was more sensitive to insulin, as given by a greater fall in TAG output during the GTT. Given the lack of an effect of post-weaning undernutrition on insulin-induced inhibition of NEFA output from adipose tissue, this effect may be largely in the liver. The reduction in adipose tissue lipid content and trend for enhanced adipose GR mRNA levels in females suggest that the relative balance between stored and circulating lipids in adipose tissue and liver could be influenced specifically by exposure only to post-weaning undernutrition. The potential mechanisms involved in this effect remain to be elucidated. Taken together, our findings suggest that changes in both glucose and lipid metabolism may be employed in CU females to enhance body mass once nutrition has been restored to normal. Even in the absence of any current effects on body weight or fatness [22], the dysregulation of lipid handling we have observed following undernutrition in the post-weaning period may increase risk of obesity or dyslipidaemia in later life [24].

In contrast to the effects of post-weaning undernutrition, undernutrition in early gestation in mature adult females, as well as in males, was associated with reduced insulin sensitivity in adipose tissue, as revealed by the insulin-induced inhibition of lipolysis (NEFA response during GTT), suggesting that this period may also influence lipid metabolism and fat accumulation and/or dyslipidaemia in the longer term. With this strategy in place, females exposed to post-weaning as well as early gestation undernutrition (UU group) may not require further alterations in adipose tissue and/or liver insulin sensitivity, as seen in the CU group, for body weight recovery.

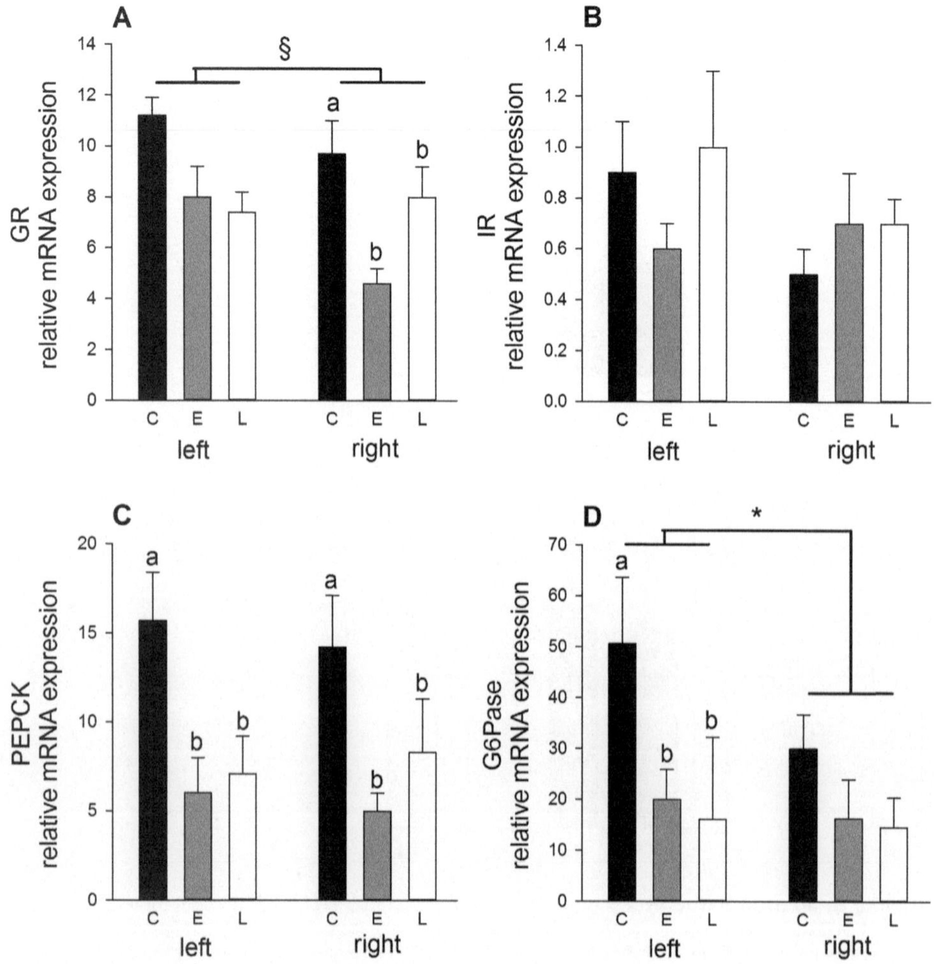

Figure 3. Factors involved in glucose homeostasis in liver of 127 dGA fetal sheep. Messenger RNA levels (normalised to geometric mean of β actin, GAPDH and RPL-19) of glucocorticoid receptor (GR; A), insulin receptor (IR; B), phosphoenolpyruvate carboxykinase (PEPCK; C) and glucose-6-phosphatase (G6Pase; D) in left and right liver lobes of control (C, $n = 8$), early gestation undernutrition (E, $n = 9$) and late gestation undernutrition (L, $n = 6$) fetuses (males and females combined). Values are mean ± S.E.M. Different letters denote significantly different values based on nutritional group ($p < 0.05$). *$p < 0.01$, § $p = 0.065$; difference between left and right liver lobes.

In male sheep, we proposed that early gestation rather than post-weaning undernutrition would have a greater impact on mechanisms regulating adiposity. Males may have a heightened sensitivity to nutrient restriction in early gestation, when their growth rate is faster than females [51], potentially causing them to make adaptations to enhance their ability to optimise growth and body composition in later nutritionally adequate times. We demonstrated previously that males exposed to early gestation undernutrition have a relatively faster growth rate in the first 12 postnatal weeks without any change in birth weight [21]. In the current study we found that insulin sensitivity in adipose tissue, as revealed by the insulin-induced inhibition of lipolysis (NEFA response during GTT), was reduced in mature adult males undernourished in early gestation alongside increases in LPL and GR mRNA levels. Although these molecular effects were small and may not be reflected in subsequent protein expression, they were also associated with faster early postnatal growth. In this cohort, we did not observe long-term effects of early nutrition on fat depth [22], although this measurement was limited to one subcutaneous region, nor was there an effect on actual lipid content in adipose tissue at 2.5 years. However, lipid content may be maintained by a balance between the actions of glucocorticoids and LPL. Changes in glucocorticoid sensitivity and the ability to hydrolyse and transport triglycerides in early gestation-undernourished males could lead to changes in fat distribution or fat deposition in other organs such as the liver, effects that may be exacerbated by a subsequent abundant diet or with ageing. Indeed, the effect of early gestation undernutrition on adipose insulin sensitivity in males only became apparent at 2.5 years of age. The possibility of an altered plasma lipid profile in these animals, alongside our previous observations that exposure to early gestation undernutrition influences cardiac morphology and coronary function in adult male sheep [21], may contribute to a risk of cardiovascular disease. For female sheep exposed to early gestation undernutrition, the insulin-induced fall in NEFA during GTT was similar to that in males however there were no changes in LPL or GR mRNA levels in adipose tissue. While this may suggest these females do not have the same risk of dyslipidaemia, the implication of these differences requires further investigation. Our molecular studies of adipose tissue utilised the perirenal depot; given the differences in metabolic profiles between fat depots [52], the possibility that early gestation or post-weaning undernutrition influenced adipose tissue metabolism and/or

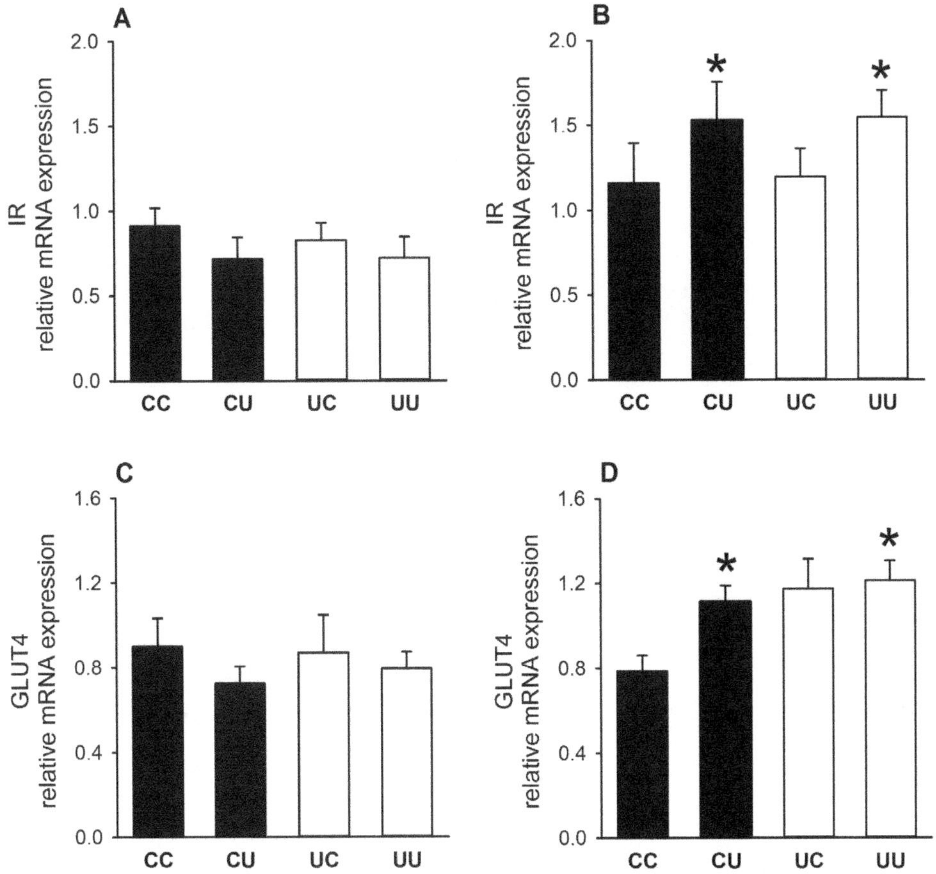

Figure 4. Components of insulin signalling in skeletal muscle of 2.5 year-old sheep. Messenger RNA levels (normalised to β actin and GAPDH) of insulin receptor (IR) and glucose transporter 4 (GLUT4) from male (A, C) and female (B, D) sheep (CC: male, *n* = 13, female, *n* = 8; CU: male, *n* = 7, female *n* = 7; UC: male, *n* = 6, female, *n* = 7; UU: male, *n* = 11, female, *n* = 10). Values are mean ± S.E.M. *p<0.05, post-weaning undernutrition groups greater than post-weaning control groups.

deposition elsewhere in the body cannot be excluded from the current study.

In the current study, as well as examining the effects of both pre- and postnatal undernutrition on adult liver, we examined fetal liver in a separate cohort of sheep exposed to maternal undernutrition at 40% of control levels (compared to a 50% reduction in the study of adult offspring). Both left and right liver lobes were examined, except for the epigenetic analyses. There is unequal provision of umbilical venous blood between the liver lobes in fetal life, with predominantly more going to the left lobe, such that each lobe may be differentially sensitive to changes in maternal nutrient provision. Nutrient restriction in both early and late gestation reduced key gluconeogenic enzymes in late gestation liver and there was differential expression between the fetal liver lobes. These effects did not persist into adult life and indeed, as with the lobar differences in gene expression patterns, appear even to switch direction over the life course. We therefore show that the developing liver makes adaptations to reductions in maternal nutritional status and there is differential expression between the lobes. However, although these hepatic effects imply potential changes in gluconeogenic capacity, as well as growth potential [53], in response to maternal undernutrition, they may not translate to significant functional significance given the absence of changes in basal glucose in either exposed fetuses or adults [22,40]. However, we must be cautious making direct comparisons between the fetal and adult cohorts reported here given the difference in the level of maternal nutritional challenge imposed. In addition, primiparous, singleton-bearing ewes were used in the fetal study, whereas older ewes carrying both singletons and twins were used in the adult study. Given findings that birth order poses a non-modifiable risk for obesity [54], the relative maternal constraint experienced by first born offspring may have imposed an additional environmental challenge to the fetuses exposed to maternal undernutrition.

The role of the liver as a sensor of maternal nutrient status is suggested in studies linking fetal liver blood flow with subsequent offspring fat mass [55,56]. Experimental manipulation of fetal liver blood perfusion and reduction in maternal diet in sheep have both been shown in sheep to influence hepatic IGF expression [57,58], with potential long term effects on offspring growth and metabolism. In addition, reduced DNA methylation at the IGF2/H19 imprinted locus has been reported in humans following the Dutch Famine [59] and in fetal and postnatal sheep in response to altered maternal diets [46,60]. Unlike findings in lamb adrenal tissue [46], no effect of early gestation undernutrition was observed at the IGF2/H19 locus in adult sheep liver. However, methylation of IGF2R in liver of early gestation undernourished males was increased, which could increase IGF2R expression. Since this receptor acts to limit circulating IGF2 availability [61], this increase may influence growth potential or muscle growth. Although we were not able to demonstrate an effect of early gestation undernutrition on hepatic IGF2R gene

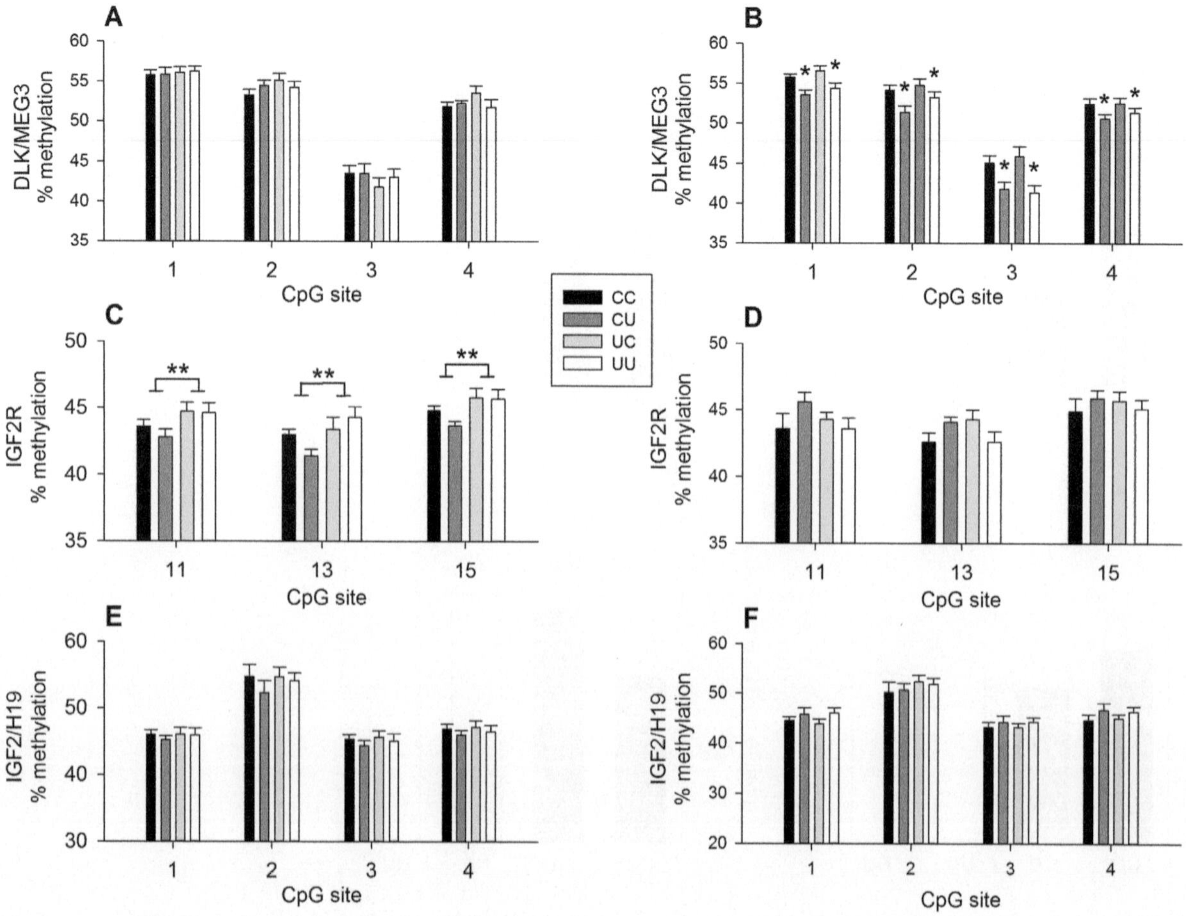

Figure 5. Epigenetic modification of genes regulating metabolic homeostasis and body composition in liver of 2.5 year-old sheep. Methylation of CpG dinucleotides within the ICRs of the DLK1/MEG3 (A, B), IGF2R (C, D) and IGF2/H19 (E, F) imprinted regions in male (A, C, E) and female (B, D, F) sheep (CC: male, $n=11$, female, $n=9$; CU: male, $n=7$, female $n=7$; UC: male, $n=8$, female, $n=9$; UU: male, $n=10$, female, $n=11$). Values are mean ± S.E.M. *p<0.05, post-weaning undernutrition less than post-weaning control; **p<0.05, early gestation undernutrition greater than early gestation control.

expression, possibly because the affected CpG dinucleotides were not contiguous, others have also shown sex-specific effects on IGF2R expression and muscle area in mature cattle exposed to a maternal low protein diet in the first trimester [62]. Whether methylation patterns of these growth factors during early life were involved in control of lean *vs.* fat mass and growth patterns prior to tissue collection at 2.5 years remains unknown.

The current study did not identify any mechanisms that would enable male sheep exposed to post-weaning undernutrition to catch up once nutrition was restored to normal. The absence of any effects of undernutrition in this period on glucose tolerance and peripheral insulin sensitivity suggests that these males must employ other mechanisms to regain body weight following the nutritional challenge. All sheep were allowed access to the same food rations after the nutritional challenge but feed intake of individual animals was not determined when group-housed. It remains possible that the regulation of appetite was influenced by the post-weaning nutrient challenge [63].

Although we [22] and others [16] have shown no influence of the early gestation nutritional environment or being a twin on whole body glucose tolerance, we observed here some differences between singleton and twin offspring e.g. glucose transporter 4 mRNA levels in muscle, that were increased following early gestation undernutrition but only in twins. Twins face an additional nutritional constraint during gestation, with lower fetal glucose levels in late gestation and reduced birth weight [64] suggesting that the double insult of being a twin and facing gestational undernutrition may be required to induce such an effect [65]. Enhanced glucose uptake in muscle of these animals may contribute to the increased insulin sensitivity observed in twins in this cohort [22]. For singleton offspring, the strongest influence on glucose transporter 4 expression was nutrient restriction in the post-weaning period.

In conclusion, undernutrition during development induces changes in mechanisms of lipid and glucose metabolism which differ between tissues and sexes contingent on the period of nutritional restriction. Such changes may increase later life obesity and dyslipidaemia risk.

Supporting Information

Figure S1 Flow diagram showing the total number of ewes and their offspring used in the study of adult sheep exposed to early gestation and/or post-weaning undernutrition.
(DOCX)

Table S1 Target gene primer and probe cDNA sequences for real-time PCR, methylation-sensitive PCR and pyrosequencing.
(DOCX)

Acknowledgments

We are grateful to D. Noakes for his long-term collaboration on these sheep studies and staff at the Biological Services Unit, Royal Veterinary College and Biological Research Facility, University of Southampton for their expert animal care. We thank J. Slater-Jefferies for the measurement of adipose GR mRNA levels, J. Jackson for the measurement of plasma NEFA concentrations, H. Whitworth for the measurement of adipose lipid content and A. Sheppard for providing the ovine express sequence tag required for analysis of GR promoter region methylation.

Author Contributions

Conceived and designed the experiments: KRP JKC KAL GCB MAH LRG. Performed the experiments: KRP LJH RJSM AW AB LF JKC LRG. Analyzed the data: KRP LJH RJSM AW AB LF LRG. Wrote the paper: KRP GCB MAH LRG.

References

1. Finucane MM, Stevens GA, Cowan MJ, Danaei G, Lin JK, et al. (2011) National, regional, and global trends in body-mass index since 1980: systematic analysis of health examination surveys and epidemiological studies with 960 country-years and 9.1 million participants. Lancet 377: 557–567.
2. Allender S, Rayner M (2007) The burden of overweight and obesity-related ill health in the UK. Obes Rev 8: 467–473.
3. Cottrell EC, Ozanne SE (2008) Early life programming of obesity and metabolic disease. Physiol Behav 94: 17–28.
4. Law CM, Barker DJ, Osmond C, Fall CH, Simmonds SJ (1992) Early growth and abdominal fatness in adult life. J Epidemiol Community Health 46: 184–186.
5. Ravelli AC, van der Meulen JH, Michels RP, Osmond C, Barker DJ, et al. (1998) Glucose tolerance in adults after prenatal exposure to famine. Lancet 351: 173–177.
6. Roseboom TJ, van der Meulen JH, Osmond C, Barker DJ, Ravelli AC, et al. (2000) Coronary heart disease after prenatal exposure to the Dutch famine, 1944–45. Heart 84: 595–598.
7. Roseboom TJ, van der Meulen JH, Osmond C, Barker DJ, Ravelli AC, et al. (2000) Plasma lipid profiles in adults after prenatal exposure to the Dutch famine. Am J Clin Nutr 72: 1101–1106.
8. Eriksson J, Forsen T, Tuomilehto J, Jaddoe V, Osmond C, et al. (2002) Effects of size at birth and childhood growth on the insulin resistance syndrome in elderly individuals. Diabetologia 45: 342–348.
9. Crowther NJ, Cameron N, Trusler J, Gray IP (1998) Association between poor glucose tolerance and rapid post natal weight gain in seven-year-old children. Diabetologia 41: 1163–1167.
10. Barker D, Osmond C, Forsen T, Kajantie E, Eriksson E (2005) Trajectories of growth among children who have coronary events as adults. N Engl J Med 353: 1802–1809.
11. Bavdekar A, Yajnik CS, Fall CH, Bapat S, Pandit AN, et al. (1999) Insulin resistance syndrome in 8-year-old Indian children: small at birth, big at 8 years, or both? Diabetes 48: 2422–2429.
12. Gonzalez-Barranco J, Rios-Torres JM, Castillo-Martinez L, Lopez-Alvarenga JC, Aguilar-Salinas CA, et al. (2003) Effect of malnutrition during the first year of life on adult plasma insulin and glucose tolerance. Metabolism 52: 1005–1011.
13. Phillips DI, Barker DJ, Hales CN, Hirst S, Osmond C (1994) Thinness at birth and insulin resistance in adult life. Diabetologia 37: 150–154.
14. Barker DJ, Winter PD, Osmond C, Margetts B, Simmonds SJ (1989) Weight in infancy and death from ischaemic heart disease. Lancet 2: 577–580.
15. Petry CJ, Ozanne SE, Hales CN (2001) Programming of intermediary metabolism. Mol Cell Endocrinol 185: 81–91.
16. Gardner DS, Tingey K, Van Bon BW, Ozanne SE, Wilson V, et al. (2005) Programming of glucose-insulin metabolism in adult sheep after maternal undernutrition. Am J Physiol Regul Integr Comp Physiol 289: R947–954.
17. Hawkins P, Steyn C, McGarrigle HH, Saito T, Ozaki T, et al. (2000) Effect of maternal nutrient restriction in early gestation on responses of the hypothalamic-pituitary-adrenal axis to acute isocapnic hypoxaemia in late gestation fetal sheep. Exp Physiol 85: 85–96.
18. Ozanne SE, Smith GD, Tikerpae J, Hales CN (1996) Altered regulation of hepatic glucose output in the male offspring of protein-malnourished rat dams. Am J Physiol Endocrinol Metab 270: E559–564.
19. Ozanne SE, Wang CL, Coleman N, Smith GD (1996) Altered muscle insulin sensitivity in the male offspring of protein-malnourished rats. Am J Physiol Endocrinol Metab 271: E1128–1134.
20. Ozanne SE, Nave BT, Wang CL, Shepherd PR, Prins J, et al. (1997) Poor fetal nutrition causes long-term changes in expression of insulin signalling components in adipocytes. Am J Physiol Endocrinol Metab 273: E46–51.
21. Cleal JK, Poore KR, Boullin JP, Khan O, Chau R, et al. (2007) Mismatched pre- and postnatal nutrition leads to cardiovascular dysfunction and altered renal function in adulthood. Proc Natl Acad Sci U S A 104: 9529–9533.
22. Poore KR, Cleal JK, Boullin JP, Noakes D, Hanson MA, et al. (2007) Nutritional challenges during development induce sex-specific changes in glucose homeostasis in the adult sheep. Am J Physiol Endocrinol Metab 292: 32–39.
23. Mericq V, Ong KK, Bazaes R, Pena V, Avila A, et al. (2005) Longitudinal changes in insulin sensitivity and secretion from birth to age three years in small- and appropriate-for-gestational-age children. Diabetologia 48: 2609–2614.
24. Morris TJ, Vickers M, Gluckman P, Gilmour S, Affara N (2009) Transcriptional profiling of rats subjected to gestational undernourishment: implications for the developmental variations in metabolic traits. PLOS ONE 4: e7271.
25. George LA, Zhang L, Tuersunjiang N, Ma Y, Long NM, et al. (2012) Early maternal undernutrition programs increased feed intake, altered glucose metabolism and insulin secretion, and liver function in aged female offspring. Am J Physiol Regul Integr Comp Physiol 302: R795–804.
26. Burdge GC, Lillycrop KA (2010) Nutrition, epigenetics, and developmental plasticity: implications for understanding human disease. Annu Rev Nutr 30: 315–339.
27. Weaver IC, Cervoni N, Champagne FA, D'Alessio AC, Sharma S, et al. (2004) Epigenetic programming by maternal behavior. Nat Neurosci 7: 847–854.
28. Lillycrop KA, Slater-Jefferies JL, Hanson MA, Godfrey KM, Jackson AA, et al. (2007) Induction of altered epigenetic regulation of the hepatic glucocorticoid receptor in the offspring of rats fed a protein-restricted diet during pregnancy suggests that reduced DNA methyltransferase-1 expression is involved in impaired DNA methylation and changes in histone modifications. Br J Nutr 97: 1064–1073.
29. Drake AJ, McPherson RC, Godfrey KM, Cooper C, Lillycrop KA, et al. (2012) An unbalanced maternal diet in pregnancy associates with offspring epigenetic changes in genes controlling glucocorticoid action and foetal growth. Clin Endocrinol (Oxf) 77: 808–815.
30. Godfrey KM, Sheppard A, Gluckman PD, Lillycrop KA, Burdge GC, et al. (2011) Epigenetic gene promoter methylation at birth is associated with child's later adiposity. Diabetes 60: 1528–1534.
31. Dudley KJ, Sloboda DM, Connor KL, Beltrand J, Vickers MH (2011) Offspring of mothers fed a high fat diet display hepatic cell cycle inhibition and associated changes in gene expression and DNA methylation. PLOS ONE 6: e21662.
32. Wiedmeier JE, Joss-Moore LA, Lane RH, Neu J (2011) Early postnatal nutrition and programming of the preterm neonate. Nutr Rev 69: 76–82.
33. O'Connell J, Lynch L, Hogan A, Cawood TJ, O'Shea D (2011) Preadipocyte factor-1 is associated with metabolic profile in severe obesity. J Clin Endocrinol Metab 96: E680–684.
34. Waddell JN, Zhang P, Wen Y, Gupta SK, Yevtodiyenko A, et al. (2010) Dlk1 is necessary for proper skeletal muscle development and regeneration. PLOS ONE 5: e15055.
35. Moon YS, Smas CM, Lee K, Villena JA, Kim KH, et al. (2002) Mice lacking paternally expressed Pref-1/Dlk1 display growth retardation and accelerated adiposity. Mol Cell Biol 22: 5585–5592.
36. Cleal JK, Poore KR, Newman JP, Noakes DE, Hanson MA, et al. (2007) The effect of maternal undernutrition in early gestation on gestation length and fetal and postnatal growth in sheep. Pediatr Res 62: 422–427.
37. Russel A, Doney J, Gunn R (1969) Subjective assessment of body fat in live sheep. Journal of Agricultural Research 72: 451–454.
38. Agricultural and Food Research Council (1993) Energy and protein requirements of ruminants. An advisory manual prepared by the AFRC Technical Committee on responses to nutrients. CAB International, Wallingford, Oxfordshire, UK.
39. Poore KR, Boullin JP, Cleal JK, Newman JP, Noakes DE, et al. (2010) Sex- and age-specific effects of nutrition in early gestation and early postnatal life on hypothalamo-pituitary-adrenal axis and sympathoadrenal function in adult sheep. J Physiol 588: 2219–2237.
40. Burrage DM, Braddick L, Cleal JK, Costello P, Noakes DE, et al. (2009) The late gestation fetal cardiovascular response to hypoglycaemia is modified by prior peri-implantation undernutrition in sheep. J Physiol 587: 611–624.
41. Costello PM, Rowlerson A, Astaman NA, Anthony FE, Sayer AA, et al. (2008) Peri-implantation and late gestation maternal undernutrition differentially affect fetal sheep skeletal muscle development. J Physiol 586: 2371–2379.
42. Lillycrop KA, Phillips ES, Torrens C, Hanson MA, Jackson AA, et al. (2008) Feeding pregnant rats a protein-restricted diet persistently alters the methylation of specific cytosines in the hepatic PPAR alpha promoter of the offspring. Br J Nutr 100: 278–282.
43. Rosa AL, Wu YQ, Kwabi-Addo B, Coveler KJ, Reid Sutton V, et al. (2005) Allele-specific methylation of a functional CTCF binding site upstream of MEG3 in the human imprinted domain of 14q32. Chromosome Res 13: 809–818.
44. Young LE, Schnieke AE, McCreath KJ, Wieckowski S, Konfortova G, et al. (2003) Conservation of IGF2-H19 and IGF2R imprinting in sheep: effects of somatic cell nuclear transfer. Mech Dev 120: 1433–1442.
45. Wylie AA, Murphy SK, Orton TC, Jirtle RL (2000) Novel imprinted DLK1/GTL2 domain on human chromosome 14 contains motifs that mimic those implicated in IGF2/H19 regulation. Genome Res 10: 1711–1718.

46. Zhang S, Rattanatray L, MacLaughlin SM, Cropley JE, Suter CM, et al. (2010) Periconceptional undernutrition in normal and overweight ewes leads to increased adrenal growth and epigenetic changes in adrenal IGF2/H19 gene in offspring. FASEB J 24: 2772–2782.
47. Thurston A, Taylor J, Gardner J, Sinclair KD, Young LE (2008) Monoallelic expression of nine imprinted genes in the sheep embryo occurs after the blastocyst stage. Reproduction 135: 29–40.
48. Burdge GC, Wright P, Jones AE, Wootton SA (2000) A method for separation of phosphatidylcholine, triacylglycerol, non-esterified fatty acids and cholesterol esters from plasma by solid-phase extraction. Br J Nutr 84: 781–787.
49. Limesand SW, Rozance PJ, Smith D, Hay WW Jr (2007) Increased insulin sensitivity and maintenance of glucose utilization rates in fetal sheep with placental insufficiency and intrauterine growth restriction. Am J Physiol Endocrinol Metab 293: E1716–1725.
50. Lee K, Villena JA, Moon YS, Kim KH, Lee S, et al. (2003) Inhibition of adipogenesis and development of glucose intolerance by soluble preadipocyte factor-1 (Pref-1). J Clin Invest 111: 453–461.
51. Pedersen JF (1980) Ultrasound evidence of sexual difference in fetal size in first trimester. Br Med J 281: 1253.
52. Wajchenberg BL (2000) Subcutaneous and visceral adipose tissue: their relation to the metabolic syndrome. Endocr Rev 21: 697–738.
53. Darp RA, de Boo HA, Phua HH, Oliver MH, Derraik JG, et al. (2010) Differential regulation of igf1 and igf1r mRNA levels in the two hepatic lobes following intrauterine growth restriction and its treatment with intra-amniotic insulin-like growth factor-1 in ovine fetuses. Reprod Fertil Dev 22: 1188–1197.
54. Ong KK, Preece MA, Emmett PM, Ahmed ML, Dunger DB (2002) Size at birth and early childhood growth in relation to maternal smoking, parity and infant breast-feeding: longitudinal birth cohort study and analysis. Pediatr Res 52: 863–867.
55. Godfrey KM, Haugen G, Kiserud T, Inskip HM, Cooper C, et al. (2012) Fetal liver blood flow distribution: role in human developmental strategy to prioritize fat deposition versus brain development. PLOS ONE 7: e41759.
56. Haugen G, Hanson M, Kiserud T, Crozier S, Inskip H, et al. (2005) Fetal liver-sparing cardiovascular adaptations linked to mother's slimness and diet. Circ Res 96: 12–14.
57. Tchirikov M, Kertschanska S, Sturenberg HJ, Schroder HJ (2002) Liver blood perfusion as a possible instrument for fetal growth regulation. Placenta 23 Suppl A: S153–158.
58. Brameld JM, Mostyn A, Dandrea J, Stephenson TJ, Dawson JM, et al. (2000) Maternal nutrition alters the expression of insulin-like growth factors in fetal sheep liver and skeletal muscle. J Endocrinol 167: 429–437.
59. Heijmans BT, Tobi EW, Stein AD, Putter H, Blauw GJ, et al. (2008) Persistent epigenetic differences associated with prenatal exposure to famine in humans. Proc Natl Acad Sci U S A 105: 17046–17049.
60. Lan X, Cretney EC, Kropp J, Khateeb K, Berg MA, et al. (2013) Maternal Diet during Pregnancy Induces Gene Expression and DNA Methylation Changes in Fetal Tissues in Sheep. Front Genet 4: 49.
61. Brown J, Jones EY, Forbes BE (2009) Keeping IGF-II under control: lessons from the IGF-II-IGF2R crystal structure. Trends Biochem Sci 34: 612–619.
62. Micke GC, Sullivan TM, McMillen IC, Gentili S, Perry VE (2011) Protein intake during gestation affects postnatal bovine skeletal muscle growth and relative expression of IGF1, IGF1R, IGF2 and IGF2R. Mol Cell Endocrinol 332: 234–241.
63. Spencer SJ (2013) Perinatal programming of neuroendocrine mechanisms connecting feeding behavior and stress. Front Neurosci 7: 109.
64. Rumball CW, Harding JE, Oliver MH, Bloomfield FH (2008) Effects of twin pregnancy and periconceptional undernutrition on maternal metabolism, fetal growth and glucose-insulin axis function in ovine pregnancy. J Physiol 586: 1399–1411.
65. MacLaughlin SM, Walker SK, Roberts CT, Kleemann DO, McMillen IC (2005) Periconceptional nutrition and the relationship between maternal body weight changes in the periconceptional period and feto-placental growth in the sheep. J Physiol 565: 111–124.

8

Phosphorus and Nitrogen Regulate Arbuscular Mycorrhizal Symbiosis in *Petunia hybrida*

Eva Nouri[1], Florence Breuillin-Sessoms[1¤], Urs Feller[2], Didier Reinhardt[1]*

1 Dept. of Biology, University of Fribourg, Fribourg, Switzerland, **2** Institute of Plant Science, University of Bern, Bern, Switzerland

Abstract

Phosphorus and nitrogen are essential nutrient elements that are needed by plants in large amounts. The arbuscular mycorrhizal symbiosis between plants and soil fungi improves phosphorus and nitrogen acquisition under limiting conditions. On the other hand, these nutrients influence root colonization by mycorrhizal fungi and symbiotic functioning. This represents a feedback mechanism that allows plants to control the fungal symbiont depending on nutrient requirements and supply. Elevated phosphorus supply has previously been shown to exert strong inhibition of arbuscular mycorrhizal development. Here, we address to what extent inhibition by phosphorus is influenced by other nutritional pathways in the interaction between *Petunia hybrida* and *R. irregularis*. We show that phosphorus and nitrogen are the major nutritional determinants of the interaction. Interestingly, the symbiosis-promoting effect of nitrogen starvation dominantly overruled the suppressive effect of high phosphorus nutrition onto arbuscular mycorrhiza, suggesting that plants promote the symbiosis as long as they are limited by one of the two major nutrients. Our results also show that in a given pair of symbiotic partners (*Petunia hybrida* and *R. irregularis*), the entire range from mutually symbiotic to parasitic can be observed depending on the nutritional conditions. Taken together, these results reveal complex nutritional feedback mechanisms in the control of root colonization by arbuscular mycorrhizal fungi.

Editor: Bas E. Dutilh, Radboud University Medical Centre, NCMLS, Netherlands

Funding: This work was supported by a grant from the National Centre of Competence in Research (NCCR) "Plant Survival". The funders had no role in study design, data collection and analysis, decision to publish, or preparation of the manuscript.

Competing Interests: The authors have declared that no competing interests exist.

* E-mail: didier.reinhardt@unifr.ch

¤ Current address: Plant Pathology Dept., University of Minnesota, St. Paul, Minnesota, United States of America

Introduction

Plant nutrition and AM symbiosis

In many environments, plant growth is limited by inadequate nutrient supply [1,2]. This condition is alleviated by a mutualistic association with soil fungi of the order *Glomeromycota* which provide the plant host with diverse mineral nutrients in exchange for assimilates [3]. This symbiosis, referred to as arbuscular mycorrhiza (AM), emerged approximately 450 Ma ago, and is thought to have facilitated the colonization of land by early vascular plants [4]. The fungal mycelium emanating from the root system reaches far beyond the rhizosphere and therefore can acquire nutrients from soil volumes to which roots have no access [5]. Furthermore, fungal hyphae are much thinner than roots [6], allowing them to explore small cracks in the micrometer range that are inaccessible to roots. Besides better nutrient supply, mycorrhizal associations provide other benefits to plants, such as increased drought tolerance and disease resistance [7–9].

The predominant nutrient element acquired through AM is phosphorus (P), which is delivered to the plant in its inorganic oxidized form phosphate (P_i) [10]. Furthermore, nitrogen (N) can be transferred to mycorrhizal plants through the fungal symbiont [11–14], involving a complex pathway that has been elucidated in considerable detail in recent years [15–17]. Apart from these central macronutrients, sulfur (S) [18,19] and several micronutrients can be delivered to plants through AM fungi [20,21].

Mycorrhizal plants have two routes of nutrient acquisition, the direct pathway (DP) through the root epidermis and its root hairs, (representing the only uptake route of non-mycorrhizal plants), and the mycorrhizal pathway (MP) through the fungal mycelium that delivers nutrients to the root cortex through the arbuscules. Surprisingly, P_i supply through the two pathways is not necessarily additive [22]. The contribution of the DP can be reduced in mycorrhizal plants, via the repression of constitutive phosphate transporter (PT) genes, to the extent that the plant becomes almost entirely dependent on the MP [23,24]. Hence, total P nutrition of mycorrhizal plants is not necessarily higher than in non-mycorrhizal plants. This effect is one possible reason for the observation that mycorrhizal colonization does not always result in a net gain of plant growth, i.e. in a positive mycorrhizal growth response (MGR). Indeed, even negative MGRs occur quite frequently depending on the pairing of host and fungal symbiont [25,26], raising the question why such interactions are tolerated by the plant. A plausible explanation for neutral or negative growth effects could be that AM confer a benefit other than growth promotion, e.g. a qualitative benefit, or that the benefit is not evident under the respective experimental conditions.

Modern agricultural practice has in many instances resulted in progressively reduced AM fungal diversity and frequency, an effect that is believed to be related to tillage methods [27] and to the use of mineral fertilizers [28,29]. In particular, P_i has long been known to negatively impact on AM [30–38]. Inhibition of AM

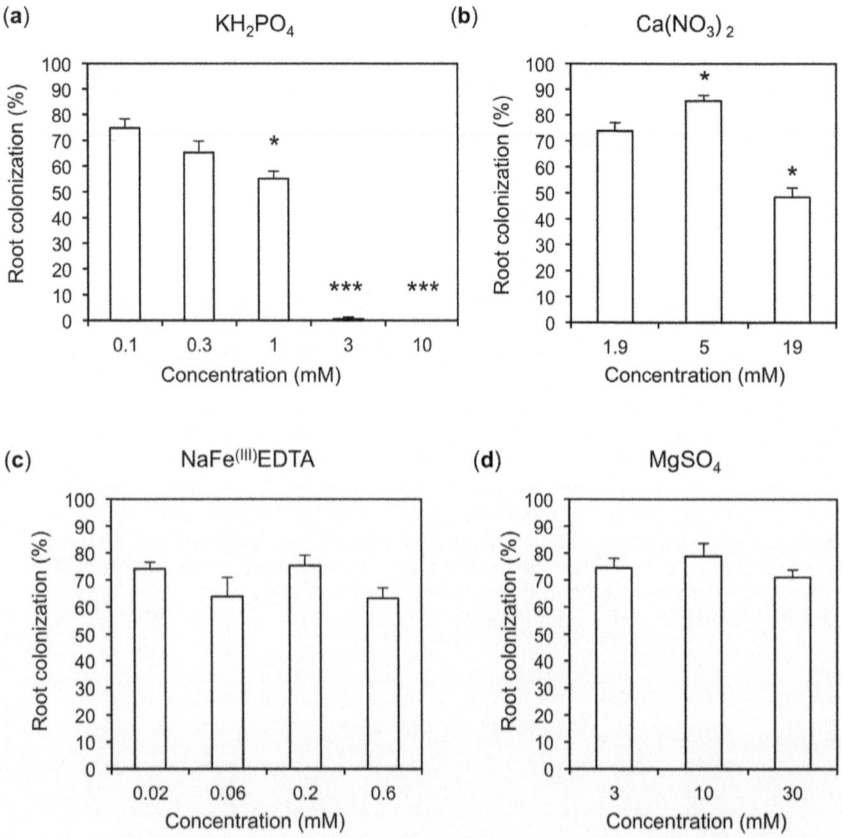

Figure 1. Exogenous phosphate and nitrate inhibit root colonization by *Rhizophagus irregularis*. Plants inoculated with *Rhizophagus irregularis* were watered with the basic nutrient solution, additionally supplemented with the indicated nutrient concentrations. The first column to the left in each graph corresponds to the concentration in the basic nutrient solution, except for KH_2PO_4 (see Table S2); the other columns represent elevated nutrient levels as indicated. Columns represent the average of four replicate plants with standard deviations.

development by P_i is a systemic effect that depends on the nutritional status of the shoot. Since AM fungi can consume a considerable fraction of the assimilates of their hosts [26,39], the suppression of AM by high P_i levels can be regarded as an energy-saving negative feedback mechanism under conditions under which the plant is optimally supplied with nutrients without the fungal symbiont. However, inhibition of AM development by P_i can potentially lead to starvation for other nutrients for which the DP is not sufficiently active, hence the P_i effect may reduce plant fitness depending on the supply with other nutrients. This raises the question whether the inhibition of AM development by P_i may become attenuated when plants are limited for other nutrients. Indeed, such nutritional interactions have been observed under natural conditions [40], however, these findings need to be substantiated under controlled conditions.

The aim of this study was to evaluate which nutrients, besides P, influence AM development, and with which nutritional pathway the P-pathway interacts. First, the major nutrient elements P, N, K, S, Mg, Ca, and Fe were tested for inhibitory effects on mycorrhizal colonization of *Petunia hybrida* by *Rhizophagus irregularis*. These experiments, together with previous findings [34], showed that strong nutritional repression of AM is specific to P. Secondly, to evaluate how the starvation for other nutrients influences the P-effect, combinatorial treatments of plants were performed with nutrient mixtures containing high P_i levels, but lacking several other nutrients alone or in combination. Our results show that the P- and N-related pathways interact, and that the AM-promoting effect of low N supply is dominant over the AM-suppressive effect of high P_i supply. These observations can serve as a basis to approach the underlying regulatory mechanisms with genetic means. Our results also show that in a given AM system (in this case *P. hybrida* and *R. irregularis*), nutrient supply has a strong influence not only on plant growth and nutrient content, but also on AM colonization and MGR. Depending on the nutritional context, AM can result in strong promotion of plant growth or in a reduction in qualitative and/or quantitative traits. Hence, the outcome of AM symbiosis is highly context-dependent.

Materials and Methods

Plant material, fungal inoculum and growth conditions

Two *Petunia hybrida* lines with indistinguishable interaction with arbuscular mycorrhizal fungi were used: Mitchell diploid (line W115) and line W138 (experiment 2; see below). Seeds were germinated on seedling substrate (Klasmann, http://www.klasmann-deilmann.com). After four weeks, plantlets were transferred to small pots (volume: 20 ml) of a sterilized mixture of 70% sand with 30% unfertilized soil (v/v; further referred to as "substrate") for another two weeks. The substrate was sterilized by heating to 90°C for 3 h with vapor. Subsequently, plantlets were transferred to larger pots (volume: 150 ml) with the same substrate and inoculated with 1 teaspoon (*ca.* 10 g) of mycorrhizal inoculum per plant directly to the root system. Inoculum of *R. irregularis* (MUCL 43204) was produced in leek pot cultures. The inoculum consisted of a mixture of soil and roots, and was tested for the presence of spores before use. In general, the plants were cultured in growth chambers with a day:night cycle (16 h day at 25°C; 8 h night at 20°C) with a photosynthetic photon flux density (PPFD) of 250 µmol m^{-2} s^{-1} (Sylvania 36 W Luxline-Plus). Nutrient composition of the substrate (Table S1) was determined by extraction of 10 g substrate in 20 ml 0.5 M $NaHCO_3$ (pH = 8.5) for 30 min under shaking. For the determination of sodium content, 10 g of substrate was extracted with 20 ml distilled water. Nutrient levels in the resulting soil extracts were determined as described below.

Experimental design and nutrient treatments

Two experiments were carried out to assess the influence of nutrient supply on the level of AM colonization (Figures 1, 2). A third experiment was designed to assess the effect of nutrient supply and mycorrhizal colonization on plant growth, nutrient content, and gene expression (Figures 3–6, Table 1). A fourth experiment was carried out to confirm gene expression results from microarray analysis by qPCR (Figure 7,8). And a final experiment tested the effect of nutrient starvation on mycorrhizal colonization (Figure 9). All experiments were carried out with the experimental system described above. After the onset of the experiments, the plants were treated once per week for five weeks with the indicated solutions (experiments 1,2,4,5). Hence, each of these plants received a total of 250 ml of the indicated solutions over the five weeks of the experiment. In experiment 3, the plants were grown in a time course for 12 d (2 treatments), 22 d (4 treatments), 29 d (5 treatments), 36 d (6 treatments), or 48 d (7 treatments), with each treatment involving 50 ml of the respective nutrient solution. In general, the watering resulted in minimal leaching from the soil, thus the plants received the entire amount of nutrients applied to the pot. If necessary, in particular at later time points when plants had grown larger, they were watered a second time per week with only tap water to avoid water stress. Composition of the basic nutrient solution, of the modified solutions with elevated P_i concentration, and of the solutions lacking individual nutrients, is listed in Table S2. In the latter case, the omitted nutrients were replaced by other nutrient salts to maintain similar osmotic conditions. The effect of increasing concentrations of individual nutrients was tested with the indicated concentrations of $MgSO_4$, Fe^{III}-EDTA, $Ca(NO_3)_2$, and KH_2PO_4, respectively, in combination with basic nutrient solution.

Determination of plant weight and AM colonization

Plants were harvested at the indicated time points to determine the fresh weight of the shoot and the root. Subsequently, root samples were taken for determination of total intraradical root colonization and, in case of experiments 3 and 4, the remaining root system was frozen in liquid N_2 for RNA extraction. The shoots were dried (overnight at 120°C) for the determination of leaf nutrient content. The shoot:root ratio was calculated by dividing the fresh weight of the shoot by the fresh weight of the root. The mycorrhizal growth response (MGR) was calculated as the ratio of the shoot fresh weights of mycorrhizal and non-mycorrhizal plants, respectively. Data shown in Figures 3 to 6 and Table 1 come from the same experiment.

Root staining and quantification of mycorrhizal colonization were carried out as described [41]. Briefly, roots were harvested, washed and stored overnight in 10% KOH (w/v) in glass tubes. Then, they were cleared for 30 min at 95°C, washed twice with water, stained for 10 min with Trypan Blue (TB) staining solution at 95°C, and rinsed twice with 30% lactic acid (v/v). TB staining

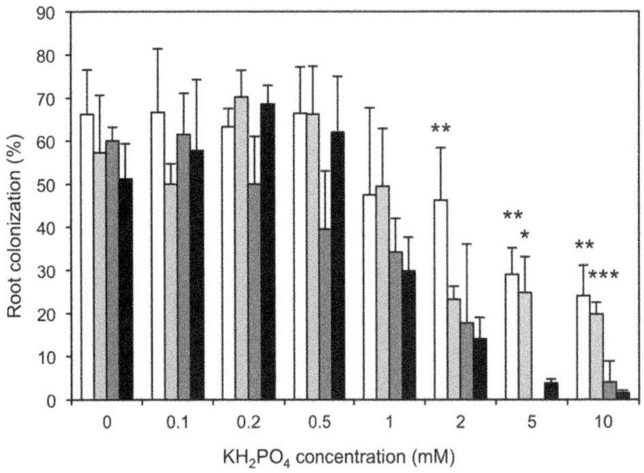

Figure 2. Inhibition of AM colonization by exogenous phosphate depends on the supply with other nutrients. KH_2PO_4 was applied to inoculated plants at the indicated concentrations either with basic nutrient solution (black columns) or alone (white columns). Additional treatments involved the application of KH_2PO_4 with only micronutrients (light grey) or only macronutrients (dark grey), respectively. Columns represent the average of four replicate plants with standard deviations. Asterisks indicate significant differences between phosphate alone (white bars) and phosphate with micronutrients (light grey bars), respectively, vs. the treatment with a combination of P_i and basic nutrient solution (black bars).

solution consisted of 20% glycerol (w/v), 30% lactic acid (v/v) and 0.01% Trypan Blue (w/v). Microscopic inspection and quantification of root colonization was carried out as described with a modified grid intersection method [41].

In general, the columns represent the mean of the values from the indicated number of biological replicates (see figure legends). Error bars represent the standard deviations. Tests for significance of differences between treatments were carried out by pairwise t-test. Significance is classified as follows: * $0.05>p>0.01$, ** $0.01>p>0.001$, *** $p>0.001$.

Determination of metal mineral nutrients

For the quantification of K, Ca, Mg, Cu, Mn, Fe, Zn and Ni by atomic absorption spectrometry, dry leaves from time point 36 d in experiment 3 were weighed, dry ashed at 550°C for 8 h and then further processed as described [42]. Briefly, the residue was dissolved in 0.2 ml 10 M HCl and 7.8 ml water. The solutions were then mixed and diluted with 1.267 g L^{-1} CsCl suprapur in 0.1 M HCl (for potassium), with 13.37 g L^{-1} $LaCl_3$-$7H_2O$ in 0.1 M HCl (for calcium and magnesium) and with 0.1 N HCl (for iron, manganese, copper, zinc, and nickel) prior to measuring the elements by atomic absorption spectrometry.

Determination of reduced nitrogen in leaves

Determination of total reduced nitrogen followed a simplified version of the micro-Kjeldahl procedure reported by [43]. Leaf material (30 mg dry matter) was homogenized in 1 ml 0.01 M KOH and 200 µl of this homogenate was transferred to micro-Kjeldahl tubes, mixed with 100 µl combustion acid (4.2 M H_2SO_4 containing 5.4 g/l $HgCl_2$) and incubated in a sand bath first at 160°C for 40 min and then for 2 h at 300°C. The samples were allowed to cool to room temperature, then 50 µl H_2O_2 (30%) were added, followed by further incubation at 160°C during 1 h and at 300°C for 2 h. After a second addition of 50 µl H_2O_2 (30%) and further incubation at 160°C for

Table 1. Microarray analysis of N-related transporter genes in relation to the nutritional status.

		Fertilized plants			*Non fertilized plants (Starved)*			
		1	**2**	**3**	**4**	**5**	**6**	**7**
		AM	**AM+Pi**	**Pi**	**water**	**AM**	**AM+Pi**	**Pi**
N/P ratio (relative to fertilized control)		0.541	0.212	0.266	0.653	0.234	0.126	0.127
Cn8666 (PhNRT2)	high-affinity nitrate transporter	1.44	18.08	21.27	18.2	11.2	16.33	37.53
CL1918 (PhNitr1)	putative nitrite transporter	7.63	13.64	10.59	6.15	26.57	27.23	23.75
cn5943 (PhNitr1)	putative nitrite transporter	6.42	19.23	15.71	6.23	41.61	41.41	17.95
cn8665	high affinity nitrate transporter	1.07	10.26	11.86	2.87	5.13	6.23	6.97
cn5272 (PhNRT1)	nitrate transporter	0.61	2.86	3.35	3.63	5.28	7.32	5.73
CL5245	nitrogen limitation adaptation	3.95	2.69	4.05	2.51	2.98	2.58	4.58
SG_SGN-U210769	nitrate transporter	1.21	1.73	1.12	1.83	4.71	10.41	3.72
cn7864	high-affinity nitrate transporter	1.32	3.01	2.96	2.83	2.69	2.85	3.51

Microarray analysis was carried out with root RNA from the plants shown in Figures 3–6 in the presence or absence of *R. irregularis* 36 d after inoculation. N/P ratio and gene expression ratios are expressed relative to reference plants supplemented with basic nutrient solution (fertilized). Relative gene induction is shown for the indicated treatments including inoculation with *R. irregularis* (AM), treatment with basic nutrient solution (fertilized plants) or water (non-fertilized plants), and treatment with 5 mM KH_2PO_4 (P_i). The list represents nitrogen-related genes among the top ten in Table S4. Values represent induction ratios between expression values from the indicated treatments divided by the expression value from the reference treatment (only nutrient solution). The individual expression values and the corresponding variation coefficients are listed in Table S3.

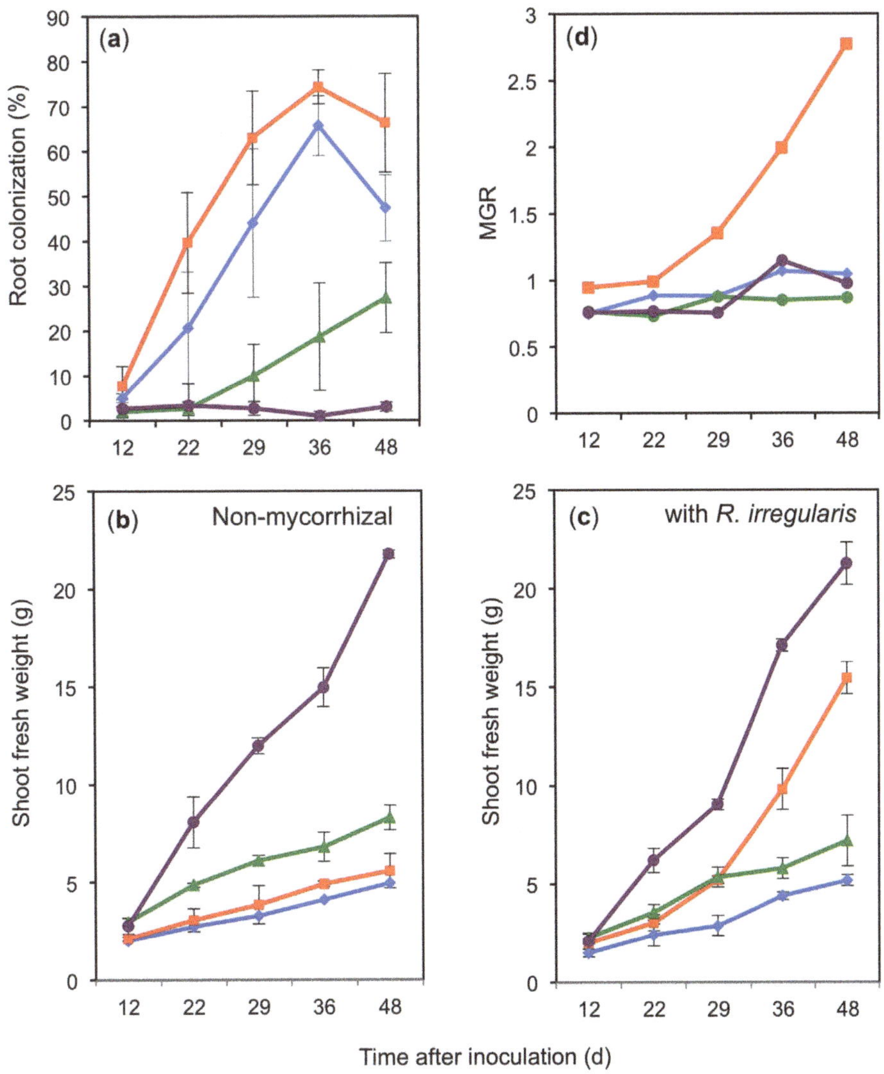

Figure 3. Dynamics of fungal root colonization and plant growth under different nutritional conditions. Plants inoculated or not with *R. irregularis* were supplied with water (blue), basic nutrient solution (red), 5 mM KH_2PO_4 (green), or with a combination of 5 mM KH_2PO_4 and basic nutrient solution (purple). Samples were harvested at the indicated time points to determine root colonization (a), shoot fresh weight (b,c), and mycorrhizal growth response (MGR; (d)). MGR is defined as the ratio of the shoot weight of mycorrhizal versus non-mycorrhizal control plants. Values are the mean of three biological replicates. Error bars represent standard deviations.

15 min, 1 ml water was added followed by colorimetric determination of the reduced nitrogen (ammonium) by mixing 50 µl of this sample solution with 100 µl 2.5% K-Na-tartrate (w/v) and 100 µl dilute Nessler reagent (1 part of Nessler Reagent Merck Nr 109028 and two parts 2.5 M NaOH). Absorbance was measured at 450 nm.

Determination of leaf phosphorus content

Dry leaf material (20 mg) was ashed overnight at 550°C in heat-resistant glass tubes. The residue was dissolved in 2 ml H_2O and 100 µl HCl (32%). 1 ml solution was then transferred to Eppendorf tubes and centrifuged in a table centrifuge (12′000 rpm for 10 min). From the supernatant, 150 µl were transferred to microtiter plates, mixed with 40 µl phosphate reagent, and absorbance was measured at 405 nm. Phosphate reagent (100 ml) was prepared by mixing 20 ml ammonium heptamolybdate (5% w/v $(NH_4)_6Mo_7O_{24}$ in water), 20 ml ammonium metavanadate (2.5% w/v NH_4VO_3 in water), 13.8 ml concentrated nitric acid, and 46.2 ml water.

Microarray analysis

Microarray analysis was performed as described [34]. Briefly, total root RNA from plants harvested at time point 36 d after inoculation (experiment 3) was extracted with the hot phenol procedure [44], pooled per treatment (equal amounts; n = 3), and sent to Nimblegen on dry ice. Array design of a four-plex microarray with 72′000 features was carried out using the ArrayScribe software from NimbleGen (http://www.nimblegen.com) to generate three optimized independent probes per gene, with an average length of 36 base pairs per probe. For shorter sequences, two probes per sequence were designed. Array design, probe synthesis, synthesis of labeled cDNA, hybridization, and data acquisition was carried out by Nimblegen as described [45]. Average expression values and a coefficient of variation for the gene expression values (Table S3) were derived by across-array quantile normalization using the Robust Multichip Average (RMA) algorithm [46]. Comparative analysis of expression data sets was carried out with Fire2.2 [47]. Table S3 compiles the entire data set resulting from microarray analysis. Gene expression ratios in Table 1 and Tables S4 and S5 represent the ratios of the expression values of the respective treatment divided by the expression values of the standard treatment (fertilized plants at low P_i levels).

Quantitative real time RT-PCR (qPCR)

For the independent assessment of gene expression by quantitative real-time polymerase chain reaction coupled to reverse transcription (qPCR), a new experiment was carried out under identical conditions as the one represented in Table 1 and Tables S4 and S5, but in this case with five biological replicates per treatment. Total RNA was extracted using the hot phenol procedure [44]. First-strand cDNA synthesis was performed with the Omniscript RT kit according to the manufacturer's guidelines. qRT-PCR was carried out with the ABsolute qPCR SYBR Green mastermix (Thermo Scientific, http://www.thermo.com) in a Rotorgene thermocycler (Corbett Life Science, http://www.corbettlifescience.com) with the primers listed in Table S6. The PCR conditions included an initial denaturation cycle for 15 min at 95°C, followed by 40 cycles of denaturation for 15 s at 95°C, annealing for 20 s at 60°C and extension for 20 s at 72°C, followed by a final extension for 5 min at 72°C. Primer design was performed with the online primer design tool primer3 (http://bioinfo.ut.ee/primer3-0.4.0/) on the entire predicted cDNA sequence derived from the genomic sequence, which had been identified using the EST sequences. For this reason, the qPCR results (Figure 8) relate to gene names (as in the case of the phylogenetic analysis on the predicted proteins; Figure 7), and not to the array IDs. (as in Tables S4 and S5). Table 1 and Figure 7 show which array ID corresponds to which gene name.

Each treatment is represented by five biological replicate plants that were analyzed with two technical replicates each. First, the relative expression value for each gene was obtained with the delta-delta-CT method [48] using GAPDH as constitutive reference gene for normalization. Then the relative expression ratios per treatment were derived by averaging the five biological replicates +/− standard deviations. Subsequently, induction ratios were calculated between the indicated treatments relative to the reference treatment (non-mycorrhizal plants with fertilizer; see Figure 8). T-test was performed for each treatment relative to the reference treatment. Standard deviations in Figure 8 were derived using the law of propagation of the error, based on the standard deviations resulting from the five biological replicates according to the following formula (for a pair of treatments a,b): $StDev = SQRT((StDev_a/Ave_a)^2 + (StDev_b/Ave_b)^2) * (Ave_b/Ave_a)$. Significance is classified as follows: * 0.05>p>0.01, ** 0.01>p> 0.001, *** p>0.001.

Phylogenetic sequence analysis

Predicted protein sequences were either retrieved from the public databases (*Arabidopsis thaliana*), or derived from genomic petunia sequences with the prediction tool Augustus (http://bioinf.uni-greifswald.de/augustus). The predicted amino acid sequences listed in File S1 were used for phylogenetic analysis (http://www.phylogeny.fr/version2).

Results

Phosphate and nitrate influence AM colonization

In order to test whether AM development is sensitive to other nutrients than phosphate (P_i), the macronutrients nitrate, sulfate, calcium, magnesium, and the micronutrient iron were applied to petunia plants inoculated with *Rhizophagus irregularis* at elevated levels in the form of $MgSO_4$, $Ca(NO_3)_2$, and $Fe^{III}EDTA$, respectively (Figure 1). The latter was used only at sub-millimolar concentrations because of its potential toxicity [49]. Apart from P_i (Figure 1a), the only nutrient salt that significantly affected AM development was $Ca(NO_3)_2$ which caused a modest reduction of colonization from approximately 80% to 50% when applied at a concentration of 19 mM, whereas at 5 mM, a small enhancement of AM colonization was observed (Figure 1b). A control experiment with $CaCl_2$ had no effect on AM (data not shown), suggesting that the effect of $Ca(NO_3)_2$ is caused by the nitrate anion rather than by the calcium cation. $Fe^{III}EDTA$ did not affect AM colonization (Figure 1c), and likewise, $MgSO_4$ as a control for osmotic effects did not interfere with AM colonization (Figure 1d; compare also with [34]).

Suppression of AM colonization by P_i depends on supply with other nutrients

To test whether the inhibition of AM development by high P_i depends on the nutritional context, inoculated plants were supplied with 5 mM KH_2PO_4 either alone or in combination with basic nutrient solution. In two additional treatments, P_i was supplied together with only micro- or macronutrients, respectively. While P_i caused a marked decrease of AM colonization in the presence of basic nutrient solution, or with only the macronutrients, inhibition reached only about 40% relative to fertilized plants (from ca. 65% colonization to ca. 25% colonization), when P_i was applied alone or with only micronutrients (Figure 2). Hence, the starvation for some macronutrient(s) generates an AM-promoting signal that counteracts the inhibitory effect of high P_i.

Dynamics of plant growth and root colonization in dependence of nutrient supply

To address the dynamics of AM colonization and plant growth in dependence of nutrient supply, a time course experiment was performed with plants treated with 5 mM KH_2PO_4 and nutrient solution in different combinations and in the presence and absence of *R. irregularis*. Shoot and root weight, as well as AM colonization, were determined 12, 22, 29, 36, and 48 days after inoculation. AM colonization increased most rapidly in plants treated with nutrient solution, reaching over 40% already after 22 d, whereas treatment with water resulted in generally lower colonization levels (Figure 3a). The treatment with 5 mM KH_2PO_4 in combination with nutrient solution strongly inhibited AM colonization, however, the inhibition was only partial in treatments with P_i alone.

P_i in combination with nutrient solution caused strong growth promotion, whereas P_i alone did only moderately stimulate growth (Figure 3b,c). This was the case irrespective of the presence of *R. irregularis*, indicating that under these conditions, fungal colonization did not provide a significant benefit. These results confirm that starvation for other nutrients reduces the inhibitory effect of P_i on AM fungal colonization (compare with Figure 2). Interestingly, a positive mycorrhizal growth response (MGR) was observed only in the presence of nutrient solution (Figure 3b-d), showing firstly that the plants could not profit from nutrient supply without the fungus, and secondly, that fungal efficiency has its limits, since plants that were not supplied with nutrient solution (and therefore relied entirely on the low nutrient concentrations in the substrate) did not show a significant MGR despite considerable colonization levels (Figure 3a,d).

R. irregularis improves plant nutrition in petunia

The marked differences in AM colonization and MGR between the nutritional treatments (Figure 3) prompted us to evaluate the nutrient status of these plants as an indicator for plant fitness and qualitative mycorrhizal benefits (Figure S1). For easier comparison, the nutrient levels of the different treatments were normalized to the respective controls that were set at 100% (Figures 4, 5). First, the effect of AM on the levels of various metal ions, phosphate and nitrate in fertilized and non-fertilized plants were determined. Fertilized plants showed an AM-related increase in several mineral nutrient levels, however, only manganese and phosphate reached the significance threshold. In contrast, potassium levels were reduced in mycorrhizal roots relative to the non-mycorrhizal controls (Figure 4a). Hence, in addition to the quantitative benefit in growth (Figure 3), mycorrhizal plants profited from a qualitative improvement in mineral nutrition (in particular of phosphorus and manganese).

Similarly, plants treated only with water exhibited increased levels of calcium, zinc, and phosphorus, (Figure 4b). These results show that mycorrhizal plants profit, in addition to the mycorrhizal growth effect, from a qualitative benefit in mineral nutrition. This qualitative benefit was also observed in the absence of a positive growth response as observed in the water-treated plants.

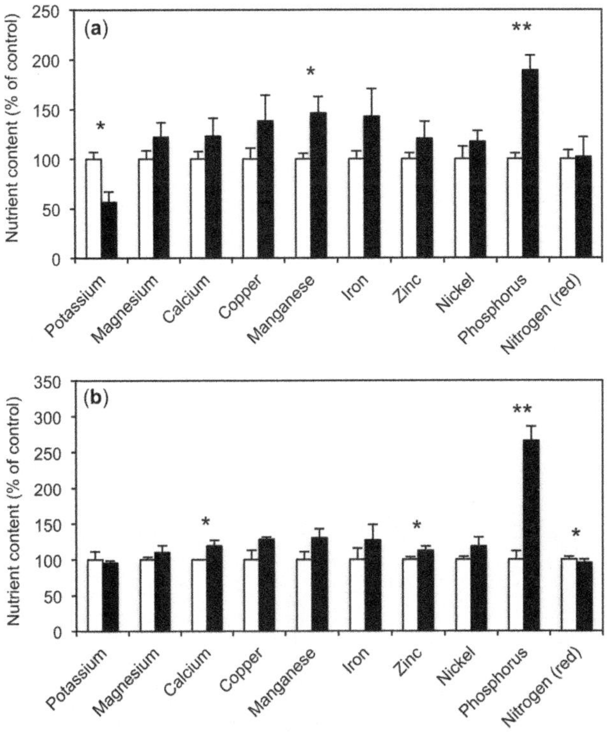

Figure 4. *R. irregularis* increases nutrient content of plants supplied with water or with nutrient solution. Nutrient levels in leaves were determined 36 days after inoculation in the plants shown in Figure 3. Values are the mean of three biological replicates. Error bars represent standard deviations. Asterisks indicate significant differences between mycorrhizal roots (black columns) and non-mycorrhizal controls (white columns). (**a**) Plants were fertilized with basic nutrient solution. Values are expressed relative to the non-mycorrhizal fertilized controls that were set to 100% for each nutrient. (**b**) As in (a), but without nutrient solution. Values are expressed relative to the non-colonized water-treated controls that were set to 100% for each nutrient.

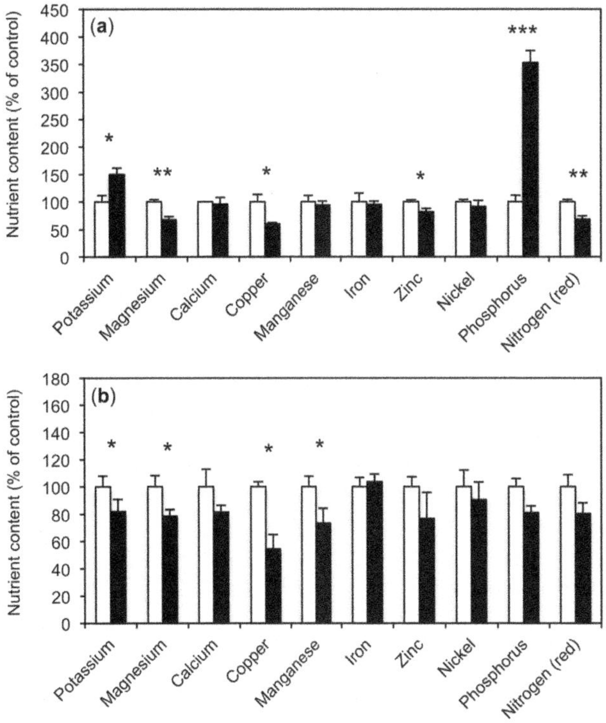

Figure 5. Treatment with KH_2PO_4 alone causes depletion of other nutrients and interferes with nutrient acquisition in mycorrhizal roots. Nutrient levels in leaves were determined 36 days after inoculation in the plants shown in Figure 3. Values are the mean of three replicates. Error bars represent standard deviations. Asterisks indicate significant differences between P_i and water treatment (a) or between mycorrhizal and non-mycorrhizal roots (b). (**a**) Treatment of non-inoculated plants with 5 mM KH_2PO_4 alone (black columns) compared to controls with water alone (white columns). Values are expressed relative to the water-treated controls that were set to 100% for each nutrient. (**b**) Nutrient content of mycorrhizal plants treated with 5 mM KH_2PO_4 (black columns) compared to non-inoculated controls treated with 5 mM KH_2PO_4 (white columns; corresponding to black columns in (a)). Values are expressed relative to the non-colonized P_i-treated controls that were set to 100% for each nutrient.

Exogenous P_i supply interferes with plant nutrition

To determine how P_i supply in the absence of other nutrients impacts on general plant nutrition, the nutrient levels in plants treated only with P_i were determined relative to plants treated with water (Figure 5a; Figure S1). As expected, supply with P_i alone resulted in a strong increase of P in the shoot, however, the levels of other nutrients, in particular Mg, Cu, Zn and nitrate, were reduced. This may reflect the dilution of these nutrients in the leaves as a result of the moderately stimulated growth in response to elevated P_i.

Examination of the effect of *R. irregularis* on mineral nutrition in plants treated with P_i alone (without fertilization) revealed a surprising trend. The levels of several nutrients were further reduced in these mycorrhizal plants relative to the respective non-mycorrhizal controls treated with only P_i (Figure 5b, compare with 4a,b). This indicates that the AM fungus did not provide a nutritional benefit, but rather acted like a parasite by consuming carbohydrates, and at the same time holding back mineral nutrients. In addition, the DP for phosphate, represented by *PhPT1* and *PhPT2*, was repressed under these conditions (Tables S4, S5).

Shoot/root ratio and N/P ratio indicate that elevated P_i levels cause N-starvation

Several lines of evidence indicated that P_i-treated plants were starved for other nutrients, in particular N (see above). Therefore, three parameters that are indicative of nutritional status in plants were compared, namely shoot weight, shoot/root (S/R) ratio, and N/P ratio. Shoot growth was significantly induced by AM in fertilized plants, and by high P_i in combination with nutrient solution, indicating that these plants experienced favorable nutrient supply (Figure 6a). The S/R ratios (Figure 6b) showed a similar trend, in particular, the supply with high P_i in combination with nutrient solution caused the S/R ratio to double compared to water and P_i alone. Similarly, the strong growth effect of mycorrhizal plants with nutrient solution (Figure 3d) translated into a pronounced increase of S/R ratio (Figure 6b). In contrast, the treatments of water or P_i alone resulted in low S/R ratio even in mycorrhizal plants, indicating that these plants were nutrient-limited despite their mycorrhizal status.

Finally, the relative levels of N and P (N/P ratio) in leaves were determined in the different treatments. Normally, the N/P ratio is in the range of 10–20 [50]. Plants treated only with water had a relatively high N/P ratio of ca. 30, and the supply with nutrient solution caused the ratio to increase to ca. 55 (Figure 6c), reflecting the effect of N supply via fertilization. Under both P_i-depleted nutrient regimes, mycorrhizal colonization dramatically reduced the N/P ratio reflecting the increased P_i supply through AM (Figure 6c). In this context, it is interesting to note that the improved P status in mycorrhizal plants supplied with only water did not translate into an MGR (Figure 3d), indicating that these plants were starved for nutrients other than P_i. As expected, the treatments with high P_i dramatically reduced the N/P ratio in particular if P_i was applied alone (Figure 6c).

Taken together, these results indicate that only fertilized mycorrhizal plants and fertilized P_i-treated plants were well supplied with nutrients, whereas the other plants were limited for some nutrients other than P_i, conceivably N. In other words, exogenous P_i caused relative N-starvation. Furthermore, the N/P ratios of mycorrhizal plants suggest that AM promote P nutrition more than N nutrition.

Microarray analysis of the P_i effect indicates N-starvation

In order to obtain further insight into the nutritional status of the plants, microarray analysis was employed to assess the expression of genes involved in nutrient acquisition, which can serve as a diagnostic tool. In order to reveal the consequences of elevated P_i levels for plant physiology, the genes that responded to a treatment with P_i alone (in the absence of additional fertilizer) were first identified. Among a total of 660 genes that were induced at least 3-fold by P_i, the first ten contained three genes encoding predicted nitrate and nitrite transporters (data not shown). Focusing on only genes involved in mineral nutrient uptake revealed 28 genes induced 2-fold and 38 genes repressed 2-fold by P_i (Table S4). Interestingly, among the genes involved in nutrient acquisition, the ten IDs with the highest induction ratio comprised eight genes with a predicted role in nitrogen acquisition (Table 1, Table S4). Functional grouping of all P_i-regulated genes involved in nutrient acquisition confirmed that N-related genes were induced to the highest levels, followed by sulfur-related genes, whereas all PTs were repressed (Table S5). Interestingly, no ammonium transporter responded to high P_i.

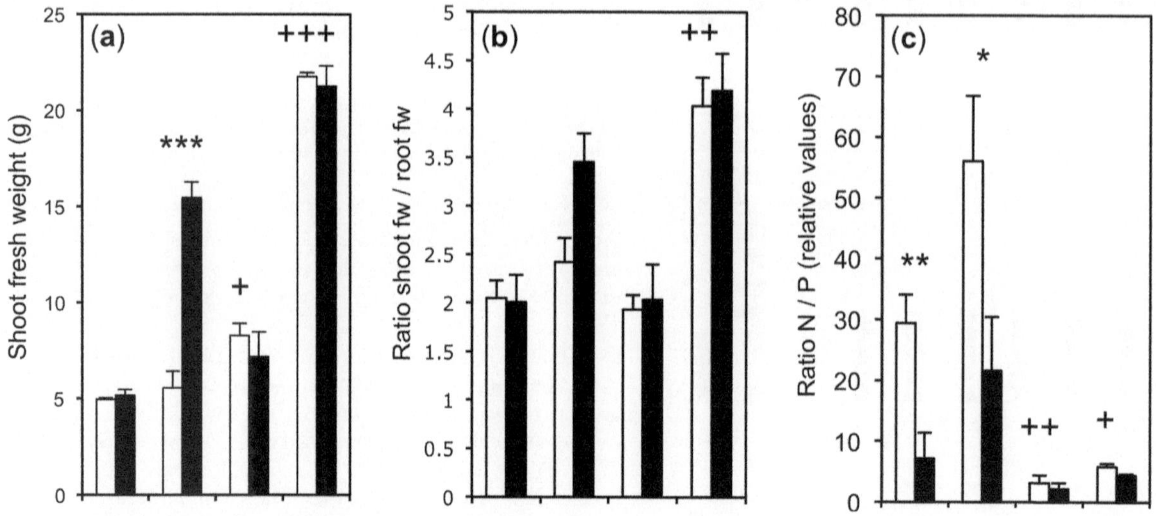

Figure 6. Shoot weight, shoot/root ratio and N/P ratio as indicators of nutritional status. Treatments were as in Figure 3, shown are the values of the final time point (48 days after inoculation). Columns represent the average of three biological replicates, error bars represent standard deviations. Asterisks indicate significant differences between mycorrhizal and non-mycorrhizal plants (white vs. black columns), crosses indicate significant differences between the non-mycorrhizal nutrient treatments vs. the non-mycorrhizal water treatment (i.e. between the different white columns). (a) Shoot weight of plants grown with *R. irregularis* (black column) or without (white columns) under different nutritional conditions. (b) Shoot/root ratio of plants inoculated with *R. irregularis* (black columns) or without (white columns) under various nutritional conditions. A ratio of 3.5–4 indicates that plants are well supplied with mineral nutrients, whereas a ratio around 2 indicates that plants are starved and allocate relatively large amounts of resources to the root system to compensate nutritional deficits. (c) N/P ratio of the same plants as in (a),(b). In the absence of exogenous P_i supply, mycorrhizal plants (black columns) exhibited lower N/P ratios than non-mycorrhizal controls, reflecting increased mycorrhizal P_i supply. Administration of 5 mM KH_2PO_4 reduced N/P ratio even stronger than AM, in particular if only P_i was supplied.

The N-related genes comprised nitrate transporters (NRTs) of both known subfamilies (NRT1 and NRT2) and a predicted nitrite transporter (Nitr1) (File S1; Figure 7). These genes were induced by P_i, irrespective of the presence of additional nutrients, and of the presence of the mycorrhizal fungus (Table 1, treatments 2, 3, 6, and 7), indicating that plants may experience relative N-limitation under all these conditions. In addition, they were induced in non-fertilized starved plants and, partially, in starved mycorrhizal roots (Table 1, treatments 4 and 5). This expression pattern is inversely correlated with the N/P ratio in the shoot (Table 1, first line; normalized to fertilized controls).

Quantitative real time RT-PCR (qPCR) analysis confirms results from microarray analysis

In order to independently evaluate the expression of the marker genes for N acquisition, a new experiment under equivalent conditions was performed and the expression of genes, identified by microarray analysis, was determined by quantitative real time RT-PCR (qPCR). Representative genes for the two NRT subfamilies and for the putative Nitr1 were selected (Figure 7), and their expression compared with the expression of the functional AM marker PT4 (Figure 8). In general, the expression of the N-related genes showed a similar trend as with microarray analysis. They were strongly induced in all treatments with KH_2PO_4 (Figures 8a–c), and, to a lesser extent, in non-fertilized plants both, in mycorrhizal roots as well as non-mycorrhizal controls. PT4 was strongly induced in mycorrhizal plants supplied with low P_i levels, but only weakly in inoculated plants treated with KH_2PO_4 (Figure 8d). Notably, the partially restored colonization in plants treated with P_i alone (28.2% colonization) was not associated with a proportional restoration of PT4 induction (Figure 8d). This indicates that the MP for P_i remained inactive, hence, the level of AM colonization and the expression of PT4 are uncoupled under these conditions.

Suppression of AM colonization by P_i depends on adequate nitrogen supply

So far, our results indicate that P caused relative N-starvation, in particular if it was applied alone (without further nutrients). Hence, it may have been the starvation for N that counteracted the inhibitory effect of high P_i and caused the recovery of root colonization. To test this possibility, several nutrients were removed individually by treating inoculated plants with high P_i together with basic nutrient solution from which individual nutrients were omitted (Figure 9; Table S2). While the treatment with all nutrients reduced AM colonization to 3%, the removal of nitrate from the nutrient solution resulted in a recovery to over 30% colonization, as in the case where all nutrients had been removed (compare with Figures 2,3). The individual removal of several other nutrient elements (S, K, Ca, Fe) also caused a partial recovery of AM colonization, although to a lesser extent.

Discussion

Genetic and nutritional control of AM symbiosis

During the past decade, genetic analysis of AM has revealed a suite of genes of the plant host that are essential for the establishment of the interaction and which are therefore referred to as symbiosis (SYM) genes [51]. They constitute a signaling pathway that triggers a characteristic calcium signal (calcium

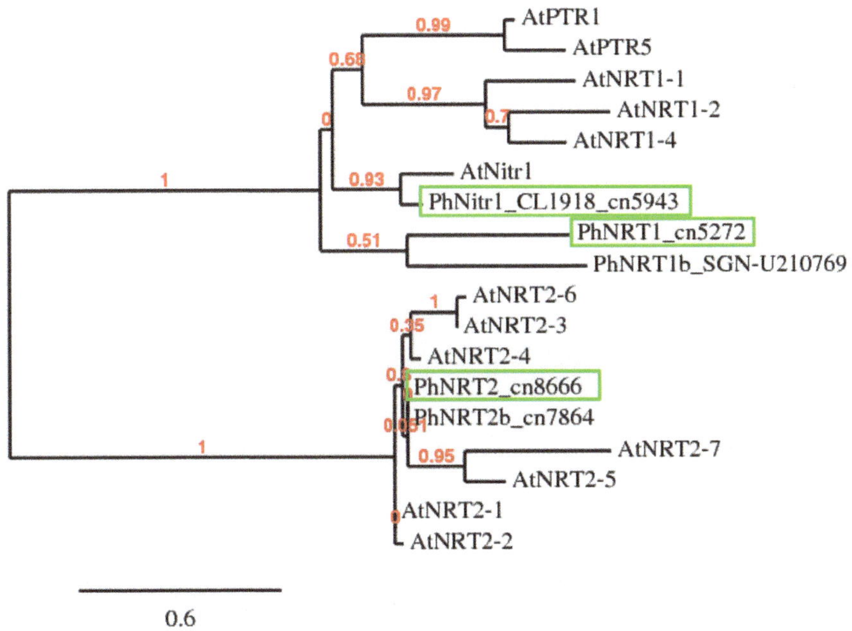

Figure 7. Phylogenetic analysis of P_i-responsive transporters of *Petunia hybrida* compared to *Arabidopsis* transporters for nitrate, nitrite, and peptides. For the EST sequences listed in Table 1 the full-length predicted cDNA sequences were derived from the petunia genome sequence. Predicted petunia protein sequences were compared with *Arabidopsis thaliana* transporters for nitrate and nitrite (NRT and Nitr1, respectively), and for peptide transporters (PTR). Note the clear separation of the nitrate transporter subfamilies NRT1 and NRT2. The NRT1 family also comprises the nitrite transporter AtNitr1 and several peptide transporters, of which only two are represented (AtPTR2 and AtPTR5). Petunia has two very closely homologous representatives of the high affinity nitrate transporter family NRT2 (cn8666 and cn7864). In addition, there is a putative nitrite transporter (corresponding to the EST sequences CL1918 and cn5943), and two additional members of the low affinity NRT1 family. Genes boxed in green were analyzed by qPCR (Figure 8). Cn8665, which is almost identical to cn8666, and CL5245, which is predicted to encode a nitrogen limitation adaptation gene (see Table 1), were omitted from phylogenetic analysis.

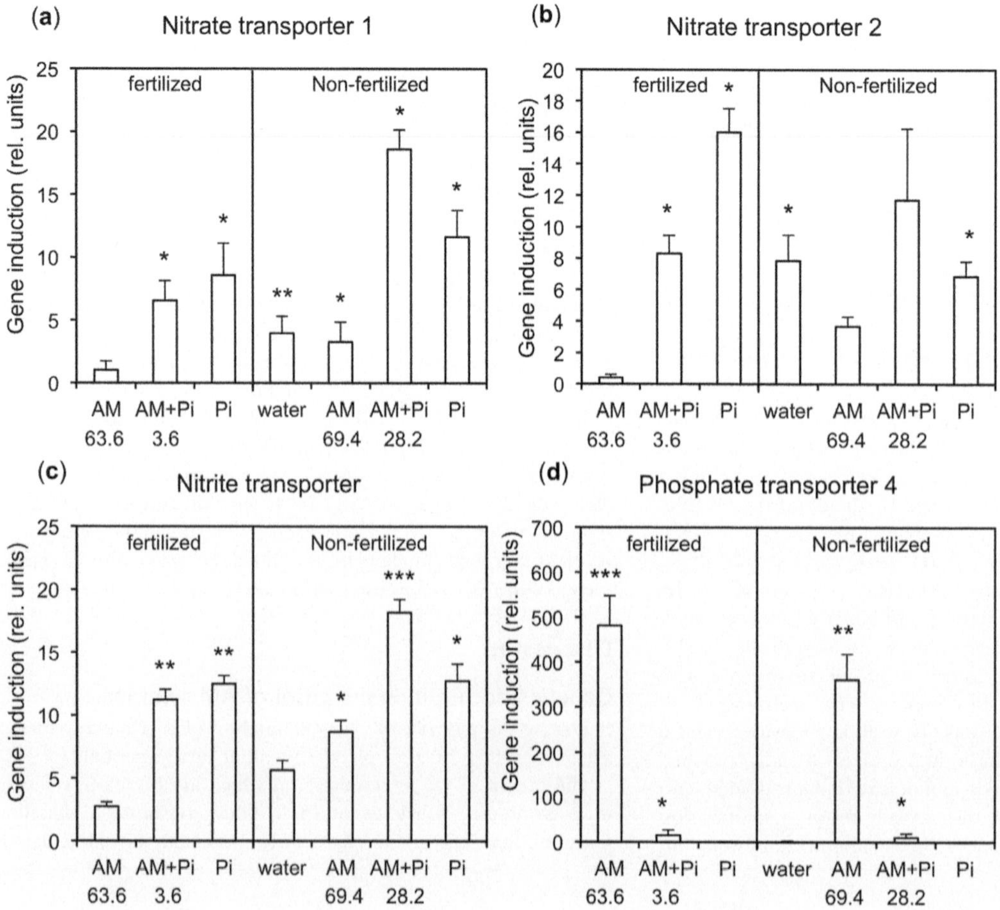

Figure 8. Quantitative real time PCR analysis (qPCR) of marker genes for nitrogen and phosphorus acquisition. qPCR analysis was performed to determine the expression of the N transporters boxed in Figure 7, and of the AM-specific phosphate transporter PhPT4. Treatments were as in Figures 3–6 and Table 1. Expression values were first normalized to GAPDH and then expressed as induction ratios for the indicated treatments relative to the standard treatment (non-mycorrhizal fertilized plants), as in Table 1. Columns represent the mean of five biological replicates. Error bars represent the standard deviations derived from the two standard deviations of the compared treatments (see Materials and Methods). Numbers below the x-axis reflect the percentage of root colonization in the respective sample.

spiking) that is required for intracellular accommodation of the endosymbiont and for reprogramming of the host cells [51–53]. Apart from these endogenous factors, environmental factors influence AM in various ways. In particular, mineral nutrients are known to influence symbiosis. In general, low nutrient levels promote symbiosis, whereas high nutrient levels are inhibitory [3]. Since the primordial benefit of AM is the acquisition of mineral nutrients, the regulatory function of nutrients may represent a feedback mechanism to coordinate AM colonization with the nutritional requirements of the plant.

Regulation of AM by phosphate

P_i is thought to be the major currency with which the obligate symbiotic AM fungi pay for assimilates of the plant [54,55]. Accordingly, plants have long been known to respond particularly sensitive to high P_i levels with suppression of the symbiosis [30–38]. Inhibition of AM development by P_i is systemic and appears to depend on the P-status of the shoot [33,34]. Although an active role of the plant in the P_i-related repression of AM is plausible, the mechanisms involved are elusive.

Transcriptomic analysis of the high P_i response showed that besides the repression of the P_i-starvation pathway, P_i repressed carotenoid biosynthetic genes and symbiosis-related genes such as PT4 [34]. Although production and secretion of the AM-promoting apocarotenoid strigolactone (SL) from the plant host is known to be inversely correlated with P_i supply [33,56–58], reduced SL secretion alone cannot explain the inhibitory action of P_i, since SL application does not alleviate the inhibition by P_i [34]. A conceivable mechanism for P-related regulation of AM is the control of fungal growth through reduced supply of assimilates to the fungus [59].

Regulation of AM by other nutrients

For optimal growth and functioning, plants rely on balanced nutrient supply, which implies some sort of coordination between the acquisition pathways for the different nutrients. In particular, the pathways for the nutrient elements required at highest amounts, namely N and P, are known to interact [50]. The present study describes a systematic analysis of the nutritional effects of P_i and other nutrients on AM, and the interactions of P_i with other nutrients. A first outcome is the finding that among all the tested nutrients, only P_i and nitrate exerted a negative influence on AM, whereas other major nutrients such as potassium (K), calcium (Ca), magnesium (Mg), sulfate (SO_4), and iron (Fe) did not influence AM at elevated concentrations (Figure 1; compare also with [34]). The relatively weak inhibitory

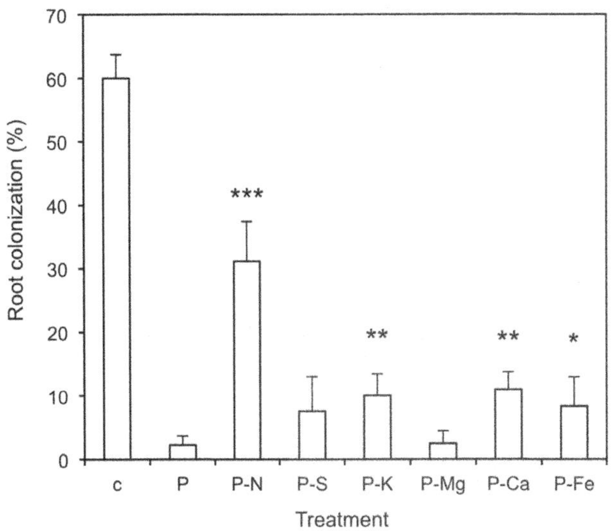

Figure 9. Withdrawal of individual nutrients interferes with the inhibitory effect of P_i. Effects of withdrawal of individual nutrients from the basic nutrient solution applied together with 5 mM KH_2PO_4. Omitted nutrients were replaced by other nutrients to maintain osmotic relationships. The strong inhibitory effect of P_i (P) was reduced particularly by removal of nitrate (P-N), but also to a lesser extent by removal of S, K, Ca, and Fe. The control treatment (c) represents fertilization with low P_i levels (0.03 mM). Columns represent the average of six biological replicates, error bars represent the standard deviations. Asterisks indicate significant differences between the treatments lacking individual nutrients and the treatment with basic nutrient solution and high P_i.

effect of nitrate suggests that this effect may not be of central importance for the regulation of AM in the case of petunia, although a significant decline of AM colonization has been associated with high nitrogen supply in other systems [60,61].

Cross-talk of P with N and other nutritional pathways

Exogenous P_i supply in the absence of other nutrients resulted in a low S/R ratio (Figure 6b), indicative of starvation for a nutritional factor that causes the plant to prioritize root growth to compensate low nutrient supply [62]. Indeed, P_i supply resulted in strongly lowered N/P ratios (Figure 6c), i.e. in relative N-starvation. Nutrient starvation often leads to the induction of nutrient transporters to compensate for low nutrient supply [63]. For example, P_i-starvation induces P_i-transporters (PT) in *Arabidopsis* and tomato [64,65], whereas N-starvation induces various nitrate transporters (NRT) in rice and Arabidopsis [66,67].

Indeed, high P_i caused a strong induction of genes with a predicted role in N acquisition (Table 1; Tables S4 and S5), while transporters for other nutrients were affected to a lesser extent (Table S5). Interestingly, the P_i-related induction of genes involved in N acquisition was also observed in mycorrhizal plants, in particular in the non-fertilized ones (Table 1, treatment 5; Figure 8), consistent with the decrease of the N/P ratio in these plants (Figure 6c). Among the induced NRTs (Table S5; Figure 7), three very similar genes encoded predicted high-affinity transporters within the NRT2 family (cn8665, cn8666 and cn7864), with cn8665 and cn8666 being 100% identical at the amino acid level. Hence, only cn8666 was analyzed phylogenetically as a representative of this group (Figure 7). Cn8666 and cn7864 are particularly closely related to AtNRT2.1, which is essential for the response to nitrate starvation in the roots of *Arabidopsis* [68], and to AtNRT2.4, which is induced by N-starvation in the root epidermis and contributes to nitrate acquisition under this condition [67]. Three further genes, represented by the EST sequences cn5272, cn5943, CL1918, and SG_SGN-U210769, fall into the NRT1 family (Figure 7). Besides low-affinity nitrate transporters, the NRT1 family of *Arabidospsis* contains a predicted plastidial nitrite transporter (AtNitr1) [69], and a so-called nitrate transceptor [70,71], which is involved in both, the transport and the perception and signaling of nitrate [72]. The petunia EST consensus sequences cn5943 and CL1918 belong to the same petunia gene, which is most closely related to the *Arabidopsis* Nitr1 [69]. While several genes involved in N acquisition were induced by N starvation, two predicted nitrate transporters (cn8317 and cn8506) behaved in the opposite way, i.e. they were repressed by N starvation (Table S4 and S5). These genes may encode nitrate transporters that are induced by their own substrate, nitrate [73,74]. Taken together, these results indicate that P_i induces the entire nitrate acquisition pathway, and possibly nitrate sensing in petunia.

Besides the induction of nitrate transporters that are involved in the DP for N uptake, N starvation caused AM colonization to be partially restored under high P_i levels (Figures 3, 6, 9), conceivably to enable symbiotic N uptake despite the inhibitory levels of P_i. Interestingly, it has been observed in a natural environment as well that the repression of AM colonization by high P_i was relieved when N became limiting [40]. A similar interaction between P and N nutrition was shown on colonization of *Allium schoenoprasum* by *Glomus caledonium* in pot cultures [75]. These results are in line with the hypothesis that AM symbiosis evolved to ensure balanced nutrient levels in both partners and a stoichiometric relationship in the exchange of C, N, and P [76].

If AM colonization at high P_i levels was promoted to enable symbiotic N acquisition, ammonium transporters (AMT) of the plant would be expected to become induced to allow N from the fungus to be taken up in the form of ammonium [16]. However, no AMT was induced by high P_i, indicating that despite the restoration of root colonization, the symbiosis does not contribute to N uptake under these conditions, an assumption that is in line with the reduced N levels in these plants (Figure 5b). Surprisingly, the recovery of AM colonization observed in plants supplied with high P_i alone was not associated with a parallel induction of symbiotic PT expression (Figure 8d), although the colonization appeared morphologically normal. PT4 is commonly regarded as a marker for functional symbiotic cells with arbuscules, however, repression of PT4 by P_i appears to be stronger than induction of PT4 by the AM fungus. Taken together, these findings suggest that AM colonization under these conditions does not confer an obvious nutritional benefit to the plant host.

Inhibition of AM development by high P_i and by mutation of P_i transporters: common mechanisms?

Interestingly, mutation of AM-related PTs in the plant causes a similar inhibitory effect on AM as high exogenous P_i supply [77–79]. However, in these cases, it is not the abundant supply, but the lack of P_i delivery that triggers inhibition. A possible explanation for this observation is that the plant can assess the costs (assimilate consumption of the fungus), and the benefits (fungal P_i supply) in the interaction, and inhibits fungal colonization if the balance is unfavorable. The fact that P_i strongly represses symbiotic PTs (Table S5) and other symbiosis-related genes [34] raises the possibility that the high P_i effect and the PT mutant phenotype may involve partially overlapping mechanisms: Although the two conditions have opposite consequences for the P status of the plant, they both result in inhibition of the symbiotic P_i uptake pathway.

Inhibition of AM development by PT mutation has been observed in legumes and rice [77–79]. Mutation of a close homologue in tomato had no AM-related phenotype [80,81], conceivably because of functional redundancy among the three symbiotic PT genes commonly found in *Solanaceae* [81–83]. In *P. hybrida*, all three PTs were strongly repressed by P_i, thus resulting in a general conditional inactivation of the symbiotic P_i uptake pathway [34], potentially contributing to inhibition of AM development as in PT mutants of legumes and rice. An interesting parallel concerning the inhibitory effects of high P_i and of PT mutation on AM development extends to the fact that both conditions can be reversed by N-starvation (Figure 9; Javot et al., 2011).

Mycorrhizal benefits depend on nutrient supply

The primary benefit of AM is thought to be the improved supply of macro- and micronutrients [21,84], in particular of P_i, which translates into increased growth rates of mycorrhizal plants, the so-called mycorrhizal growth response (MGR). Indeed, a robust MGR and enhanced nutrient levels in mycorrhizal plants were observed upon fertilization with basic nutrient solution (Figures 3d, 4a; Figure S1). Taking into account both the MGR and the increased nutrient content per gram of leaf tissue, mycorrhizal plants contained approximately 6-fold the amount of P_i compared to fertilized plants without AM, and approximately 4-fold the amount of the other nutrients.

Unfertilized mycorrhizal plants also had increased nutrient levels compared to non-mycorrhizal control plants, although to a lesser extent, and only P_i accumulation was substantial (Figure 4b), showing that despite the lack of an MGR (Figures 2, 3), these plants had gained a qualitative benefit from AM symbiosis. Although the growth of these plants was apparently limited by some factor, the higher nutrient content represents a potential advantage in fitness that can be translated into growth or in the production of additional offspring at a later stage of development.

On the other end of the scale, plants treated with only P_i alone were colonized to 30% but had no positive MGR and no induction of the symbiotic P_i uptake machinery. Notably, these plants even contained lower nutrient levels than non-mycorrhizal control plants treated with P_i only, hence, under these conditions, the interaction exhibited characteristics of a parasitic interaction.

MGR varies considerably with some plant species showing spectacular increases of >10-fold. Such cases are usually based on the bad performance of the plant in the absence of the fungal partner, a phenomenon that is expressed as 'dependency' of the plant on AM [85]. In contrast, many species, in particular cereals, show no (or even negative) MGR, and therefore are considered non-responsive [85,86]. However, it has been pointed out that such classifications represent an oversimplification [26], since the outcome of an interaction depends on both partners and involves environmental factors [87]. Indeed, our study shows that the environment has a strong influence on the MGR of *Petunia hybrida* with *R. irregularis*. Although plants in natural environments may experience less extreme conditions than in our experiments, our results show that depending on the nutritional conditions, an AM interaction can represent a range of outcomes along the continuum between strongly mutualistic and parasitic [88]. However, it should be kept in mind that mycorrhizal plants with neutral or negative MGR may profit from other benefits than improved nutrition, for example increased drought tolerance or disease resistance [7–9].

Conclusions

Nutrient-dependent regulation of AM colonization provides an important feedback mechanism for plants to promote or limit fungal colonization according to their needs. We show here that the nutrients P_i and nitrate can potentially exert negative regulation on AM, whereas sulfate and the cations Mg^{2+}, Ca^{2+}, and Fe^{3+} have no effect. On the other hand, starvation for several mineral nutrients, in particular for nitrate, reversed the inhibitory effect of P_i on AM, indicating that nutrient starvation triggers a dominant AM-promoting signal that counteracts the effects of high P_i. Future research should address the interplay of exogenous and endogenous factors in AM, in particular, how nutrients impinge on symbiotic signaling and on the subsequent cellular program in host cells.

Supporting Information

Figure S1 Nutrient content of mycorrhizal and non-mycorrhizal plants under different nutritional treatments. Nutrient levels were determined in the leaves of plants treated with only water, with basic nutrient solution (Nutr.), with 5 mM KH_2PO_4 (P), or with a combination of nutrient solution and 5 mM KH_2PO_4 (Nutr.+P). Plants were harvested 36 days after inoculation with *R. irregularis* (black columns) or mock inoculation (white columns). Columns represent the average of three biological replicates, error bars represent the standard deviations.
(TIF)

File S1 Predicted amino acid sequences of nitrate and nitrite transporters of *Arabidopsis thaliana* and *Petunia hybrida* used for phylogenetic analysis.
(DOCX)

Table S1 Nutrient content of plant growth substrate.
(XLSX)

Table S2 Composition of nutrient solutions.
(XLSX)

Table S3 Microarray data after first level analysis by Nimblegen. Mean gene expression values (Exprs) and variation coefficients (SE_Exprs) resulting from the three probes per sequence ID are listed for the different nutritional regimes. All the induction ratios shown in Tables S4 and S5, and Table 1, are derived from the data listed in Table S3.
(XLSX)

Table S4 Genes regulated by high P_i supply. Gene expression ratios above 2-fold and below 0.5-fold of genes with a predicted role in mineral nutrient acquisition are shown. Expression ratios were obtained by dividing the expression values from the treatment of interest (indicated combinations of basic nutrient solution, 5 mM KH_2PO_4, and *R. irregularis*) by the expression values of the reference treatment, i.e. non-mycorrhizal fertilized plants (see Table S3 for individual expression values). Expression ratios were sorted according to the treatment with high P_i alone (treatment 7). Note that the ten genes induced at highest levels comprise eight N-related genes (in bold), in particular transporters (see also Table 1).
(XLS)

Table S5 Nutritional regulation of genes involved in nutrient acquisition. Expression ratios as in Table S4 but ordered according to predicted function.
(XLS)

Table S6 Primers for quantitative real time RT-PCR (qPCR). (XLSX)

Acknowledgements

We thank Thomas L. Sims and the *Petunia* community for access to the *P. axillaris* draft genome sequence. We would like to express our thanks to Abbas KHANI for his suggestions on the experimental work and his comments on the manuscript. We thank Michael Stumpe for statistical analysis, Christine Jakob and Joseph Schoepfer for taking care of the plants, and Jonathan Schramm and Patrick Favre for experimental support. This study would not have been possible without the longstanding promotion of petunia as a model system by Tom Gerats. This paper is dedicated to mark his retirement.

Author Contributions

Conceived and designed the experiments: DR EN FBS UF. Performed the experiments: DR EN FBS UF. Analyzed the data: DR EN FBS UF. Contributed reagents/materials/analysis tools: DR UF. Wrote the paper: DR EN FBS UF.

References

1. Elser JJ, Bracken MES, Cleland EE, Gruner DS, Harpole WS, et al. (2007) Global analysis of nitrogen and phosphorus limitation of primary producers in freshwater, marine and terrestrial ecosystems. Ecology Letters 10: 1135–1142.
2. Hell R, Hillebrand H (2001) Plant concepts for mineral acquisition and allocation. Current Opinion in Biotechnology 12: 161–168.
3. Smith S, Read D (2008) Mycorrhizal Symbiosis. New York: Academic Press.
4. Brundrett MC (2002) Coevolution of roots and mycorrhizas of land plants. New Phytologist 154: 275–304.
5. Friese CF, Allen MF (1991) The spread of VA mycorrhizal fungal hyphae in the soil – Inoculum types and external hyphal architecture. Mycologia 83: 409–418.
6. Bago B, Azcon-Aguilar C, Goulet A, Piche Y (1998) Branched absorbing structures (BAS): a feature of the extraradical mycelium of symbiotic arbuscular mycorrhizal fungi. New Phytologist 139: 375–388.
7. Augé RM (2001) Water relations, drought and vesicular-arbuscular mycorrhizal symbiosis. Mycorrhiza 11: 3–42.
8. Conrath U, Beckers GJM, Flors V, Garcia-Agustin P, Jakab G, et al. (2006) Priming: Getting ready for battle. Molecular Plant-Microbe Interactions 19: 1062–1071.
9. Jung SC, Martinez-Medina A, Lopez-Raez JA, Pozo MJ (2012) Mycorrhiza-induced resistance and priming of plant defenses. Journal of Chemical Ecology 38: 651–664.
10. Karandashov V, Bucher M (2005) Symbiotic phosphate transport in arbuscular mycorrhizas. Trends in Plant Science 10: 22–29.
11. Fellbaum CR, Gachomo EW, Beesetty Y, Choudhari S, Strahan GD, et al. (2012) Carbon availability triggers fungal nitrogen uptake and transport in arbuscular mycorrhizal symbiosis. Proceedings of the National Academy of Sciences of the United States of America 109: 2666–2671.
12. Hodge A, Fitter AH (2010) Substantial nitrogen acquisition by arbuscular mycorrhizal fungi from organic material has implications for N cycling. Proceedings of the National Academy of Sciences of the United States of America 107: 13754–13759.
13. Mäder P, Vierheilig H, Streitwolf-Engel R, Boller T, Frey B, et al. (2000) Transport of N-15 from a soil compartment separated by a polytetrafluoroethylene membrane to plant roots via the hyphae of arbuscular mycorrhizal fungi. New Phytologist 146: 155–161.
14. Müller A, George E, Gabriel-Neumann E (2013) The symbiotic recapture of nitrogen from dead mycorrhizal and non-mycorrhizal roots of tomato plants. Plant and Soil 364: 341–355.
15. Govindarajulu M, Pfeffer PE, Jin HR, Abubaker J, Douds DD, et al. (2005) Nitrogen transfer in the arbuscular mycorrhizal symbiosis. Nature 435: 819–823.
16. Guether M, Neuhauser B, Balestrini R, Dynowski M, Ludewig U, et al. (2009) A mycorrhizal-specific ammonium transporter from *Lotus japonicus* acquires nitrogen released by arbuscular mycorrhizal fungi. Plant Physiology 150: 73–83.
17. Tian CJ, Kasiborski B, Koul R, Lammers PJ, Bucking H, et al. (2010) Regulation of the nitrogen transfer pathway in the arbuscular mycorrhizal symbiosis: Gene characterization and the coordination of expression with nitrogen flux. Plant Physiology 153: 1175–1187.
18. Allen JW, Shachar-Hill Y (2009) Sulfur transfer through an arbuscular mycorrhiza. Plant Physiology 149: 549–560.
19. Sieh D, Watanabe M, Devers EA, Brueckner F, Hoefgen R, et al. (2013) The arbuscular mycorrhizal symbiosis influences sulfur starvation responses of Medicago truncatula. New Phytologist 197: 606–616.
20. Clark RB, Zeto SK (2000) Mineral acquisition by arbuscular mycorrhizal plants. Journal of Plant Nutrition 23: 867–902.
21. George E (2000) Nutrient uptake – Contributions of arbuscular mycorrhizal fungi to plant mineral nutrition. In: Kapulnik Y, Douds DD, editors. Arbuscular mycorrhizas: Physiology and function. Dordrecht: Kluwer Academic Publishers. 307–343.
22. Smith SE, Smith FA (2011) Roles of arbuscular mycorrhizas in plant nutrition and growth: New paradigms from cellular to ecosystem scales. Annual Review of Plant Biology 62: 227–250.
23. Smith SE, Smith FA, Jakobsen I (2003) Mycorrhizal fungi can dominate phosphate supply to plants irrespective of growth responses. Plant Physiology 133: 16–20.
24. Smith SE, Smith FA, Jakobsen I (2004) Functional diversity in arbuscular mycorrhizal (AM) symbioses: the contribution of the mycorrhizal P uptake pathway is not correlated with mycorrhizal responses in growth or total P uptake. New Phytologist 162: 511–524.
25. Klironomos JN (2003) Variation in plant response to native and exotic arbuscular mycorrhizal fungi. Ecology 84: 2292–2301.
26. Smith FA, Grace EJ, Smith SE (2009) More than a carbon economy: nutrient trade and ecological sustainability in facultative arbuscular mycorrhizal symbioses. New Phytologist 182: 347–358.
27. Alguacil MM, Lumini E, Roldan A, Salinas-Garcia JR, Bonfante P, et al. (2008) The impact of tillage practices on arbuscular mycorrhizal fungal diversity in subtropical crops. Ecological Applications 18: 527–536.
28. Lin XG, Feng YZ, Zhang HY, Chen RR, Wang JH, et al. (2012) Long-term balanced fertilization decreases arbuscular mycorrhizal fungal diversity in an arable soil in north China revealed by 454 pyrosequencing. Environmental Science & Technology 46: 5764–5771.
29. Liu YJ, Shi GX, Mao L, Cheng G, Jiang SJ, et al. (2012) Direct and indirect influences of 8 yr of nitrogen and phosphorus fertilization on Glomeromycota in an alpine meadow ecosystem. New Phytologist 194: 523–535.
30. Abbott LK, Robson AD, De Boer G (1984) The effect of phosphorus on the formation of hyphae in soil by the vesicular arbuscular mycorrhizal fungus, *Glomus fasciculatum*. New Phytologist 97: 437–446.
31. Amijée F, Tinker PB, Stribley DP (1989) Effects of phosphorus on the morphology of VA mycorrhizal root-system of leek (*Allium porrum* L). Plant and Soil 119: 334–336.
32. Amijée F, Tinker PB, Stribley DP (1989) The development of endomycorrhizal root systems .7. A detailed study of effects of soil-phosphorus on colonization. New Phytologist 111: 435–446.
33. Balzergue C, Puech-Pagès V, Bécard G, Rochange SF (2011) The regulation of arbuscular mycorrhizal symbiosis by phosphate in pea involves early and systemic signalling events. Journal of Experimental Botany 62: 1049–1060.
34. Breuillin F, Schramm J, Hajirezaei M, Ahkami A, Favre P, et al. (2010) Phosphate systemically inhibits development of arbuscular mycorrhiza in *Petunia hybrida* and represses genes involved in mycorrhizal functioning. Plant Journal 64: 1002–1017.
35. Hepper CM (1983) The effect of nitrate and phosphate on the vesicular arbuscular mycorrhizal infection of lettuce. New Phytologist 93: 389–399.
36. Jasper DA, Robson AD, Abbott LK (1979) Phosphorus and the formation of vesicular-arbuscular mycorrhizas. Soil Biology & Biochemistry 11: 501–505.
37. Menge JA, Steirle D, Bagyaraj DJ, Johnson ELV, Leonard RT (1978) Phosphorus concentrations in plants responsible for inhibition of mycorrhizal infection. New Phytologist 80: 575–578.
38. Thomson BD, Robson AD, Abbott LK (1986) Effects of phosphorus on the formation of mycorrhizas by Gigaspora calospora and Glomus fasciculatum in relation to root carbohydrates. New Phytologist 103: 751–765.
39. Douds DD, Pfeffer PE, Shachar-Hill Y (2000) Carbon partitioning, cost, and metabolism of arbuscular mycorrhizas. In: Kapulnik Y, Douds DD, editors. Arbuscular Mycorrhizas: Physiology and Function. Dordrecht: Kluwer Academic Publishers.
40. Blanke V, Renker C, Wagner M, Fullner K, Held M, et al. (2005) Nitrogen supply affects arbuscular mycorrhizal colonization of Artemisia vulgaris in a phosphate-polluted field site. New Phytologist 166: 981–992.
41. Sekhara Reddy DMR, Schorderet M, Feller U, Reinhardt D (2007) A petunia mutant affected in intracellular accommodation and morphogenesis of arbuscular mycorrhizal fungi. Plant Journal 51: 739–750.
42. Stieger PA, Feller U (1994) Nutrient accumulation and translocation in maturing wheat plants grown on waterlogged soil. Plant and Soil 160: 87–95.
43. Bohley P (1967) Reihenbestimmungen von Stickstoff im Ultramikromassstab – Kjeldahlveraschung und Phenol-Hypochlorit-Reaktion. Hoppe-Seylers Zeitschrift für Physiologische Chemie 348: 100–110.
44. Verwoerd TC, Dekker BMM, Hoekema A (1989) A small-scale procedure for the rapid isolation of plant RNAs. Nucleic Acids Research 17: 2362–2362.
45. Nuwaysir EF, Huang W, Albert TJ, Singh J, Nuwaysir K, et al. (2002) Gene expression analysis using oligonucleotide arrays produced by maskless photolithography. Genome Research 12: 1749–1755.
46. Irizarry RA, Hobbs B, Collin F, Beazer-Barclay YD, Antonellis KJ, et al. (2003) Exploration, normalization, and summaries of high density oligonucleotide array probe level data. Biostatistics 4: 249–264.

47. Garcion C, Metraux JP (2006) FiRe and microarrays: a fast answer to burning questions. Trends in Plant Science 11: 320–322.
48. Schmittgen TD, Livak KJ (2008) Analyzing real-time PCR data by the comparative C-T method. Nature Protocols 3: 1101–1108.
49. Nagajyoti PC, Lee KD, Sreekanth TVM (2010) Heavy metals, occurrence and toxicity for plants: a review. Environmental Chemistry Letters 8: 199–216.
50. Güsewell S (2004) N:P ratios in terrestrial plants: variation and functional significance. New Phytologist 164: 243–266.
51. Parniske M (2008) Arbuscular mycorrhiza: the mother of plant root endosymbioses. Nature Reviews Microbiology 6: 763–775.
52. Charpentier M, Oldroyd GE (2013) Nuclear calcium signaling in plants. Plant Physiology 163: 496–503.
53. Seddas P, Gianinazzi-Pearson V, Schoefs B, Kuster H, Wipf D (2009) Communication and signaling in the plant-fungus symbiosis: The mycorrhiza. In: Baluska F, editor. Plant-Environment Interactions: From Sensory Plant Biology to Active Plant Behavior. 45–71.
54. Javot H, Pumplin N, Harrison MJ (2007) Phosphate in the arbuscular mycorrhizal symbiosis: transport properties and regulatory roles. Plant, Cell and Environment 30: 310–322.
55. Bucher M (2007) Functional biology of plant phosphate uptake at root and mycorrhiza interfaces. New Phytologist 173: 11–26.
56. Lopez-Raez JA, Charnikhova T, Gomez-Roldan V, Matusova R, Kohlen W, et al. (2008) Tomato strigolactones are derived from carotenoids and their biosynthesis is promoted by phosphate starvation. New Phytologist 178: 863–874.
57. Yoneyama K, Yoneyama K, Takeuchi Y, Sekimoto H (2007) Phosphorus deficiency in red clover promotes exudation of orobanchol, the signal for mycorrhizal symbionts and germination stimulant for root parasites. Planta 225: 1031–1038.
58. Yoneyama K, Xie XN, Kusumoto D, Sekimoto H, Sugimoto Y, et al. (2007) Nitrogen deficiency as well as phosphorus deficiency in sorghum promotes the production and exudation of 5-deoxystrigol, the host recognition signal for arbuscular mycorrhizal fungi and root parasites. Planta 227: 125–132.
59. Olsson PA, Rahm J, Aliasgharzad N (2010) Carbon dynamics in mycorrhizal symbioses is linked to carbon costs and phosphorus benefits. FEMS Microbiology Ecology 72: 123–131.
60. Egerton-Warburton LM, Graham RC, Allen EB, Allen MF (2001) Reconstruction of the historical changes in mycorrhizal fungal communities under anthropogenic nitrogen deposition. Proceedings of the Royal Society B-Biological Sciences 268: 2479–2484.
61. van Diepen LTA, Lilleskov EA, Pregitzer KS, Miller RM (2007) Decline of arbuscular mycorrhizal fungi in northern hardwood forests exposed to chronic nitrogen additions. New Phytologist 176: 175–183.
62. Hermans C, Hammond JP, White PJ, Verbruggen N (2006) How do plants respond to nutrient shortage by biomass allocation? Trends in Plant Science 11: 610–617.
63. Amtmann A, Blatt MR (2009) Regulation of macronutrient transport. New Phytologist 181: 35–52.
64. Muchhal US, Pardo JM, Raghothama KG (1996) Phosphate transporters from the higher plant Arabidopsis thaliana. Proceedings of the National Academy of Sciences of the United States of America 93: 10519–10523.
65. Muchhal US, Raghothama KG (1999) Transcriptional regulation of plant phosphate transporters. Proceedings of the National Academy of Sciences of the United States of America 96: 5868–5872.
66. Cai HM, Lu YG, Xie WB, Zhu T, Lian XM (2012) Transcriptome response to nitrogen starvation in rice. Journal of Biosciences 37: 731–747.
67. Kiba T, Feria-Bourrellier AB, Lafouge F, Lezhneva L, Boutet-Mercey S, et al. (2012) The Arabidopsis nitrate transporter NRT2.4 plays a double role in roots and shoots of nitrogen-starved plants. Plant Cell 24: 245–258.
68. Remans T, Nacry P, Pervent M, Girin T, Tillard P, et al. (2006) A central role for the nitrate transporter NRT2.1 in the integrated morphological and physiological responses of the root system to nitrogen limitation in Arabidopsis. Plant Physiology 140: 909–921.
69. Sugiura M, Georgescu MN, Takahashi M (2007) A nitrite transporter associated with nitrite uptake by higher plant chloroplasts. Plant and Cell Physiology 48: 1022–1035.
70. Bouguyon E, Gojon A, Nacry P (2012) Nitrate sensing and signaling in plants. Seminars in Cell & Developmental Biology 23: 648–654.
71. Gojon A, Krouk G, Perrine-Walker F, Laugier E (2011) Nitrate transceptor(s) in plants. Journal of Experimental Botany 62: 2299–2308.
72. Wang RC, Xing XJ, Wang Y, Tran A, Crawford NM (2009) A genetic screen for nitrate regulatory mutants captures the nitrate transporter gene NRT1.1. Plant Physiology 151: 472–478.
73. Dechorgnat J, Nguyen CT, Armengaud P, Jossier M, Diatloff E, et al. (2011) From the soil to the seeds: the long journey of nitrate in plants. Journal of Experimental Botany 62: 1349–1359.
74. Tsay YF, Chiu CC, Tsai CB, Ho CH, Hsu PK (2007) Nitrate transporters and peptide transporters. FEBS Letters 581: 2290–2300.
75. Baath E, Spokes J (1989) The effect of added nitrogen and phosphorus on mycorrhizal growth-response and infection in *Allium schoenoprasum*. Canadian Journal of Botany 67: 3227–3232.
76. Johnson NC (2010) Resource stoichiometry elucidates the structure and function of arbuscular mycorrhizas across scales. New Phytologist 185: 631–647.
77. Javot H, Penmetsa RV, Terzaghi N, Cook DR, Harrison MJ (2007) A *Medicago truncatula* phosphate transporter indispensable for the arbuscular mycorrhizal symbiosis. Proceedings of the National Academy of Sciences of the United States of America 104: 1720–1725.
78. Maeda D, Ashida K, Iguchi K, Chechetka SA, Hijikata A, et al. (2006) Knockdown of an arbuscular mycorrhiza-inducible phosphate transporter gene of Lotus japonicus suppresses mutualistic symbiosis. Plant and Cell Physiology 47: 807–817.
79. Yang SY, Gronlund M, Jakobsen I, Grotemeyer MS, Rentsch D, et al. (2012) Nonredundant regulation of rice arbuscular mycorrhizal symbiosis by two members of the PHOSPHATE TRANSPORTER1 gene family. Plant Cell 24: 4236–4251.
80. Nacry P, Canivenc G, Muller B, Azmi A, Van Onckelen H, et al. (2005) A role for auxin redistribution in the responses of the root system architecture to phosphate starvation in Arabidopsis. Plant Physiol 138: 2061–2074.
81. Nagy F, Karandashov V, Chague W, Kalinkevich K, Tamasloukht M, et al. (2005) The characterization of novel mycorrhiza-specific phosphate transporters from *Lycopersicon esculentum* and *Solanum tuberosum* uncovers functional redundancy in symbiotic phosphate transport in solanaceous species. Plant Journal 42: 236–250.
82. Chen A, Hu J, Sun S, Xu G (2007) Conservation and divergence of both phosphate- and mycorrhiza-regulated physiological responses and expression patterns of phosphate transporters in solanaceous species. New Phytologist 173: 817–831.
83. Wegmüller S, Svistoonoff S, Reinhardt D, Stuurman J, Amrhein N, et al. (2008) A transgenic dTph1 insertional mutagenesis system for forward genetics in mycorrhizal phosphate transport of Petunia. Plant Journal 54: 1115–1127.
84. Clark RB, Zeto SK (1996) Mineral acquisition by mycorrhizal maize grown on acid and alkaline soil. Soil Biology & Biochemistry 28: 1495–1503.
85. Tawaraya K (2003) Arbuscular mycorrhizal dependency of different plant species and cultivars. Soil Science and Plant Nutrition 49: 655–668.
86. Angelard C, Colard A, Niculita-Hirzel H, Croll D, Sanders IR (2010) Segregation in a mycorrhizal fungus alters rice growth and symbiosis-specific gene transcription. Current Biology 20: 1216–1221.
87. Sawers RJH, Gebreselassie MN, Janos DP, Paszkowski U (2010) Characterizing variation in mycorrhiza effect among diverse plant varieties. Theoretical and Applied Genetics 120: 1029–1039.
88. Johnson NC, Graham JH, Smith FA (1997) Functioning of mycorrhizal associations along the mutualism–parasitism continuum. New Phytologist 135: 575–586.

9

Nutritional Transition in Children under Five Years and Women of Reproductive Age: A 15-Years Trend Analysis in Peru

Christian Loret de Mola[1,2]*, Renato Quispe[1,3], Giancarlo A. Valle[1], Julio A. Poterico[1]

1 CRONICAS Center of Excellence in Chronic Diseases, Universidad Peruana Cayetano Heredia, Lima, Peru, **2** Post-Graduate Program in Epidemiology, Federal University of Pelotas, Pelotas, Rio Grande do Sul, Brazil, **3** CONEVID Unidad de Conocimiento y Evidencia, Universidad Peruana Cayetano Heredia, Lima, Peru

Abstract

Background: Rapid urbanization, increase in food availability, and changes in diet and lifestyle patterns have been changing nutritional profiles in developing nations. We aimed to describe nutritional changes in children under 5 years and women of reproductive age in Peru, during a 15-year period of rapid economic development and social policy enhancement.

Materials and Methods: Trend analyses of anthropometric measures in children of preschool age and women between 15–49 years, using the Peruvian National Demographic and Family Health Surveys (DHS) from 1996 to 2011. WHO growth curves were used to define stunting, underweight, wasting and overweight in children <5y. We employed the WHO BMI-age standardized curves for teenagers between 15–19y. In women >19 years, body mass index (BMI) was analyzed both categorically and as a continuous variable. To statistically analyze the trends, we used regression models: Linear and Poisson for continuous and binary outcomes, respectively.

Results: We analyzed data from 123 642 women and 64 135 children, from 1996 to 2011. Decreases over time were evidenced for underweight ($p<0.001$), wasting ($p<0.001$), and stunting ($p<0.001$) in children under 5y. This effect was particularly noted in urban settings. Overweight levels in children reduced ($p<0.001$), however this reduction stopped, in urban settings, since 2005 (~12%). Anemia decreased in children and women ($p<0.001$); with higher reduction in urban (↓43%) than in rural children (↓24%). BMI in women aged 15–19 years increased ($p<0.001$) across time, with noticeable BMI-curve shift in women older than 30 years. Moreover, obesity doubled during this period in women more than 19y.

Conclusion: Nutrition transition in Peru shows different patterns for urban and rural populations. Public policies should emphasize targeting both malnutrition conditions—undernutrition/stunting, overweight/obesity and anemia—considering age and place of residence in rapid developing societies like Peru.

Editor: Victor Alberto Laguna-Torres, US Naval Medical Research Center Detachment Research Unit 6, Peru

Funding: The authors have no support or funding to report.

Competing Interests: The authors have declared that no competing interests exist.

* E-mail: chlmz@yahoo.com

Introduction

Since the 1960s, worldwide economic growth, has been accompanied by an increase in food availability, animal fat intake, less physical activity and urbanization [1]. This nutritional transition has been changing anthropometric and health patterns throughout populations, having special impact in low and middle-income countries (LMIC) [2].

Underweight and stunting have been dropping in LMIC, mainly in children under 5 years [3]; but overweight depicts diverse distribution and rates between children populations [3,4]. Since 1990, overweight rates have been raising in children from high and low-income countries. However, children from some upper-middle income societies depict a slight decrease in over-nutritional indicators, suggesting a diverse nutritional transition in children of preschool age [3]; and that country's development and economic growth may play an important role.

In the last 30 years, body mass index (BMI) in adults has been increasing in the world [5], and during this period global age-standardized obesity prevalence has nearly doubled [6] and developing countries appear to be at the forefront of this trend [7,8], and rapid nutritional changes in urban settings might explain the over-nutrition climb [2,7].

Previous studies have reported nutritional characteristics and trends of Peruvian children and adults through population-based datasets. For instance, a recent publication reported a high prevalence of over-nutrition (overweight or obesity) in Peruvians between 30–59 years (62.3%), where women had higher rates compared to males [9]. From 1991 to 2005, stunting decreased but overweight increased in children of preschool age [10]. Similar analyses from 2007 to 2010 showed that overweight in children under five years was related to: first year of life, male gender, birth weight more than 2.5 kg and living in high urbanized areas (i.e. Lima and the Coast region) [11]. However, these studies lacked of nutrition characterization during the entire period of economic development and social policy enhancement in Peru.

Anemia represents another malnutrition indicator in children and women. Global estimates show a concentration of this condition in low socioeconomic groups, and anemia in children correlates strongly to maternal anemia [12]. In Peru, factors associated with anemia in children of preschool age are: lack of prenatal care, adolescent mother and poor socioeconomic position [13].

Peru, as other Latin-American countries, has experienced a rapid economic growth in the last two decades. According to the World Bank, in 1996, Peru had a Gross Domestic Product (GDP) of $55.9 billion (current $) and a Gross National Income (GNI) per capita of $2200; whereas, in 2011, GDP was reported as $176.9 billion and GNI per capita reached to $5150 (http://data.worldbank.org/country/peru). Since 2006, social programs directed to aiding poor populations have enhanced nutritional programs in Peru [14]. Information of the Peruvian situation would help to better understand how combined economic growth with social policy targeting could affect nutritional transition in rapid developing nations.

We aimed to analyze in this study the nutritional transition of the Peruvian population through anthropometric measures—and anemia levels—of children under 5 years and women in childbearing age; using Peruvian Demographic Health Surveys during a 15-year period and stratifying analyses by urban and rural settings.

Methods

Ethics Statement

During data collection, INEI was responsible for obtaining an informed consent from all participants for the survey information, anthropometric measures and hemoglobin test. Using an information sheet, the research team explained to the participants the nature of the study and what kind of question they were going to answer as well as what kind of measure they were going to take. For survey and anthropometric data, verbal informed consent was obtained for all women, including adolescents, which, in addition, required their parents' or legal guardian's consent. For children under five years, verbal consent was obtained directly from their parents or legal guardians. For hemoglobin tests a written informed consent was required and in the case of adolescents and children under 5 years, their parents or legal guardian had to sign the consent and the adolescent give their assent. The consent forms stated that this was a national survey sponsored by the Peruvian Government and explaining its nature and importance, that all collected information would be confidential and that the person could stop answering the questions or reject to continue participating in this research at any time, explained the kind of questions they were going to answer, the measures that were going to be taken and the time this survey would take, depending on the amount of children under 5 and women in reproductive age living in the house, it also explained the nature and procedures they would use for the hemoglobin test, including a detailed explanation, which included showing the materials they were going to use for the test, as well as explaining that only one drop of blood was going to be taken from them, in addition it explained to them what anemia was, its signs and symptoms. The acceptance or rejection to answer the survey, give their anthropometric measures or do the hemoglobin test, was documented by the field worker in the response sheet. ENDES methodological procedures were reviewed and approved by the IRB from the Peruvian National Institute of Health and the "Centro de Alimentacion y Nutricion" (CENAN). In addition, the study protocol, specifically for this secondary analysis, was sent to the ethics committee of the Universidad Peruana Cayetano Heredia. They considered that this secondary analysis and the original research did not violate any ethics procedure, and approved further analysis and publication (SIDISI Code 61753).

Study Design

Secondary analysis, evaluating the trends of anthropometric measures in children under 5 years and women of reproductive age using the Peruvian National Demographic and Family Health Surveys (DHS), from 1996 to 2011. We also included percentages of anemia as other malnutrition indicator in both children and women.

DHS were cross-sectional surveys performed by the National Institute of Statistics and Informatics (INEI) in Peru; each being a nationally representative, multi-staged, and probabilistic study. Each wave included participants from rural and urban areas. These surveys formed part of the Monitoring and Evaluation to Assess and Use Results Demographic and Health Surveys (MEASURE DHS), until 2008. Since then, the Peruvian government and INEI have supported, conducted and monitored the surveys—using similar methodologies used in previous DHS (http://www.measuredhs.com/Data/).

Participants and Settings

Each DHS recruited women between 15 to 49 years and children aged 5 years or younger who lived in the same household. In rural areas, villages of 500–2,000 people were the primary sampling units, and households within each of these clusters were the secondary sampling units. In urban areas, primary sampling units consisted of blocks or groups of blocks with more than 2,000 people (with 100 houses on average), and secondary sampling units were the same as in rural settings. More details about the methodology for each survey are available publicly (http://desa.inei.gob.pe/endes/).

For some waves, the total sampling goal was achieved in more than one year (namely continuous DHS), but the annual-based sample remained representative of the Peruvian population in that specific year. We used all available surveys from 1996 to 2011, having eight waves: 1996, 2000, 2004–2006 (which only had children anthropometric data for 2005), 2007–2008, and 2009–2011. Household response rates, were above 93% in all surveys.

For this analysis, we included all children under 5 years and non-pregnant women with anthropometric and hemoglobin information. We had available data for 93.1% of children <5y and 64.7% of all interviewed women. Anthropometry in 1996 was measured in a subsample of women (29.8%), afterwards, 90% of non-pregnant women had available data.

Measurements and Variables

Anthropometric measures were recorded by trained personnel in all eight waves (1996, 2000, 2005, 2007, 2008, 2009, 2010, and 2011). Participants' weight was measured using solar-powered mother-baby scales with an accuracy of ±100 g. Since 2007, an electric scale (SECA model 881-872) has been used, having a maximum load of 150 kg. Previously, a similar scale (SECA model 874) was employed, which had a maximum load of 200 kg. Height was evaluated using a wooden stadiometer—an adjustable board calibrated in millimeters—following international standards for DHS [15]; measuring adults and children older than 2 years in a standing position, whereas children younger than 2 years lying down.

We evaluated three under-nutritional variables in children under 5 years: stunting, wasting, and underweight. We defined these indicators as: having a height for age, weight for height, and weight for age in Z score less than 2 standard deviations (SD) below the mean of the World Health Organization (WHO) international reference standards, respectively. Overweight (including obesity) in children <5y was defined as having a BMI-for-age more than 2 SD above the mean of the WHO international standards [16].

In women between 19 and 49 years, nutritional status was based on BMI, which was subsequently analyzed as a continuous and categorical variable. Using WHO standards, we used the following definitions in women older than 19y: underweight (BMI≤18.5 kg/m^2), normal (18.5-<25 kg/m^2), overweight (25-<30 kg/m^2), and obese (≥30 kg/m^2) [17]. Available information of these definitions can be found at: http://apps.who.int/bmi/index.jsp. For women between 15 and 19 years, we used WHO standardized growth curves because BMI cut-off points for obesity and overweight in this age range may differ from adults. Thus, we defined a BMI-for-age of more than 1 SD but less than 2 SD above the mean as overweight, and more than 2 SD as obese [18].

We also evaluated trends in women and children socio-demographic variables: age, years of education, child sex and place of residence—all information was asked to children's mothers. Anemia was defined using WHO cut-offs for non-pregnant women (hemoglobin count <12 g/dl) and children aged 5 to 59 months(hemoglobin count<11 g/dl)[19]. We used years of education as a proxy for socioeconomic status (SES) because the wealth and assets indexes constructed by INEI did not maintain standard variables across waves, making comparability and standardization difficult. In addition, it has been shown that for rural populations' assets index are not a good SES indicator [20], so for our analysis we used women education as a proxy of SES.

Statistical Analysis

Descriptive analyses were conducted for all DHS waves calculating prevalence and mean values for the evaluated variables, as appropriate. Moreover, we plotted women's BMI curves of 1996 and 2011 to compare general BMI changes—stratifying by age range (15–19; 20–29; 30–39; 40–49). We divided women in age-groups due to different BMI shifts by age. Our intention was to show the secular trend in BMI and women's age temporary effect modification. Children BMI curves standardized for age and sex were plotted according to WHO growth curves [21], in urban and rural comparing 1996 and 2011.

We performed trend analysis, stratifying by place of residence (urban or rural), using linear regression models for continuous variables (e.g. BMI); and Poisson regression for binary outcomes calculating prevalence ratios (PR) [22]. We analyzed every anthropometric variable independently in a regression model: each category of women's BMI (Poisson regression), continuous BMI (linear regression), each nutritional variable in children (Poisson regression), anemia (Poisson regression), and socio-demographic variables.

The year of survey was employed as a continuous independent variable, evaluating any linear increase or decrease across years. When data showed a visual non-linear trend, we analyzed total rise or decrease using the survey-year as a dummy variable. When this happened, we tried to analyze smaller periods in which trends appeared to be linear. For instance, if we evidenced a linear decline from 1996 to 2005, but a flattened pattern since then or inverse direction of the trend, we analyzed separately the periods 1996–2005 and 2005–2011.

We also compared in some cases differences in point prevalence (for any specific year) between urban versus rural populations using regression models (Poisson). Since BMI cut-off points were different for adult (20–49 years) and adolescent (15–19 years) women, we performed separated analyses to evaluate trends of categorized BMI (obesity, overweight, normal, underweight). Adolescents' analyses were not stratified by place of residence due to small sample sizes in some periods.

STATA version 11.2 software (STATA Corp, College Station, TX, US) was employed for our analyses. Given surveys' multistage random samples, we used the *svy* set of commands. Accounting sampling units and stratification of the samples, we calculated weights of the analyzed individuals in the household and linearized standard errors (SE). We calculated 95% confidence intervals and p<0.05 was considered significant in our analyses.

Results

We analyzed data from 123,642 women—78,408 urban and 45,234 rural—and 64,135 children under 5 years—33,304 urban and 30,831 rural—in all DHS waves (1996 to 2011). Table 1 shows a detailed description of populations' socio-demographic characteristics and sample size for each wave.

Overall, 73% of women were from urban areas maintaining this percentage throughout years (p = 0.132). Women's mean age, across waves, was 30.3 years SE[0.03]; with 19.7% from 15 to 19 years old, 30.5% from 20 to 29 years, 27.3% from 30 to 39 years, and 22% from 40 to 49 years. Mean years of education in women increased in both settings (p<0.001), especially from 1996 to 2000 with a greater upsurge among urban women over time. Anemia among women declined significantly from 1996 to 2011 (p<0.001), with similar reductions in rural (decrease of 48% SE [2.7]) and urban (decrease of 43% SE [2.8]) areas. In 2011, we found that rural women had higher prevalence of anemia compared to their urban counterparts (p = 0.005) (Table 1). Conversely, children from urban areas (decrease of 43%, from 1996 to 2011) depicted a higher anemia diminution compared to rural counterparts (decrease of 24%, from 1996 to 2011, p<0.001).

Children's mean age, across waves, was 2.5 years SE [0.01] with similar values across all waves and no differences between urban and rural areas. The number of evaluated male and female children across time was constant (~1:1 proportion). A declining trend of anemia in children was observed in both settings (p<0.001). Comparing 2000 to 2011, children with anemia in the overall analysis had a 48% reduction (PR = 0.62 SE [0.02]), decreasing more in urban (PR = 0.57 SE [0.03]) than in rural settings (PR = 0.73 SE [0.03]). Moreover, the prevalence of anemia among rural children was 46% higher than in their urban counterparts (p<0.001) in 2011 (Table 1).

Nutritional Trends for Children

Between 1996 and 2011, stunting, wasting, and underweight decreased (p<0.001 for all three). A small decrease in overweight prevalence was also observed (p<0.001) (Figure 1).

Stratifying by place of residence, we observe a deeper decline of stunting in urban (51.5%) than rural (19.6%) areas (p<0.001) over time. Figure 1 shows that stunting decrease started in 2007 for rural children, having a significant reduction from 2007 to 2011 (p<0.001), but not from 1996 to 2007 (p = 0.973).

During the analyzed period, wasting declined in urban (p<0.001) and rural (p<0.001) children, with no significant reductions from 2007 to 2011 in the rural areas (p = 0.979). In 2011, wasting prevalence was 0.22% SE [0.08] and 0.64% SE

Table 1. Age, education, anemia, sex and BMI description of Women and children under five years old in Urban and Rural Areas of Peru between years 1996–2011.

	Urban								**Rural**							
	Mean/Proportion								**Mean/Proportion**							
	1996	*2000*	*2005*	*2007*	*2008*	*2009*	*2010*	*2011*	*1996*	*2000*	*2005*	*2007*	*2008*	*2009*	*2010*	*2011*
Women	6,128	15,715	3,479	3,101	9,121	13,842	13,520	13,502	4,715	9,791	2,198	2,129	4,073	7,334	7,509	7,485
Age *	29.5	29.5	30.0	30.4	30.4	30.3	30.5	30.5	29.6	29.8	30.5	30.6	31.1	30.7	30.7	30.9
Education*	8.4	10.2	10.9	10.7	10.6	10.6	10.7	10.8	4.0	5.8	6.1	6.4	6.3	6.4	6.5	6.5
BMI	25.61	26.15	25.59	26.22	26.31	26.35	26.40	26.97	24.27	24.55	24.69	24.96	24.92	25.09	25.07	25.29
Anemia**	ND	28.9%	27.1%	27.2%	25.2%	20.7%	20.1%	16.5%	ND	36.6%	31.2%	30.0%	25.4%	22.0%	24.7%	19.0%
Children	7938	5337	1066	1086	3257	5115	4731	4774	7171	6384	1248	1308	2465	4257	4038	3960
Male	50.5%	50.5%	51.4%	50.1%	49.7%	51.2%	50.5%	51.2%	50.3%	51.1%	51.8%	49.7%	50.3%	52.2%	49.2%	49.1%
Age*	2.5	2.5	2.4	2.5	2.5	2.5	2.5	2.5	2.4	2.5	2.5	2.5	2.6	2.5	2.5	2.5
Anemia**	ND	45.8%	ND	37.2%	39.9%	32.8%	33.2%	25.9%	ND	52.3%	ND	49.6%	47.2%	43.7%	45.9%	40.0%

ND = No Data.
*Mean of years of education and age.
**Percentage of anemic children/women.

[0.02] in urban and rural children, respectively. On the other hand, underweight has also been dropping in both settings, having a constant reduction in urban children, going from 2.9% to 1.9% ($p<0.001$). In the rural children, underweight dropped from 10.1% to 8.2% in an irregular way ($p<0.001$) (Figure 1).

In urban children, overweight prevalence declined from 1996 to 2011 ($p<0.001$), but this trend seemed to have flattened since 2005 ($p = 0.235$); depicting in 2011 an overweight prevalence of 12.0% SE [0.73], surpassing stunting levels (10.3% SE [0.66]). In rural children, overweight declined between 1996 and 2011 ($p<0.001$).

Women Nutritional Trends

We observe an overall increase in the prevalence of overweight from 1996 to 2011 ($p<0.001$), in women between 20–49 years. However, the curve flattened since 2008. Percentages of women with normal BMI have been declining over time ($p<0.001$), especially since 2005; showing similar percentages of normal (39.6% SE [0.56]) and overweight (39.4% SE [0.52]) women in 2011 (Figure 2).

Obesity levels depict a constant increase over time ($p<0.001$). In 2011, the prevalence of overweight/obese women was higher than the normal BMI-category ($p<0.001$); and underweight maintained constant across years with a prevalence of ~1% in most waves for urban and rural settings.

Overweight did not show a clear trend in urban women ($p = 0.796$), but percentages of normal women declined, especially since 2005 ($p<0.001$). We evidenced for 2011 similar percentages of overweight (39.3% SE [0.63]) and normal-BMI women (37.4% SE [0.67]) (Figure 2). Furthermore, obesity increased 1.78 (SE [0.09]) times in 2011 compared to 1996 ($p<0.001$) (increase of 0.65% points per/year). In 2011, 22.3% adult women (SE [0.06]) were obese, and 61.6% SE [1.03] had a BMI ≥ 25 kg/m^2.

Rural areas depicts a decrease of normal-BMI women ($p<0.001$), meanwhile overweight prevalence increased over time ($p<0.001$), specially since 2005 (Figure 2). Obesity shows a constant increase during the analyzed period ($p<0.001$) and its prevalence in 2011 was 2.75 (SE [0.35]) times higher than in 1996. On the other hand, for rural women in 2011, the prevalence of normal-BMI (45.9%) was higher than overweight (39.7%) women ($p<0.001$); but lower than obese/overweight females (53.2%) ($p<0.001$).

Teenagers between 15 to 19 years, showed a slight increment in obesity since 2005 ($p = 0.020$) (Figure 3).

In Table 1, we observe that women's mean BMI has been constantly increasing from 1996 to 2011 ($p<0.001$): ↑ 0.09 kg/m^2 per year. Mean BMI augmented for urban and rural women ($p<0.001$ in both settings), with a higher increase per year in urban (↑ 0.19%/year SE [0.04]) than rural (↑ 0.09%/year SE [0.04]) settings.

BMI Curves

In figure 4, when comparing women's BMI curves of 1996 and 2011, we can see a slight shift to the right and flattening of the curve in 2011 in adult women between 30–39 and 40–49 years. When looking only at the curves from 1996, data suggests that older populations had very little increase in overall BMI. However, in 2011 this changed, and we evidence that older populations tend to increase their overall BMI more than in 1996; consequently, women from 1996 increased their BMI in 2011 more than expected. Women between 20–30 years in 1996 and 2011 did not have differences in BMI curves, however, those from 1996, which would be in the 30–40/40–49 age groups in 2011 had more flattened BMI curves with an evident shift to the right, when compared with the same age groups from 1996. Suggesting, therefore, a temporary modification of the effect of age on the risk of BMI increase.

We plotted the BMI distribution for children under 5y, noticing that rural and urban children's curves maintained constant between1996 to 2011 (Figure 5).

Discussion

Peru has experienced a rapid nutritional transition in a short period of time with remaining malnutrition associated with stunting and anemia; and increasing rates of obesity in adult women.

We found declining levels of chronic malnutrition (stunting) in children under 5 years since 2007, with greater reduction in urban

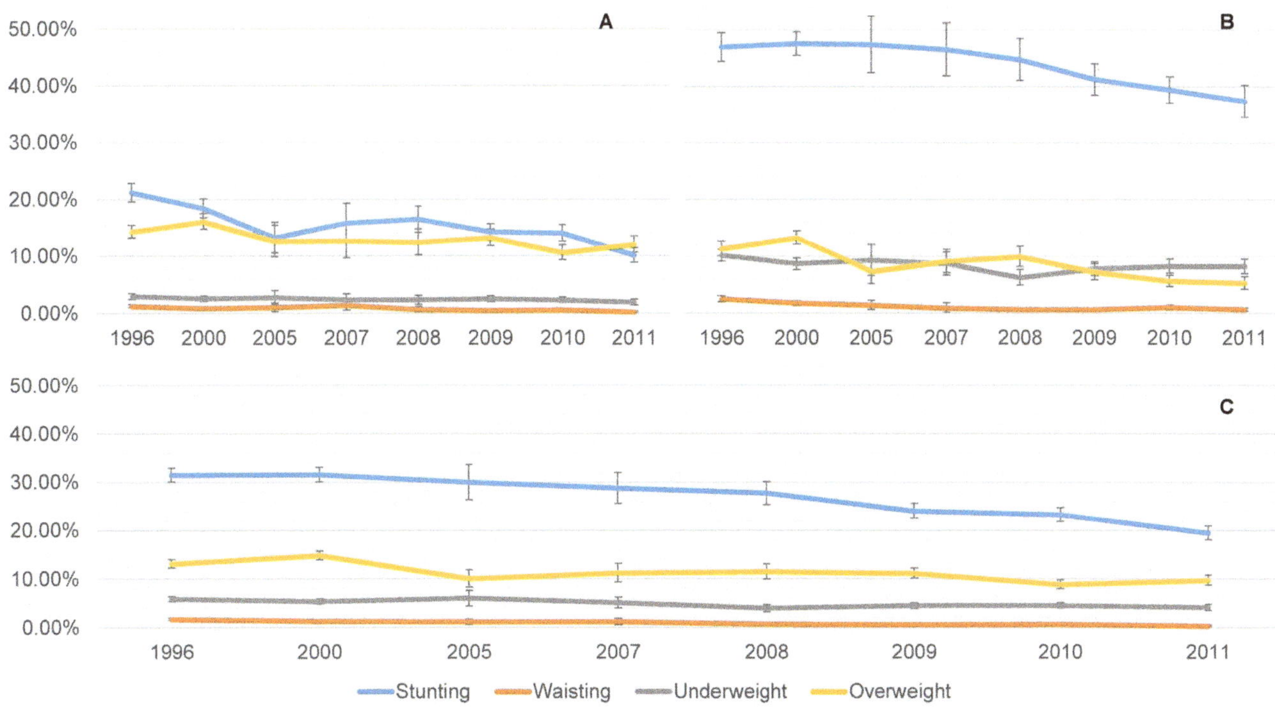

Figure 1. Stunting, wasting, underweight, and overweight trends of urban and rural children under five years, 1996–2011. A. Urban children (n = 33,304). B. Rural Children (n = 30,831). C. All Children (n = 64,135).

(↓ 51.5%) than rural (↓ 19.6%) areas from 1996 to 2011; with similar patterns of wasting and underweight. Overweight in children have declined in both rural and urban settings, but since 2005, the overall decrease levelled off.

Women's mean BMI increased over time, especially in females older than 30 years. In addition, not just the overall BMI of adult women augmented, but also the risk of increasing their BMI with older age.

Furthermore, obesity doubled during this15 year-period in both urban and rural adult women. Anthropometric profile of rural women in 2011 resembled to what urban counterparts presented in 1996; reflecting a 15-year nutritional gap between these two settings.

The prevalence of anemia has been decreasing in Peruvian women in both settings from 2000 to 2011; with greater reduction in rural women (↓ 43%). Conversely, anemia reduced more in urban children (↓ 48%); maintaining high levels of anemia in rural areas.

Similarities in proportions of urban women and mean age across the studied waves, shown in table 1, suggests that sample populations were comparable and trends are not an artifact of sampling.

Children from other developing countries have shown decreasing levels of chronic malnutrition [23]; and underweight [3]. In Peru, Mispireta *et al* [10] reported slight decreasing stunting levels, from 38.9% to 31.7% during 1991 to 2005. They also found that stunting prevalence in Peruvian rural areas remained high, but urban areas evidenced a more prominent reduction. These findings agree with ours, but our analysis included later years and we were able to demonstrate that chronic malnutrition reduction was greater beyond 2005.

Social factors enhancement might have contributed to reduce chronic malnutrition levels in Peru, such as: reduction in maternal mortality [24], increasing access to water and sanitation [13,25], and improvement of breastfeeding rates [13] and education in women. The latter statement could support any beneficial effect of mother's education in chronic malnutrition in children under five years between 1996 and 2011. We show in this period a 27% and 62.5% increase in the mean of years of education for urban and rural women, respectively. Other Latin American countries have reduced their stunting levels improving maternal schooling, health care, sanitation, purchasing power of families [26]; and fortified supplements and cash transfer interventions [27]. Thus, improving Peruvian families living conditions might have been associated with reductions in stunting levels through social programs [14].

Peru has experienced a particular scenario regarding its nutritional and social programs, which may explain declining stunting levels after 2005 reported in this manuscript.

It seemed that Peruvian feeding programs had not being contributing to chronic malnutrition levels until 2005 [14]. Therefore, the Peruvian Government with other national and international institutions joined to form in 2006 the Children Malnutrition Initiative (CMI), placing nutrition in the priority agenda. With CMI, strong political commitment and technical support helped to struggle against stunting. Social programs such as CRECER (National Strategy for Poverty Reduction and Economic Opportunities, implemented in 2007) and JUNTOS (the Government's target cash transfer program) may have improved stunting levels in a short period—since [14]. The former program focused on children and pregnant women in poor areas; and the latter targeted on the reduction of children malnutrition and increase in families' use of children and maternal health care services. Thus, social policy enhancement seems to play a role in the fight against stunting.

Acosta [14] suggested that socioeconomic growth and the commodities boom did not affect stunting level, but poverty reduction did. Despite the Peruvian development, social programs have faced challenges in rural areas until more recently in mid

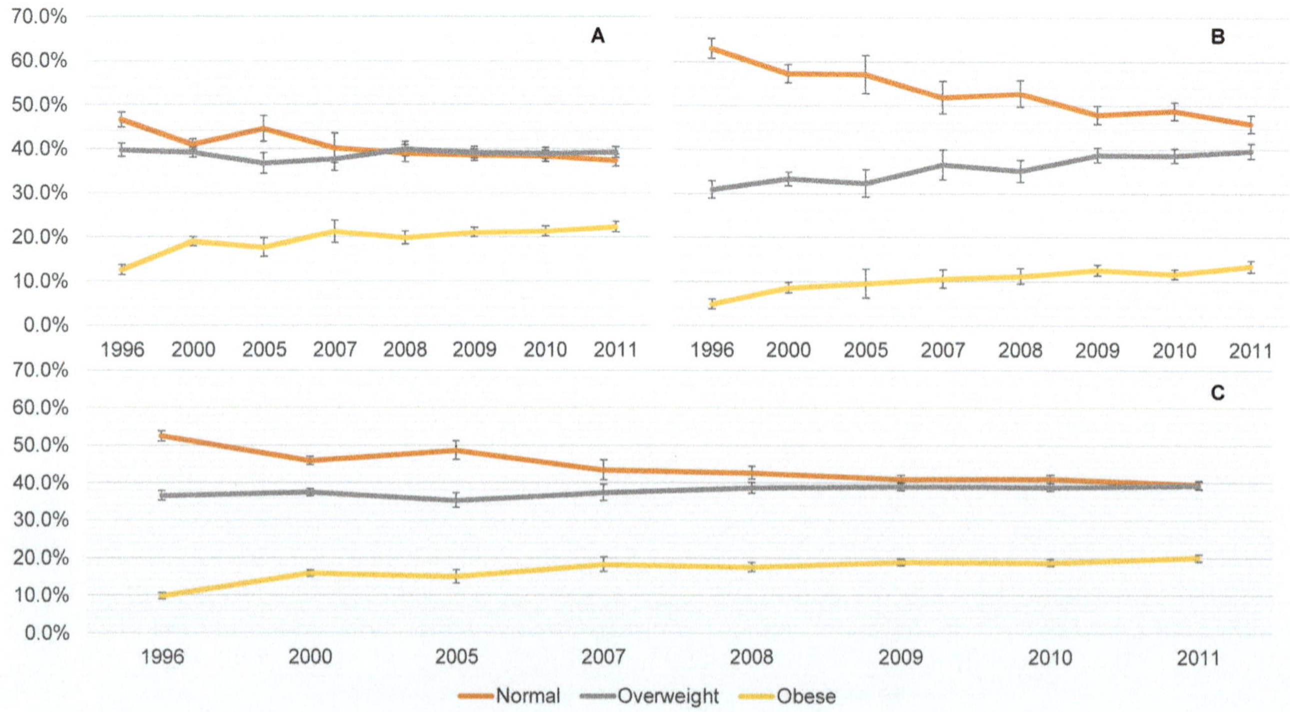

Figure 2. Categorical BMI trends for Peruvian urban and rural adult women (20–49 years), 1996–2011. A. Urban adult women (n = 63,895). B. Rural adult women (n = 37,088). C. All adult women (20–49 years) (n = 100,983).

2000's because of internal conflict (i.e. terrorism) in 1980's and early 1990's. These challenges might have maintained stunting disparities between urban and rural areas, supported by our results. Between 1996 and 2011, social and nutritional programs intensified rural malnutrition targeting; and enhanced of social programs focused in vulnerable groups after 2007 [14].

Education improvement in mothers might have affected levels of children with overweight in Peru, because more educated women could have less overweight children [28]; and nutritional

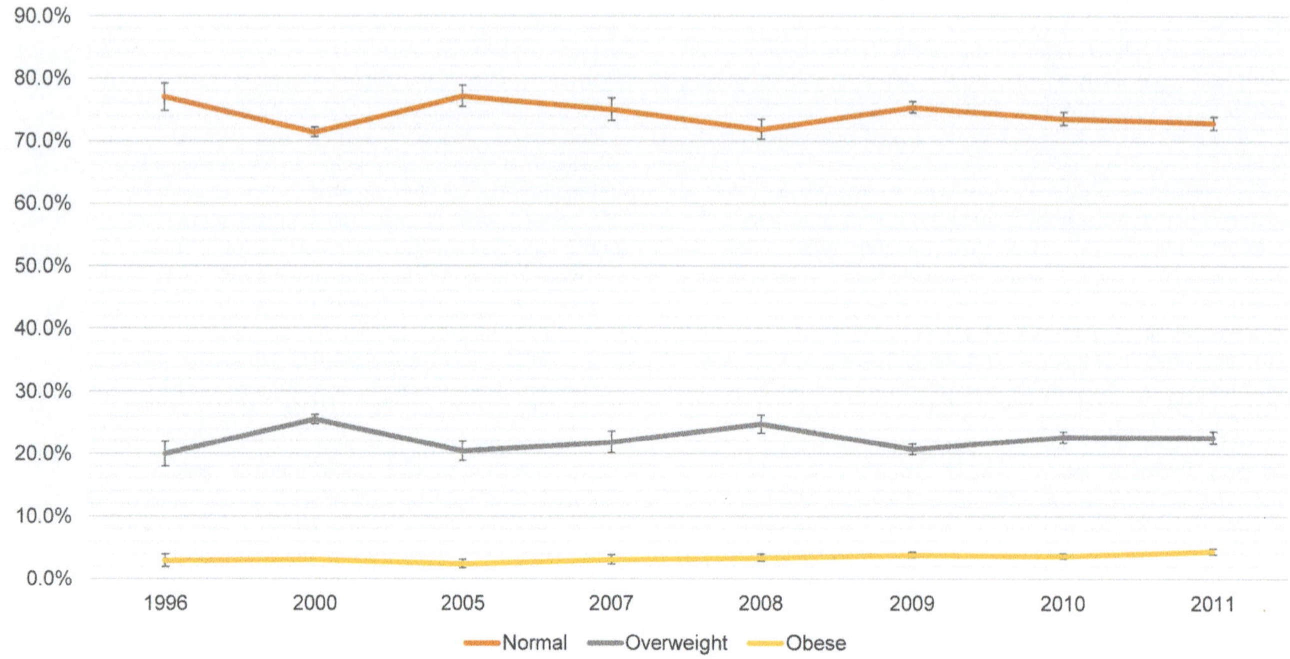

Figure 3. Categorical BMI trends for Peruvian adolescent women (15–19 years), 1996–2011. Total n = 22,659; 1996 n = 717; 2000 n = 5,340; 2005 n = 1,154; 2007 n = 1,001; 2008 n = 2,462; 2009 n = 4,021; 2010 n = 4,038; 2011 n = 3,926.

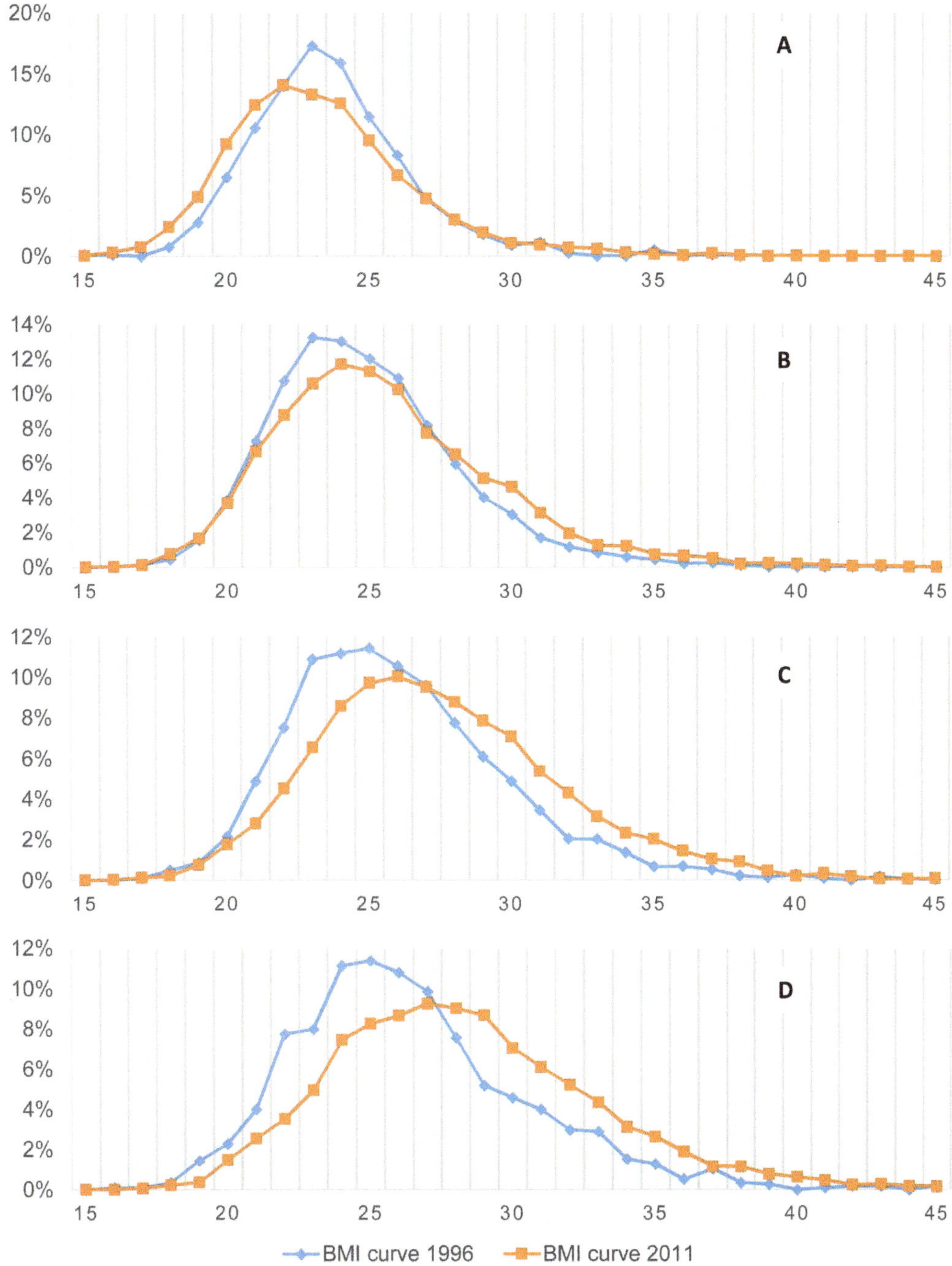

Figure 4. Peruvian women BMI curves, 1996–2011, stratified by age. A. 15–19 years (1996 n = 717/2011 n = 3,926) **B.** 20–29 years (1996 n = 5,141/2011 n = 6,058) **C.** 30–39 years (1996 n = 3,836/2011 n = 5,928) **D.** 40–49 years (1996 n = 1,149/2011 n = 5,075). Y-axis Percentage of women with a given BMI in each age group; X-axis Women BMI.

programs and subsidized meals in low income populations might have exerted an unintentional impact in overweight of children under 5y [29]. Our declining pattern in overweight in children under 5y resemble to what WHO-UNICEF-World Bank have reported since 1990 in upper-middle income countries [3]. Although overweight and obesity levels in preschool children of some Latin American countries appear to be low [30], de Onis *et al* have reported an overall increase in this region from 1990 to 2010 [21]. Moreover, augmenting rates in LMIC are projected [21], mainly affecting urban areas and privileged groups [9,31].

Several factors for malnutrition control have been reported in rapid-growing societies of the Latin American region. For instance, in Brazil, 4 factors contributed with two-thirds of stunting decrease between 1996 to 2007: 25.7% to improved maternal schooling; 21.7% to an increase in the purchasing power of families; 11.6% to the expansion of health care; and 4.3% to improved sanitation [26]. Meanwhile, Mexico has been succeeding the fight against stunting with supplemented fortified supplements, health-care, education and cash transfer interventions [27].

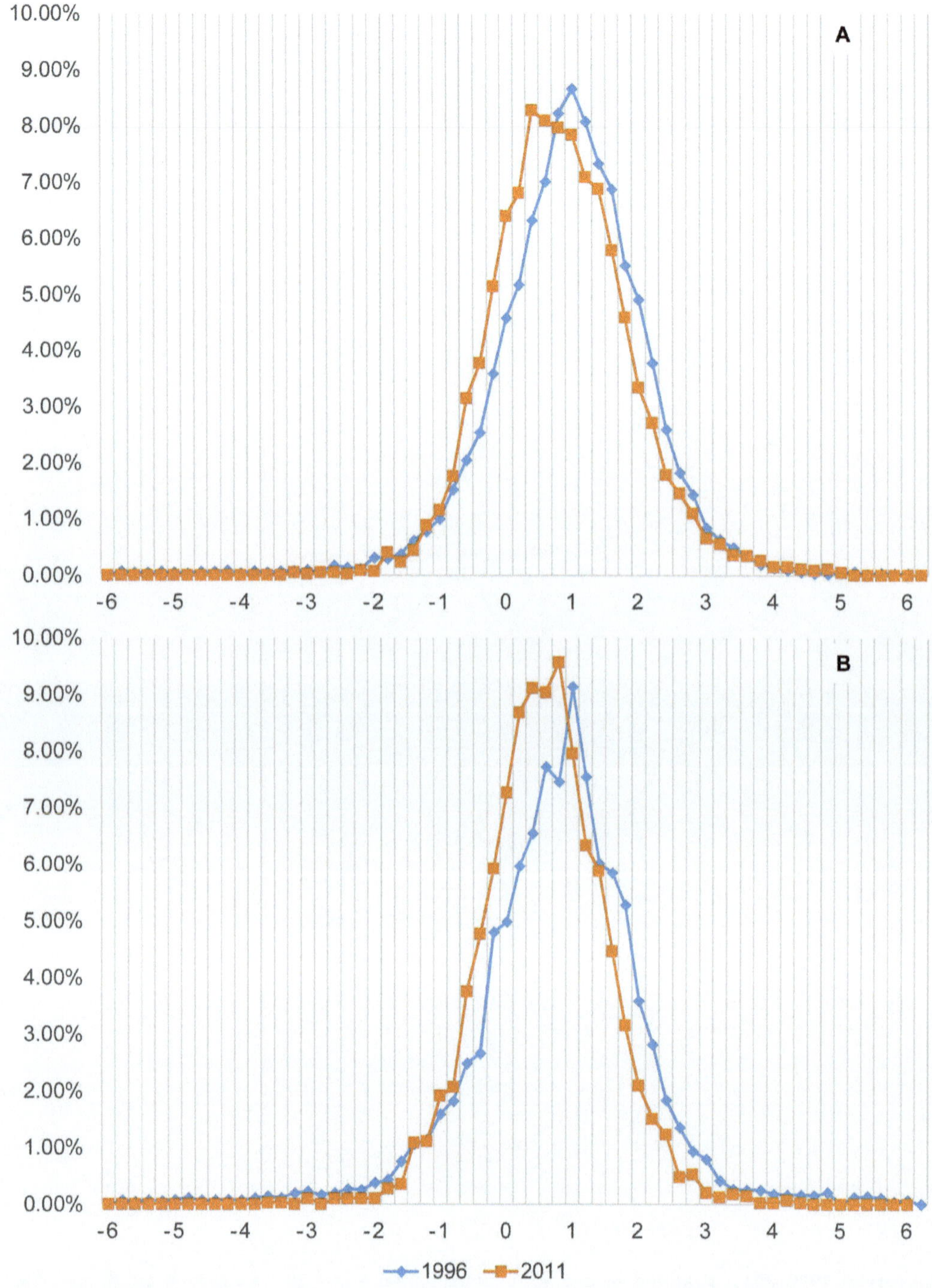

Figure 5. Peruvian Children BMI curves standardized for age and sex using WHO reference, 1996–2011. A. Urban Children (1996 n = 7,938/2011 n = 4,774) **B.** Rural children (1996 n = 7,171/2011 n = 3,960). Y-axis Percentage of children with a given BMI; X-axis WHO age-sex Standardized BMI.

Peruvian women have increased their BMI in 1.3 kg/m^2 between 1996 and 2011 (with a rate of 0.09 kg/m^2 per year), surpassing—and almost doubling—global women trend rate reported by Finucane *et al.* [5]; but supporting the fact that Latin American countries are facing a rapid nutritional transition. Worldwide, adult BMI has increased: 0.4 kg/m^2 and 0.5 kg/m^2 per decade in males and females, respectively, from 1980 to 2008, with Latin America presenting the second highest BMI rise after Oceania [5]. Moreover, adult global age-standardized obesity and overweight levels have augmented, from 6.4% to 12.0%, and from 24.6% to 34.4%, respectively [6].

Mendez *et al.* showed that more urbanized and developed LMIC tend to have higher levels of over-nutrition, and women of most developing societies reflect more overweight than underweight [7]. In a previous study with nationally representative data from Peruvian women of reproductive age, over-nutrition reached 44.7% in 2005, with concomitant raising levels of obesity from 1991 to 2005 (8,9% to 10,9%, respectively) [10]. Climbing numbers of overweight and obese women in our study could be explained by rapid nutritional transition, where changes in diet and lifestyle pattern through years contributed to over-nutrition, like other Latin American countries [32]. Growing economies in Latin America have been experiencing this transition, augmenting adult obesity rates explained by change in dietary pattern [33]: more intake of fats and carbohydrates (including raising consumption of refined foods), and less vegetables and fruits consumption. In addition, sedentary lifestyles and physical inactivity due to rapid urbanization have been contributing to escalating levels of over-nutrition [32].

As suggested by data of the Food and Agriculture Organization (FAO: http://faostat.fao.org/), Peruvian population increased their caloric intake during the studied years—from 2280 kcal/day in 1996 to 2563 kcal/day in 2009 (12% increase)—mainly coming from refine products, animal raw fat, vegetable fat and products rich in simple carbohydrates. Recent evidence suggests high prevalence of physical inactivity in Peruvian urban population [34], which added to inactive hobbies [35] and weight underestimation [36], among other factors, might have hastened the nutritional transition in Peru, starting in adult populations—supported by a recent nationally representative study of the Peruvian population, highlighting high levels of obesity in males and females between 30 to 59 years old [9].

Obesity and overweight vary within and between countries, reflecting social determinants in adult obesity burden [37]. Monteiro *et al.* [38], and Dinsa *et al.*[39] suggested that poor women start suffering from the burden of obesity when a nation's GNI reach $2500 and $1000, respectively.

According to the World Bank, Peru has accomplished a rapid economic development from 1996 to 2011, with a total GDP (Constant LCU) augmentation of 104.4% and GNI per capita (constant LCU) increase of 60.0% in this period. Moreover, Peru declined poverty levels from 58.7% in 2004 to 27.8% in 2011.

This rapid economic growth in Peru has brought little decrease in GNI index (e.g. 0.56 in 1998 and 0.48 in 2010), suggesting remaining inequalities. The relationship between SES and obesity changes according to which SES indicator is analyzed, and by place of residence; having that wealthier rural women seem to have more chance of being obese, with unclear association in the urban areas [40]. Conversely, Peruvian women with more education seem to have less odds of obesity, more noticeable in urban settings [40]. Further evidence should address when (if happened) obesity burden went towards people in less advantaged SES groups—including different SES indicators—in Peru; for understanding the effect of rapid national macroeconomic progress on obesity inequality.

On the other hand, Latin American countries showed declining rates of anemia, where their government entities have taken emphasized strategies to reduce this condition in children, including dietary supplements with ferrous sulfate and fortified foods [41], and even when this intervention might be dubiously effective in the short term [42], this could partially explain the decreasing trend of anemia percentage that we present in our manuscript for Peruvian children [13]. On the other hand, high levels of anemia have been reported in overweight or obese women from 3 developing countries (including Peru) [43], telling us that individuals from LMIC can be malnourished even if they appear in ranges of over-nutrition.

Remaining high levels of anemia in Peruvian children of preschool age and women of reproductive age could be explained by incomplete targeting of these vulnerable populations, mainly affecting children of rural settings [14]. Additional explanations may arise, such as the effect of Peruvian economic development on anemia, but stay beyond the objective of this manuscript. Further studies and interventions assessment should be performed to determine why Peruvian children and women still manifest current anemia figures.

Our study presents some limitations. First, it is a descriptive study and any apparent relationship interpreted from figures or tables between anthropometric measures variations and/or socio-demographic variables would only imply an ecologic association and readers should take this findings with precaution—since it could reflect an ecologic fallacy [44]. We must emphasize that our hypotheses regarding macroeconomic growth, change in diet, and/or enhancement of social programs on nutritional transition in Peru, represent also an ecological relation. In this manuscript we postulate that these factors seem the more plausible reasons behind our depicted trends. Formal studies assessing impact of interventions should be carried out, to evaluate nutritional programs among SES groups and settings in Peru. We were unable to evaluate the effect of other variables like wealth, diet or breastfeeding due to lack of comparability in measurement methodologies across waves or because unavailable data, nevertheless data from other sources, like FAO and World Bank, has been discussed in this section, for a better explanation of the probable causes of the trends.

On the other hand we should point-out that population-based surveys, used in this study, were representative of the entire Peruvian pre-school children and women in reproductive age (15–49 years) between1996 to 2011. We can assure with high certainty that our results depict the nutritional transition in Peru, which rapidly became an upper-middle income country in the last 20 years.

Our findings support the fact that Peru is on track to meet the Millennium Development Goals (MDG) (http://www.un.org/millenniumgoals), which include reduction of extreme poverty and hunger. However, Peru has been facing persistent malnutrition profiles, being over-nutrition dramatically escalating in adult women.

Even when under-nutritional indicators, in children under five have dropped, same as for overweight, and women's obesity have increased, the nutritional transition in Peru shows different patterns for urban and rural populations. Public policies should emphasize targeting both malnutrition conditions—under-nutrition/stunting, overweight/obesity and anemia—considering age and place of residence in rapid progressing societies like Peru.

Acknowledgments

We would like to thank Dr Jaime Miranda and Dr Carlos Delgado, for their valuable comments and suggestions. We also appreciate editorial support from Lena Shah. We appreciate the effort of the Peruvian National Institute of Statistics and Informatics (INEI), for collecting this rich and vital data every year and for supporting us on DHS details. We also acknowledge the valuable participation of Peruvian women and their children in DHS survey.

Author Contributions

Analyzed the data: CL. Contributed reagents/materials/analysis tools: CL JAP. Wrote the paper: CL JAP GAV RQ.

References

1. Drewnowski A, Popkin BM (1997) The nutrition transition: new trends in the global diet. Nutr Rev 55: 31–43.
2. Popkin BM, Adair LS, Ng SW (2012) Global nutrition transition and the pandemic of obesity in developing countries. Nutr Rev 70: 3–21.
3. WHO U, World Bank (2012) Level & Trends in Child Malnutrition. UNICEF-WHO-The World Bank: Joint child malnutrition estimates - Levels and trends.
4. Wang Y, Monteiro C, Popkin BM (2002) Trends of obesity and underweight in older children and adolescents in the United States, Brazil, China, and Russia. Am J Clin Nutr 75: 971–977.
5. Finucane MM, Stevens GA, Cowan MJ, Danaei G, Lin JK, et al. (2011) National, regional, and global trends in body-mass index since 1980: systematic analysis of health examination surveys and epidemiological studies with 960 country-years and 9.1 million participants. Lancet 377: 557–567.
6. Stevens GA, Singh GM, Lu Y, Danaei G, Lin JK, et al. (2012) National, regional, and global trends in adult overweight and obesity prevalences. Popul Health Metr 10: 22.
7. Mendez MA, Monteiro CA, Popkin BM (2005) Overweight exceeds underweight among women in most developing countries. Am J Clin Nutr 81: 714–721.
8. Popkin BM, Gordon-Larsen P (2004) The nutrition transition: worldwide obesity dynamics and their determinants. Int J Obes Relat Metab Disord 28 Suppl 3: S2–9.
9. Alvarez-Dongo D, Sanchez-Abanto J, Gomez-Guizado G, Tarqui-Mamani C (2012) [Overweight and obesity: prevalence and determining social factors of overweight in the Peruvian population (2009-2010)]. Rev Peru Med Exp Salud Publica 29: 303–313.
10. Mispireta M, Rosas A, Velásquez J, Lescano A, Lanata CF (2007) [Nutrition Transition in Peru, 1991–2005]. Rev Peru Med Exp Salud Publica 24: 129–135.
11. Pajuelo-Ramirez J, Miranda-Cuadros M, Campos-Sanchez M, Sanchez-Abanto J (2011) [Prevalence of overwight and obesity among children under five years in Peru 2007-2010]. Rev Peru Med Exp Salud Publica 28: 222–227.
12. Balarajan Y, Ramakrishnan U, Ozaltin E, Shankar AH, Subramanian SV (2011) Anaemia in low-income and middle-income countries. Lancet 378: 2123–2135.
13. Instituto Nacional de Salud (2012) Evolución de los Indicadores del Programa Articulado Nutricional y los factores asociados a la Desnutrición Crónica y Anemia. In: Centro Nacional de Alimentación y Nutrición, editor. Lima, Peru: Ministerio de Salud.
14. Acosta AM (2011) Analysing Success in the Fight against Malnutrition in Peru. IDS Working Papers 2011: 2–49.
15. Macro ORC (2006) Demographic and Health Survey interviewer's manual. Calverton, MD.
16. WHO Multicentre Growth Reference Study Group (2006) WHO Child Growth Standards: Methods and development: Length/height-for-age, weight-for-age, weight-for-length, weight-for-height and body mass index-for-age. World Health Organization.
17. WHO (1995) Physical status: the use and interpretation of anthropometry. Report of a WHO Expert Committee. Geneva: World Health Organization. 460 p.
18. de Onis M, Onyango AW, Borghi E, Siyam A, Nishida C, et al. (2007) Development of a WHO growth reference for school-aged children and adolescents. Bull World Health Organ 85: 660–667.
19. World Health Organization (2008) Worldwide prevalence of anemia 1993–2005: WHO global database on anemia. Geneva.
20. Howe LD, Galobardes B, Matijasevich A, Gordon D, Johnston D, et al. (2012) Measuring socio-economic position for epidemiological studies in low- and middle-income countries: a methods of measurement in epidemiology paper. Int J Epidemiol 41: 871–886.
21. de Onis M, Blossner M, Borghi E (2010) Global prevalence and trends of overweight and obesity among preschool children. Am J Clin Nutr 92: 1257–1264.
22. Barros AJ, Hirakata VN (2003) Alternatives for logistic regression in cross-sectional studies: an empirical comparison of models that directly estimate the prevalence ratio. BMC Med Res Methodol 3: 21.
23. Stevens GA, Finucane MM, Paciorek CJ, Flaxman SR, White RA, et al. (2012) Trends in mild, moderate, and severe stunting and underweight, and progress towards MDG 1 in 141 developing countries: a systematic analysis of population representative data. Lancet 380: 824–834.
24. Hogan MC, Foreman KJ, Naghavi M, Ahn SY, Wang M, et al. (2010) Maternal mortality for 181 countries, 1980–2008: a systematic analysis of progress towards Millennium Development Goal 5. Lancet 375: 1609–1623.
25. WHO-UNICEF (2013) Progress on sanitation and drinking-water - 2013 update.
26. Monteiro CA, Benicio MH, Konno SC, Silva AC, Lima AL, et al. (2009) Causes for the decline in child under-nutrition in Brazil, 1996-2007. Rev Saude Publica 43: 35–43.
27. Rivera JA, Sotres-Alvarez D, Habicht JP, Shamah T, Villalpando S (2004) Impact of the Mexican program for education, health, and nutrition (Progresa) on rates of growth and anemia in infants and young children: a randomized effectiveness study. JAMA 291: 2563–2570.
28. Baughcum AE, Chamberlin LA, Deeks CM, Powers SW, Whitaker RC (2000) Maternal perceptions of overweight preschool children. Pediatrics 106: 1380–1386.
29. Kimbro RT, Rigby E (2010) Federal food policy and childhood obesity: a solution or part of the problem? Health Aff (Millwood) 29: 411–418.
30. Kain J, Vio F, Albala C (2003) Obesity trends and determinant factors in Latin America. Cad Saude Publica 19 Suppl 1: S77–86.
31. Adel el T, Marie-Francoise RC, Mahmud Salaheddin M, Najeeb E, Ahmed AM, et al. (2008) Nutritional status of under-five children in libya; a national population-based survey. Libyan J Med 3: 13–19.
32. Uauy R, Albala C, Kain J (2001) Obesity trends in Latin America: transiting from under- to overweight. J Nutr 131: 893S–899S.
33. Bermudez OI, Tucker KL (2003) Trends in dietary patterns of Latin American populations. Cad Saude Publica 19 Suppl 1: S87–99.
34. Masterson Creber RM, Smeeth L, Gilman RH, Miranda JJ (2010) Physical activity and cardiovascular risk factors among rural and urban groups and rural-to-urban migrants in Peru: a cross-sectional study. Rev Panam Salud Publica 28: 1–8.
35. Jacoby E, Goldstein J, Lopez A, Nunez E, Lopez T (2003) Social class, family, and life-style factors associated with overweight and obesity among adults in Peruvian cities. Prev Med 37: 396–405.
36. Loret de Mola C, Pillay TD, Diez-Canseco F, Gilman RH, Smeeth L, et al. (2012) Body mass index and self-perception of overweight and obesity in rural, urban and rural-to-urban migrants: PERU MIGRANT study. PLoS One 7: e50252.
37. McLaren L (2007) Socioeconomic status and obesity. Epidemiol Rev 29: 29–48.
38. Monteiro CA, Moura EC, Conde WL, Popkin BM (2004) Socioeconomic status and obesity in adult populations of developing countries: a review. Bull World Health Organ 82: 940–946.
39. Dinsa GD, Goryakin Y, Fumagalli E, Suhrcke M (2012) Obesity and socioeconomic status in developing countries: a systematic review. Obes Rev 13: 1067–1079.
40. Poterico JA, Carrillo-Larco RM, Quispe R (2012) [Obesity in Peru: recommendations for a surveillance system]. Rev Peru Med Exp Salud Publica 29: 581.
41. World Health Organization (2001) Iron Deficiency Anemia Assessment, Prevention and Control: A Guide for Programme Managers. Geneva: WHO;.
42. Assuncao MC, Santos IS, Barros AJ, Gigante DP, Victora CG (2007) Effect of iron fortification of flour on anemia in preschool children in Pelotas, Brazil. Rev Saude Publica 41: 539–548.
43. Eckhardt CL, Torheim LE, Monterrubio E, Barquera S, Ruel MT (2008) The overlap of overweight and anaemia among women in three countries undergoing the nutrition transition. Eur J Clin Nutr 62: 238–246.
44. Robinson WS (2009) Ecological correlations and the behavior of individuals. Int J Epidemiol 38: 337–341.

10

Descriptive Characteristics and Health Outcomes of the Food by Prescription Nutrition Supplementation Program for Adults Living with HIV in Nyanza Province, Kenya

Jason M. Nagata[1]*, Craig R. Cohen[2], Sera L. Young[3], Catherine Wamuyu[4], Mary N. Armes[4], Benard O. Otieno[4], Hannah H. Leslie[5], Madhavi Dandu[6], Christopher C. Stewart[7], Elizabeth A. Bukusi[4], Sheri D. Weiser[8]

1 School of Medicine, University of California, San Francisco, San Francisco, California, United States of America, 2 Department of Obstetrics, Gynecology and Reproductive Sciences, University of California, San Francisco, San Francisco, California, United States of America, 3 Division of Nutritional Sciences, Cornell University, Ithaca, New York, United States of America, 4 Family AIDS Care and Education Services, Center for Microbiology Research, Kenya Medical Research Institute, Nairobi, Kenya, 5 Division of Epidemiology, University of California, Berkeley, Berkeley, California, United States of America, 6 Division of Hospital Medicine, University of California, San Francisco, San Francisco, California, United States of America, 7 Department of Pediatrics, University of California, San Francisco, San Francisco, California, United States of America, 8 Division of HIV/AIDS, University of California, San Francisco, San Francisco, California, United States of America

Abstract

Background: The clinical effects and potential benefits of nutrition supplementation interventions for persons living with HIV remain largely unreported, despite awareness of the multifaceted relationship between HIV infection and nutrition. We therefore examined descriptive characteristics and nutritional outcomes of the Food by Prescription (FBP) nutrition supplementation program in Nyanza Province, Kenya.

Methods: Demographic, health, and anthropometric data were gathered from a retrospective cohort of 1,017 non-pregnant adult patients who enrolled into the FBP program at a Family AIDS Care and Education Services (FACES) site in Nyanza Province between July 2009 and July 2011. Our primary outcome was FBP treatment success defined as attainment of BMI>20, and we used Cox proportional hazards to assess socio-demographic and clinical correlates of FBP treatment success.

Results: Mean body mass index was 16.4 upon enrollment into the FBP program. On average, FBP clients gained 2.01 kg in weight and 0.73 kg/m^2 in BMI over follow-up (mean 100 days), with the greatest gains among the most severely undernourished (BMI <16) clients ($p<0.001$). Only 13.1% of clients attained a BMI>20, though 44.5% achieved a BMI increase ≥0.5. Greater BMI at baseline, younger age, male gender, and not requiring highly active antiretroviral therapy (HAART) were associated with a higher rate of attainment of BMI>20.

Conclusion: This study reports significant gains in weight and BMI among patients enrolled in the FBP program, though only a minority of patients achieved stated programmatic goals of BMI>20. Future research should include well-designed prospective studies that examine retention, exit reasons, mortality outcomes, and long-term sustainability of nutrition supplementation programs for persons living with HIV.

Editor: Javier R. Lama, Asociacion Civil Impacta Salud y Educacion, Peru

Funding: This study was funded by the University of California, San Francisco Pathways Explore Grant, the University of California, San Francisco Library Open Access Publishing Fund, and the Phi Beta Kappa, Northern California Association, Scholarship (JN), the National Institutes of Health R01 MH095683 (SW), and the National Institute of Mental Health K01 MH098902 (SY).

Competing Interests: The authors have declared that no competing interests exist.

* E-mail: jasonmnagata@gmail.com

Introduction

The human immunodeficiency virus (HIV), undernutrition, and food insecurity remain leading causes of morbidity and mortality in sub-Saharan Africa despite increases in international funding for care and improved access to highly active antiretroviral therapy (HAART) [1,2]. Undernutrition and food insecurity converge to exacerbate the detrimental health consequences of HIV through complex feedback cycles [1,3] and disproportionately affect the estimated 22.5 million persons living with HIV/AIDS in sub-Saharan Africa [4]. HIV infection amplifies undernutrition by weakening metabolic function through impaired storage and utilization of nutrients, reduced absorption of carbohydrates and fats (including fat-soluble vitamins), and recurrent diarrhea from compromised immunity [1,5]. In addition, persons living with HIV have increased protein and energy requirements due to increased resting energy expenditure as a function of HIV load [6,7]. Weight loss [8] and undernutrition [9,10] are well-established predictors of mortality in HIV-infected patients, independent of CD4 lymphocyte counts.

Various nutritional interventions have been developed for persons living with HIV, including food-based supplement interventions, oral supplements with specific micronutrients, enteral or total parenteral therapy, and appetite stimulants [11]. In sub-Saharan Africa, food-based nutrition supplementation is regularly used to complement locally available foods to provide adequate daily macronutrient and micronutrient intake for persons living with HIV [2]. One study found that 90% of HIV programs across nine African countries provided some form of nutrition support [12]. Common supplements include corn-soy blends, fortified blended foods, and high-energy ready-to-use therapeutic foods [2].

In spite of knowledge of the multifaceted relationship between HIV infection and nutrition [1] as well as funding for supplementation programs [13], the quantitative clinical effects and potential benefits of macronutrient supplementation interventions to persons living with HIV remain largely unknown [14,15]. Indeed, a 2007 Cochrane systematic review on the effect of macronutrient supplementation on morbidity and mortality in persons living with HIV found no relevant clinical trials that reported on mortality, morbidity, or HIV disease progression [11]. The review did identify studies evaluating BMI change and found no significant effects of macronutrient supplementation on BMI or weight gain [11,16]. However, one recent trial in Malawi demonstrated that patients receiving ready-to-use fortified spread had significantly greater increase in BMI than patients receiving corn-soy blend over a 14-week intervention period, though there was no control study arm without nutritional supplementation [17]. One Haitian study found that food assistance was associated with significantly improved BMI and adherence to clinic visits at 12 months [18]. Limited data exist to guide targeted food programs to identify individuals with the greatest potential to benefit, appropriate enrollment criteria, optimal duration, and appropriate exit criteria for nutrition supplementation programs for persons living with HIV/AIDS. Multiple review articles have highlighted the critical importance of additional research in these areas [1,2,11].

In response to these calls, we examined the Food by Prescription (FBP) program, a nutrition supplementation program for persons living with HIV/AIDS in Nyanza Province, Kenya. The objectives of this study were to: 1) describe the demographic and health characteristics of patients enrolled in the FBP program, 2) describe programmatic outcomes including duration of enrollment in FBP, weight change, BMI change, and attainment of BMI≥20; and 3) identify demographic and health factors associated with attainment of BMI≥20.

Materials and Methods

Study setting and program description

Nyanza Province has the highest HIV prevalence in Kenya, at 15.1% [19]. Nearly universal food insecurity among persons living with HIV/AIDS has been reported in rural Nyanza Province [20,21]. Furthermore, 34% of men and 25% of women living with HIV in Nyanza Province are underweight (BMI<18.5) [22].

FBP was established in 2006 as a public-private partnership among the National AIDS and STI Control Programme in the Kenyan Ministry of Health, the United States Agency for International Development, and Insta Products Ltd., a Kenyan food manufacturing company. FBP operates in all regions of Kenya and reached 27,913 clients by 2007 [23]. The program includes nutritional screening, assessment, education, counseling, and provision of fortified corn-soy flour supplements to malnourished adults living with HIV, HIV-positive pregnant and postpartum women, and malnourished orphans and vulnerable children. The FBP adult supplement, called *Foundation Plus*, consists of nutrient-dense, pre-cooked whole maize, soybeans, vegetable oil, and cane sugar, fortified with vitamins and minerals in varying quantities that is rehydrated in boiling water and consumed as porridge by participants. This provides the majority of patients' daily micronutrient requirements and approximately one-half of clients' average daily energy requirement (450 kcal total and 15 g of protein per 100 g of *Foundation Plus*).

Adult (defined as age 15 or older) enrollment criteria for this FBP program study included having a body mass index (BMI) <18.5 kg/m^2 among patients enrolling into HIV care. The goal of the program is to restore patients to healthy nutritional status; FBP program guidelines state that adults should be discharged when their BMI improves to ≥ 20 kg/m^2 [23]. The program discharge criteria of BMI>20 was designed to help clients accrue buffer weight above BMI of 18.5 to prevent relapse in the FBP program [23].

For this retrospective cohort study, we obtained electronic FBP program encounter records for all non-pregnant adult patients who enrolled into the FBP program with BMI <18.5 kg/m^2 at all 48 Family AIDS Care and Education Services (FACES) sites in Nyanza Province between 1 July 2009 and 31 July 2011. We limited inclusion to those with a minimum of one follow-up visit.

Data collection

This study was conducted at FBP distribution sites supported by FACES, a collaboration between the Kenya Medical Research Institute (KEMRI) and the University of California, San Francisco (UCSF) that provides HIV prevention, care, and treatment services in Nyanza Province. At all FACES-supported sites offering FBP, trained community and clinic health assistants collected demographic information including gender, age, marital status, and household size using a standardized intake form upon enrollment. Patients' weight and height, World Health Organization (WHO) adult staging category [24], CD4 T-cell count, and HAART status were also determined at enrollment and at follow-up visits, generally scheduled one month apart. Patients were classified as severely underweight (< 16), moderately underweight (≥16.5 to <17), mildly underweight (≥17 to <18.5), normal weight (≥18.5 to <25), or overweight (BMI ≥ 25) using criteria from the Food and Agriculture Organization of the United Nations [25].

Ethics statement

The study was approved by the Ethical Review Committee at the Kenya Medical Research Institute and the Committee on Human Research at the University of California, San Francisco. The data were analyzed anonymously. A waiver of informed consent for adults and minors was specifically granted by the approving institutional review boards.

Data management and statistical analysis

Patient FBP encounter records were entered and stored in Microsoft Access 2007, subsequent data management was performed using STATA 12 (StataCorp LP, College Station, TX), and analysis was conducted using SPSS 12.0 (SPSS Inc., Chicago, IL). Any individual with at least two visits within a six month timeframe was included in analyses. If there was a more than six month gap between two visits, the latter visit and all subsequent visits were considered part of a new entry and all data (baseline values, duration, BMI change) were calculated separately for each entry. Duration of FBP was defined as days from FBP enrollment to attainment of BMI >20 or time of censoring. Individuals not reaching BMI >20 were censored at date of exit or last recorded appointment.

Differences in selected programmatic outcomes of FBP participants (including duration of FBP, weight change, BMI change, and attainment of BMI>20 as well as other BMI values) were analyzed by baseline BMI using ANOVA and Pearson's chi square tests, and by HAART status using independent samples t-tests. Cox proportional hazards regression was used to build a model in which the outcome was time until event, in this case, time in the FBP program until a participant achieved a BMI >20. For this evaluation our goal was to determine how long a patient spent in the program before achieving the desired outcome, as well as the clinical and demographic predictors of the outcome. Survival curves were used to evaluate factors associated with time to FBP treatment success. The associations between predictors and time to treatment success were analyzed using bivariate and multivariate Cox proportional hazards regression. Predictor variables were measured at baseline and included age (continuous), gender (male versus female), household size (continuous), marital status (categorical: single, married, divorced, widowed), BMI classification (categorical: severely, moderately, or mildly underweight, normal weight), antiretroviral therapy status (receiving or not receiving HAART during the study period, eligibility based on immunologic criteria of CD4 <350 to receive HAART), CD4 count (continuous), and WHO Stage (categorical: stages 1, 2, 3, and 4) [24]. All predictor variables were included in adjusted models. Hazard ratios (HR) and 95% confidence intervals (CI) were calculated from the Cox proportional hazards regression model. All variables were checked for multicollinearity and had a variance inflation factor <2. Models were tested for violations of the proportional hazards assumption and time varying covariates were used when the proportional hazards assumption was not met. All p values were two-tailed, with the level of significance set at $p<0.05$.

Results

Overall, 1,017 individuals met the study eligibility criteria. Mean age was 36, a majority of the sample were female, approximately half were married, and mean household size was four (Table 1). The average BMI was 16.4 at the time of entry into the FBP program. Mean CD4 count was 259 at baseline and a majority of the sample received HAART during the study period.

Mean and median duration of FBP were 100 and 62 days, respectively. Differences in FBP duration varied by baseline BMI (Table 2). The mean weight gain was 2.01 kg during FBP treatment. Patients classified as severely underweight gained significantly more weight than moderately underweight and mildly underweight patients (Figure 1). Overall, 13.1% of participants reached a BMI of 20, the threshold for discharge from the FPB program, while nearly half of participants achieved a BMI increase ≥0.5. Overall, FBP participants experienced an increase in CD4 count of 54 cells/mm^2. Participants enrolling with lower BMI had lower baseline CD4 counts; however, there was no statistically significant difference in CD4 count change by BMI category over the study period.

Patients not requiring HAART per CD4 guidelines as well as those receiving HAART both gained weight with no significant differences based on HAART status ($t=-0.848$, $p=0.40$, Figure 2). Patients not attaining BMI >20 exited without a recorded reason (60.3%), were still active in treatment (14.4%), deceased (3.0%), considered treatment failure (1.7%), or referred to another facility (0.8%).

In the multivariate model, younger age, male sex, greater BMI, and not requiring HAART during the study period were strongly associated with an increased rate of attaining a BMI>20 (Table 3). For each additional year of age, patients had a decreased rate of attaining a BMI>20 while receiving FBP. Compared with men, women had a decreased rate of attaining BMI>20, controlling for all other predictor variables.

Higher baseline BMI was associated with a higher rate of attaining BMI>20 (Table 3, Figure 3). Compared to patients receiving HAART, patients who did not qualify for and therefore did not receive HAART during the study period had an increased rate of attaining BMI>20 (Table 3, Figure 4). Household size, marital status, CD4 count, and WHO stage were not significantly associated with time to attainment of BMI>20 in bivariate and multivariate Cox proportional hazards regression models.

Discussion

Patients receiving FBP had significant increases in weight and BMI, with the greatest gains among the most severely undernourished clients. Yet only 13.1% of clients attained a BMI >20, the program criteria for discharge. Higher nutritional status at baseline, younger age, male sex, and not requiring HAART during the study period were associated with a higher rate of attainment of BMI>20.

FBP program participants gained an average of 2 kg during the duration of their FBP treatment and increased their BMI by 0.73 kg/m^2. This is consistent with the findings of weight and BMI gains from a corn-soy supplementation trial in Malawi [17] and a food assistance program in Haiti [18], but stands in contrast to studies in Europe [26] and the USA [27,28] that did not find significant effects of macronutrient supplementation on BMI or weight gain [11,16].

The most severely underweight clients had the greatest gains in weight and BMI, given that they had the most opportunity for improvement. This may argue for prioritization of food supplements to participants with the lowest BMIs if food supplementation is limited. However, because participants in the severely underweight category also started with the lowest BMI at baseline, they never attained an absolute BMI as high as those who started in higher BMI categories. Therefore, those who started with the highest BMI had the best endpoint weights. Severely malnourished clients also received the longest duration of therapy compared to other less undernourished groups. This suggests that FBP programs might consider a longer duration or higher calorie content of nutritional supplementation for severely malnourished clients.

Overall, 13% of clients attained the FBP program discharge criteria of BMI>20. The program discharge criteria of BMI>20 was designed to help clients accrue buffer weight above BMI of 18.5 to prevent relapse in the FBP program [23]. Therefore, a larger percentage (22.2% attaining BMI>18.5) of clients attained a "normal weight" status than were actually discharged from the program (13.1% attaining BMI>20). These low rates of attainment may indicate that the program's set discharge criteria are unrealistic to attain for most participants. However, nearly half of participants achieved a BMI increase of ≥0.5, which may be a more attainable target outcome. Alternative BMI outcome goals may be considered in the future.

There are several potential reasons for low rates of attainment of program discharge criteria. Patients living in households with less food availability may be more likely to share their FBP with

Table 1. Selected demographic and health characteristics of study participants at enrollment to Food by Prescription in Nyanza Province, Kenya.

	n	Mean or %	SD	Range
Demographic characteristics				
Age (years)	1017	36.4	11.4	16–81
Gender	998			
Male	355	34.8%		
Female	643	63.1%		
Household size	869	4.4	2.3	0–42
Marital status	990			
Single	146	14.3%		
Married	528	51.8%		
Divorced	96	9.4%		
Widowed	220	21.6%		
Health characteristics				
BMI at baseline (kg/m^2)	987	16.4	1.5	11.0–18.5
BMI classification	987			
Severely underweight (BMI <16)	361	35.4%		
Moderately underweight (16 ≤ BMI <17)	244	23.9%		
Mildly underweight (17 ≤ BMI <18.5)	382	37.5%		
CD4 at baseline (cells/mm^3)	712	258.8	237.5	1–1848
WHO stage at baseline	932			
Stage 1	86	8.4%		
Stage 2	242	23.7%		
Stage 3	459	45.0%		
Stage 4	145	14.2%		
Highly active antiretroviral therapy (HAART) status	1015			
Pre-HAART	339	33.3%		
Received HAART during study period	676	66.3%		

children and other members of their household, reducing the effect of supplementation on their own BMI. Furthermore, the FBP intervention was designed to supplement an existing diet, rather than to provide a primary food source [13], but participants living with severe food insecurity may not have regular access to other adequate food. Longer duration or higher caloric content of supplementation may also be considered. In addition, many patients exited before achieving target outcomes. Some potential reasons for exiting or lost to follow-up reported in other FBP studies include health workers and participants being unclear of the protocol (clients discharged after gaining some weight or after certain duration of time), lack of documentation in the medical record, patient dislike of the product, and the burden of transportation costs [13]. Additional exit reasons identified in the present study included lost to follow-up, nutritional deterioration, food allergies, transfer of care to another facility, or death. Participants receiving HAART had lower rates of lost to follow-up than participants not receiving HAART, even while receiving food supplementation. Furthermore, high rates of lost to follow-up have been reported in other FBP programs, at 50.1% in Kenya [23] and 70.6% in Ethiopia [13]. Future research should further explore clients' reasons for exiting the FBP program prior to attainment of program goals to guide future policies and ensure program objectives are consistent with what is being practiced in the field.

Clients not receiving HAART during the study period had a higher rate of attainment of BMI >20 compared with clients receiving HAART. This may be because individuals on HAART had more advanced disease at study enrollment (CD4<350 was eligibility criteria for receiving HAART) or alternatively that individuals on HAART had poorer adherence to FBP due to gastrointestinal side effects as reported elsewhere [23]. Though many nutrition support programs often specifically target individuals receiving HAART [1], our data suggest that nutrition supplementation can be beneficial for persons not yet requiring HAART by potentially increasing CD4 count.

Younger age was significantly associated with a greater rate of achievement of BMI>20. Younger persons may be more resilient and responsive to nutritional supplementation than the elderly. Several studies have reported higher food insecurity levels among the elderly due to challenges in completing agricultural labor, difficulty accessing alternate sources of food, dependence on others for food, and having additional medical co-morbidities [20,29–31]. The elderly who are physically weak or disabled may also have a greater challenge carrying and transporting large amounts of heavy food supplements [23]. They may additionally have lower success rates due to compromised immunity and reluctance to follow the FBP instructions. Though FBP is intended only for the individual client, there may be differences in how persons at different stages of life share and allocate their food within their

Table 2. Programmatic outcomes of Food by Prescription nutrition intervention by BMI classification.

			BMI classification at baseline				
			Severely underweight	**Moderately underweight**	**Mildly underweight**		
	Overall	**Range**	**BMI <16**	**BMI ≥16.5 to <17**	**BMI ≥17 to <18.5**	**Test statistic**	**p value**
Number of subjects	965		361	244	382		
Outcome, mean (SD)							
Duration of FBP (days)	99.90 (112.90)	30 - 583	103.43 (119.05)	105.36 (122.40)	94.27 (100.95)	0.92[a]	0.399
Weight change during FBP (kg)	2.01 (4.67)	−18.00 - 30.00	3.06 (5.30)	1.64 (4.89)	1.26 (3.62)	14.99[a]	<0.001
BMI change during FBP (kg/m^2)	0.73 (1.69)	− 5.56 - 11.02	1.09 (1.90)	0.61 (1.76)	0.46 (1.33)	13.76[a]	<0.001
Achieved BMI>20, n (%)	129 (13.1%)		30 (8.3%)	34 (13.9%)	65 (17.0%)	12.59[b]	0.002
Achieved BMI≥18.5, n (%)	215 (22.2%)		38 (10.8%)	45 (19.1%)	132 (34.9%)	63.52[b]	<0.001
Achieved BMI increase ≥5%, n (%)	359 (37.1%)		162 (45.9%)	87 (36.9%)	110 (29.1%)	22.06[b]	<0.001
Achieved BMI increase ≥0.5, n (%)	430 (44.5%)		180 (51.0%)	101 (42.8%)	149 (39.5%)	10.08[b]	0.006
CD4 count, mean (SD)							
CD4 count at baseline (cells/mm^3)	258.83 (237.48)	1 - 1848	226.02 (230.06)	242.72 (229.28)	295.54 (244.80)	6.13[a]	0.002
CD4 change during FBP (cells/mm^3)	54.33 (217.52)	−1440 - 1041	28.28 (243.65)	81.53 (211.40)	63.30 (204.07)	0.662[a]	0.518

a F test from ANOVA
b Pearson's chi square test

household based on level of perceived social responsibility for others, seniority in the household, capacity to perform labor and generate income, or other factors [1,23].

Men had a higher rate of achieving BMI>20 than women. Men on average enroll later into HIV care with more advanced HIV progression and lower BMI than women [22], which one would expect to predict poorer nutritional outcomes. However, women may be more likely to be non-adherent to FBP due to sharing of food at home with other family members, particularly to young dependents or HIV-positive spouses, due to their central role in household food resource allocation and perceived social obligation [23,32]. Sharing of food supplements at home may be the most important contributor to non-adherence with FBP and the reason for inadequate nutrient intake [23] particularly among women. The issue of food sharing should be carefully explored in future studies and addressed in nutrition guidelines. In particular, future household-level research could investigate the impact of FBP on individuals living in households in which single versus multiple members were receiving FBP.

Though this study only included FBP participants who enrolled based on strict BMI criteria (BMI <18.5), participants may also qualify with a mid-upper arm circumference (MUAC) <22 cm if

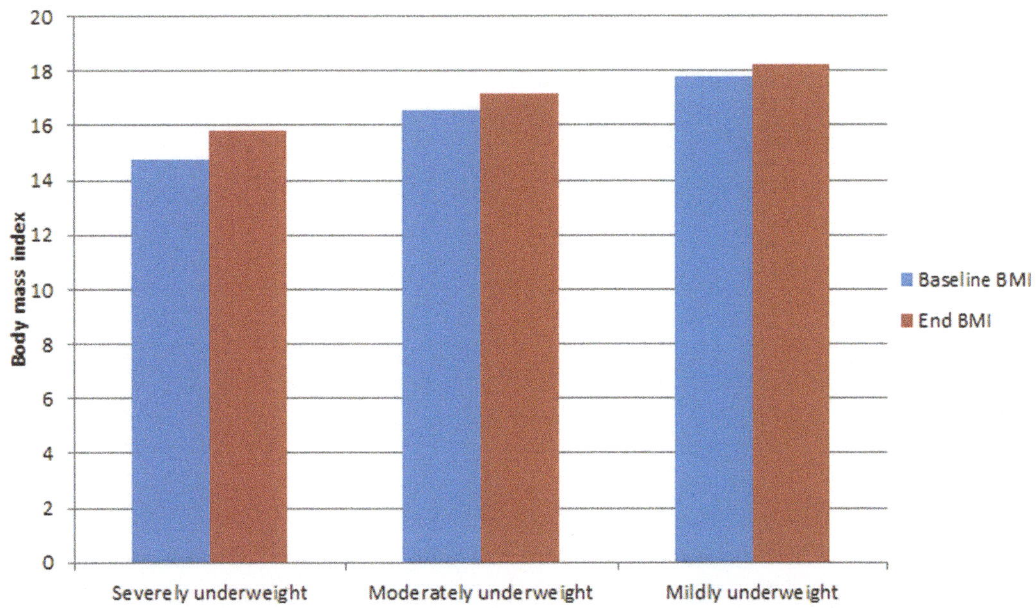

Figure 1. BMI at baseline and end of FBP, stratified by baseline BMI classification.

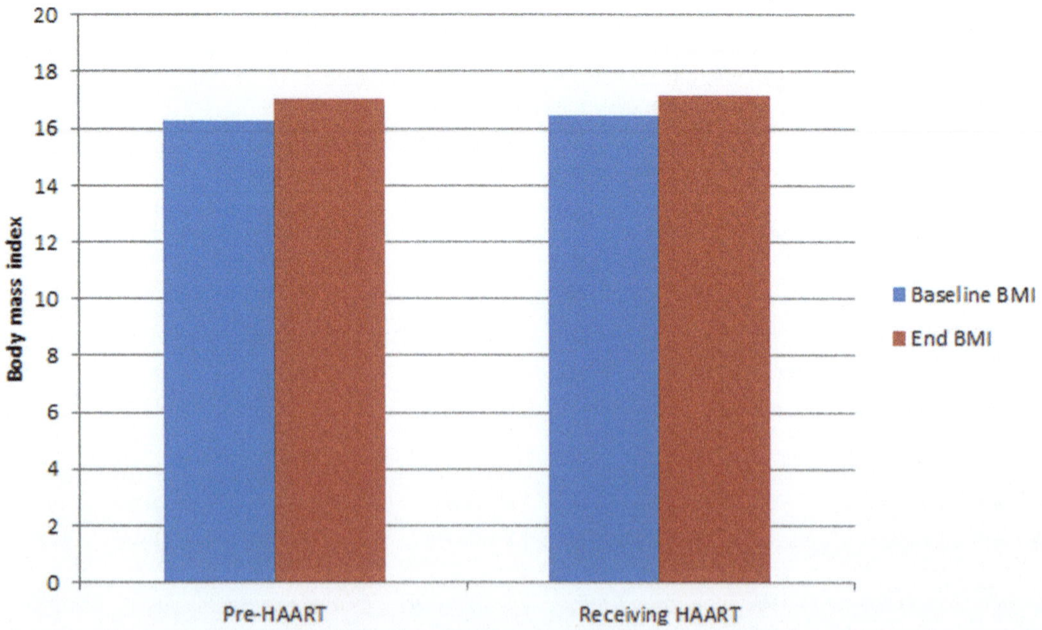

Figure 2. BMI at baseline and end of FBP, stratified by HAART status.

BMI is not available. Clinics in resource-limited settings may not have access to well calibrated scales and height measuring boards. MUAC is an alternate measurement used by the FBP program for enrollment in the absence of BMI data and may be a viable alternative to BMI as it does not require expensive equipment or mathematical calculations for assessment of nutritional status [33]. Future research should examine nutritional and health outcomes of participants who enroll using MUAC criteria in comparison to

Table 3. Factors associated with time to attainment of BMI>20 for patients receiving Food by Prescription.

		Bivariate analysis		Multivariate analysis	
Variable	n (%)	HR (95% CI)	p value	AHR (95% CI)	p value
Age	1017	0.98 (0.96–0.99)	0.008	0.97 (0.94–1.00)	0.029
Gender	998				
Male	355 (34.8%)	1 [Reference]		1 [Reference]	
Female	643 (63.1%)	0.57 (0.40–0.81)	0.002	0.51 (0.30–0.86)	0.012
Household size	869	0.97 (0.88–1.07)	0.568	1.00 (0.87–1.14)	0.954
Marital status	990		0.970		0.480
Single	146 (14.3%)	0.98 (0.55–1.73)	0.932	0.82 (0.36–1.86)	0.63
Married	528 (51.8%)	0.92 (0.59–1.43)	0.71	0.61 (0.31–1.21)	0.158
Divorced	96 (9.7%)	1.03 (0.53–2.04)	0.914	0.87 (0.31–2.43)	0.796
Widowed	220 (21.6%)	1 [Reference]		1 [Reference]	
Baseline BMI	987	1.29 (1.12–1.48)	<0.001	1.52 (1.23–1.86)	<0.001
CD4[a]	712	1.00 (1.00–1.00)	0.202	1.00 (1.00–1.00)	0.093
WHO stage	932		0.51		0.075
Stage 1	86 (8.4%)	0.82 (0.41–1.63)	0.566	0.63 (0.23–1.69)	0.356
Stage 2	242 (23.7%)	0.67 (0.39–1.15)	0.142	0.34 (0.15–0.80)	0.013
Stage 3	459 (45.0%)	0.75 (0.47–1.21)	0.235	0.76 (0.39–1.49)	0.422
Stage 4	145 (14.2%)	1 [Reference]		1 [Reference]	
HAART status	1015				
Pre-HAART	339 (33.3%)	2.54 (1.77–3.64)	<0.001	4.18 (2.42–7.22)	<0.001
Receiving HAART	676 (66.3%)	1 [Reference]		1 [Reference]	

Abbreviations: HR, Hazard ratio; AHR, Adjusted hazard ratio; CI, Confidence interval; HAART, Highly active antiretroviral therapy
[a]Time-varying covariate used in multivariate model.

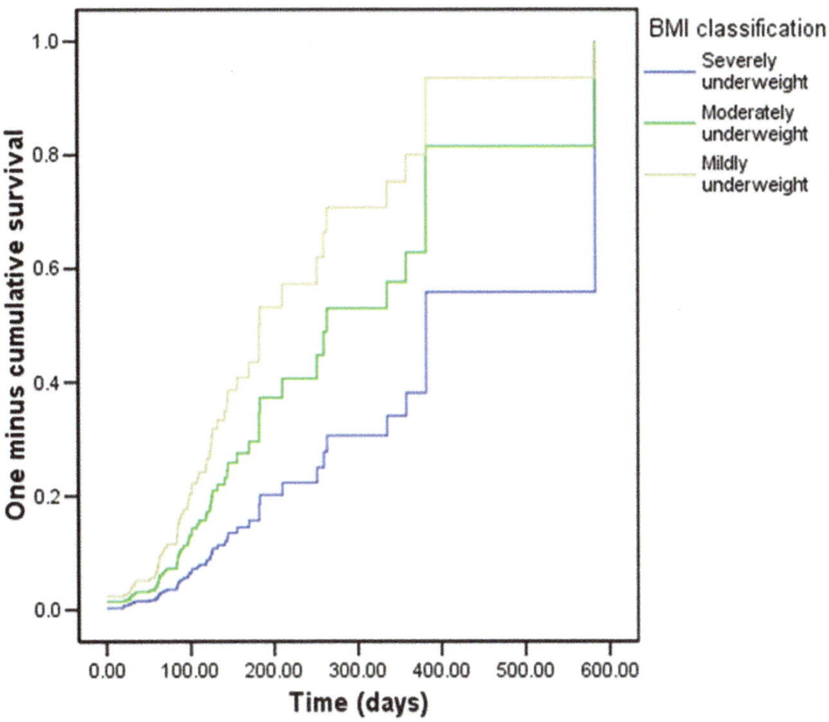

Figure 3. Survival curve of time to BMI > 20, by BMI classification.

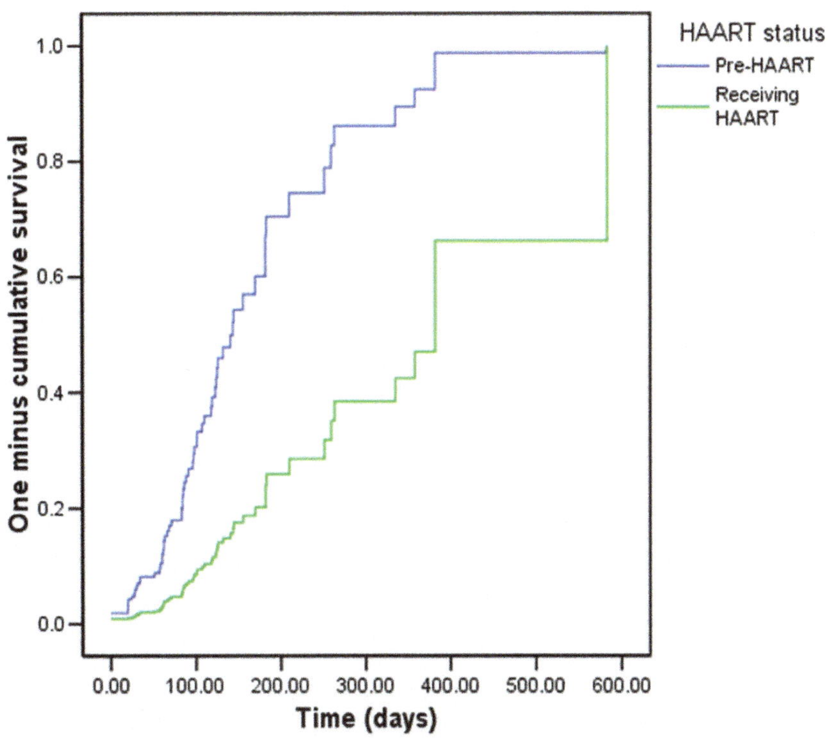

Figure 4. Survival curve of time to BMI > 20, by HAART status.

those who enroll with BMI criteria. Furthermore, in practice, patients with a BMI ≥18.5 deemed to be clinically malnourished are occasionally enrolled for FBP nutrition support, a phenomenon that should additionally be explored in future investigations.

This study has several limitations. Not all patient charts were complete, which led to missing data. Selection bias may have occurred as we only included patients with longitudinal data (minimum of one follow-up visit); however, there were no significant differences in demographic or health characteristics between patients who only had one recorded visit and those with more than one visit (data not shown). Patients were followed through their last recorded appointment; however, many patients did not have a recorded exit reason and therefore were lost to follow-up before attaining program discharge criteria of BMI >20. Though participants' demographics ranged widely in terms of age and household size, these variables were overall normally distributed and likely represented true variation possibly seen in other parts of sub-Saharan Africa. Due to regular shortages in FBP supply, it is possible that some patients did not receive FBP for their entire recorded duration of treatment. Although useful for international comparison, BMI has limitations in measuring undernutrition, body fat, and visceral adipose tissue, particularly among non-European populations [34,35]. Finally, there was no comparison group of persons who did not receive FBP nutrition supplementation, and thus our longitudinal findings remain descriptive.

Despite these limitations, the relatively large sample size, the demographic similarities of FBP clientele to the overall HIV patient population in Nyanza Province [22], and the implementation of the FBP program throughout Kenya and other parts of sub-Saharan Africa in regions with similar documented rates of undernutrition [22,36,37] supports the generalizability of this study's findings.

In sum, athough we found weight and BMI gain among FBP participants, only 13% of participants met stated program goals. Thus, there is critical need for well-designed and adequately-powered studies evaluating the effect of nutrition supplementation on clinical outcomes and mortality for adults living with HIV in order to guide global policy. Future research should examine the longer-term effects and sustainability of nutrition supplementation programs. Furthermore, understanding the complementary role of agricultural, educational, and poverty reduction interventions may be imperative to the success and longevity of sustainable nutrition programs for persons living with HIV.

Acknowledgments

The authors thank Lusine Mehrabyan, David Guzman, Starley Shade, Cinthia Blat, Jayne Kulzer, Lisa Dillabaugh, Chris Stewart, Irene Achieng, and the Family AIDS Care and Education Services (FACES) and Kenya Medical Research Institute staff for their assistance with study design and data management. The content is solely the responsibility of the authors and does not necessarily represent the official views of the National Institute of Mental Health or the National Institutes of Health. This study is published with the permission of the Director, KEMRI.

Author Contributions

Conceived and designed the experiments: JN CC SY CW MA BO MD CS EB SW. Analyzed the data: JN CC SY MA BO HL MD CS SW. Contributed reagents/materials/analysis tools: JN CC SY MA BO HL MD CS SW. Wrote the paper: JN CC SY MA HL SW.

References

1. Ivers LC, Cullen KA, Freedberg KA, Block S, Coates J, et al. (2009) HIV/AIDS, undernutrition, and food insecurity. Clinical Infectious Diseases 49: 1096–1102.
2. Koethe JR, Chi BH, Megazzini KM, Heimburger DC, Stringer JS (2009) Macronutrient supplementation for malnourished HIV-infected adults: A review of the evidence in resource-adequate and resource-constrained settings. Clinical Infectious Diseases 49: 787–798.
3. Weiser SD, Young SL, Cohen CR, Kushel MB, Tsai AC, et al. (2011) Conceptual framework for understanding the bidirectional links between food insecurity and HIV/AIDS. The American Journal of Clinical Nutrition 94: 1729S–1739S.
4. Joint United Nations Programme on HIV/AIDS (UNAIDS) (2010) UNAIDS report on the global AIDS epidemic. Geneva: World Health Organization.
5. de Waal A, Whiteside A (2003) New variant famine: AIDS and food crisis in southern Africa. The Lancet 362: 1234–1237.
6. World Health Organization (WHO) (2003) Nutrient requirements for people living with HIV/AIDS: Report of a technical consultation. Geneva: World Health Organization.
7. Shevitz AH, Knox TA, Spiegelman D, Roubenoff R, Gorbach SL, et al. (1999) Elevated resting energy expenditure among HIV-seropositive persons receiving highly active antiretroviral therapy. AIDS 13: 1351–7.
8. Tang AM, Forrester J, Spiegelman D, Knox TA, Tchetgen E, et al. (2002) Weight loss and survival in HIV-positive patients in the era of highly active antiretroviral therapy. Journal of Acquired Immune Deficiency Syndromes 31: 230–6.
9. Argemi X, Dara S, You S, Mattei JF, Courpotin C, et al. (2012) Impact of malnutrition and social determinants on survival of HIV-infected adults starting antiretroviral therapy in resource-limited settings. AIDS 26: 1161–1166.
10. van der Sande MAB, van der Loeff MFS, Aveika AA, Sabally S, Togun T, et al. (2004) Body mass index at time of HIV diagnosis: A strong and independent predictor of survival. Journal of Acquired Immune Deficiency Syndromes 37: 1288–1294.
11. Mahlungulu S, Grobler LA, Visser ME, Volmink J (2007) Nutritional interventions for reducing morbidity and mortality in people with HIV. Cochrane Database Syst Rev: CD004536.
12. Anema A, Zhang W, Wu Y, Elul B, Weiser SD, et al. (2012) Availability of nutritional support services in HIV care and treatment sites in sub-Saharan African countries. Public Health Nutr 15: 938.
13. Sadler K, Bontrager E, Rogers B, Coates J, Ghosh S, et al. (2012) Food by Prescription: Measuring the impact and cost-effectiveness of prescribed food on recovery from malnutrition and HIV disease progression among HIV+ adult clients in Ethiopia. Boston: Feinstein International Center, Tufts University.
14. Marchione TJ (2005) Interactions with the recipient community in targeted food and nutrition programs. The Journal of Nutrition 135: 886–889.
15. Agnarson AM, Ericson J, Ekström AM, Thorson A (2007) Antiretroviral therapy: What about food? AIDS 21: 1225–6.
16. Cantrell RA, Sinkala M, Megazinni K, Lawson-Marriott S, Washington S, et al. (2008) A pilot study of food supplementation to improve adherence to antiretroviral therapy among food-insecure adults in Lusaka, Zambia. Journal of Acquired Immune Deficiency Syndromes 49: 190–5.
17. Ndekha MJ, van Oosterhout JJ, Zijlstra EE, Manary M, Saloojee H, et al. (2009) Supplementary feeding with either ready-to-use fortified spread or corn-soy blend in wasted adults starting antiretroviral therapy in Malawi: Randomised, investigator blinded, controlled trial. BMJ 338.
18. Ivers L, Chang Y, Gregory Jerome J, Freedberg K (2010) Food assistance is associated with improved body mass index, food security and attendance at clinic in an HIV program in central Haiti: A prospective observational cohort study. AIDS Research and Therapy 7: 33.
19. National AIDS and STI Control Programme (2013) Kenya AIDS Indicator Survey 2012: Preliminary report. Nairobi: Ministry of Health, Kenya.
20. Nagata JM, Magerenge RO, Young SL, Oguta JO, Weiser SD, et al. (2011) Social determinants, lived experiences, and consequences of household food insecurity among persons living with HIV/AIDS on the shore of Lake Victoria, Kenya. AIDS Care 24: 728–736.
21. Nagata JM, Jew AR, Kimeu JM, Salmen CR, Bukusi EA, et al. (2011) Medical pluralism on Mfangano Island: Use of medicinal plants among persons living with HIV/AIDS in Suba District, Kenya. J Ethnopharmacol 135: 501–509.
22. Nagata JM, Fiorella KJ, Young SL, Otieno OD, Ijaa K, et al. (2013) Socio-demographic and health associations with body mass index at the time of enrollment in HIV care in Nyanza Province, Kenya. AIDS Care 25: 1491–1498.
23. Food and Nutrition Technical Assistance II Project (FANTA-2) (2009) Review of Kenya's Food by Prescription Program. Washington, D.C.: Academy for Educational Development.
24. World Health Organization (WHO) (2007) WHO case definitions of HIV for surveillance and revised clinical staging and immunological classification of HIV-related disease in adults and children. Geneva: World Health Organization.
25. Food and Agriculture Organization (FAO) (2000) The state of food insecurity in the world 2000. Rome, Italy: Food and Agriculture Organization of the United Nations.

26. Schwenk A, Steuck H, Kremer G (1999) Oral supplements as adjunctive treatment to nutritional counseling in malnourished HIV infected patients: Randomized controlled trial. Clinical Nutrition 18: 371–374.
27. Rabeneck L, Palmer A, Knowles JB, Seidehamel RJ, Harris CL, et al. (1998) A randomized controlled trial evaluating nutrition counseling with or without oral supplementation in malnourished HIV-infected patients. J Am Diet Assoc 98: 434–438.
28. Keithley J, Swanson B, Zeller J, Sha B, Cohen M, et al. (2002) Comparison of standard and immune-enhancing oral formulas in asymptomatic HIV-infected persons: A multicenter randomized controlled clinical trial. Journal of Parenteral and Enteral Nutrition 26: 6–14.
29. Knueppel D, Demment M, Kaiser L (2010) Validation of the household food insecurity access scale in rural Tanzania. Public Health Nutr 13: 360–367.
30. Leyna GH, Mmbaga EJ, Mnyika KS, Hussain A, Klepp K (2010) Food insecurity is associated with food consumption patterns and anthropometric measures but not serum micronutrient levels in adults in rural Tanzania. Public Health Nutr 13: 1438.
31. Laraia BA, Siega-Riz AM, Gundersen C, Dole N (January 2006) Psychosocial factors and socioeconomic indicators are associated with household food insecurity among pregnant women. The Journal of Nutrition 136: 177–182.
32. Nagata JM, Valeggia CR, Barg FK, Bream KDW (2009) Body mass index, socio-economic status and socio-behavioral practices among Tz'utujil Maya women. Economics & Human Biology 7: 96–106.
33. Powell-Tuck J, Hennessy EM (2003) A comparison of mid upper arm circumference, body mass index and weight loss as indices of undernutrition in acutely hospitalized patients. Clinical Nutrition 22: 307–312.
34. Lear SA, Humphries KH, Kohli S, Chockalingam A, Frohlich JJ, et al. (2007) Visceral adipose tissue accumulation differs according to ethnic background: Results of the multicultural community health assessment trial (M-CHAT). The American Journal of Clinical Nutrition 86: 353–359.
35. Rothman KJ (2008) BMI-related errors in the measurement of obesity. Int J Obes 32: S56–S59.
36. Kuria EN (2010) Food consumption and nutritional status of people living with HIV/AIDS: A case of Thika and Bungoma Districts, Kenya. Public Health Nutr 13: 475.
37. Leathers H, Foster P (2009) The World Food Problem: Toward Ending Undernutrition in the Third World, 4th ed. Boulder, CO: Lynne Rienner Publishers, Inc.

11

Protein Malnutrition Impairs the Immune Response and Influences the Severity of Infection in a Hamster Model of Chronic Visceral Leishmaniasis

Eugenia Carrillo[1]*, MªAngeles Jimenez[2], Carmen Sanchez[1], Joana Cunha[3], Camila Marinelli Martins[4], Anaiá da Paixão Sevá[4], Javier Moreno[1]

1 WHO Collaborating Centre for Leishmaniasis, Centro Nacional de Microbiología, Instituto de Salud Carlos III, Madrid, Spain, **2** Departamento Medicina y Cirugía Animal, Facultad de Veterinaria, Universidad Complutense de Madrid, Madrid, Spain, **3** Instituto de Biología Molecular e Celular, Instituto de Ciências Biomédicas Abel Salazar e Faculdade de Medicina, Universidade do Porto, Porto, Portugal, **4** Departamento Medicina Veterinária Preventiva e Saúde Animal, Faculdade de Medicina Veterinária e Zootecnia da Universidade de São Paulo, São Paulo, Brazil

Abstract

Leishmaniasis remains one of the world's most devastating neglected tropical diseases. It mainly affects developing countries, where it often co-exists with chronic malnutrition, one of the main risk factors for developing the disease. Few studies have been published, however, on the relationship between leishmaniasis progression and malnutrition. The present paper reports the influence of protein malnutrition on the immune response and visceral disease development in adult hamsters infected with *Leishmania infantum* fed either standard or low protein diets. The low protein diet induced severe malnutrition in these animals, and upon infection with *L. infantum* 33% had severe visceral leishmaniasis compared to only 8% of animals fed the standard diet. The infected, malnourished animals showed notable leukocyte depletion, mild specific antibody responses, impairment of lymphoproliferation, presence of parasites in blood (16.67% of the hamsters) and significant increase of the splenic parasite burden. Animals fed standard diet suffered agranulocytosis and monocytopenia, but showed stronger specific immune responses and had lower parasite loads than their malnourished counterparts. The present results show that protein malnutrition promotes visceral leishmaniasis and provide clues regarding the mechanisms underlying the impairment of the immune system.

Editor: Simona Stager, INRS – Institut Armand Frappier, Canada

Funding: This work was funded by project PI10/00829 from the Fondo de Investigación Sanitaria, http://www.isciii.es/. The funders had no role in study design, data collection and analysis, decision to publish, or preparation of the manuscript.

Competing Interests: The authors have declared that no competing interests exist.

* E-mail: ecarrillo@isciii.es

Introduction

Malnutrition is a serious health problem that remains common in many parts of the world. Protein energy malnutrition is the most frequent form of malnutrition, and globally affects some 800 million people, including over 150 million children under 5 years of age, most of them in developing countries [1]. Much of the excess morbidity and mortality associated with malnutrition is owed to the impairment of sufferers' defence mechanisms, which predisposes them to infectious diseases [2]. Leishmaniasis, a vector-transmitted, poverty-related disease – the second and fourth most important among tropical diseases in terms of mortality and morbidity rates [3] – is commonly encountered where protein malnutrition is also prevalent. Visceral leishmaniasis (VL), the most severe clinical manifestation, is generally fatal if not treated.

Although there is strong evidence that malnutrition is one of the major factors influencing the outcome of visceral leishmaniasis [4,5], few studies have measured the effects of this condition on the development of the disease. Anstead et al. (2001) reported that mice fed a protein-, iron- and zinc-deficient diet, were at increased risk of visceral disease following intradermal inoculation into both hind footpads with *L. donovani* [6]. Malafaia et al. (2009) also described that protein-deficient diets increased splenic parasitism in a BALB/c model of infection after intravenous challenge with *L. chagasi* [7]. Although it is clear that protection against *L. infantum* is dependent upon cellular immunity [8], which is known to be diminished by protein calorie malnutrition [9], the specific, cell-mediated mechanisms compromised in malnourished persons with visceral leishmaniasis remain unclear. In fact, the impact of infection or protein malnutrition on the host immune response, as well as the progression of the infection towards chronic visceral disease, have never been addressed with standardized experimental models.

Unlike in certain murine models, in which *Leishmania* infection tends to be self-limiting [10], golden hamsters (*Mesocricetus auratus*) develop a progressive, severe disease similar to visceral leishmaniasis seen in humans and dogs [8,11]. The effects of low protein and standard diets on certain parasitic infections have been reported in hamsters [12], but their effects on the course of chronic visceral leishmaniasis are unknown. The aim of the present work was to examine the relationship between protein malnutrition and visceral leishmaniasis in a hamster model. The results showed prolonged protein deprivation to be associated with a weakened immune response and severe visceral disease following *L. infantum* infection.

Materials and Methods

Ethics statement

The research ethics and animal welfare committee of the Instituto de Salud Carlos III ("Comité de Ética de la Investigación y de Bienestar Animal, Instituto de Salud Carlos III") approved this study (Report CBA PA 77_2010) that was carried out in accordance with Spanish law on the protection of animals used for experimentation and other scientific purposes (Royal Decree 1201/2005 and Law 32/2007). The Spanish legislation is a transposition of the Directive 86/609/EEC.

Parasites

L. infantum promastigotes (MCAN/ES/98/LLM-722, JPC strain) were grown in NNN medium and complete RPMI medium (RPMI1640, Gibco, Paisley, UK) supplemented with 100 UI/ml of penicillin, 100 µg/ml of streptomycin, 2 mM L-glutamine, 5×10^{-5} M 2-mercaptoethanol and 10% heat inactivated foetal calf serum (Lonza, Spain) as liquid phase for 2 weeks.

Animals and infection

Forty-eight 12 week-old male golden hamsters (*Mesocricetus auratus*), purchased from Janvier (France), were randomly assigned to isocaloric diets (Harlan Laboratories, Indianapolis, Indiana) containing either 14% (TD.00168) or 3% (TD.97138) protein (Table 1) but identical micronutrient content. Quantity of food given to hamsters from 14% group was adjusted to the 3% group to confirm comparable feed consumption [13]. Once total body weights in the low protein diet group showed statistical differences with those fed standard protein diet (day 53), 12 hamsters from both diet groups were inoculated with 2×10^{7} promastigotes by intracardiac route (i.e., the 14%INF and 3%INF groups). The remaining, non-infected hamsters were maintained on the initially assigned diets (14%NI and 3%NI groups). At 113 days post-infection, all animals were anesthetized with isoflurane and euthanized by cervical dislocation.

Haematology and biochemistry

Blood samples were collected from all animals by cardiac puncture (under anaesthesia with isoflurane) on day 113 post-infection. 300 µL were placed in Ca^{2+}-EDTA tubes for haematological, flow cytometry and PCR determinations. Haematocrit and total erythrocyte, leukocyte, lymphocyte and platelet (PLT) counts were recorded using an automated blood cell counter (VetABC, Scil, France). The mean corpuscular volume (MCV), mean corpuscular haemoglobin (MCH) and red blood cell distribution width (RDW) were then calculated. The remaining fraction of the blood samples was placed in sodium heparin tubes. The plasma was then isolated, frozen and stored for subsequent biochemical and immunological analysis. Plasma alanine aminotransferase (ALT), aspartate aminotransferase (AST), blood urea nitrogen (BUN), creatinine, alkaline phosphatase (ALkP), glucose, globulins and total protein concentrations were determined using a Biochemistry Serum Analyzer (IDDEX, Netherlands).

Table 1. Nutrients and kilocalories in the 3% and 14% protein diets used in the study.

Nutrient	% by weight		% kilocalories	
	3% Diet	14% Diet	3% Diet	14% Diet
Protein	3.1	14.2	3.3	15.2
Carbohydrates	78.6	66.6	83.6	71.5
Fat	5.5	5.5	13.2	13.3
Kcalories/g	3.8	3.7		

Control diet (14% protein diet) and low protein diet (3% protein diet) were purchased from Harlan Laboratories. Both diets contained similar amounts of corn oil (54.3 g/kg in 3% diet, 53 g/kg in 14% diet), cellulose (62.43 g/kg in 3% diet, 56.23 g/kg in 14% diet), Teklad vitamin mix 40060 (10 g/kg), ethoxyquin antioxidant (0.01 g/kg), calcium (0.7%) and phosphorous (0.54%).

Cell isolation and proliferation assay

PBMCs from blood collected in sodium heparin tubes were separated on a Ficoll-Hypaque density gradient (Lymphocyte Isolation Solution, Rafer, Spain) and washed twice in phosphate-buffered saline (PBS, pH7.4). These cells were then cultured in flat-bottomed 96-well plates (1×10^{5} cells/well) at 37°C for 5 days in RPMI medium. After further incubation with 10 µg/ml soluble *Leishmania* antigen (SLA) or 10 µg/ml concanavalin A (CONA) (Sigma) (performed in triplicate), the plates were pulsed with 5-bromo-2′ deoxyuridine (BrdU) and lymphocytes proliferation examined using the BrdU Cell Proliferation Assay Kit (GE Healthcare Life Sciences, UK) according to the manufacturer's instructions.

Delayed type hypersensitivity response

The delayed type hypersensitivity (DTH) response was determined by inoculating the left forepaw pad of each hamster with 5×10^{4} formalin-inactivated promastigotes (Leishmanin, Institute Pasteur, Teheran). The right forepaw was injected with PBS and used as a control. Oedema/inflammation was assessed by measuring paw pad thickness in the dorsal-plantar axis at 48 h post-inoculation.

Flow cytometry analysis

50 µl of blood (from the samples collected in the Ca^{2+}-EDTA tubes) were incubated with rat anti-mouse CD4 (clone 520 GK1.5, eBioscience, UK) and mouse-anti-mouse/rat MHCII (I-Ek) (clone 14-4-4S, eBioscience, UK); these have previously been shown to identify hamster CD4+ T cells [14] and B cells respectively [15]. The cells were then fixed in 1% p-formaldehyde-PBS solution and analysed by flow cytometry using a FACSCalibur (Becton Dickinson, Spain).

Enzyme immunoassay (ELISA) and immunofluorescence antibody (IFAT) tests

Maxisorp microtitre plates (Nunc, Roskilde, Denmark) were coated overnight with 1 µg SLA in carbonate buffer (1 mM Na_2CO_3, 28 mM $NaHCO_3$, pH9.6) and blocked for 1 h at 37°C with 200 µL of 1% BSA and 0.1% Tween20 in PBS. Plates were washed three times using PBS containing 0.01% Tween20, and then incubated for 30 min with 100 µL of plasma diluted 1:100 with dilution buffer (0.1% BSA and 0.1% Tween20 in PBS). The plates were then washed and incubated for 30 min with 1:250 horseradish peroxidase-conjugated goat anti-hamster IgG (Abd Serotec, Oxford, UK). ELISA was revealed using o-phenylenediamine dihydrochloride tablets (Sigma, Spain), quenching with 50 µL of 1M H_2SO_4. IFAT was performed using *L. infantum* promastigotes (MCAN/ES/98/LLM-722). Plasma was assayed in two-fold serial dilutions from 1/20 to ≥1/640 in PBS to determine total IgG levels using FITC-conjugated goat anti-hamster IgG (Abd Serotec, Oxford, UK) diluted 1/100. Antigen-antibody reactions in dilutions >1/40 were considered positive.

Histopathology

After collecting circulating blood by cardiac puncture, necropsies were performed on all hamsters at day 113 post-infection at the *Centro Nacional de Microbiología, Instituto de Salud Carlos III* (n = 48). Sections from the liver, spleen, right and left kidney, skin, ear, forelimbs, tongue and diaphragm were collected from each animal, placed in 10% buffered formalin and processed for histopathological analysis at the histology laboratory of the *Hospital Clínico Veterinario Complutense* (Madrid, Spain). Fixed tissues were embedded in paraffin, sectioned (4 μm), and stained with haematoxylin-eosin (H-E) following standard laboratory procedures. All samples were examined under the light microscope. Inflammatory and degenerative lesions in each tissue were qualitatively described and scored semi-quantitatively according to their severity as either non-existent (0), mild (+), moderate (++) or severe (+++).

DNA extraction and real time PCR (qPCR)

Blood, ear skin, mesenteric lymph nodes, bone marrow, liver and spleen were aseptically collected during necropsy. Bone marrow cells were isolated by flushing the bone marrow from the left femur with RPMI medium. Liver and spleen samples from each animal were individually homogenised through a 40 μm stainless steel tissue grinder in RPMI, and 1×10^6 cells used for total DNA isolation. 200 μL of blood from the samples collected in the Ca^{2+}-EDTA tubes were also used.

400 μL of NET10 buffer (10 mM NaCl, 10mM EDTA, 10 mM Tris-HCl pH 8.0) and 40 μL of 10% SDS were added to each sample following incubation at 70°C for 1 h and DNA purification using traditional phenol/chloroform extraction and ethanol precipitation. Total DNA was resuspended in 100 μL of distilled water and quantified using an ND-1000 UV-V Spectrophotometer (NanoDrop Technology, USA). *Leishmania* DNA was quantified using a LightCycler high speed thermocycler and the LightCycler FastStart DNA Master SYBR Green I kit (Roche Diagnostics, Spain) as previously described [16].

Evaluation of the severity of *L.infantum* infection

The evaluation of haematological and biochemical values, humoral and cellular responses, parasite load and histopathological damage of spleen and liver were assessed for each hamster and a disease score was performed. Altered parameters compatible with visceral leishmaniasis were scored with the maximum grade. Visceral leishmaniasis status was recorded as: Mild, Moderate, and Severe.

Statistical analysis

To analyse weight variations between the groups, the area under the curve for each animal was calculated and the results subjected to two-way ANOVA [17].

Haematological, biochemical, immunological, parasitological data and the disease score were tested for normality using the Shapiro-Wilk test. Since some parameters were not normally distributed, non-parametric tests were chosen to compare groups. When comparing 3%INF, 14%INF, 3%NI and 14%NI, Kruskal-Wallis one-way analysis of variance was used followed by pair wise comparison of groups using Mann-Whitney U test. When comparing two groups, Mann-Whitney U test was used. For the analysis of the score, two multiple comparisons were performed. First, we studied 3%INF, 14%INF, 3%NI and 14%NI groups by using Kruskal-Wallis and Mann-Whitney U tests. Second, we grouped the hamsters based on their mild, moderate, and severe infection, analysed differences among them using the Kolmogorov-Smirnov test and determined statistical significance by Mann-Whitney U test. Significance of the means was set at $p < 0.05$. All calculations were performed using SPSS version 20 (SPSS Inc., Chicago).

Results

The 3% protein diet induced weight loss and, ultimately, severe malnutrition

Feeding the animals a diet poor in protein content led to significant alterations in their body weight (Figure 1). These differences were significant ($p<0.05$) at the moment of infection and throughout the study. Following 166 days of dietary restriction and 113 days after *L. infantum* infection, the weight change percentages were (mean ± standard error) −35.81%±16.38% for the 3%INF group, 10.21%±19.63% for the 14%INF, −37.38%±12.64% for the 3%NI group, and 12.64%±13.77% for the 14%NI group. The hamsters' weight change could, therefore, be considered unrelated to *L. infantum* infection.

The degree of malnutrition of the hamsters, according to Gomez's classification of human malnutrition [18], was determined based on their weight-for-age (WA) results, using the 14%NI group as the control. The WA was calculated according to Anstead et al. [6] as: *(weight of the animals [by group]/expected weight of these animals if they had followed the diet of the 14%NI animals) x 100%.*

The mean WA was 55.59% for 3%NI group, 97.85% for 14%INF, and 56.98% for 3%INF. Animals following the 3% protein diet, irrespectively of the presence of *L. infantum* (groups 3%NI and 3%INF), showed severe malnutrition (WA<60%).

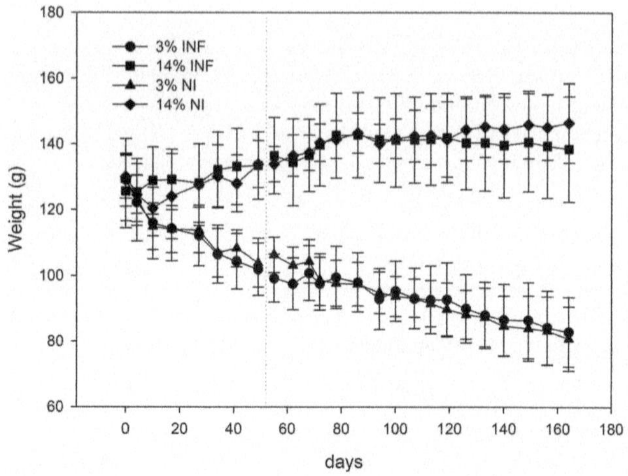

Figure 1. Growth of infected and non-infected hamsters fed the standard (14%) and protein-deficient (3%) diets. Changes in body weight were assessed every seven days. The dotted vertical line indicates the moment of intracardiac infection. Data show means of one representative experiment of two independent assays. The differences in mean body weight between hamsters on the different diets were statistically significant: *p<0.05, **p<0.01, ***p<0.001.

Protein malnutrition and visceral leishmaniasis induced haematological and biochemical alterations

The 3% protein diet was associated with a significant reduction in the number of leukocytes (p = 0.001) (Table 2). Non-infected malnourished hamsters (3%NI) showed significantly reduced numbers of monocytes, granulocytes and lymphocytes, especially $CD4^+$ (p = 0.0112) and B cells (p = 0.007), compared to the 14%NI animals. White blood cells depletion, mainly of monocytes (p = 0.007) and granulocytes (p = 0.031), was also seen in the 14%INF animals compared to non-infected animals on the same diet (14%NI) (Table 2). The low protein diet was also associated with reduced MCV and MCH values ($p<0.001$), as well as increased RDW values.

L. infantum infection was associated with a significant increase in ALkP levels, regardless of the diet followed (Table 3). ALT levels were also increased in both infected groups, but only statistically significant in the 14%INF group (p = 0.023). High levels of AST were found in all groups compared to the 14%NI group, but differences were not significant. The 3%NI animals showed reduced levels of albumin and globulin ($p<0.001$), but infection in the malnourished animals (3%INF) promoted a significant increase in globulins (p = 0.002). However, the infection induced a reduction of albumin levels in those fed with the standard protein diet (14%INF). A significant increase of creatinine was found between infected animals fed with 3% or 14% protein diet (p = 0.006). Malnourished hamsters (3%NI and 3%INF) also showed significantly reduced total proteins and blood urea nitrogen levels compared to the standard protein diet groups (14%NI and 14%INF); however, the reduction in total proteins was less pronounced in the 3%INF animals than in the 3%NI animals ($p<0.007$). Both the 3% protein diet and *L. infantum* infection were associated with increased glucose levels (p = 0.028 and p = 0.002, respectively).

The cellular response to leishmanial stimulation was impaired in malnourished animals

The response to concanavalin A (CONA) and soluble *Leishmania* antigen (SLA) was assessed using PBMCs from all groups. A statistically significant lymphoproliferative response to SLA was found in well-nourished infected hamsters (P = 0.005). Malnourished animals infected with *L.infantum* (3%INF) showed reduced lymphoproliferative response to both stimuli (Figure 2A and 2B, respectively) ($p<0.05$). However, infection alone is responsible for decreasing the unspecific lymphoproliferation in hamsters independently of the protein diet consumed (14%INF). Malnutrition also induced a reduced lymphoproliferative response to CONA (3%NI), similar to that showed for the infected well-nourished hamsters (14%INF).

Skin reactivity in response to leishmanin increased significantly in the 14%INF animals (p = 0.022; Figure 2C). Although no significant differences were found, infected 14% hamsters display a more robust DTH response, as compared to infected 3% hamsters.

Protein malnutrition was associated with a weaker *Leishmania*-specific humoral response

Anti-SLA antibody levels detected by ELISA were high in both infected groups (Figure 3A). However, the mean IgG level of the 14%INF animals was significantly higher than in the 3%INF group (p = 0.0009). Similar results were obtained in IFAT analysis. Most of the 3%INF animals (8/12) had a 1/80 positive titre, while four had values of 1/160, the maximum titre detected for this group (Figure 3 B). However, higher antibody levels were detected in the 14%INF group; four animals had values of 1/80, five had 1/160 and three had 1/320. IFAT titres of non-infected animals were <1/40.

Table 2. Haematological variables (mean ± SD) evaluated in infected (INF) and non-infected (NI) hamsters following the 14% and 3% protein diets.

Haematological variables	Groups: 3%INF	14%INF	3%NI	14%NI	Physiological values
Erythrocytes ($\times10^6/mm^3$)	8.42±2.37	8.6±1.72	9.35±1.32	8.85±0.72	3.96–10.60
Haemoglobin (g/dL)	12.69±3.32	14.31±2.62	14.63±1.76	14.49±1.35	10.00–19.20
Haematocrit (%)	43.20±12.02	47.22±9.91	48.20±6.72	49.24±4.65	32.90–59.00
MCV (fL)	$71.42\pm3.26^{A***}$	$74.83\pm1.19^{A***}$	$71.67\pm0.65^{D***}$	$75.92\pm1.68^{D***}$	64.00–77.60
MCH (pg)	$21.22\pm1.22^{A**}$	$22.71\pm0.59^{A**}$	$21.70\pm0.52^{D**}$	$22.53\pm0.55^{D**}$	20.00–25.80
PLT ($\times10^3/mm^3$)	474.00±277.69	377.00±176.55	477.42±149.60	482.50±105.36	200–590
RDW (%)	$15.83\pm1.39^{A***,B*}$	$12.79\pm0.48^{A***}$	$14.77\pm0.58^{B*,D***}$	$12.82\pm0.23^{D***}$	
Leukocytes ($\times10^3/mm^3$)	4.12±2.06	5.28±2.65	$3.94\pm1.29^{D***}$	$6.53\pm1.74^{D***}$	3.00–15.00
Lymphocytes	$2.15\pm1.00^{A*}$	$3.23\pm1.53^{A*}$	$2.14\pm1.00^{D**}$	$3.35\pm0.92^{D**}$	50–96%
CD4	0.86±0.42	1.16±0.72	$0.80\pm0.36^{D*}$	$1.21\pm0.35^{D*}$	
$I\text{-}E^{k+}$ (IgG/IgM^+)	0.94±0.69	1.28±0.73	$0.89\pm0.38^{D**}$	$1.46\pm0.45^{D**}$	
Monocytes	0.19±0.14	$0.23\pm0.15^{C**}$	$0.21\pm0.09^{D***}$	$0.41\pm0.12^{C**,D***}$	0–3%
Granulocytes	1.78±1.06	$1.83\pm1.07^{C*}$	$1.48\pm0.56^{D***}$	$2.83\pm0.85^{C*,D***}$	17–35%

The comparison of the groups showed at least one significant difference among the averages of MCV ($p<0.0001$), MCH (p = 0.001), RDW ($p<0.0001$), leukocytes (p = 0.008), lymphocytes (p = 0.013), CD4 (p = 0.05), $I\text{-}E^{k+}$ (p = 0.029), monocytes (p = 0.002) and granulocytes (p = 0.005). Statistically significant differences are indicated by (A) for 3%INF vs. 14%INF; (B) for 3%INF vs. 3%NI; (C) for 14%INF vs. 14%NI; and (D) for 3%NI vs. 14%NI. Letters with * indicate $p<0.05$; letters with ** indicate $p<0.01$; letters with *** indicate $p<0.001$. Abbreviations: PLT- platelets, MCV- mean corpuscular volume, MCH- mean corpuscular haemoglobin, RDW- red blood cell distribution width.

Table 3. Biochemical profiles (mean ± SEM) of the infected (INF) and non-infected (NI) hamsters fed 14% and 3% protein diets.

Biochemical variables	Groups:				Physiologi-cal values
	3%INF	14%INF	3%NI	14%NI	
ALKP (IU/L)	$91.73 \pm 36.79^{B***}$	$97.00 \pm 41.93^{C***}$	$45.25 \pm 19.95^{B***}$	$46.50 \pm 15.75^{C***}$	8–187
ALT (IU/L)	70.73 ± 21.21	$79.73 \pm 17.18^{C*}$	56.83 ± 17.67	$61.75 \pm 14.65^{C*}$	22–128
AST (IU/L)	95.75 ± 43.53	103.27 ± 48.46	100.75 ± 31.18	75.58 ± 22.92	28–122
Creatinine (mg/dl)	$0.57 \pm 0.14^{A**}$	$0.39 \pm 0.16^{A**}$	0.46 ± 0.10	0.41 ± 0.16	0.40–1.00
Glucose (mg/dl)	121.45 ± 49.28	$121.83 \pm 26.12^{C***}$	$108.75 \pm 36.14^{D*}$	$80.75 \pm 24.82^{C***,D*}$	37–198
Total proteins (g/dL)	$5.95 \pm 0.42^{A**,B***}$	$6.58 \pm 0.55^{A**}$	$4.92 \pm 0.34^{B***,D***}$	$6.65 \pm 0.67^{D***}$	5.20–7.00
BUN (mg/dL)	$7.09 \pm 3.51^{A***}$	$24.75 \pm 9.99^{A***}$	$6.92 \pm 6.36^{D***}$	$23.92 \pm 9.26^{D***}$	12–26
Albumin (g/dL)	2.47 ± 0.75	$2.69 \pm 0.46^{C*}$	$2.10 \pm 0.23^{D***}$	$3.03 \pm 0.34^{C*,D***}$	2.60–4.10
Globulin (g/dL)	$3.47 \pm 0.61^{B**}$	3.79 ± 0.33	$2.83 \pm 0.28^{B**,D***}$	$3.61 \pm 0.40^{D***}$	2.70–4.20

There was at least one significant difference among the averages of all biochemical parameters, except AST ($p<0.02$). Statistical differences are indicated by (A) for 3%INF vs. 14%INF; (B) for 3%INF vs. 3%NI; (C) for 14%INF vs. 14%NI; and (D) for 3%NI vs. 14%NI. Letters with * indicate $p<0.05$; letters with ** indicate $p<0.01$; letters with *** indicate $p<0.001$. Abbreviations: ALkP – alkaline phosphatase, ALT – alanine aminotransferase, AST – aspartate aminotransferase, BUN – blood urea nitrogen.

L. infantum infection induced granulomatous splenitis and hepatitis

Infected hamsters (3% INF and 14% INF) had granulomatous inflammatory infiltrates in liver and spleen. In the liver, these infiltrates were random, multifocal and arranged in either discrete granulomas or sheets of inflammatory cells within the same individual (Figure 4A and 4B). Inflammatory cells consisted of macrophages, lesser lymphocytes, plasma cells, and few giant multinucleated cells (GMCs) that mildly disrupted the parenchyma, and were additionally surrounded by epithelioid macrophages when arranged in granulomas (Figure 4D). Some giant multinucleated cells contained variably sized lamellar concentric mineral concretions often surrounded by a colorless halo (Shaumann's bodies) (Figure 4C). The extent and severity of the granulomatous hepatitis was variable among infected individuals (Table 4). Most of the 3% INF hamsters had mild hepatitis (7/12), while animals in

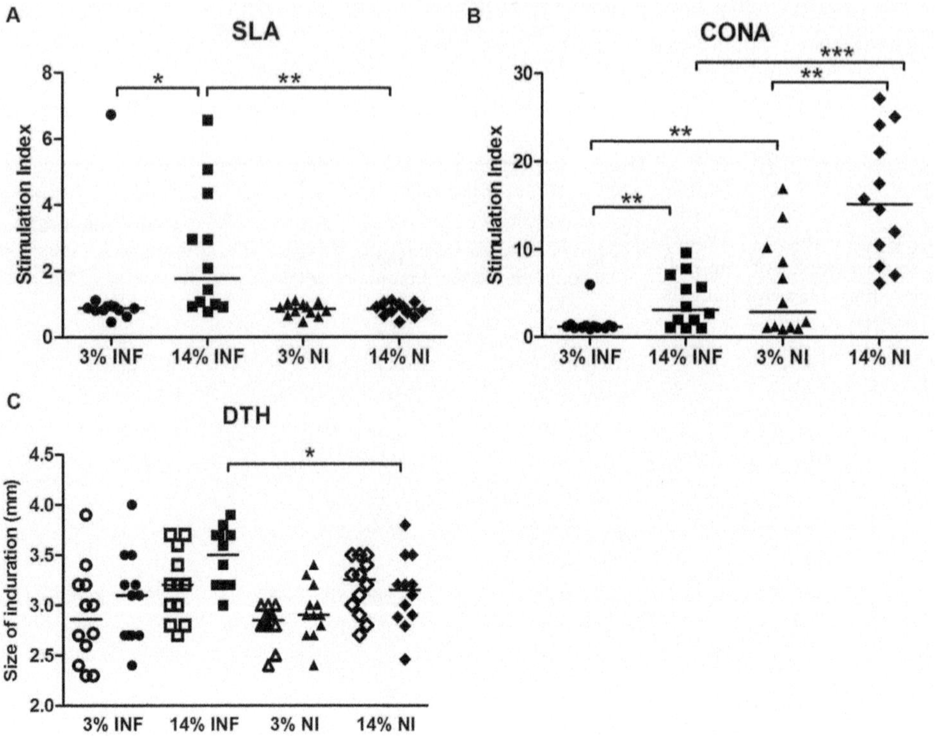

Figure 2. Evaluation of the cellular response and leishmanin test. Lymphoproliferative response to specific SLA (A) and non-specific CONA (B) stimuli, at 113 days post-infection, of PBMCs from infected and non-infected hamsters following the 14% and 3% protein diets. (C) Measurements of the footpads inoculated with PBS (open symbols) and leishmanin (close symbols), taken at 48 h. *$p<0.05$, **$p<0.001$. Two independent experiments were performed, one representative experiment is shown.

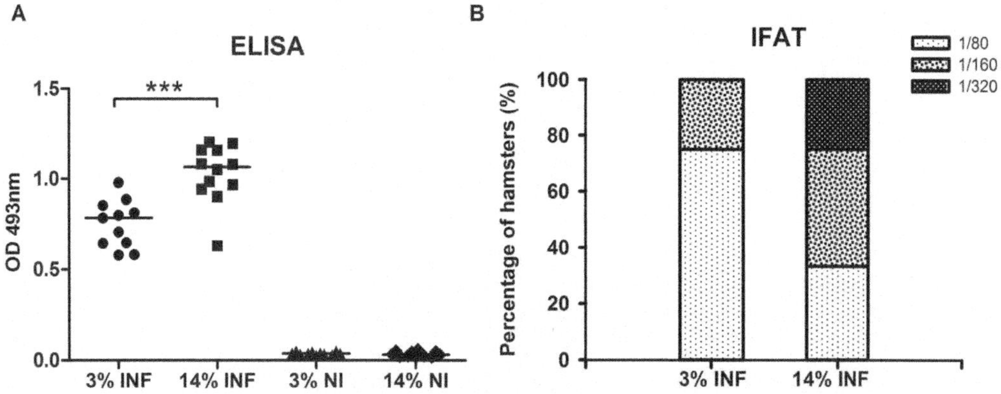

Figure 3. Serum antibodies detected by SLA ELISA (A) and IFAT (B). The difference in response, as measured by ELISA, of the hamsters fed the 3% and 14% protein diets was significantly different. ***p<0.001. Data show medians of one representative experiment of two independent assays.

the 14%INF group had moderate inflammation (7/12). In spleens from both infected groups inflammatory infiltrates were either multifocal or diffuse disrupting the totality of the red pulp in more severe cases (Figure 4E). Inflammation was predominantly moderate in both groups (9/12 animals in the 3%INF group versus 7/12 in the 14% INF group). Intralesional *Leishmania* amastigotes were difficult to discern in either organ tissues with routine H-E staining (Figure 4F).

Malnourishment contributed to higher parasite loads and favoured the development of visceral leishmaniasis

Parasite loads of blood, skin, bone marrow, lymph node, liver and spleen were measured in all groups (Figure 5). All skin samples were negative for parasites (data not shown). Two out of 12 hamsters in the 3%INF group had parasites in the blood, while no parasites were detected in the blood of any of the 14%INF animals (data not shown). Lymph node's parasite loads were similar in both infected groups, regardless of the diet. In the visceral organs, the 3%INF animals presented higher parasite loads than the 14%INF, with calculated two-fold increase in the liver and seven-fold increase in the spleen ($p = 0.0026$). However, in the bone marrow, though not statistically significant, the well-nourished hamsters revealed to harbour more parasites than the animals fed with the 3% protein diet.

Different numbers of animals in the 3%INF and 14%INF groups suffered severe visceral leishmaniasis. By day 165, the 3%INF group had 4 severe, 4 moderate and 4 mild visceral disease; while the 14%INF group had 1 severe, 3 moderate and 8 mild leishmaniasis (Figure 6). The multiple comparison of the total score showed differences among the 3%INF, 14%INF, 3%NI and 14%NI groups ($p<0.0001$). Particularly, the detailed analysis of the parameters of the score showed that 3%INF and 14%INF presented significant differences in the biochemical parameters, cellular and humoral response ($p<0.01$). The evaluation of the score classification showed that the proportion of animals with mild visceral leishmaniasis was significantly higher in 14%INF group ($p = 0.039$). There was at least one significant difference among the averages of the groups mild, moderate and severe on biochemical parameters, cellular response and qPCR ($p<0.01$). Mildly and moderately infected groups had different biochemical parameters and cellular responses ($p<0.02$), while mild and severe infections had differences in these two factors and also in the parasite load ($p<0.01$). Moderately and severely infected hamsters differed statistically in their *Leishmania* burdens ($p = 0.007$).

Discussion

In the present study we evaluated for the first time haematological, biochemical, humoral and cellular immune responses, and parasitism in malnourished (3% protein diet) and well-nourished (14% protein diet) hamsters experimentally infected with *L. infantum* after 4 months post-infection.

In the 14%INF group, one severely, three moderately and eight mildly *L.infantum* infected hamsters were recorded. These infected hamsters showed minimal changes in their serum biochemistry in relation to non-infected animals, with the exception of a significant increase of ALT levels. ALKP was also elevated in these well-nourished infected hamsters as it was in the malnourished animals, thus we correlate this parameter to *L. infantum* infection independently of the diet followed. As it is known, most naturally infected persons and dogs are asymptomatic or show subclinical signs of disease [19–21]. The opportunity to experimentally mimic some conditions present in the real scenario makes our hamster model a valuable tool for studying the pathological aspects of chronic visceral leishmaniasis, as previously described [22,23].

It is well known that a state of malnutrition increases the severity of the clinical outcome of leishmaniasis [4,24]. Using a hamster model of protein malnutrition, we have found that most of the infected animals (3%INF) had a worse manifestation of the disease with four severely and four moderately infected hamsters. This clearly demonstrates the low protein diet ingestion was associated with a higher development of patent visceral leishmaniasis. Although in these infected animals total protein and globulin levels suffered changes in relation to well-nourished hamsters, severe malnourishment produced in non-infected animals most of the alterations of the biochemical parameters, such as reduced total protein, urea, albumin and globulin levels. Low serum albumin and total protein levels are good markers for the protein status of the organism, as previously found in severe malnourished humans and dogs [25–26]. Based on these observations, this model provides an excellent opportunity to address the study of the factors implicated in severe malnutrition and, in extension, as showed in this work, in both severe malnutrition and visceral leishmaniasis interaction.

Low white blood cell count is one of the main signs of humans and dogs suffering from visceral leishmaniasis [21,27]. In our

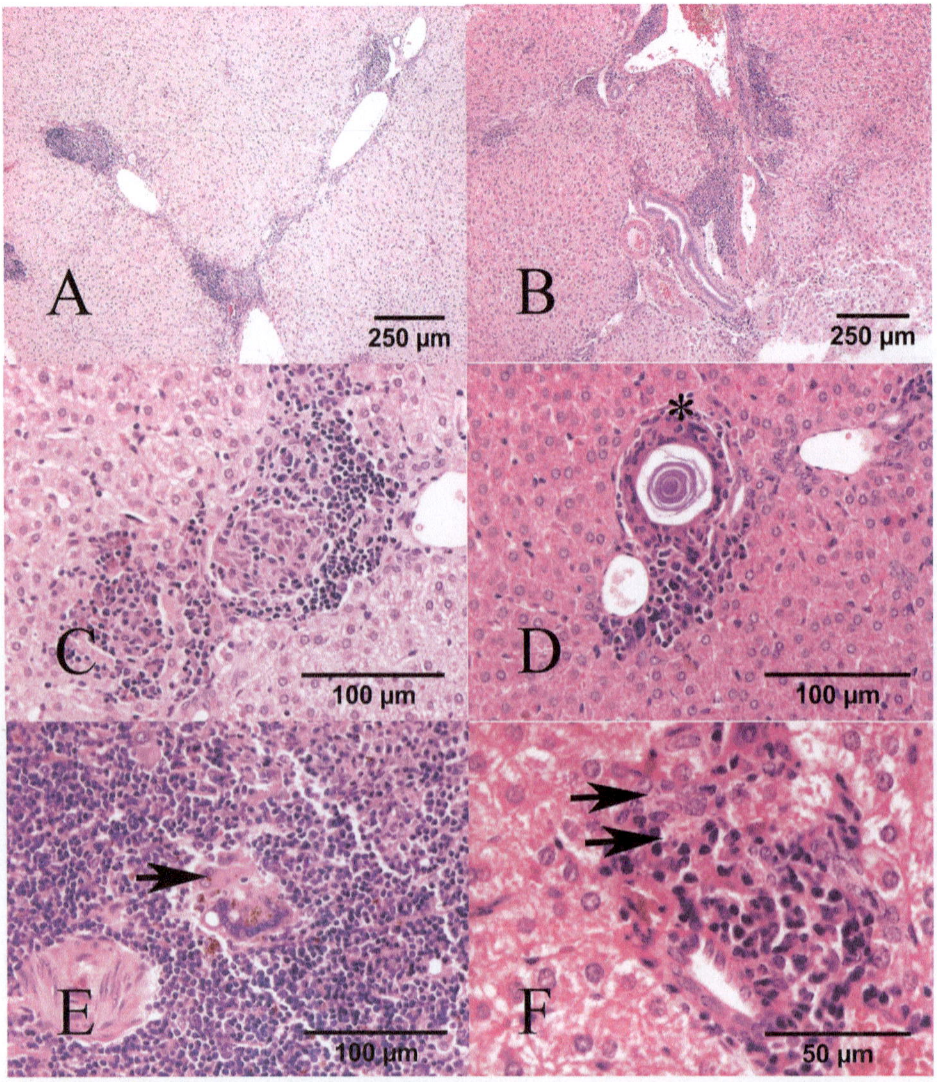

Figure 4. Granulomatous inflammation in liver and spleen of infected hamsters on 3% and 14% protein diets. H–E. (A) 3%INF and (B) 14%INF: Severe, multifocal to coalescing granulomatous hepatitis. (C) Liver, 3%INF: Giant multinucleated cell containing a Shaumanns body (asterisk) within a granuloma. (D) Liver, 14%INF: two discrete granulomas containing macrophages, cell debris, epitheliod macrophages, surrounded by few lymphocytes and plasma cells. (E) Spleen, 3%INF: Giant multinucleated cell (arrow) with intracytoplasmic cell debris and hemosiderin. (F) Liver, 14%INF: Granuloma with few macrophages containing rare intracytoplasmic amastigotes (arrows).

model, *L. infantum* infection caused leukocyte depletion, mainly in monocytes and granulocytes numbers. Furthermore, we found that severe leukopenia was strongly linked to malnourishment, affecting the numbers of all the white cell subsets, including $CD4^+$ T lymphocytes and B cells. The malnourished animals – regardless to infection status – also had reduced MCV and MCH values, which are indicative of chronic non-regenerative anaemia. Haematopoiesis is known to be strongly impaired by protein energy malnutrition [28], and the present results suggest that severe protein malnutrition induces bone marrow dysfunction in the hamster, as it does in mice [29]. The presence of *Leishmania* in the bone marrow might also influence haematopoiesis. The inability to develop an efficient, demand-adapted haematopoiesis due to such an infection [30] would influence the final immune response and, therefore, the ability of the host to fight back.

The persistence of *Leishmania* parasites in the lymph nodes was not influenced by protein malnutrition. Increased rates of systemic spread are reported not to depend on higher parasite burdens in the lymph nodes [6]; indeed, the latter authors reported that dissemination was more evident when the total lymph node's parasite burden was lower. However, in our hamsters, protein malnutrition was associated with the presence of circulating parasites and increased parasite burdens, mainly in spleen.

Infected animals had granulomatous hepatitis and splenitis associated with *Leishmania* infection, with only mild insignificant variations in severity between the 3% INF and the 14% INF groups, and regardless of the parasite burdens detected in either tissue. The mere presence of granulomatous inflammation does not necessarily imply an active infection or an effective cellular immune response. As an example, the presence of hepatic granulomas in human visceral leishmaniasis is associated with the maintenance of subclinical infections [31]. Granulomatous inflammation is regulated by multiple factors -such as poorly degradable or persistent antigens and the host's immune response- that determine the effectiveness and type of granulomatous reaction. We could speculate that perhaps some of the immune

Table 4. Relevant histopathological findings.

Observations	Tissue	Groups:			
		3%INF	**14%INF**	**3%NI**	**14%NI**
Multifocal to coalescing granulomatous infiltrates	Liver	+ (7/12)	+ (3/12)	0 (12/12)	0 (12/12)
		++ (3/12)	++ (7/12)		
		+++ (2/12)	+++ (2/12)		
	Spleen	+ (2/12)	+ (2/12)	0 (12/12)	0 (12/12)
		++ (9/12)	++ (7/12)		
		+++ (1/12)	+++ (3/12)		
Giant multinucleated cells with intra-cytoplasmic concentric lamellar mineral	Liver	0 (3/12)	0 (4/12)	0 (12/12)	0 (12/12)
		+ (9/12)	+ (8/12)		

Severity of the histopathological findings: non-existant (0), mild (+), moderate (++), severe (+++).
(n/n) – Number of animals with the given severity of the histopathological feature within each group.

mechanisms involved against the parasite might have been impaired in the malnourished group, given that a more severe cellular infiltration would have been expected considering the higher parasite loads detected in this group.

Schaumann's bodies are a common finding in granulomatous lesions associated with *Leishmania* [32], to the point that some authors claim that the mere presence of these Schaumann's bodies in the absence of amastigotes is strongly suggestive of *Leishmania* infection in hamsters [33]. These structures were consistently detected in our infected animals in concordance with these observations. The mechanisms involved in the formation of these structures did not appear to be influenced by the protein malnutrition, but by factors related to the infection only.

It is well known that severe protein malnutrition causes functional abnormalities in host defence systems [34,35], and that the depression of T cell responses following long-term protein malnutrition renders the host unable to prevent the systemic spread of *L. infantum*. Although *Leishmania* infection is known to impair the immune system [5,36], only two studies have examined the adaptative immune response to *Leishmania* in conjunction with

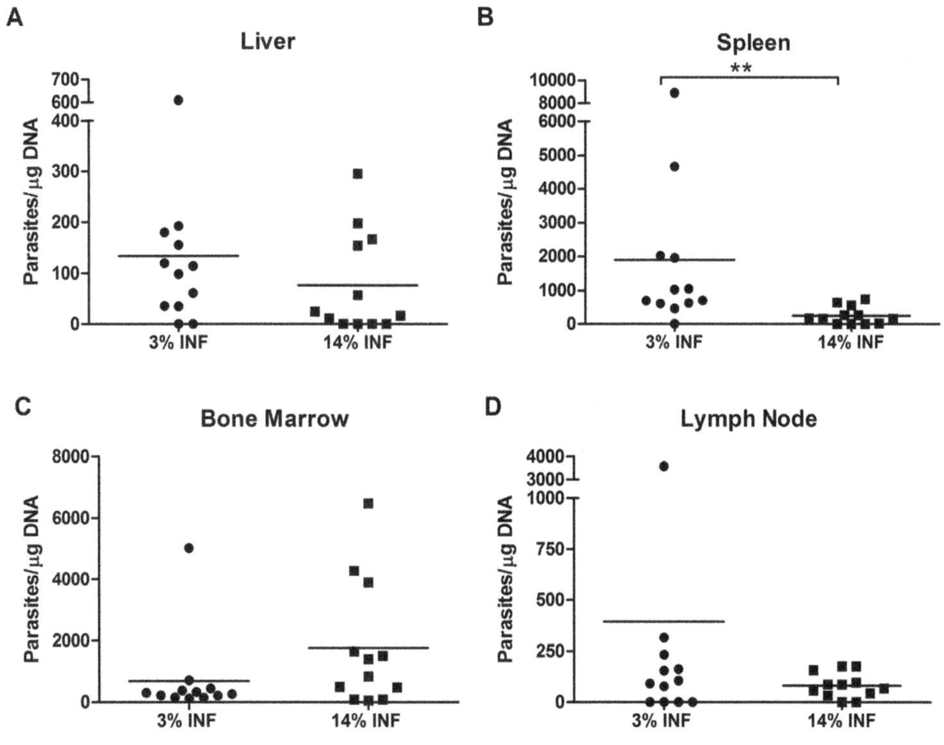

Figure 5. Quantitative distribution of *L. infantum* in malnourished and well-nourished hamsters. The parasite burden was quantified on the (A) liver, (B) spleen, (C) bone marrow, and (D) lymph node. Data represent means ± SD of 12 animals per group of a representative experiment of two independent assays. Splenic parasite loads were significantly increased in malnourished animals. The presence of parasites in blood was detected only in hamsters fed the 3% protein diet (2/12, data not shown).

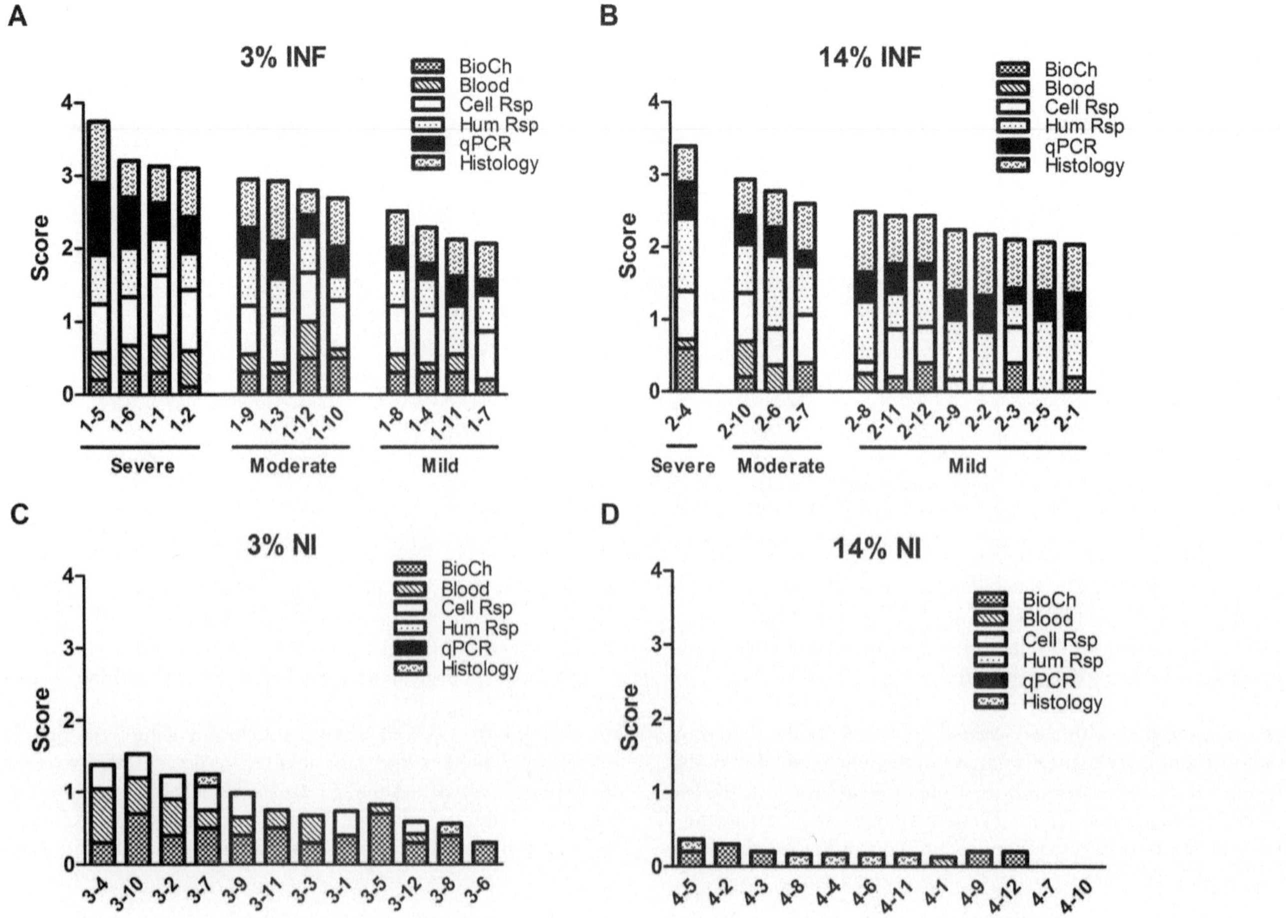

Figure 6. Disease score for visceral leishmaniasis. A score to measure the grade of severity of the disease was performed for 3%INF (A), 14%INF (B), 3%NI (C) and 14%NI (D). For each hamster, a score of 2 was given to values below normal for leukocytes, lymphocytes, PLT and albumin; and to values above normal for total proteins, BUN, AST, globulin and erythrocytes. Other abnormalities in these biochemical (BioCh) or blood variables were scored as 1. Lymphoproliferative responses for SLA and CONA were scored as: 3 for a stimulation index (SI) <0.60; 2 for $0.60\leq SI<2.00$; 1 for $2.00\leq SI<4.00$; and 0 for $SI\geq4.00$. The humoral response as determined by ELISA was scored as: 1 for $0.10\leq$ OD 430 nm <0.60; 2 for $0.60\leq$ OD 430 nm <1.00; 3 for OD 430 nm≥1.00. As determined by IFAT, the humoral response was scored as: 1 for 1/80 titre; 2 for 1/160 titre; 3 for 1/320 titre. Spleen and bone marrow parasite loads as determined by qPCR were scored as: 1 for $35\leq$ parasites/μg/ml<1000; 2 for $1000\leq$ parasites/μg/ml<5000; 3 for parasites/μg/ml≥5000. Liver and lymph node parasite loads were scored as: 1 for $35\leq$ parasites/μg/ml<600; 2 for parasites/μg/ml≥600. Presence of *Leishmania* DNA in the blood was given a disease score of 2. Histopathology for liver and spleen was scored from 0 to 3. A corrective factor was applied to the 6 categories of data to compensate the global score. Visceral leishmaniasis status was recorded as: Mild, when the total score for an animal was 2–2.5; Moderate, when between 2.6–3.0; and Severe, when >3.1. The bars represented each hamster and showed the contribution of each parameter to the total score. Abbreviations: BioCh- serum biochemistry profile, Blood- haematological alterations, Cell Rsp- lymphoproliferative response to SLA and CONA, Hum Rsp- ELISA and IFAT results, qPCR- parasite load (blood, lymph node, spleen, liver and bone marrow), and Histology- grade of alterations in spleen and liver.

protein restriction. Malafaia et al. [7] reported a reduction in IFN-γ production from SLA-stimulated splenocytes in malnourished mice infected with *L. chagasi* for 4 weeks, while Perez et al. [37] found that protein-deprived mice infected with *L. mexicana* showed a depressed DTH response and a low *in vitro* splenic cell response to SLA and mitogens. In the present work, the 14%INF animals showed a patent specific cellular response, while the 3%INF animals showed an impaired response to leishmanial antigen and lower lymphocyte counts, particularly of $CD4^+$ T cells. A DTH response was detected in both the 3%INF and 14%INF animals, but statistically significant differences were only seen between the 14%INF and 14%NI groups. Although most authors report protein energy malnutrition to affect DTH after BCG vaccination [38], some present similar skin test results for malnourished and well-nourished individuals [39].

The ability of the hamsters to mount a cell-mediated immune response when faced with severe malnutrition and visceral leishmaniasis was determined by examining the lymphocyte response to mitogens. In the present hamster model, chronic infection by *L. infantum* induced a decline in T-cell functionality similar in severity to that caused by protein malnutrition, but this condition plus infection dramatically reduced T cell functionality, as reported in a cutaneous leishmaniasis mice model [37]. The humoral immune response was also affected by protein malnutrition, manifested in the form of B cell depletion. Although protein energy malnutrition has been described to affect B cell and antibody responses less profoundly than T cell responses [40], studies on malnutrition in infectious diseases have shown an important depletion of the B cell population [41] as well as antibody production by B cells [42].

Conclusion

In conclusion, the present work suggests that the nutritional status of individuals infected with *Leishmania* spp. has an important effect on the immune response they can mount, and therefore on the development of visceral leishmaniasis. The present results corroborate epidemiological observations that malnutrition is an important risk factor in the development of severe visceral leishmaniasis. The importance of nutrition as part of immunoprophylactic and therapeutic measures, especially in developing countries, deserves further study.

Acknowledgments

We thank the members of the veterinary facilities at the *Instituto de Salud Carlos III* for their help, especially Enrique Viguera. Javier Nieto, also from the *Instituto de Salud Carlos III*, is thanked for performing the IFAT tests.

Author Contributions

Conceived and designed the experiments: EC JM. Performed the experiments: EC CS JC APS MAJ. Analyzed the data: EC APS JC JM CMM. Contributed reagents/materials/analysis tools: EC CS APS MAJ CMM. Wrote the paper: EC MAJ JC.

References

1. WHO website. The World Health Report 2002: reducing risks, promoting healthy life, chapter 4. Available: http://www.who.int/whr/2002/en/. Accessed 2014 Jan 27.
2. Gross RL, Newberne PM (1980) Role of nutrition in immunologic function. Physiol Rev 60: 188–302.
3. Mathers CD, Ezzati M, Lopez AD (2007) Measuring the burden of neglected tropical diseases: the global burden of disease framework. PLoS Negl Trop Dis 1: e114.
4. Cerf BJ, Jones TC, Badaro R, Sampaio D, Teixeira R, et al. (1987) Malnutrition as a risk factor for severe visceral leishmaniasis. J Infect Dis 156: 1030–1033.
5. Harrison LH, Naidu TG, Drew JS, de Alencar JE, Pearson RD (1986) Reciprocal relationships between undernutrition and the parasitic disease visceral leishmaniasis. Rev Infect Dis 8: 447–453.
6. Anstead GM, Chandrasekar B, Zhao W, Yang J, Perez LE, et al. (2001) Malnutrition alters the innate immune response and increases early visceralization following *Leishmania donovani* infection. Infect Immun 69: 4709–4718.
7. Malafaia G, Serafim TD, Silva ME, Pedrosa ML, Rezende SA (2009) Protein-energy malnutrition decreases immune response to *Leishmania chagasi* vaccine in BALB/c mice. Parasite Immunol 31: 41–49.
8. Goto H, Lindoso JA (2004) Immunity and immunosuppression in experimental visceral leishmaniasis. 37: 615–623.
9. Redmond HP, Shou J, Kelly CJ, Schreiber S, Miller E, et al. (1991) Immunosuppressive mechanisms in protein-calorie malnutrition. Surgery 110: 311–317.
10. Trotter ER, Peters W, Robinson BL (1980) The experimental chemotherapy of leishmaniasis, IV. The development of a rodent model for visceral infection. Ann Trop Med Parasitol 74: 127–138.
11. Melby PC, Chandrasekar B, Zhao W, Coe JE (2001) The hamster as a model of human visceral leishmaniasis: progressive disease and impaired generation of nitric oxide in the face of a prominent Th1-like cytokine response. J Immunol 166: 1912–1920.
12. Flavell DJ, Pattanapanyasat K, Lucas SB, Vongsangnak V (1980) *Opisthorchis viverrini*: liver changes in golden hamsters maintained on high and low protein diets. Acta Trop 37: 337–350.
13. Yan L, Combs GF Jr, DeMars LC, Johnson LK (2011) Effects of the physical form of the diet on food intake, growth, and body composition changes in mice. J Am Assoc Lab Anim Sci 50: 488–494.
14. Liu H, Steiner BM, Alder JD, Baertschy DK, Schell RF (1990) Immune T cells sorted by flow cytometry confer protection against infection with *Treponema pallidum* subsp. *pertenue* in hamsters. Infect Immun 58: 1685–1690.
15. Dondji B, Bungiro RD, Harrison LM, Vermeire JJ, Bifulco C, et al. (2008) Role for nitric oxide in hookworm-associated immune suppression. Infect Immun 76: 2560–2567.
16. Cunha J, Carrillo E, Sanchez C, Cruz I, Moreno J, et al. (2013) Characterization of the biology and infectivity of *Leishmania infantum* viscerotropic and dermotropic strains isolated from HIV+ and HIV− patients in the murine model of visceral leishmaniasis. Parasit Vectors 6: 122.
17. Jungersen G, Jensen L, Rask MR, Lind P (2002) Non-lethal infection parameters in mice separate sheep Type II *Toxoplasma gondii* isolates by virulence. Comp Immunol Microbiol Infect Dis 25: 187–195.
18. Gomez F, Galvan RR, Cravioto J, Frenk S, Santaella JV, et al. (1956) Fat absorption in chronic severe malnutrition in children. Lancet 271: 121–2.
19. Chappuis F, Sundar S, Hailu A, Ghalib H, Rijal S, et al. (2007) Visceral leishmaniasis: what are the needs for diagnosis, treatment and control? Nat Rev Microbiol 5: 873–882.
20. Sideris V, Papadopoulou G, Dotsika E, Karagouni E (1999) Asymptomatic canine leishmaniasis in Greater Athens area, Greece. Eur J Epidemiol 15: 271–276.
21. Abranches P, Silva-Pereira MC, Conceicao-Silva FM, Santos-Gomes GM, Janz JG (1991) Canine leishmaniasis: pathological and ecological factors influencing transmission of infection. J Parasitol 77: 557–561.
22. Requena JM, Soto M, Doria MD, Alonso C (2000) Immune and clinical parameters associated with *Leishmania infantum* infection in the golden hamster model. Vet Immunol Immunopathol 76: 269–281.
23. Garg R, Dube A (2006) Animal models for vaccine studies for visceral leishmaniasis. Indian J Med Res 123: 439–454.
24. Gomes CM, Giannella-Neto D, Gama ME, Pereira JC, Campos MB, et al. (2007) Correlation between the components of the insulin-like growth factor I system, nutritional status and visceral leishmaniasis. Trans R Soc Trop Med Hyg 101: 660–667.
25. Pointer E, Reisman R, Windham R, Murray L (2013) Starvation and the clinicopathologic abnormalities associated with starved dogs: a review of 152 cases. J Am Anim Hosp Assoc 49: 101–107.
26. Dusingize JC, Hoover DR, Shi Q, Mutimura E, Kiefer E, et al. (2012) Association of serum albumin with markers of nutritional status among HIV-infected and uninfected Rwandan women. PLoS One 7: e35079.
27. Dedet JP, Pratlong F (2003) Leishmaniasis. In: Cook G ZA, editor. Manson's Tropical Diseases. London: Elsevier Science.
28. Xavier JG, Favero ME, Vinolo MA, Rogero MM, Dagli ML, et al. (2007) Protein-energy malnutrition alters histological and ultrastructural characteristics of the bone marrow and decreases haematopoiesis in adult mice. Histol Histopathol 22: 651–660.
29. Fock RA, Vinolo MA, Blatt SL, Borelli P (2012) Impairment of the hematological response and interleukin-1beta production in protein-energy malnourished mice after endotoxemia with lipopolysaccharide. Braz J Med Biol Res 45: 1163–1171.
30. Takizawa H, Boettcher S, Manz MG (2012) Demand-adapted regulation of early hematopoiesis in infection and inflammation. Blood 119: 2991–3002.
31. Murray HW (2001) Tissue granuloma structure-function in experimental visceral leishmaniasis. Int J Exp Pathol 82: 249–267.
32. Laurenti MD, Sotto MN, Corbett CE, da Matta VL, Duarte MI (1990) Experimental visceral leishmaniasis: sequential events of granuloma formation at subcutaneous inoculation site. Int J Exp Pathol 71: 791–797.
33. Gomes-Silva A, Valverde JG, Ribeiro-Romao RP, Placido-Pereira RM, Da-Cruz AM (2013) Golden hamster (*Mesocricetus auratus*) as an experimental model for *Leishmania* (Viannia) *braziliensis* infection. Parasitology 140: 771–779.
34. Faulk WP, Mata LJ, Edsall G (1975) Effects of malnutrition on the immune response in humans: a review. Trop Dis Bull 72: 89–103.
35. Scrimshaw NS, SanGiovanni JP (1997) Synergism of nutrition, infection, and immunity: an overview. Am J Clin Nutr 66: 464S–477S.
36. Carvalho EM, Bacellar O, Barral A, Badaro R, Johnson WD Jr (1989) Antigen-specific immunosuppression in visceral leishmaniasis is cell mediated. J Clin Invest 83: 860–864.
37. Perez H, De La Rosa M, Malave I (1984) The effect of protein restriction on the development of protective immunity to *Leishmania mexicana*. Parasite Immunol 6: 285–294.
38. Chandra RK (1983) Nutrition, immunity, and infection: present knowledge and future directions. Lancet 1: 688–691.
39. Satyanarayana K, Bhaskaram P, Seshu VC, Reddy V (1980) Influence of nutrition on postvaccinial tuberculin sensitivity. Am J Clin Nutr 33: 2334–2337.
40. Keusch GT (1981) Host defense mechanisms in protein energy malnutrition. Adv Exp Med Biol 135: 183–209.
41. Taylor AK, Cao W, Vora KP, De La Cruz J, Shieh WJ, et al. (2013) Protein energy malnutrition decreases immunity and increases susceptibility to influenza infection in mice. J Infect Dis 207: 501–510.
42. Law DK, Dudrick SJ, Abdou NI (1973) Immunocompetence of patients with protein-calorie malnutrition. The effects of nutritional repletion. Ann Intern Med 79: 545–550.

12

The Effect of Gender and Social Capital on the Dual Burden of Malnutrition: A Multilevel Study in Indonesia

Masoud Vaezghasemi[1,2,3]*, Ann Öhman[1,2,3], Malin Eriksson[1,2], Mohammad Hakimi[4], Lars Weinehall[1,2], Hari Kusnanto[5], Nawi Ng[1,2]

1 Department of Public Health and Clinical Medicine, Division of Epidemiology and Global Health, Umeå University, Umeå, Sweden, **2** Umeå Centre for Global Health Research, Umeå University, Umeå, Sweden, **3** Umeå Centre for Gender Studies, Umeå University, Umeå, Sweden, **4** Centre for Health and Nutrition Research Laboratory, Faculty of Medicine, Gadjah Mada University, Yogyakarta, Indonesia, **5** Centre for Environmental Studies, Faculty of Medicine, Gadjah Mada University, Yogyakarta, Indonesia

Abstract

Introduction: The paradoxical phenomenon of the coexistence of overweight and underweight individuals in the same household, referred to as the "dual burden of malnutrition", is a growing nutrition dilemma in low- and middle-income countries (LMICs).

Aims: The objectives of this study were (i) to examine the extent of the dual burden of malnutrition across different provinces in Indonesia and (ii) to determine how gender, community social capital, place of residency and other socio-economic factors affect the prevalence of the dual burden of malnutrition.

Methods: The current study utilized data from the fourth wave of the Indonesian Family Life Survey (IFLS) conducted between November 2007 and April 2008. The dataset contains information from 12,048 households and 45,306 individuals of all ages. This study focused on households with individuals over two years old. To account for the multilevel nature of the data, a multilevel multiple logistic regression was conducted.

Results: Approximately one-fifth of all households in Indonesia exhibited the dual burden of malnutrition, which was more prevalent among male-headed households, households with a high Socio-economic status (SES), and households in urban areas. Minimal variation in the dual burden of malnutrition was explained by the community level differences (<4%). Living in households with a higher SES resulted in higher odds of the dual burden of malnutrition but not among female-headed households and communities with the highest social capital.

Conclusion: To improve household health and reduce the inequality across different SES groups, this study emphasizes the inclusion of women's empowerment and community social capital into intervention programs addressing the dual burden of malnutrition.

Editor: Abdisalan Mohamed Noor, Kenya Medical Research Institute - Wellcome Trust Research Programme, Kenya

Funding: The project has been funded through a grant from the Swedish International Development Cooperation Agency (Sida) (Grant number: AKT-2010-048). The funders had no role in study design, data collection and analysis, decision to publish, or preparation of the manuscript.

Competing Interests: The authors have declared that no competing interests exist.

* Email: masoud.vaezghasemi@umu.se

Introduction

As the gross national product (GNP) of low- and middle-income countries (LMICs) increases, the overweight burden shifts to the populations with a low socio-economic status (SES), among whom the underweight burden still remains high [1]. The coexistence of both overweight and underweight individuals in the same household, referred to as the "dual burden of malnutrition", is a growing nutritional dilemma in LMICs. This dilemma is most prevalent in countries experiencing the chronic disease phase of the nutrition transition because of rapid social, economic, and technological changes [2–4].

The global burden of overweight mothers and stunted children demonstrates a critical situation in middle-income countries. The highest prevalences of this phenomenon were observed in Guatemala (Latin America), Egypt (Africa), and Uzbekistan (Asia). These results consistently confirm a higher prevalence of a dual burden of malnutrition in rural areas compared with urban areas [5]. Only two studies have observed the dual burden of malnutrition in Indonesia. The first study used data from the 1993 Indonesian Family Life Survey (IFLS) and reported that 11% of households had both overweight and underweight members [2]. The second study analyzed data from the Indonesian Nutrition Surveillance System (NSS) in 2000–2003. This study investigated households with overweight mothers and stunted children and reported a prevalence of 11% in rural areas [6].

The dual burden of malnutrition has been associated with economic factors such as higher SES, household wealth, income, and GDP and socio-demographic characteristics such as family size, age difference between the underweight and overweight members, maternal support, and urban residency [2,5,7–9]. Despite explicit recognition of the dual burden of malnutrition, knowledge on how gender relations and social capital influence the extent of the dual burden of malnutrition is lacking. Gender is commonly used as a variable for controlling significant differences between men and women in epidemiological studies. However, gender has greater potential to address health issues if this variable is used within a theoretical framework [10]. Gender relations are defined as the relations of power and dominance that structure the life chances of women and men in specific social contexts [11]. Moreover, to complete the theory of justice, Okin argues that equal participation of both men and women in all spheres of human life is remarkably important regardless of whether it is principally the women's or men's domain [12]. Therefore, it is essential to analyze the effect of gender when women take on a typically male role.

In Indonesia, women play a minor role in policy and government decision-making processes [13]. The lack of a female provincial governor and the fact that fewer than 2% of village heads are female indicate that women's representation is even lower at lower levels of government [14]. However, in many parts of Indonesia, women play a critical role in their households, especially in the management of household finances [15]. Although the common perception is that female-headed households are primarily poor and subordinated and encounter numerous social and political discriminations, many of the women generate income through formal employment or informal activities. An active economic role inside and outside the household empowers women to control the finances and authority in the home, which is in contrast with many other predominantly Muslim societies that highly restrict women's economic roles [16]. Therefore, such a culturally, socially, and geographically diverse context provides a unique opportunity to investigate gender and possible inequalities and inequities involved in expanding or diminishing the dual burden of malnutrition in the same households.

Numerous studies have reported a potential link between social capital and health outcomes, including non-communicable diseases (NCDs) [17,18]. Social capital is generally considered to play an important role in influencing the well being of individuals and households and the development of communities, whether it is an individual attribute or a collective feature. Individual approaches view social capital as something individuals can have more or less access to and describe it as "*the ability of actors to secure benefits by virtues of memberships in networks and other social structures*" [19]. The collective approach views social capital as something characterizing whole communities by levels of trust and civic engagement (e.g., community social capital). This approach defines social capital as "*social networks, the reciprocity that arise from them, and the value of these for achieving mutual goals*" [20]. Collective social capital is often measured as aggregated measures of trust and social participation that does not evidently relate to the living area and therefore the need for a clearer place related measures have been raised [21,22]. As a country with a long-standing local tradition of community involvement, Indonesia is a unique setting to study social capital. The majority of adult Indonesian women have only elementary education and community participation and social interaction have a huge potential for enriching Indonesian women (as well as men) with additional knowledge that was not received from formal schooling.

Aims

The objectives of this study were (i) to explore the extent of the dual burden of malnutrition in Indonesia across different provinces and (ii) to determine how gender, community social capital, place of residency and other socio-economic factors affect the dual burden of malnutrition.

Methods

Study setting

Indonesia is an archipelago in Southeast Asia with a population of 247 million living in its 34 provinces. Approximately half of the Indonesians live on Java Island. Sixty-nine percent of the population live in rural areas. Muslims form the largest religious group, which accounts for 89% of the population [23].

Data source

This study utilized the IFLS dataset, which is the only large-scale longitudinal survey available for Indonesia (*http://www.rand.org/labor/FLS/IFLS.html*). The survey was conducted by the RAND Corporation and consists of four waves that were conducted in 1993, 1997, 2000, and 2007–2008. Thirteen out of 27 provinces, which contain 83% of the population, were selected. Enumeration areas (EAs), the primary sampling unit, were randomly selected within each of the provinces. In total, 321 EAs were selected. We used the term "community" to refer to EAs in this study. Households were randomly selected within the EAs. Although the IFLS is a longitudinal survey, weights were constructed both at the individual and household level treating the IFLS as a cross-sectional survey. Therefore, the IFLS was representative of the Indonesian population living in the 13 IFLS provinces in each wave [24]. Only data from the fourth wave (IFLS4) that was collected from 2007–2008 were used in this study. This dataset contains information from 12,048 households and 45,306 individuals of all ages who lived in 13 of the 27 provinces in Indonesia.

Outcome variables

(i) Assessment of overweight and underweight at the individual level. Children less than two years old and pregnant women were excluded. As a result, 12,037 households and 42,749 individuals remained in the study (Figure 1). Two trained nurses recorded physical health measurements of the household members, including their height and weight [24]. For adults, we calculated the body mass index (BMI) and used the cut-offs of $<$ 18.5 and $\geq$25 kg/m^2 to categorize individuals as underweight, normal weight, and overweight/obese [25]. We calculated BMI based on the definition of World Health Organization (WHO) to facilitate the comparison of the findings with other studies conduced in different Asian and African countries. It has been shown that Asian population such as Indonesians (Malays and Chinese ancestry), Singaporean Chinese, Malays and Indians, and Hong Kong Chinese have a higher body fat percent at a lower BMI compared to Caucasians that might lead to higher risk of chronic diseases [26]. For children and adolescents aged 2–18 years old, age- and sex-specific cut-off points established by Cole et al. [27,28] that correspond to an adult BMI of 18.5 and 25 at the age of 18 were used to determine underweight and overweight, respectively. In these studies the same method (LMS) were used to define overweight and obesity as well as thinness or underweight using data from nationally representative surveys of children in six high and middle-income countries. The LMS method summarizes the distribution of BMI by age and sex in terms of three curves called L (lambda), which expresses the Skewness of BMI distribution, M (mu), which is median BMI by age, and S (sigma), which is the coefficient of variation of BMI. Accordingly, any required BMI centile curve is defined as follows: $\mathbf{M(1+L\times S\times z)^{1/L}}$. Where z is the z score corresponding to the required centile and the values of L, M, and S vary with age and sex. The reverse process, of converting a child's BMI to a z score, involves the equation: $\mathbf{z = ((BMI/M)^{L}-1)/(L\times S)}$. The values of L, M, and S are for the child's age and sex.

(ii) Assessment of the dual burden of malnutrition at the household level. A household with a dual burden of malnutrition was identified if there was at least one underweight and one overweight member in the household. Households with only one member and households without BMI data or only one available BMI measurement were excluded. Finally, 9,743 households consisting of 38,237 individuals were included in the analysis (Figure 1).

Households were classified into four distinct groups, including (i) "underweight households" with at least one underweight member and no overweight member (28%), (ii) "normal households" without underweight or overweight members (21%), (iii) "overweight households" with at least one overweight and no underweight member (32%), and (iv) "dual burden households" with at least one underweight and one overweight member (19%). In this study, we focus on comparing the "dual burden households" with the other types of households combined.

Household level variables

(i) Male- and female-headed households. Households were classified as male- and female-headed households based on the sex of the household's head reported in the survey. Statistics Indonesia (BPS) defined a head of the household as (i) the person who is actually responsible for the daily needs of a household or (ii) the person who is considered the head of the household [29].

(ii) Education level of the household heads. The education level of the household head is based on their highest education level and was categorized into "no schooling", "elementary", "secondary", and "university/college".

(iii) Socio-economic status of households (SES). We used asset and housing variables to create SES quintiles (1 = poorest and 5 = richest) using a Principal Component Analysis (PCA) [30]. The variables included households' ownership of durable assets (e.g. TV, refrigerator, jewelry, vehicles, and savings certificates or disposal stocks) and infrastructure and housing characteristics (e.g. source of water, drainage, toilet, cooking, type of walls, roof, and floor).

(iv)Under 15- and over 60-year-olds. We controlled for the influence of age in the analysis by accounting for the proportion of household members less than 15 years old and greater than 60 years old.

Community level variables

(i) Community social capital. In this study, the collective feature of social capital was measured based on the existence of programs and activities in the community, such as village cooperatives, neighborhood watch programs, village improvements, child development, teen development, elderly programs, youth and family groups, village loans, and health funds in the communities. The responses to each of these indicators were used and summarized with a PCA and the resulting index was divided into tertiles, including lowest, middle, and highest community social capital.

(ii) Place of residency. In addition, households were categorized based on living in urban or rural areas to control for the effect of residency on the analysis.

Statistical analysis

To account for the multistage/cluster sampling design, we used the individual and household weights in all the analyses of individual and household level data, respectively. This was performed using the svyset and svy commands in Stata Version 12.1 (StataCorp, 4905 Lakeway Drive, College Station, Texas 77845, USA). The individual level data were used to calculate the prevalence of underweight and overweight individuals. The data were further collapsed into household level data for subsequent analyses on the dual burden of malnutrition. The results of the descriptive analysis were presented as numbers and weighted percentages with their 95% confidence interval (CI). Prevalences were presented for each province and provinces were ranked based on their 2008 Human Development Index (HDI) [29]. Simple and multiple logistic regression analyses were used to

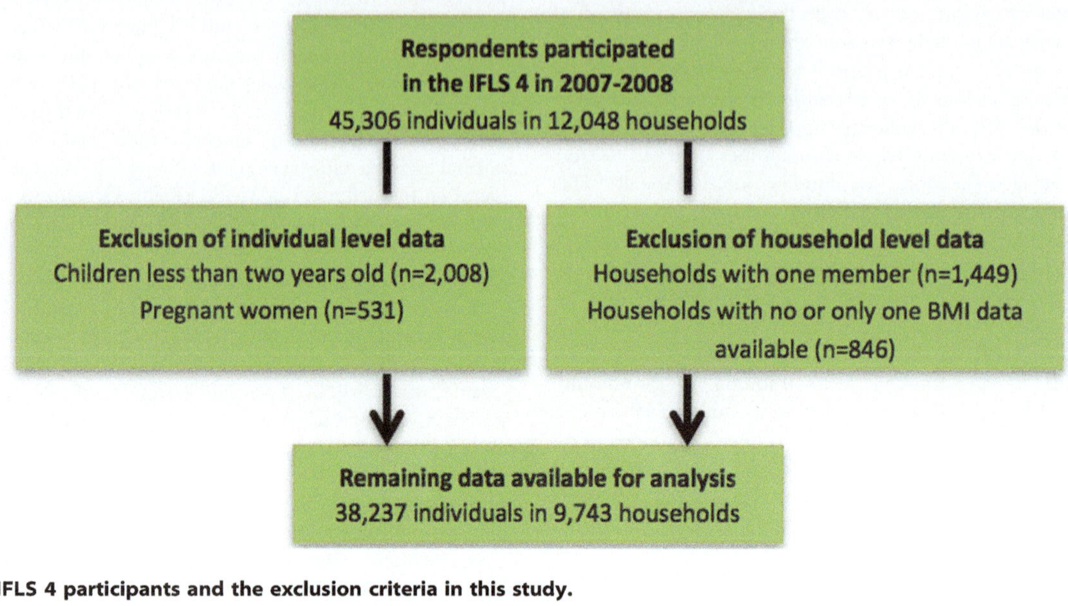

Figure 1. IFLS 4 participants and the exclusion criteria in this study.

evaluate associations between household and community level factors with the dual burden of malnutrition. The results were expressed as odds ratios (ORs) with a 95% CI. Variables were considered significant at the 0.05 level. To account for the multilevel nature of the data (households within communities), we conducted a multilevel multiple logistic regression to assess the interclass correlation and variations of the outcome variables at a higher level [31]. We estimated a random intercept model to investigate the extent that the dual burden of malnutrition could be explained by community level determinants. The data were stratified by household type (female- or male-headed), community level of social capital (lowest or highest), and place of residency (urban or rural).

Results

A total of 45,306 individuals within 12,048 household participated in the IFLS4 with a female/male ratio of 0.96. In this study, complete data were obtained from 38,237 individuals within 9,743 households.

Prevalence of underweight and overweight individuals

The prevalence of underweight and overweight were significantly different among provinces ($p<0.001$). Underweight was more common in rural areas (20% in rural vs. 18% in urban, $p<0.001$) and in provinces with a lower HDI. In contrast, overweight was more prevalent in provinces with a higher HDI and in urban areas (25% in urban vs. 17% in rural, $p<0.001$) (Table 1). Additionally, we determined that underweight was more prevalent among children and overweight/obesity was more prevalent among women (Appendix 1).

Prevalence of the dual burden of malnutrition among households

The percentage of households with a dual burden of malnutrition in Indonesia was 19% and significantly different among provinces ($p<0.01$). Jakarta (25%), South Sulawesi (23%), and Lampung (22%) had the highest prevalences. North Sumatra (15%), Central Java (17%), and Yogyakarta (17%) had the three lowest percentages of households with a dual burden of malnutrition (Figure 2).

The differences in the prevalence of the dual burden of malnutrition across provinces were more prominent among female-headed households compared with male-headed households (Figure 3A and 3B) and in urban compared to rural areas (Figure 3E and 3F). No significant difference was observed across provinces when we compared households living in communities with the lowest and highest social capital (Figure 3C and 3D). In Jakarta, no differences in the prevalence of the dual burden of malnutrition across these population subgroups were observed, which is in contrast with Central Java, where large differences were observed.

Determinants of the dual burden of malnutrition

The univariate logistic regression revealed that the dual burden of malnutrition was more prevalent (i) among male-headed households than female-headed households, with prevalences of 20% and 16%, respectively, (ii) among households for which head had a higher education level, and (iii) among households with a high socio-economic status. There was no significant difference between households with less than 50% and more than 50% less than 15- and greater than 60-year-old members. When we analyzed community level characteristics, the prevalence was higher in urban areas compared with rural areas, 23% and 17%, respectively. Although the prevalence was slightly higher in

Table 1. Prevalence (and 95% confidence interval/CI) of underweight and overweight at the individual level in the 13 provinces of Indonesia in 2007.

Provinces (ranked based on their human development index)	Sample size (n = 42755)		Underweight % (95% CI)		Overweight % (95% CI)	
	Rural (n)	Urban (n)	Rural	Urban	Rural	Urban
Jakarta	NA	3199	NA	17 (15–19)	NA	30 (27–32)
Yogyakarta	526	1719	23 (20–27)	18 (15–21)	15 (12–16)	24 (20–28)
North Sumatra	1534	1629	12 (10–15)	15 (12–18)	19 (13–25)	26 (22–29)
West Sumatra	1211	965	20 (16–24)	15(12–18)	20 (14–25)	27 (22–31)
South Sumatra	1449	723	22 (18–26)	20 (17–23)	14 (10–17)	30 (27–33)
Central Java	3052	2328	17 (14–19)	18 (14–21)	18 (16–20)	24 (20–27)
West Java	2415	4172	22 (18–26)	17(15–19)	17 (14–20)	24 (22–26)
Bali	939	1281	15 (11–19)	13 (11–15)	23 (17–30)	27 (22–32)
East Java	3335	2969	23 (19–26)	18 (16–20)	18 (15–21)	25 (22–27)
Lampung	1302	598	20 (18–23)	23 (20–26)	16 (13–19)	17 (12–22)
South Sulawesi	1323	1180	21 (19–24)	23 (18–29)	16 (11–22)	19 (15–23)
South Kalimantan	1199	878	24 (20–28)	22 (17–27)	16 (14–19)	27 (22–31)
West Nusa Tenggara	1704	1125	29 (22–36)	27 (23–30)	9 (7–12)	19 (15–23)
Total	**19989**	**22766**	**20 (19–22)***	**18 (17–19)***	**17 (16–18)**	**25 (24–26)***

Note: NA = There is no rural area in the province of Jakarta. The 1990 Census declared this city as a fully urbanized area. To adapt to the growth of Jakarta, all non-urban areas were converted to urban areas.
Provinces were ranked by the human development index from 77.03 in Jakarta to 64.12 in West Nusa Tenggara (35).
*p-value <0.05 (difference among provinces).

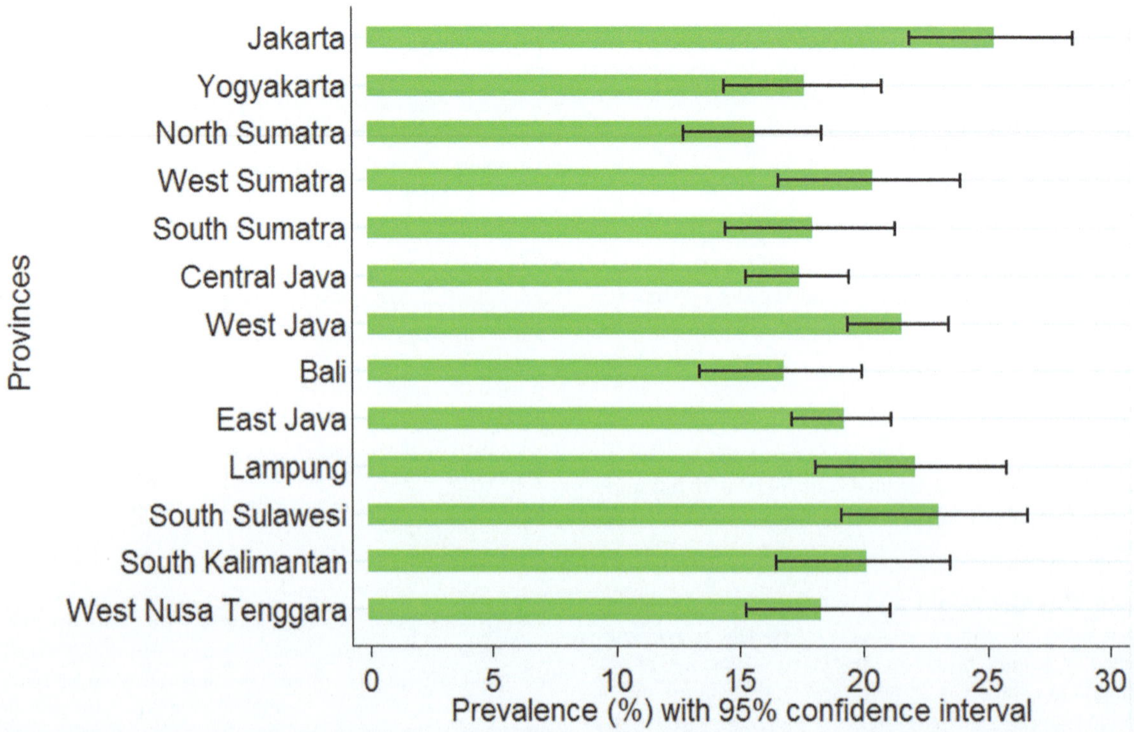

Figure 2. Prevalence of dual burden of malnutrition by province, sorted based on their Human Development Index (Jakarta and West Nusa Tenggara were the provinces with the highest and lowest HDI, respectively.

communities with the highest social capital compared with communities with lowest social capital, 20% and 18%, respectively, the difference was not statistically significant (Table 2).

The multilevel multiple logistic regression (only fixed-effect) analysis revealed that being in a female-headed household and living in a rural area was significantly associated and had a protective effect. The odds of having a dual burden of malnutrition were higher in households with a higher SES. Community social capital was not significantly associated with the dual burden of malnutrition in any of the regression analyses (Table 2).

The results from the random-effect portion of the multilevel multiple logistic regression models indicated that (i) a small amount of the variation in the prevalence of the dual burden of malnutrition (VPC 2%) was explained by the community level differences and the place of residency, (ii) the proportional change in variance (PCV) was 34%, (iii) the median odds ratio (MOI) was 1.26, (iv) the interval odds ratio (IOR) was 0.49–1.20, and (v) the sorting out index was 22%. Additionally the differences in province level were controlled for in this model, but no significant change was observed.

After stratifying the multilevel multiple logistic regression analyses by household head, community social capital, and place of residency, the results from the fixed-effect portion of Table 3 illustrate that (i) being in a female-headed household exhibited a protective effect regardless of community social capital and place of residency, (ii) being in a household in the highest SES quintiles was not significantly associated with the dual burden of malnutrition in female-headed households and households having the highest community social capital, (iii) among households in communities with the lowest social capital, being in the highest SES quintiles increased the odds of a household having a dual burden of malnutrition (2.07, 1.45–2.96) compared with those in the lowest SES quintiles, (iv) living in households with the highest SES quintiles also increased the odds of having a dual burden of malnutrition by 54% in urban areas and by 67% in rural areas compared with those in the lowest SES quintiles.

The random-effect portion of Table 3 indicates that less than 4% of the variation in the prevalence of the dual burden of malnutrition is explained by community level differences in the regression analyses for all the sub-groups.

Discussion

The main findings of this study include the following: (i) approximately one-fifth of all households in Indonesia exhibit a dual burden of malnutrition with significant differences in the prevalence across provinces; (ii) only a small amount of the variation in the dual burden of malnutrition could be explained by the community level differences (<4%), while the remaining 96% could be explained by differences between households; and (iii) the main determinants of the dual burden of malnutrition are having a male head of the household, living in households with a higher SES, and living in an urban area. Moreover, the level of community social capital is not significantly associated with the prevalence of the dual burden of malnutrition, and households with higher SES levels are positively associated with a dual burden of malnutrition regardless of whether the household is located in an urban or a rural area. However, these associations are only significant in male-headed households and households in communities with the lowest social capital.

The prevalence of a dual burden of malnutrition has nearly doubled during the last fifteen years according to data from another conducted study in Indonesia using the 1993 IFLS data, which had reported a prevalence of 11% [2]. Moreover, studies in other LMICs have revealed that this phenomenon is not unique for Indonesia. In 2006, the Food and Agriculture Organization of

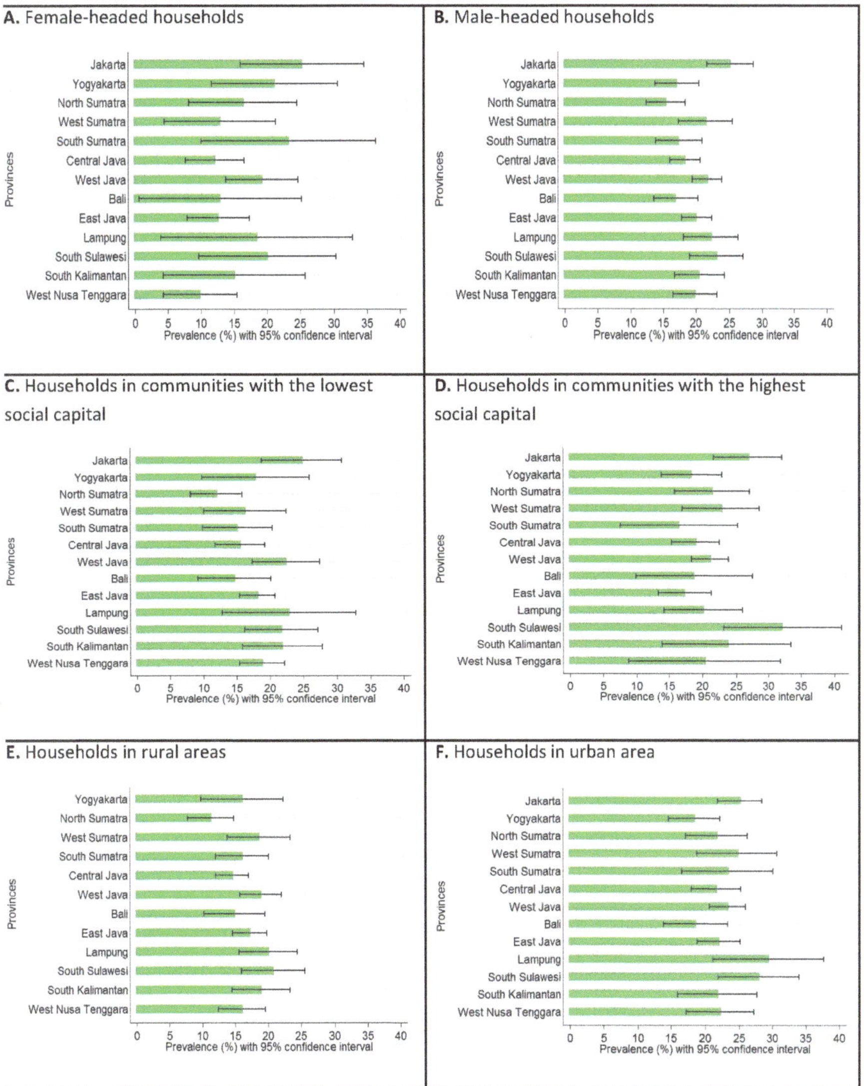

Note: There is no rural area in the province of Jakarta. The 1990 Census declared this city as a fully urbanized area. Provinces were ranked by the human development index from 77.03 in Jakarta to 64.12 in West Nusa Tenggara.

Figure 3. The prevalence of dual burden of malnutrition across provinces in Indonesia in households with different characteristics based on the head of household gender, community social capital, and type of area.

the United Nations (FAO) documented the dual burden of malnutrition in six LMICs, including China, Egypt, India, Mexico, the Philippines, and South Africa. India and the Philippines exhibited the highest prevalence of underweight, while over nutrition is an emerging problem, especially in urban areas. In the Philippines, 27% of children under five years of age are underweight, while 27% of women are overweight or obese [32]. In this study, interventions aimed at the dual burden should be prioritized in India and the Philippines, while overweight and obesity should be targeted in Egypt, Mexico, and, to a lesser degree, China and South Africa. Because India and the Philippines have the lowest GDPs among these countries, comparing the GDP may reveal that when the economy develops, the problem of dual burden of malnutrition arises in countries with low GDP, while it disappears in countries with a higher GDP as the transition moves toward overnutrition and an obesity epidemic [8].

In agreement with our findings, several other studies have reported the association between a higher SES, income or GDP and urban residency with a dual burden of malnutrition in LMICs [2,5,7,8]. In LMICs, as the country's GDP increases, overweight emerges while underweight remains a prominent health problem resulting in the dual burden of malnutrition [1]. Therefore, at a macro level, the population's diet structure shifts combined with decreased physical activity and increased sedentary jobs, the introduction of labor-saving technology as well as urbanization deteriorates the current situation [3,33]. At the micro level, as the economic development proceeds, households' per capita income and expenditures increase. Consequently, an increase in total calorie intake and higher consumption of carbohydrates, proteins, and fats results in unbalanced dietary habits [34]. However, improvement in the spouse's education has a positive and significant influence on the consumption of some nutrients, including protein, vitamins, and the substitution of fat for carbohydrates [34].

Table 2. Household and community level characteristics associated with the dual burden of malnutrition in Indonesia in 2007.

Household characteristics	Total number of households with dual burden n (%)	Simple single level logistic regression	Multilevel multiple logistic regression
Overall (n = 9743 households)	1940 (19)		
Fixed-effects model **(OR with 95% CI)**			
Household level variables			
Household head			
Male (n = 8498)	1739 (20)	1	1
Female (n = 1232)	199 (16) *	0.74 (0.62–0.88)	0.74 (0.62–0.88)
Household head education			
No schooling (n = 693)	114 (15)	1	1
Elementary school (n = 3905)	750 (19)	1.29 (0.94–1.78)	1.06 (0.85–1.33)
Secondary school (n = 3520)	737 (20)	1.40 (1.01–1.93)	0.99 (0.78–1.25)
University/college (n = 851)	204 (24) *	1.74 (1.21–2.51)	1.07 (0.80–1.42)
Household SES			
1 poorest (n = 1969)	275 (13)	1	1
2 (n = 1932)	353 (18)	1.40 (1.14–1.72)	1.29 (1.08–1.56)
3 (n = 2011)	435 (21)	1.76 (1.44–2.16)	1.61 (1.34–1.93)
4 (n = 1897)	438 (22)	1.85 (1.49–2.30)	1.65 (1.36–1.99)
5 richest (n = 1930)	437 (23) *	1.95 (1.57–2.41)	1.61 (1.31–1.99)
Less than 15- and greater than 60-year-olds			
< 50% (n = 5787)	1115 (19)	1	1
≥50% (n = 3956)	825 (20)	1.09 (0.98–1.22)	1.16 (1.04–1.29)
Community level variables			
Community social capital			
1 Lowest (3490)	651 (18)	1	1
2 Middle (3042)	609 (20)	1.13 (0.94–1.36)	1.05 (0.90–1.22
3 Highest (3211)	680 (20)	1.16 (0.98–1.38)	1.02 (0.88–1.18)
Residency			
Urban (n = 5002)	1139 (23)	1	1
Rural (n = 4741)	801 (17) *	0.69 (0.60–0.78)	0.77 (0.68–0.88)
Random effects			
Null model community random variance (SE)			0.092
Community random variance (SE)	--------	--------	0.061
Variance Partition Coefficient (%)	--------	--------	2%
Proportional changes in the variance (PCV)	--------	--------	34%
Median Odds Ratio (MOR)	--------	--------	1.26
Interval Odds Ratio (IOR) for residency	--------	--------	0.49–1.20
Sorting out index for residency	--------	--------	22%

*p-value<0.05.
Variables were considered significant at the 0.05 level.

To our knowledge, no study has investigated the societal aspect of dual burden of malnutrition such as female-headed households and community social capital as well as applying related theories in explaining the statistical significances. In this study, we identify the inequality in the distribution of double burden of malnutrition across different provinces in Indonesia, and the prevalence ranges from 15% in North Sumatera province to 25% in Jakarta province. We also use multilevel approach and identify that only 4% of the variation in dual burden of malnutrition could be attributed to the unobserved factors at community level. These are novice knowledge that has not been addressed in previous research. A recently published article, however, examined the association between intra-household inequalities and dual burden of malnutrition in Indonesia using longitudinal IFLS data [35]. This study reported lower nutritional inequality among households with female-headed households and suggested follow-up research on more detailed data in order to understand the gender role in male-headed households. Another study in the Andhra Pradesh State of India reported a protective effect of maternal social capital and dual burden of malnutrition [9]. This study argues that a larger number of people available to supports mothers results in an increased possibility of information sharing and financial, mater-

Table 3. Household and community level characteristics associated with dual burden of malnutrition in Indonesia in 2007 across households with different characteristics.

	Model stratified by household head		Model stratified by community social capital		Model stratified by place of residency	
	Female	**Male**	**Lowest**	**Highest**	**Rural**	**Urban**
Fixed-effects (OR with 95% CI)						
Household level variables						
Household head						
Male (n = 8498)	--------	--------	1	1	1	1
Female (n = 2332)	--------	--------	0.68 (0.51–0.92)	0.76 (0.57–1.00)	0.74 (0.57–0.96)	0.74 (0.59–0.93)
Household head education						
No schooling (n = 693)	1	1	1	1	1	1
Elementary school (n = 3905)	1.04 (0.67–1.60)	1.06 (0.81–1.38)	1.22 (0.85–1.74)	0.84 (0.56–1.27)	1.00 (0.75–1.34)	1.12 (0.78–1.61)
Secondary school (n = 3520)	1.03 (0.63–1.70)	0.99 (0.75–1.30)	1.06 (0.73–1.55)	0.83 (0.55–1.27)	0.94 (0.69–1.29)	1.04 (0.72–1.49)
University/college (n = 851)	1.27 (0.58–2.79)	1.04 (0.76–1.44)	0.95 (0.58–1.55)	1.02 (0.64–1.64)	1.15 (0.73–1.80)	1.07 (0.71–1.60)
Household SES						
1 poorest (n = 1969)	1	1	1	1	1	1
2 (n = 1932)	0.93 (0.54–1.60)	1.36 (1.12–1.66)	1.26 (0.93–1.69)	1.26 (0.90–1.77)	1.28 (1.02–1.60)	1.26 (0.91–1.75)
3 (n = 2011)	1.09 (0.65–1.82)	1.70 (1.40–2.07)	1.78 (1.32–2.40)	1.29 (0.92–1.79)	1.57 (1.24–1.99)	1.56 (1.14–2.13)
4 (n = 1897)	1.48 (0.88–2.50)	1.68 (1.37–2.06)	1.85 (1.35–2.54)	1.36 (0.97–1.91)	1.70 (1.30–2.22)	1.54 (1.13–2.10)
5 richest (n = 1930)	1.28 (0.71–2.33)	1.68 (1.34–2.09)	2.07 (1.45–2.96)	1.20 (0.84–1.72)	1.67 (1.18–2.37)	1.54 (1.12–2.10)
Less than 15- and greater than 60-year-olds						
<50% (n = 5787)	1	1	1	1	1	1
≥50% (n = 3956)	0.68 (0.50–0.94)	1.25 (1.11–1.40)	1.25 (1.04–1.51)	1.07 (0.90–1.29)	1.15 (0.98–1.36)	1.17 (1.01–1.34)
Community level variables						
Community Social Capital						
1 Lowest (3490)	1	1	--------	--------	1	1
2 Middle (3042)	1.21 (0.82–1.79)	1.03 (0.88–1.21)	--------	--------	1.07 (0.85–1.34)	1.00 (0.83–1.20)
3 Highest (3211)	1.12 (0.76–1.66)	1.00 (0.86–1.17)	--------	--------	1.10 (0.87–1.39)	0.94 (0.79–1.12)
Residency						
Urban (n = 5002)	1	1	1	1	--------	--------
Rural (n = 4741)	0.82 (0.57–1.17)	0.77 (0.67–0.88)	0.74 (0.59–0.94)	0.79 (0.65–0.98)	--------	--------
Random effects						
Null model community random variance (SE)	1.36	0.096	0.177	0.005	0.094	0.016
Community random variance (SE)	1.51	0.065	0.137	4.030	0.090	0.011
Variance Partition Coefficient (%)	0%	2%	4%	0%	3%	0%
PCV	−11%	32%	22%	-------[1]	4%	31%
MOR	1.00	1.27	1.42	1.00	1.33	1.10
IOR (residency)	0.09–7.58	0.48–1.22	0.38–1.45	0.071–8.84	--------	--------
Sorting out index (residency)	45%	23%	28%	42%	--------	--------

[1]Not Available.
Variables were considered significant at the 0.05 level.

nal, and psychological support. These events lead to better childcare and have a protective effect against underweight child and overweight mother households. Moreover, the results from a case study by Quisumbing and Maluccio in Bangladesh, Indonesia, Ethiopia, and South Africa revealed a positive and significant effect on expenditure allocation to the next generation, including education and children's clothing, when the households' assets are controlled by women [36]. While the authors did not investigate the nutritional status of children, they determined that children are better off in households where women have bargaining power and decision-making power.

Several studies emphasize the positive influence on children's health and condition when women are empowered in the households. Additionally, underweight children contribute significantly to the dual burden phenomenon; thus, if empowerment of women improves children's health, this empowerment will also, in turn, protect households against the dual burden of malnutrition. This hypothesis may explain the protective effect of the female-headed households on the dual burden of malnutrition reported in the present study even after controlling for the head's education and household SES. Taken together, it is "gendered power relations" within the households that affect household health when women take the position that is typically a male role [11,37]. This theoretical model might be useful in describing and analyzing how power structure functions in a specific context, as well as in exploring how gender theory may explain the intricate relationship between gender and health. However, the mechanisms of how "gendered power relations" affect the dual burden of malnutrition have not been elucidated further.

Additionally, this study presents the effects of different household SES on the dual burden of malnutrition at the household level compared with the household head gender and the level of community social capital where the households were located. Household SES does not significantly affect the dual burden of malnutrition in households with a female head and situated in communities with a high social capital. These results suggest that empowering women and improving community social capital could reduce inequalities across different SES groups. These findings are supported by studies in Indonesia [15,38] and in other developing countries [39,40]. Putnam emphasized the relationship between social capital and economic development [41]. He argues that the dense social networks in the rapidly growing economies of East Asia are based on the extended family or close-knit ethnic communities that foster trust, lower transaction costs, and increased information and innovation, which can also be used as a form of financial capital. However, in the present study, understanding how community social capital functions in reducing the harmful effects of high SES on the dual burden of malnutrition requires further examination.

The current study has several strengths, including a large sample size, a low percentage of missing data and a high response rate, which provide sufficient statistical power to make robust inferences of the extent of the dual burden of malnutrition in Indonesia. Therefore, the probability of bias in estimating the odds ratios is reduced. Conducting a multilevel analysis at the country level on a novel research topic, such as the dual burden of malnutrition, is an additional strength of the present study. Considering the role of gender and community social capital with other household and community level factors provides an opportunity to examine the dual burden of malnutrition from different societal angles and to identify niches for potential interventions from a social perspective.

Some limitations of this study need to be considered when interpreting the results. Drawing conclusions about causality was not possible because of the cross-sectional study design. Dual burden of malnutrition was not separately compared with other types of households such as overweight, underweight, and normal weight. Even though, such comparisons were not within the scope of the current study, further detailed analyses could better help understanding the determinants of the dual burden of malnutrition. For instance, in the study by Roemling and Qaim, fewer significant effects were observed when they compared dual burden households with overweight households, separately. This indicates that dual burden households are more similar to overweight households compared to normal weight households [35]. In addition, the reported relationships may arise from the influence of unobserved household and community level factors associated with both the dependent and independent variables. Factors such as household diets and nutritional intake as well as community level strategies and measurements to prevent malnutrition were not available in this study. Children less than two years old were excluded because information on age based on month was not available. Therefore, it was not possible to assess their nutritional status. As children less than two years old generally constitute the majority of underweight members in households, exclusion of this group might influence the estimates reported in this study.

Conclusion

The dual burden of malnutrition in Indonesia doubled between 1993 and 2008 and is unequally distributed. Inequalities in the dual burden of malnutrition in Indonesia exist across populations with different economic developments. However, these gaps are decreased in populations with access to community social capital. Furthermore, the sex of household's head as a proxy for gender relations plays a significant role in influencing the existing problem at the household level. Therefore, to address the dual burden of malnutrition in Indonesia, this study emphasizes the importance of women's empowerment and improvement of community social capital in community intervention programs.

Acknowledgments

This study has been conducted within the Evidence for Policy and Implementation (EPI-4) project, set up by leading Swedish global health-oriented institutions with the purpose to contribute to capacity-building to make evidence-informed decisions on policies and implementations for health for disadvantaged groups in relation to MDG 4, 5 and 6 in China, India, Indonesia and Vietnam.

Author Contributions

Conceived and designed the experiments: MV AÖ ME NN LW HK. Analyzed the data: MV NN. Contributed reagents/materials/analysis tools: MV AÖ ME NN LW HK MH. Wrote the paper: MV.

References

1. Monteiro CA, Moura EC, Conde WL, Popkin BM (2004) Socioeconomic status and obesity in adult populations of developing countries: a review. Bull World Health Organ 82: 940–946.
2. Doak CM, Adair LS, Bentley M, Monteiro C, Popkin BM (2005) The dual burden household and the nutrition transition paradox. Int J Obes (Lond) 29: 129–136.
3. Popkin BM (1994) The nutrition transition in low-income countries: an emerging crisis. Nutr Rev 52: 285–298.
4. Dans A, Ng N, Varghese C, Tai ES, Firestone R, et al. (2011) The rise of chronic non-communicable diseases in southeast Asia: time for action. Lancet 377: 680–689.
5. Garrett JL, Ruel MT (2005) Stunted child-overweight mother pairs: prevalence and association with economic development and urbanization. Food Nutr Bull 26: 209–221.
6. Oddo VM, Rah JH, Semba RD, Sun K, Akhter N, et al. (2012) Predictors of maternal and child double burden of malnutrition in rural Indonesia and Bangladesh. Am J Clin Nutr 95: 951–958.
7. Doak C, Adair L, Bentley M, Fengying Z, Popkin B (2002) The underweight/overweight household: an exploration of household sociodemographic and dietary factors in China. Public Health Nutr 5: 215–221.
8. Doak CM, Adair LS, Monteiro C, Popkin BM (2000) Overweight and underweight coexist within households in Brazil, China and Russia. J Nutr 130: 2965–2971.
9. VanderKloet M (2008) Dual burden of malnutrition in Andhra Pradesh, India: identification of independent predictors for underweight and overweight in adolescents with overweight mothers. London: University of London. 25 p.
10. Ohman A (2008) Global public health and gender theory: the need for integration. Scand J Public Health 36: 449–451.
11. Connell RW (1987) Gender and power. Stanford, CA: Stanford University Press.
12. Okin SM (1989) Justice, gender, and the family. United States of America: Basic Books, Inc.
13. International IDEA Institute for Democracy and Electorial Assistance (2000) Gender. Democratization in Indonesia: An Assesment. Stockholm: International IDEA.

14. The Asia Foundation ADB, Canadian International Development Agency, National Democratic Institute TWB (2006) Indonesia - country gender assessment. Manila, Philippines.
15. Papanek H, Schwede L (1988) Women are good with money: earning and managing in an Indonesian city. Econ Polit Weekly 23: WS73–84.
16. Manderson L (1983) Women's work and women's roles: economics and everyday life in Indonesia, Malasia and Singapore. Canberra: Australian University Press, Development Studies Center.
17. Kim D, Subramanian SV, Gortmaker SL, Kawachi I (2006) US state- and county-level social capital in relation to obesity and physical inactivity: a multilevel, multivariable analysis. Soc Sci Med 63: 1045–1059.
18. Eriksson M (2010) Social capital, health and community action: implications for health promotion. Umeå University: Umeå.
19. Portes A (1998) Social capital: Its origins and applications in modern sociology. Annu Rev Sociol 24: 1–24.
20. Schuller T, Baron S, Field J (2000) Social capital: a review and critique. In: Baron S, Field J, Schuller TE, editors. Social capital: Critical perspectives. New York: Oxford University Press. pp. 1–38.
21. Harpham T (2002) Measuring child poverty and health: a new international study. J Trop Pediatr 48: 128–130.
22. Poortinga W (2006) Social relations or social capital? Individual and community health effects of bonding social capital. Soc Sci Med 63: 255–270.
23. Statistics Indonesia Statistical Yearbook of Indonesia 2012.
24. Strauss J, Witoelar F, Sikoki B, Wattie AM (2009) The fourth wave of the Indonesia Family Life Survey: overview and field report. RAND. WR-675/1-NIA/NICHD WR-675/1-NIA/NICHD.
25. World Health Organization (2000) Obesity: preventing and managing the global epidemic. Report of a WHO consultation. World Health Organ Tech Rep Ser 894: i–xii, 1–253.
26. Deurenberg P, Deurenberg-Yap M, Guricci S (2002) Asians are different from Caucasians and from each other in their body mass index/body fat per cent relationship. Obes Rev 3: 141–146.
27. Cole TJ, Bellizzi MC, Flegal KM, Dietz WH (2000) Establishing a standard definition for child overweight and obesity worldwide: international survey. BMJ 320: 1240–1243.
28. Cole TJ, Flegal KM, Nicholls D, Jackson AA (2007) Body mass index cut offs to define thinness in children and adolescents: international survey. BMJ 335: 194.
29. Statistics Indonesia (May 2012) Trends of selected socio-economic indicators of Indonesia
30. Vyas S, Kumaranayake L (2006) Constructing socio-economic status indices: how to use principle component analysis. Health Policy Plan 21: 459–468.
31. Merlo J, Chaix B, Ohlsson H, Beckman A, Johnell K, et al. (2006) A brief conceptual tutorial of multilevel analysis in social epidemiology: using measures of clustering in multilevel logistic regression to investigate contextual phenomena. J Epidemiol Community Health 60: 290–297.
32. Food and Agriculture Organization of the United Nations (2006) The double burden of malnutrition. Case studies from six developing countries. FAO Food Nutr Pap 84: 1–334.
33. Popkin BM (2004) The nutrition transition: an overview of world patterns of change. Nutr Rev 62: S140–143.
34. Rae AN (1999) Food consumption patterns and nutrition in urban Java households: the discriminatory power of some socioeconomic variables. Aust J Agr Resour Ec 43: 359–383.
35. Roemling C, Qaim M (2013) Dual burden households and intra-household nutritional inequality in Indonesia. Econ Hum Biol http://dxdoiorg/101016/jehb201307001.
36. Quisumbing AR, Maluccio JA (1999) Intrahousehold allocation and gender relations: new empirical evidence. The World Bank.
37. Connell RW (1995) Masculinities. Berkeley: University of California Press.
38. Miller DL, Scheffler R, Lam S, Rosenberg R (2006) Social capital and health in Indonesia. World Development 34: 1084–1098.
39. Buvinić M, Gupta GR (2012) Female-headed households and female-maintained families: are they worth targeting to reduce poverty in developing countries? Econ Devel Cult Change 45: 259–280.
40. Gillespie S, Haddad L (2001) Attacking the double burden of malnutrition in Asia and the Pacific. Manila, Philippines: Asian Development Bank.
41. Putnam RD (1993) The prosperous community: social capital and public life. The American Prospect 13: 35–42.

Gut Microbiomes of Indian Children of Varying Nutritional Status

Tarini Shankar Ghosh[1]◑, Sourav Sen Gupta[2]◑, Tanudeep Bhattacharya[1], Deepak Yadav[1], Anamitra Barik[3], Abhijit Chowdhury[3,4], Bhabatosh Das[2], Sharmila S. Mande[1]*, G. Balakrish Nair[2]*

1 Bio Sciences R&D, TCS Innovation Labs, Pune, India, 2 Center for Human Microbial Ecology, Translational Health Science and Technology Institute, Gurgaon, India, 3 Society for Health and Demographic Surveillance, West Bengal, India, 4 Department of Hepatology, School of Digestive and Liver Diseases, Institute of Post Graduate Medical Education and Research, Kolkata, India

Abstract

Background: Malnutrition is a global health problem affecting more than 300 million pre-school children worldwide. It is one of the major health concerns in India since around 50% of children below the age of two suffer from various forms of malnutrition. The gut microbiome plays an important role in nutrient pre-processing, assimilation and energy harvest from food. Consequently, dysbiosis of the gut microbiota has been implicated in malnutrition.

Methodology/Principal Findings: Metagenomics approach was adopted to investigate the gut microbiome sampled from 20 rural Indian children with varying nutritional status. The changes in the abundances of various taxonomic and functional groups were investigated across these gut microbiomes. A core set of 23 genera were observed across samples, with some showing differential abundances with varying nutritional status. One of the findings of the current study is the positive/negative associations of specific taxonomic and functional groups with the nutritional status of the children. Notable alterations in the architecture of the inter-microbial co-occurrence networks were also observed with changes in nutritional status. A key example is the clustering of potentially pathogenic groups into a distinct hub in severely malnourished gut. Our data does not demonstrate causality with the microbiome patterns that we observed, rather a description of some interesting patterns, whose underlying mechanism remains to be uncovered.

Conclusions: The present study envisioned interrelationships between the pattern of gut microbiome and the nutritional status of children. The cause of this pattern needs to be explored. However, insights obtained from the present study form the basis for further metagenomic investigations on larger population of children. Results of such studies will be useful in identifying the key microbial groups that can be utilized for targeted therapeutic interventions for managing severe acute malnutrition.

Editor: Michael Edward Zwick, Emory University School Of Medicine, United States of America

Funding: This work was supported by the financial grant from the Department of Biotechnology, Govt. of India, for the establishment of Center for Human Microbial Ecology (Grant No. BT/MB/THSTI/HMC-SFC/2011). The funders had no role in study design, data collection and analysis, decision to publish, or preparation of the manuscript.

Competing Interests: Although some of the authors are employed by a commercial company (TCS Innovation Labs, Pune, India), this does not alter the authors' adherence to all the PLOS ONE policies on sharing data and materials.

* E-mail: sharmila.mande@tcs.com (SSM); nairgb@thsti.res.in (GBN)

◑ These authors contributed equally to this work.

Introduction

In its journey down the human alimentary canal, food is intercepted by trillions of microbes (10^{13}–10^{14}) residing in the human gut. The human gut microbiome, collective genomes of all the microbes residing in the gastrointestinal tracts, provides several metabolic functions that are not encoded in our own genome. Examples of these functions include fermentation of dietary polysaccharides, anaerobic metabolism of proteins and peptides, biosynthesis of vitamins, absorption of ions and regulation of a number of host metabolic pathways [1]. These functions facilitate the pre-processing of dietary nutrients and efficient harvest of dietary energy for the host. Aberrations in the composition of the gut microbiome are thus likely to affect the nutritional status of the hostand lead to over/under-nutrition.

Malnutrition is a major health problem in developing countries and is characterized by symptoms like delayed growth, deficiencies in vital nutritional components, namely proteins, vitamins, minerals, essential fatty acids and others. Malnutrition can be broadly attributed to lack of food, and inability to successfully digest and use food that is available. Around 314 and 258 million children under the age of five in low and middle income countriesare estimated to suffer from stunting and wasting respectively [2]. Poor nutrition accounts for more than one-third of child deaths worldwide [3] and associated with half of all child deaths in India [4]. An estimated 42% and 58% of children in India (under the age of two) suffer from stunting and wasting respectively [5]. Linear growth retardation and low weight (for height or age) in children in developing countries like India cannot be attributed to food insecurity alone. Sub-clinical conditions like tropical/environmental enteropathy, widely prevalent in developing countries,have been reported to be responsible for nutrient malabsorption [6,7]. A few recent studies have also indicated the association of the gut microbial community with malnutrition [8–10]. Dysbiosis of the gut microbiomeis likely to decrease the efficacy of nutritional interventions aimed at improving growth, thereby rendering them ineffective.

The gut microbiomes are observed to be heterogeneous across populations [11,12]. Although previous studies have focused on the characterization of gut microbiota sampled from individuals belonging to diverse geographies, similar investigations on the Indian population are currently limited. Given the environment and unique socio-economic-cultural set up within India, the gut microbiome of the Indian population is expected to be different from those reported for other geographies.

Three public health indicators are commonly used for quantifying the extent of malnourishment in children [13–15]. These are: (1) Stunting (short height for age); (2) Wasting (low weight for height) and; (3) Underweight (low weight for age). Although a few studies have indicated the association of gut microbiota with malnutrition, the question of how gut microbial community structure changes with nutritional status remains unanswered till date. In order to obtain insights into this aspect, we have analyzed the gut microbiome from twenty Indian children of varying nutritional status (ranging from healthy to severe acute malnutrition).

Materials and Methods

The details of the 20 subjects considered for this study, along with the methodology for sample collection, DNA extraction, pyrosequencing and quality filtering of sequenced metagenomic reads are described in Supporting Information S1 in File S1. All data were submitted to the NCBI Sequence Read Archive (SRA, http://www.ncbi.nlm.nih.gov/Traces/sra) with the following accession numbers SRR1067674, SRR1087919, SRR1068216, SRR1067721, SRR1068217, SRR1068218, SRR1068219, SRR1068596, SRR1068597, SRR1067720, SRR1067719, SRR1087910, SRR1087911, SRR1067716, SRR1087913, SRR1087914, SRR1087915, SRR1087916, SRR1067717, SRR1087918. Data was anonymized immediately after collection of the samples. The study was approved by the institutional review board of the Society for Health and Demographic Surveillance. Written informed consent was obtained from parents of the children in presence of another third person. The process of obtaining consent was not documented. The institutional review board had approved the procedurefor obtaining consent.

The nutritional status of each of the 20 children considered in this study was quantified using the WHO recommended (2009) three nutritional Z-scores namely, height for age (referred to in this study as Z-score1); weight for age (referred as Z-score2) and weight for height (referred as Z-score3). The formulae used for the calculation of these Z-scores, as recommended by WHO [15], are provided in Table S1 in File S1. Further, in order to obtain an overall measure of the nutritional status of these children, a cumulative Z-score was computed as the sum total of the above mentioned three Z-scores and was referred to as 'Cumulative Nutritional Index'.

Based on the cumulative nutritional index, the 20 gut metagenomes were divided into three groups. These groups were (a) apparently healthy (AH) (or mild malnourished) with cumulative nutritional indices greater than -6, (b) borderline malnourished (BL) ($-9<$cumulative nutritional indices <-6) and (c) severely malnourished (SM) (cumulative nutritional index <-9).

Taxonomic classification of metagenomic sequences

A database containing taxonomic information on known bacterial groups was created from the available data from the fully sequenced genomes at the NCBI database as well as from the bacterial/archaeal genomes sequenced as part of the Meta-HIT and the Human Microbiome Project consortiums. The database contained 2352 fully/partially sequenced bacterial genomes. Reads in each metagenome were subjected to BLASTN search [16] against this database (with thresholds of identity greater than 65%, query coverage >70% and minimum alignment length >75 base pairs). Subsequently, the reads were taxonomically classified using DiScRIBinATE [17]. DiScRIBinATE is a similarity-based taxonomic classification method that uses a two-step approach. Based on the alignment parameters (between a hit and its corresponding BLAST hit), the method first identifies an appropriate taxonomic level the read has to be assigned. In this study, the thresholds of alignment parameters used by Arumugamet *al.* [18] were utilized (by DiScRIBinATE) for identifying the appropriate taxonomic level. In the second step, DiScRIBinATE uses a bit-score/distance based approach to finally assign the read to a taxonomic group.

Profiling the abundance of different taxonomic groups in the gut microbiomes

The abundances of different taxonomic groups (at the level of genus, family, order, class and phylum) in each gut microbiome were obtained by normalizing the number of reads assigned to the group in the corresponding gut metagenome by the number of sequenced reads in the entire metagenome [18]. The normalized abundance values of the taxonomic groups obtained were subsequently ranked across the 20 samples.

In order to identify taxonomic groups having positive or negative influence on nutritional status, Spearman rank correlations were computed between the ranked abundances of different groups in each metagenome and the cumulative nutritional index of the corresponding child. Taxonomic groups showing statistically significant correlations with at least one Z-score measure were suggested to influence the nutritional status of the children. The statistical significances of these associations were judged using the ReBoot Method [19]. The power associated with the correlation values was computed using the arctanh transformation method [20]. Additionally the multivariate analysis of taxonomic profiles of the 20 gut microbiomes were also performed using Principal Component Analysis (PCA) and Principal Least Square Discriminant Analysis (PLS-DA).

In order to identify taxonomic groups that were specifically over-abundant in one of the three groups of microbiomes (AH, BL or SM), the abundances of the microbiota across the three groups were compared, using both parametric (ANOVA) and non-parametric (Kruskal-Wallis-H) tests. Furthermore, to reduce the chances of Type I error, multiple test corrections were performed using the Benjamini-Hochberg FDR method. Given the lower sample size in the current study, this method was chosen over the Bonferroni method since the power of Bonferroni corrections (for datasets with limited sample size) is usually low and is likely to miss out on bona fide relationships. Further, Tukey-Kramer's test was used for post-hoc analysis of difference of means (for the relationships with significant p-values) in ANOVA. This method considers all possible pairs of means while controlling the family-wise error rate (i.e., accounting for multiple comparisons). The Effect size (measured by η^2), which can be defined as the proportion of variance associated with or accounted for each of the main effects, interactions, and error in an ANOVA study, was also measured.

Profiling the abundances of different functional categories in the gut microbiomes

Sequences in each metagenome were first subjected to a BLAST search (with thresholds of identity >65% and query coverage >90%) against the eggNOG database [21]. Based on the hits obtained, these sequences were assigned to different Clusters of Orthologous Groups (COGs) and subsequently to higher level functional categories.

The relative abundances of the different COG groups in each gut microbiome were obtained by dividingthe number of reads assigned to the group in the corresponding gut metagenome by the metagenome size. These abundance values were then rank normalized across the 20 samples.

In order to identify functional groups showing positive or negative associations with nutritional status, Spearman Rank correlations were calculated between the abundances of functional groups in each metagenome and the nutritional indices of the corresponding child. The COG groups showing significant positive or negative correlations (with $P<0.05$) were further analyzed.

The abundances of the various carbohydrate active enzyme families [22] as well as virulent factors [23] were then profiled across the 20 gut microbiomes. The details of the methodology adopted are provided in Supporting Information S2 in File S1.

Identification of networks of co-occurring genera

For the metagenomes under study, pairwise correlations betweenthe rank normalized abundances of different genera were first obtained. Subsequently, pairs of genera having a correlation coefficients of P-value less than 0.05 (obtained using the ReBoot method) were linked by edges. Using this strategy, networks of co-occurring genera were generated and visualized using Cytoscape [24]. Finally various graph properties of the generated networks were computed using the Network-Analyzer plugin of Cytoscape. These properties included average number of neighbors, average path length, clustering co-efficient, network centralization, network density, network heterogeneity, number of nodes and shortest path. The networks of co-occurring genera (with $P<0.01$) were obtained separately for each of the three groups of children (AH, BL and SM). In order to study the transitions of the network architecture of co-occurring genera across the nutritional indices, the above mentioned graph properties were also calculated on a continuously evolving landscape, across varying nutritional indices, rather than as three discrete snapshots (corresponding to AH, BL and SM). For this purpose, a 'sliding window' approach was used. The 20 gut microbiomeswere first arranged in increasing order of their cumulative nutritional indices. Subsequently, 14 overlapping windows, each containing seven microbiomes,were considered. Pairwise correlation coefficients between the abundances of various genera were computed for each window. For each of the 14 windows, networks of co-occurring genera were then built following the above described procedure. The variations in the various graph properties werethen correlated with the average nutritional indices of the microbiomesin each of these windows.

Results

Anthropometric information and metadata of the subjects

The anthropometric data along with the sample metadata corresponding to the 20 children are provided in Table S2 in File S1. The overall variations in the three Z-scores (Z-score1, Z-score2 and Z-score3) corresponding to the nutritional status of the children constituting the study population were observed to range from −0.63 to −4.16, −1.07 to 4.32 and, 1.6 to −3.10, respectively. The above distribution indicates that the nutritional status of the children ranged from mild (i.e. apparently healthy) to severe malnourishment [14]. Cumulative Z-score ranged from −11.58 to −2.18. Overall the sizes of the gut metagenomes (in terms of the amount of nucleotide base pair data per sample) varied from 391 to 791 Mbps.

Taxonomic composition inthe gut microbiomes

Across the 20 microbiomes, 72% of the sequences (ranging from 61.8% to 86.6%) could be assigned at the phylum level (Table S3 in File S1). Approximately 36.2% of the sequences (ranging from 21.8% to 50.7%) could be assigned to taxa at the genus level (Table S3 in File S1), while only around 4.2% of the sequences (ranging from 1.4–12.4%) could be assigned at the species level.

Eight phyla (Bacteroidetes, Firmicutes, Proteobacteria, Actinobacteria, Spirochaetes, Fusobacteria, Synergistetes and Euryarchaeota) were observed to be present across all 20 gut microbiomes (Table S4, S5, in File S1; Figure 1). Out of these, a core set of 23 genera belongingto four phyla (Bacteroidetes, Firmicutes, Proteobacteria and Actinobacteria) were observed to be present (with normalized abundance ratio greater than 0.01) in at least 50% (i.e. 10 out of 20) of the gut microbiomes (Figure 1). One of the key observations was the overall dominance of Prevotellaacross the metagenomes (Table S4, S5, in File S1; Figure 2), indicating that the majority of the gut microbiomes in the children under study were similar to the *Prevotella* enterotype gut microbial community previously studied by Arumugam*et al.* [18].

Variation of microbial groups with nutritional status

Figure 3 shows the variations of the rank normalized abundances of the 23 core genera and the 8 phyla across the 20 gutmicrobiomes (arranged in order of their cumulative nutritional indices). A closer inspection reveals that the taxa could be divided into four groups (G1–G4) based on similarities in their abundance patterns. Taxa belonging to G4 were observed to have a progressive increase in their abundances with the decreasing nutritional index (Figure 3). The five genera belonging to this group namely, *Escherichia* ($R=-0.59$, $P<0.032$, Power at P-value<0.05: 0.85), *Streptococcus* ($R=-0.70$, $P<0.019$, Power at P-value<0.05: 0.97), *Shigella* ($R=-0.62$, $P<0.04$), *Enterobacter* ($R=-0.75$, $P<0.032$, Power at P-value<0.05: 0.97) and *Veillonella* ($R=-0.80$, $P<0.005$, Power at P-value<0.05: 0.99), wereobserved to have significant negative correlation with the nutritional index of the children (Table S6 in File S1). Taxa belonging to G2 and G3 do not show any significant correlation in their abundance patterns with the nutritional index of the study subjects.

The taxa belonging to the group G1 showed a progressive decrease in their rank normalized abundances with decreasing nutritional status (Figure 3). It was alsoobserved that several genera belonging to the group G1, namely *Roseburia* ($R=0.51$, $P<0.048$, Power at P-value<0.05: 0.63), *Faecalibacterium* ($R=0.49$, $P<0.003$, Power at P-value<0.05: 0.62), *Butyrivibrio* ($R=0.52$, $P<0.027$, Power at P-value<0.05: 0.63) had significant positive correlations with nutritional index (Table S6 in File S1). Among the phyla, while Proteobacteria (belonging to G4) wasobserved to show a decrease with increasing nutritional status, Synergistetes (belonging to G1) was observed to havea positive correlation with nutritional status. Interestingly, the dominant genus in the analyzed gut microbiomes, namely *Prevotella*, was not observed to have significant correlations with nutritional indices. Unexpectedly, the probiotic genera like *Lactobacillus* and *Bifidobacterium* were

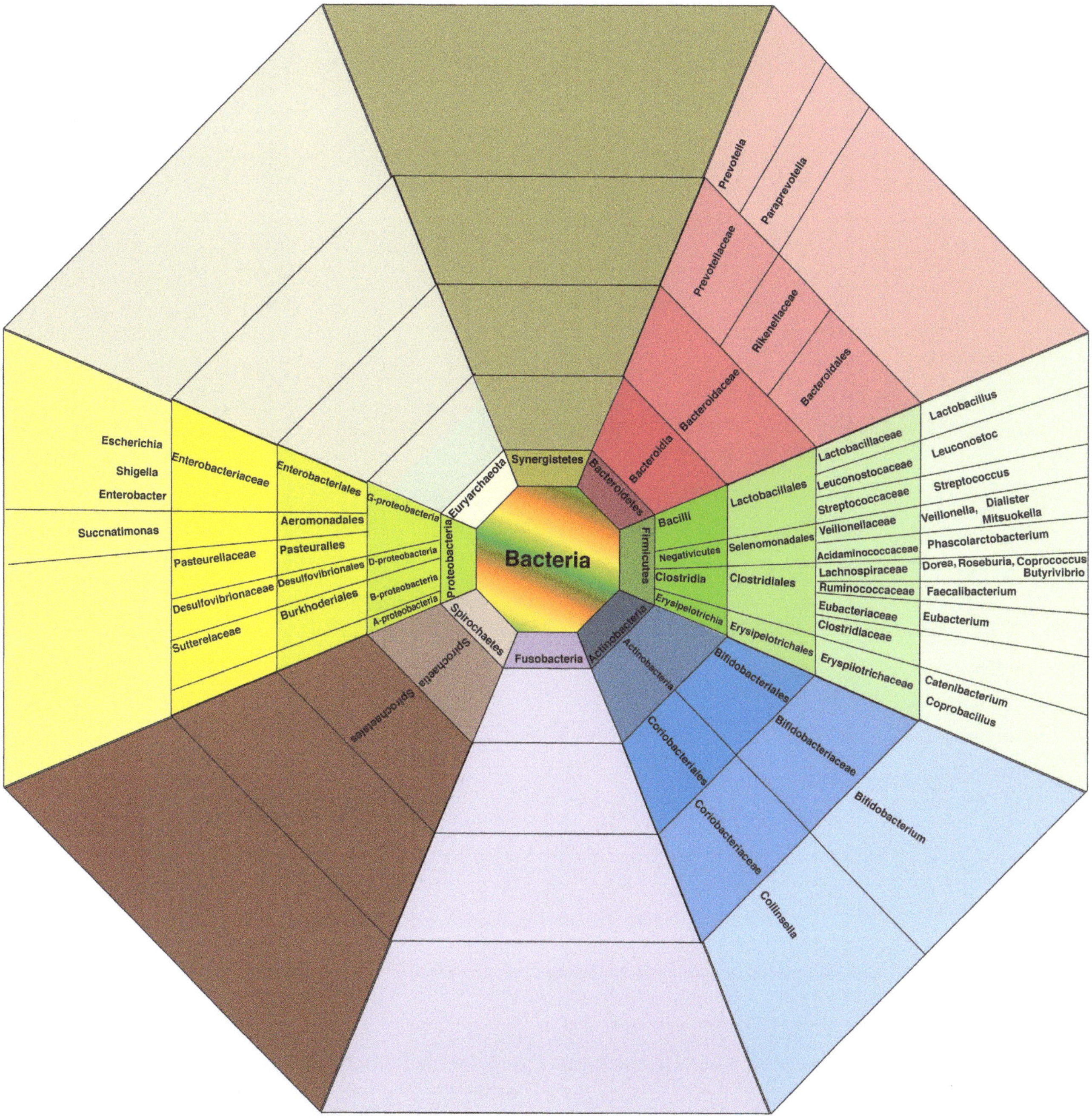

Figure 1. Distribution of taxonomic groups at various levels (including the core set of 23 genera) commonly present across at least 50% metagenomes with normalized abundance ratios of more than 0.01.

also not observed to have any significant correlation with nutritional indices.

Comparison of microbial groups across the three categories (AH, BL and SM)

The results of the comparative analysis, using ANOVA, Kruskal-Wallis-H test (along with multi-test corrections), indicated five taxonomic groups that were significantly different across the three categories (AH, BL and SM) of microbiome (Figure 4, Table S7 in File S1). Several genera belonging to the group G4, namely *Escherichia*, *Streptococcus* and *Shigella*, were observed to be significantly over-abundant in the SM categories as compared to AH. These results are in line with those obtained using the correlation-based analysis (Table S6 in File S1, Figure 3). Further, although individual genera belonging to the group G1 did not show any significant differences across the three groups, the combined abundances of all the genera belonging to this group was observed to be significantly higher in the AH category (Figure 4, Table S7 in File S1). This result suggests that, not all members of a particular group of genera (having similar characteristics) may be required for conferring a specific phenotype. Multivariate analysis using PCA as well as PLS-DA also indicated a distinct separation between the AH and SM categories of microbiomes, with the BL

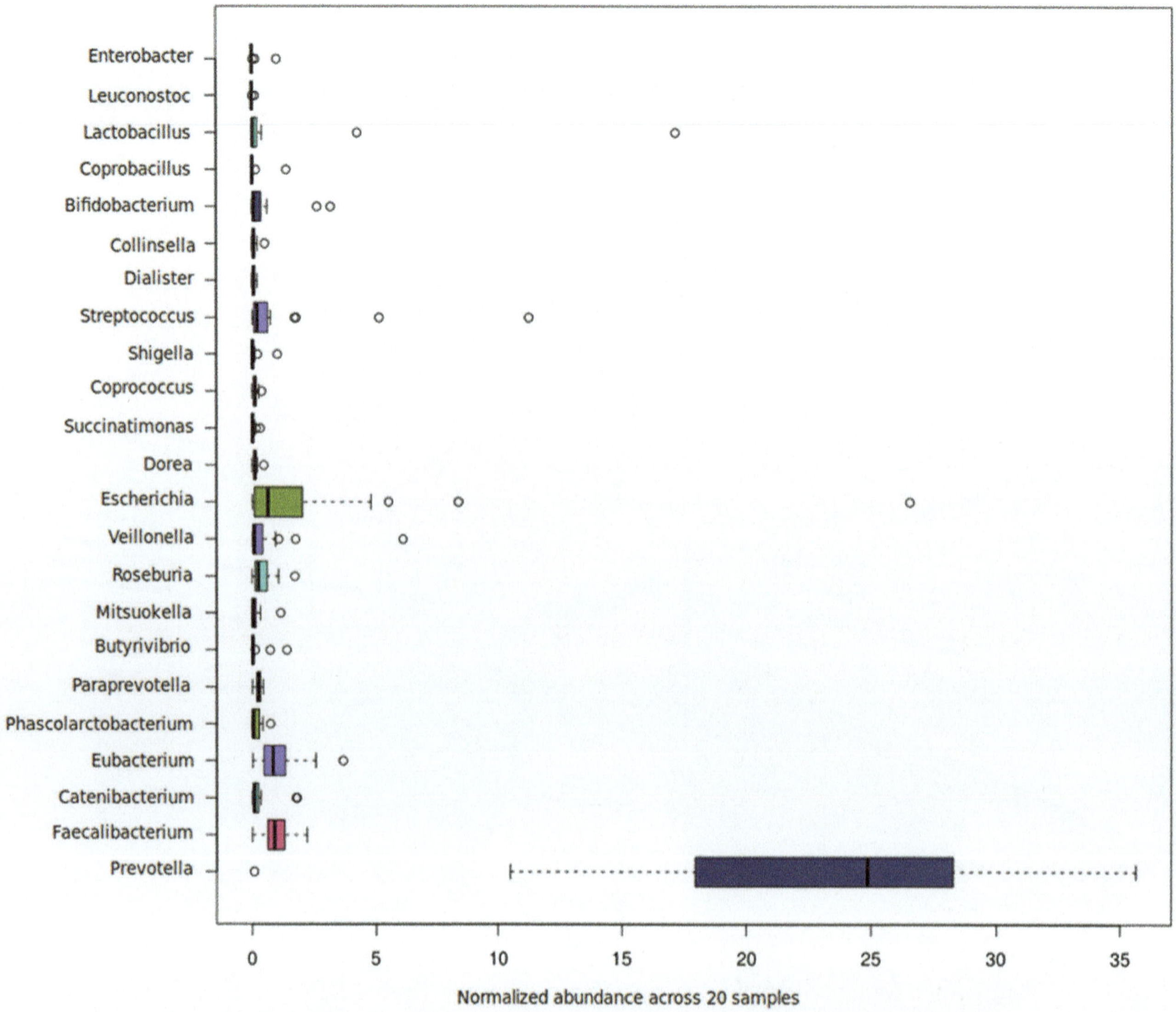

Figure 2. Variation of the normalized abundances (expressed as percentages) of the 23 core genera across the 20 gut metagenomes.

categories of microbiomes interspersed in between (Figure S1 in File S1).

Functional profiles ofthe gut microbiomes

64 and 112 COG groups were observed to have significant positive (ReBoot Z-value>1.97; P<0.05) and negative correlation (ReBoot Z-value<−1.97; P<0.05) with the cumulative nutritional indices, respectively (Tables S8 and S9 in File S1). These two COG groups were referred to as Positively Correlated (PC) and Negatively Correlated (NC) COG groups. The COGs belonging to the PC and NC groups were then mapped to their respective higher level functional categories. The relative abundances of the different functional categories in the two groups were then compared (Figure 5).

Several functional categories associated with nutrient uptake and metabolism was observed to be either over-represented or present only in the PC COG groups (Figure 5). These functional categories included secondary metabolites biosynthesis, transport and catabolism; energy production and conversion; amino acid transport and metabolism and carbohydrate transport and metabolism. The only exception to the above trend was lipid transport and metabolism which was observed to be over-represented in the NC COG group.

In contrast to the PC COG groups, the NC COG group was observed to have an over-representation of functional categories that have been associated with virulence and bacterial pathogenesis [8]. These included intracellular trafficking; secretion and vesicular transport; cell motility and inorganic ion transport and metabolism (Figure 5).

Profiles of carbohydrate active enzyme families in the gut microbiomes

The results of the analysis indicated that none of the CAZyme families were significantly correlated with the cumulative nutritional index (Figure S2 in File S1). In order to evaluate whether groups of CAZyme families worked in tandem and showed significant correlation with the nutritional index, CAZyme families having similar abundance patterns were grouped together and

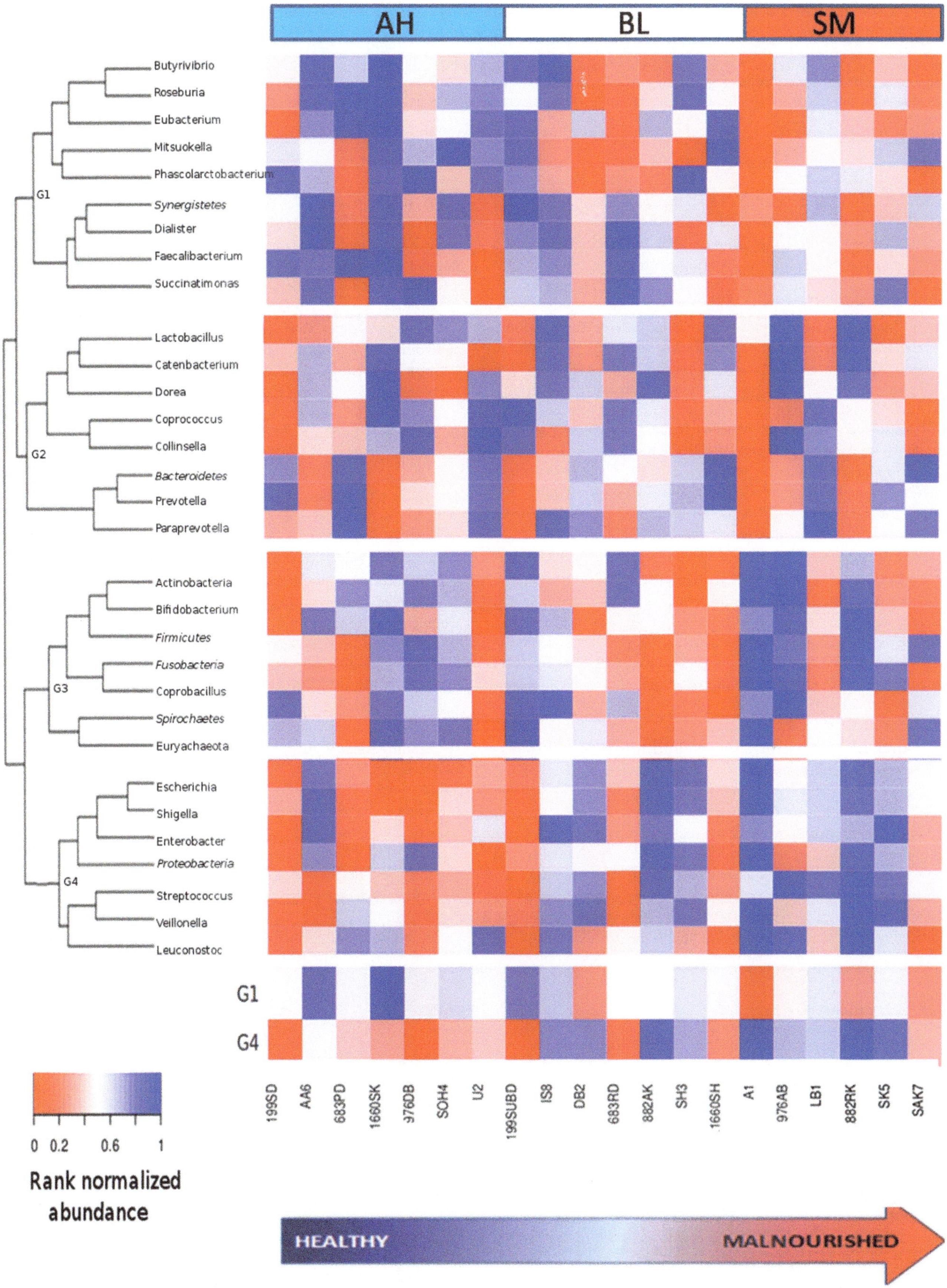
AH
BL
SM
Butyrivibrio
Roseburia
Eubacterium
Mitsuokella
Phascolarctobacterium
Synergistetes
Dialister
Faecalibacterium
Succinatimonas
Lactobacillus
Catenbacterium
Dorea
Coprococcus
Collinsella
Bacteroidetes
Prevotella
Paraprevotella
Actinobacteria
Bifidobacterium
Firmicutes
Fusobacteria
Coprobacillus
Spirochaetes
Euryachaeota
Escherichia
Shigella
Enterobacter
Proteobacteria
Streptococcus
Veillonella
Leuconostoc
G1
G2
G3
G4
G1
G4
199SD
AA6
683PD
1660SK
976DB
SOH4
U2
199SUBD
IS8
DB2
683RD
882AK
SH3
1660SH
A1
976AB
LB1
882RK
SK5
SAK7
0 0.2 0.6 1
Rank normalized abundance
HEALTHY
MALNOURISHED

Figure 3. Variation of the rank normalized abundances of the 23 genera and 8 phyla (in italics) across the 20 gut metagenomes. The metagenomes are arranged in the bottom panel (from left to right) in decreasing order of their cumulative nutritional scores. The groups of microbiomes belonging to Apparently Healthy (AH), Borderline (BL) and Severely Malnourished (SM) children are also indicated. The taxa are arranged vertically on the left panel as a hierarchical tree based on the similarities in their abundance patterns. The four groups of taxa (G1–G4) with similar abundance patterns across the metagenomes are also demarcated. The cumulative rank normalized abundances of groups G1 (showing progressive increase with nutritional scores) and G4 (showing a progressive decrease with nutritional scores) across the 20 samples are provided in the bottom most panel.

analysed (Figure 6, Supporting Information S2 in File S1). The constituent CAZyme families within each of these groups are provided in Table S10 in File S1.

It was observed that CAZyme families belonging to groups 3 and 7 had significant ($P<0.05$) positive correlations with at least one of the nutritional indices (Figure 6, Table S11 in File S1). While most of the CAZyme families belonging to group 3 are known for degrading complex plant carbohydrates, those belonging to group 7 are mostly peptidoglycan degraders. In addition, group 6 was observed to have marginal positive correlations ($P<0.10$) with Z-score2 as well as with the overall nutritional index. CAZyme families belonging to group 6 are chiefly responsible for degradation of complex plant carbohydrates. When the CAZyme families belonging to groups 3, 6 and 7 were combined together, their cumulated abundances were found to have an even stronger correlation with the overall nutritional index ($R=0.583$, $P<0.007$). Interestingly, none of the groups were observed to have significant negative correlation with nutritional indices.

Profiles of virulence factors in the gut microbiomes

The number of virulence factor homologs detected in the microbiomes was observed to show a progressive increase with decreasing cumulative nutritional index ($R=-0.498$, $P<0.02$) (Figure S3 in File S1). Thus, the presence of higher number of virulence genes in children with lower nutritional index indicates the presence of more pathogenic species.

Networks of co-occurringgenera and nutritional indices

The symptomatic characteristics of the gut environment depend not only on the presence of specific microbial groups but also on the inherent inter-microbial co-occurrence networks present therein. The network of co-occurring genera, obtained for the three groups of gut microbiomes (AH, BL and SM), were observed to be characterized by distinct network architecture.

The co-occurrence network of the AH group of metagenomes were characterized by four distinct connected groups of genera. Interestingly, although genera belonging to the groups G1 and G4 were observed to have contrasting trends in their abundance patterns, some of themshowed strong positive associations amongst each other (Figure 7). For example, the genus *Streptococcus* (belonging to the group G4) was observed to be associated with beneficial genera like *Faecalibacterium* (belonging to group G1). Similarly the genera *Enterobacter* (belonging to G4) was observed to be associated with genera *Eubacterium*, *Roseburia* and *Dorea* (from group G1).

Distinct changes were observed in the genera co-occurrence network with a progressive decrease in the nutritional status. For example, in the borderline (BL) group of metagenomes, genera belonging to the group G4 (namely, *Esherichia*, *Shigella*, *Streptococcus*, *Veillonella*) were observed to be placed together in a single connected hub. Furthermore, the average node density of the co-occurrence networks obtained for the borderline metagenomes was also observed to be higher as compared to that obtained for the apparently healthy metagenomes. This probably indicates that with a progressive decrease in nutritional status, there may be an increasing degree of functional interdependence among genera (especially those belonging to the group G4).

The increasing interdependence among the genera is observed to be even more pronounced in the co-occurrence networks obtained for the severely malnourished group of metagenomes. The networks of co-occurring generain the severely malnourished (SM) microbiomes were observed to contain two dominant hubs of genera. While one hub was primarily constituted by the likely pathogenic genera (e.g. *Shigella*, *Escherichia* and *Enterobacter*) belonging to the group G4, the second hub was constituted by the commensal and the beneficial genera (e.g. *Roseburia*, *Butyrivibrio* and *Faecalibacterium*), belonging to G1, in addition to *Prevotella* and *Paraprevotella*. These results suggest that the gut microbial community in SM group is likely to be characterized by the presence of two (functionally opposing) groups of genera. The average node degree within these two hubs were also observed to be high (28 nodes for 20 genera; average node degree: 2.61), indicating a strong inter-dependency within the members in each group.

Analysis of graph properties of co-occurrence networks obtained for the 14 overlapping groups of metagenomes (described in the

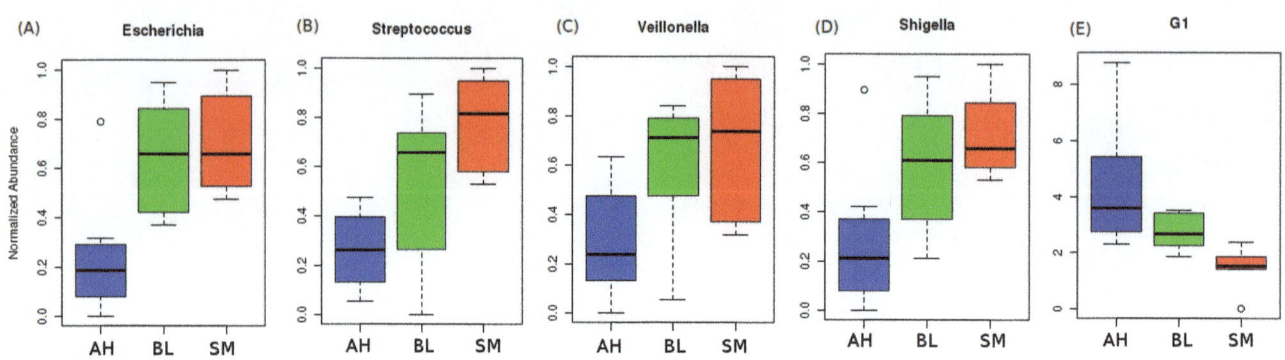

Figure 4. Box-plots showing the abundances of the taxonomic groups significantly differing across the three groups (AH, BL and SM) of gut microbiomes.

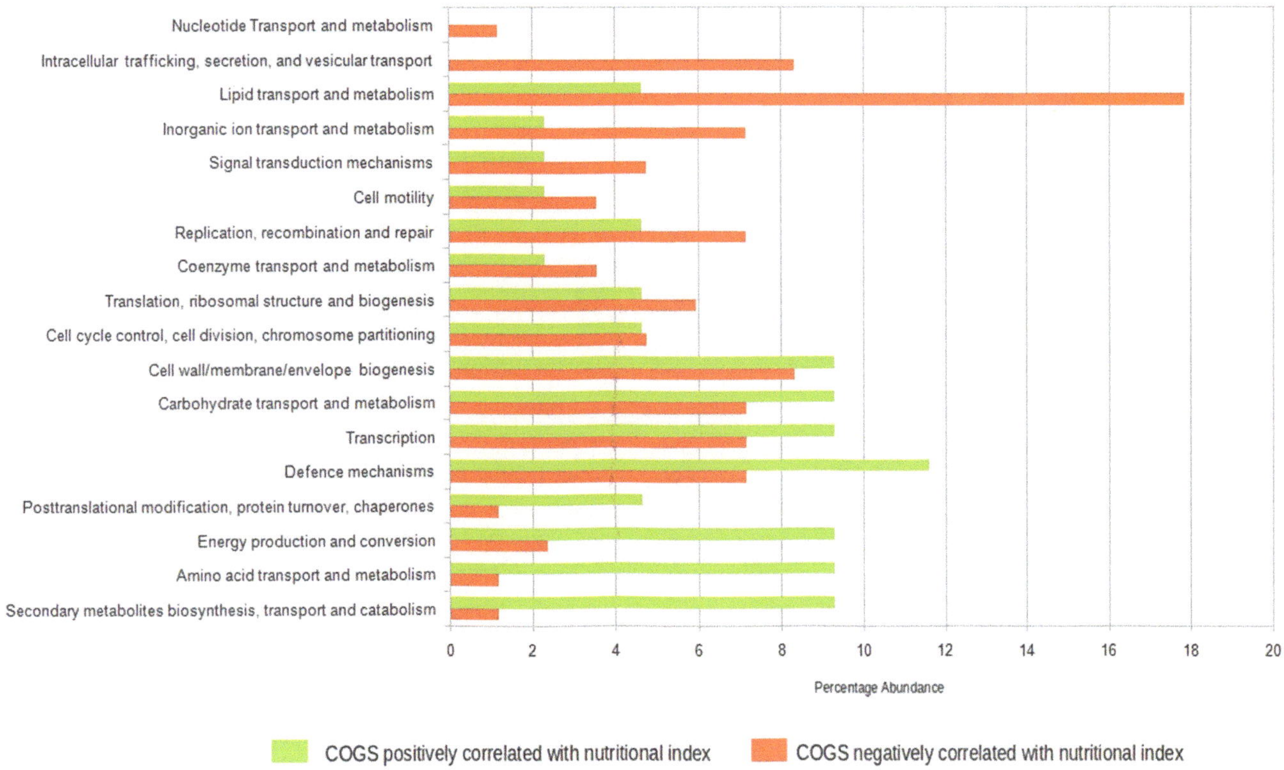

Figure 5. Percentage abundances of the different functional categories corresponding to the COGs identified either as positively correlated (shown in green) or as negatively correlated (shown in red) with nutritional indices.

Methods section) identified the average number of neighbors to have significant negative correlation with the nutritional status (Figure 8a, Figure S4 in File S1) indicating that with an increase in the nutritional status, the inter-dependence amongst microbial groups shows a progressive decrease. This result is in line with that obtained for the three discrete groups of metagenomes (Figure 7). Similarly, Figure 8b shows the variation of the average number of neighbors across COG co-occurrence networks obtained for the groups of gut microbiomes with progressively increasing status. The average number of neighbours obtained in each of the COG co-occurrence networks also showed a similar pattern to that obtained using the microbial genera. This further indicates a likely decrease in functional inter-dependence with an increase in nutritional status.

Discussion

The onset and progression of malnutrition has been attributed to a variety of causal factors. These include inadequate nutrient intake, prolonged enteric infections due to sub-standard hygiene, metabolic disorders and the variations in the taxonomic and functional composition of the gut microbiota. Previous studies have provided the early snapshots of the taxonomic and functional dysbiosis in the gut microbiome of malnourished children [8,9]. A separate study by Smith *et al.* [10] implicated the gut microbiome as a causal factor in kwashiorkor, an enigmatic form of severe acute malnutrition. These studies have provided the first insights into the role of the gut microbiome in this global health problem. Several pathogenic bacteria, typically associated with enteric infections, were reported in the gut of a malnourished child [8] Such aberrations in gut microbiome are expected to lead to sub-clinical disorders like inflammation and nutrient malabsorption. Infection has been known to adversely affect nutritional status and also malnutrition can predispose children to infections [25]. The current study has attempted to deepen these insights further by performing a comprehensive investigation of gut microbiomes obtained from a larger population of children from rural India with varying nutritional status.

The present study indicates that the impaired nutritional status is not only due to the abundances of likely pathogenic microbial groups, but also a result of depletion of several commensal genera. These genera, namely, *Roseburia*, *Faecalibacterium*, *Butyrivibrio*, *Eubacterium* and *Phascolarctobacterium*, have been suggested to have positive influence on the nutritional status of the children. These genera have earlier been reported to be a part of the normal commensal microflora of the human gut [26–32]. Several studies have indicated the beneficial and probiotic properties of these genera in either nutrition harvest from the food or in maintaining the immune stability of the gut. For example, genera like *Roseburia* and *Butyrivibrio* are known producers of short chain fatty acids (SCFA) in the intestine [27,28]. The production of SCFA from the dietary fibers has been reported to be crucial factor for improved harvest and intake of carbohydrates [29,30]. Furthermore, genera like *Faecalibacterium*, *Roseburia* and *Eubacterium* have been shown to possess anti-inflammatory properties [27–32]. Studies have suggested that depletion of species belonging to these genera could be associated with low grade inflammation and onset of inflammatory bowel diseases [31,32]. Inflammation has also been associated with malabsorption of nutrients and subsequent decline in the nutritional status [33].

The present study revealed that certain functional categories (COG groups) are positively/negatively correlated with nutritional status. The identified positively correlated functional groups are

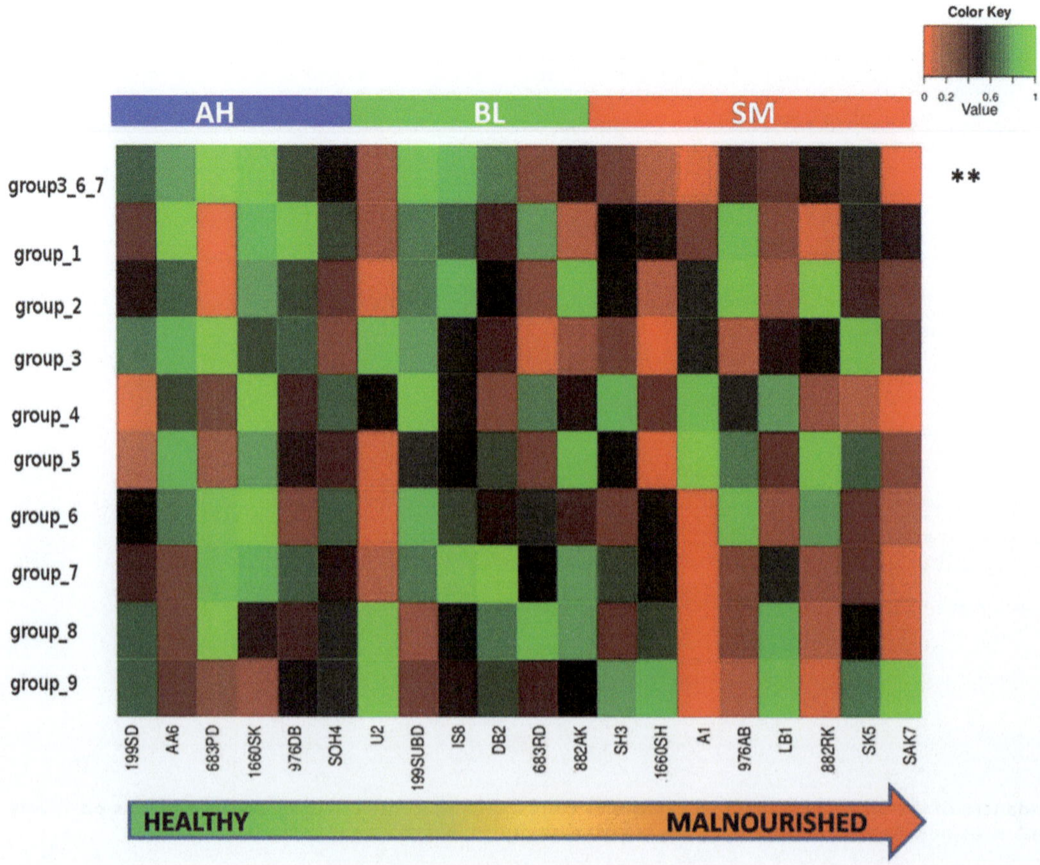

Figure 6. Abundance patterns of different groups of CAZyme families across gut metagenomes with varying nutritional status. The metagenomes are arranged in the bottom panelin decreasing order of their cumulative nutritional scores. The groups of microbiomes belonging to Apparently Healthy (AH), Borderline (BL) and Severely Malnourished (SM) children are also indicated. "**"indicates the variation of the cumulated abundances of members belonging to groups 3, 6 and 7.

likely to aid in better utilization of the nutrients in the gut, thereby helping in maintenance of the overall well-being of the child. On the other hand, the negatively correlated functional groups may initiate the infection process which might indirectly lead to malabsorption of nutrients. The higher number of virulence genes identified in the children with lower nutritional index further corroborates this finding.

A key finding of the current study is the identification of three groups of carbohydrate active enzymes (called CAZymes) families (in the gut microbiomes) showing positive associations with the nutritional status of the children. These groups were observed to be dominated by CAZyme families that preferentially degrade peptidoglycans and complex plant carbohydrates. Dietary fibers, chiefly constitutedby complex carbohydrates, cannot be completely degraded by enzymes coded by the human genome. These complex carbohydrates can only be degraded by the enzymes encoded by the gut microbiota. The human host can harvest energy from such recalcitrant carbohydrates only after bacterial enzymes have pre-processed them. Such 'energy harvest' in the gut becomes particularly crucial for subjects with lower nutritional status.

Identification of distinct changes in genera co-occurrence networks with progressive decrease in the nutritional status of the children is a key finding in the current study. The results indicate that with decrease in the nutritional status, there is a likely increase in functional interdependence among the various microbes residing in the gut. It was also interesting to observe the associations of probable pathogenic groups with potentially beneficial ones in healthy gut microbiomes. Clustering of potentially pathogenic groups into a distinct hub in severely malnourished gut probably suggests how these groups may help each other in a cooperative manner to a create an imbalance in microbial populations. This in turn may lead to the creation of milieu that is progressively detrimental in maintaining the nutritional homeostasis of the gut. Functional associations within microbial groups may modulate specific functional behaviors of its constituent members in terms of their expressed genes and proteins. Thus, the observed changes in the architecture and composition of networks of co-occurring microbial groups under different nutritional settings add further insights into the gut microbial environments associated with the nutritional status. The functional interdependence of the network could be used in future for therapeutic interventions to address the challenge of clinical management of severe acute malnutrition. The network analysis suggests that one can modulate the gut microbiome by disrupting certain key players (genera) in order to achieve conditions that could result in the regression of the disease phenotype.

Considering the pilot nature of the study and the limited sample size, the results obtained in the study should be interpreted with due caution. However, the present findings open up an interesting premise which furthers our understanding of the role of gut microbiota in causation of malnutrition under nutrient limited

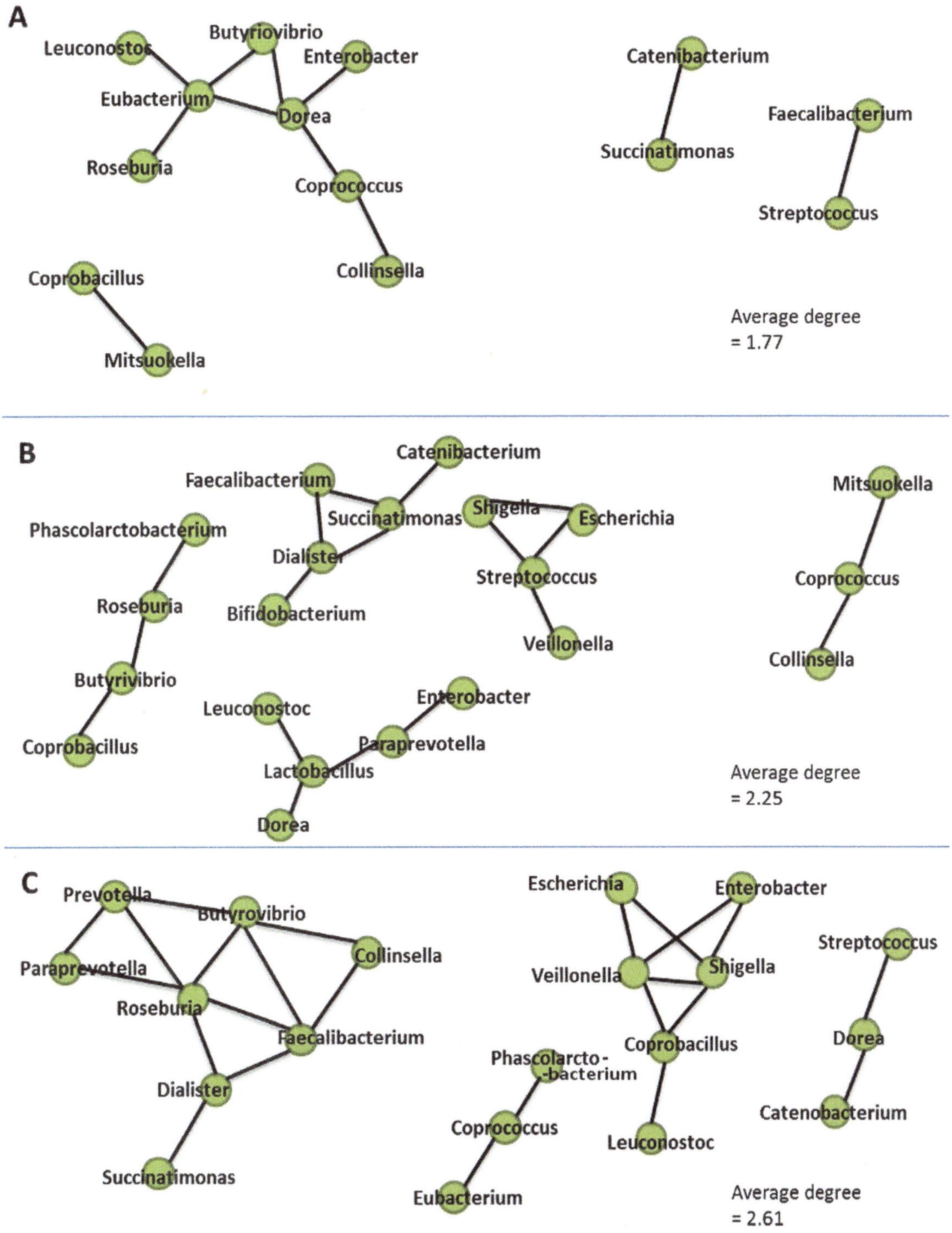

Figure 7. Genera co-occurrence networks obtained for gut microbiomes from (A) Apparently Healthy, AH, (B) Borderline, BL and, (C) Severely Malnourished, SM children.

conditions. Further, given that the geographical location, age and diet of most of the children (considered in the current study) were similar, it was assumed that the observed trends (of either increasing/decreasing functional interdependence) could provide a rough indication of the changes in the microbiome with varying nutritional status. However, in order to obtain a definitive picture of the underlying changes associated with either increase or decrease of nutritional status, a longitudinal study is absolutely necessary. We further acknowledge that 'unacknowledged heterogeneity' remains as there could be numerous genetic and environmental factors affecting the composition of the gut microbiome [12]. Additionally, other unmeasured epidemiological factors could be influencing our findings and this warrants replication in a larger population. It is virtually impossible to

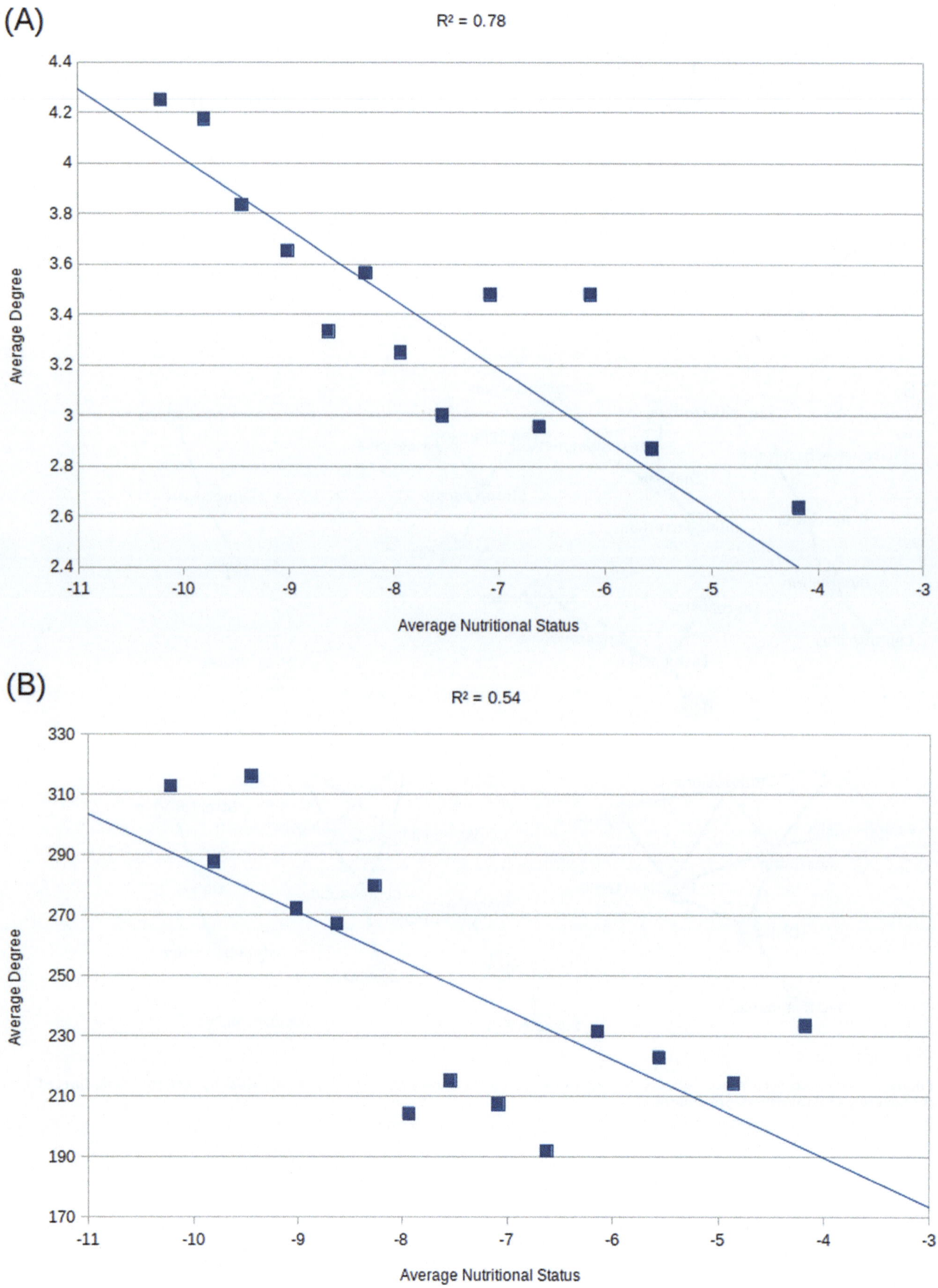
(A)
R² = 0.78
Average Degree
4.4
4.2
4
3.8
3.6
3.4
3.2
3
2.8
2.6
2.4
-11
-10
-9
-8
-7
-6
-5
-4
-3
Average Nutritional Status
(B)
R² = 0.54
Average Degree
330
310
290
270
250
230
210
190
170
-11
-10
-9
-8
-7
-6
-5
-4
-3
Average Nutritional Status

Figure 8. Variations of graph properties (of the genera co-occurrence networks obtained for the overlapping groups of metagenomes) namely, (A) Average number of neighbors and, (B) Shortest path with the average nutritional index.

consider all the factors in a single analysis. However, we have tried to obtain samples from a similar age-geography-economy strata (all children from eastern part of India from a low economic strata which are supposed to be the key factors in influencing gut microbiota composition). Thus, we have tried to reduce the number of variables in our analysis as much as possible. We expect that, considering the pilot nature of the study, the results provide a rough picture of microbial community dynamics, at least at the basic level.

Conclusion

The present study describes patterns wherein the gut microbiome varies in response to nutritional status. Although the biological bases of such patterns may be inferred to a certain extent, the universality and the biological mechanisms governing the occurrence of these patterns remains to be experimentally verified. Although limited by sample size and range of nutritional status of selected subjects, the present study opens up avenues for in-depth analyses of gut microbiomes on much larger populations belonging to diverse geographies as well as nutritional status. Such studies will help in better understanding the role of microbial groups in host nutrient assimilation and how they interact, which are evolving as important determinants of systemic conditions like malnutrition. Much comprehensive and well designed functional studiesare required for formulating a microbial basis of therapy for severe acute malnutrition.

Supporting Information

File S1 Combined supporting information. Additional data including details of study population, sample collection, DNA extraction, pyrosequencing, quality filtering, abundances of carbohydrate active enzyme families and virulence factors in the gut microbiomes are provided in supporting information in File S1. Supplementary Figures and supplementary Tables are also available in File S1.
(PDF)

Acknowledgments

We would sincerely like to acknowledge Dr. Partha Pratim Majumder and Dr. Arindam Maitra from National Institute of Biomedical Genomics, Kalyani, West Bengal, for their help related to metagenomic sequencing. We would also like to thank Kuntal Kumar Bhusan, from TCS Innovation Labs, for his help during the course of this study.

Author Contributions

Conceived and designed the experiments: GBN SSM AC. Performed the experiments: SSG TSG. Analyzed the data: TSG SSG TB DY BD SSM GBN. Wrote the paper: TSG SSG TB DY BD SSM GBN. Identification of subjects and collection of faecal samples: AC AB SB. Read and approved the manuscript: TSG SSG TB DY AB AC BD SSM GBN.

References

1. Guarner F, Malagelada JR (2003) Gut flora in health and disease. Lancet 361: 512–519.
2. Black RE, Victora CG, Walker SP, Bhutta ZA, Christian P, et al. (2013) Maternal and child undernutrition and overweight in low-income and middle-income countries. Lancet 382: 427–451.
3. UN (2012) Estimation Levels & Trends in Child Mortality. UN Inter-agency Group for Child Mortality.
4. Gragnolati M SM, Das Gupta M, Bredenkamp C, Lee YK (2005) India's undernourished children: A call for reform and action.
5. Report of Association of Voluntary Agencies for Rural Development ND, India (2012) Hunger and malnutrition in India: Status, Causes and Cures.
6. Dewey KG, Mayers DR (2011) Early child growth: how do nutrition and infection interact? Matern Child Nutr 7 Suppl 3: 129–142.
7. Gordon JI, Dewey KG, Mills DA, Medzhitov RM (2012) The human gut microbiota and undernutrition. Sci Transl Med 4: 137ps112.
8. Gupta SS, Mohammed MH, Ghosh TS, Kanungo S, Nair GB, et al. (2011) Metagenome of the gut of a malnourished child. Gut Pathog 3: 7.
9. Monira S, Nakamura S, Gotoh K, Izutsu K, Watanabe H, et al. (2011) Gut microbiota of healthy and malnourished children in bangladesh. Front Microbiol 2: 228.
10. Smith MI, Yatsunenko T, Manary MJ, Trehan I, Mkakosya R, et al. (2013) Gut microbiomes of Malawian twin pairs discordant for kwashiorkor. Science 339: 548–554.
11. De Filippo C, Cavalieri D, Di Paola M, Ramazzotti M, Poullet JB, et al. (2010) Impact of diet in shaping gut microbiota revealed by a comparative study in children from Europe and rural Africa. Proc Natl Acad Sci U S A 107: 14691–14696.
12. Yatsunenko T, Rey FE, Manary MJ, Trehan I, Dominguez-Bello MG, et al. (2012) Human gut microbiome viewed across age and geography. Nature 486: 222–227.
13. Picot J, Hartwell D, Harris P, Mendes D, Clegg AJ, et al. (2012) The effectiveness of interventions to treat severe acute malnutrition in young children: a systematic review. Health Technol Assess 16: 1–316.
14. Shoham J, Duffield A (2009) Proceedings of the World Health Organization/UNICEF/World Food Programme/United Nations High Commissioner for Refugees Consultation on the management of moderate malnutrition in children under 5 years of age. Food Nutr Bull 30: S464–474.
15. WHO (2009) WHO Child Growth Standards. Growth Velocity Based on Weight, Length and Head Circumference. Methods and Development. WHO, Geneva, WHO Press.
16. Altschul SF, Gish W, Miller W, Myers EW, Lipman DJ (1990) Basic local alignment search tool. J Mol Biol 215: 403–410.
17. Ghosh TS, Monzoorul Haque M, Mande SS (2010) DiScRIBinATE: a rapid method for accurate taxonomic classification of metagenomic sequences. BMC Bioinformatics 11 Suppl 7: S14.
18. Arumugam M, Raes J, Pelletier E, Le Paslier D, Yamada T, et al. (2011) Enterotypes of the human gut microbiome. Nature 473: 174–180.
19. Faust K, Sathirapongsasuti JF, Izard J, Segata N, Gevers D, et al. (2012) Microbial co-occurrence relationships in the human microbiome. PLoS Comput Biol 8: e1002606.
20. Cohen J (1988) Statistical Power Analysis for the Behavioral Sciences: L. Erlbaum Associates.
21. Powell S, Szklarczyk D, Trachana K, Roth A, Kuhn M, et al. (2012) eggNOG v3.0: orthologous groups covering 1133 organisms at 41 different taxonomic ranges. Nucleic Acids Res 40: D284–289.
22. Cantarel BL, Coutinho PM, Rancurel C, Bernard T, Lombard V, et al. (2009) The Carbohydrate-Active EnZymes database (CAZy): an expert resource for Glycogenomics. Nucleic Acids Res 37: D233–238.
23. Chen L, Yang J, Yu J, Yao Z, Sun L, et al. (2005) VFDB: a reference database for bacterial virulence factors. Nucleic Acids Res 33: D325–328.
24. Smoot ME, Ono K, Ruscheinski J, Wang PL, Ideker T (2011) Cytoscape 2.8: new features for data integration and network visualization. Bioinformatics 27: 431–432.
25. Brown KH (2003) Diarrhea and malnutrition. J Nutr 133: 328S–332S.
26. Gevers D, Knight R, Petrosino JF, Huang K, McGuire AL, et al. (2012) The Human Microbiome Project: a community resource for the healthy human microbiome. PLoS Biol 10: e1001377.
27. Benus RF, van der Werf TS, Welling GW, Judd PA, Taylor MA, et al. (2010) Association between Faecalibacterium prausnitzii and dietary fibre in colonic fermentation in healthy human subjects. Br J Nutr 104: 693–700.
28. Van den Abbeele P, Gerard P, Rabot S, Bruneau A, El Aidy S, et al. (2011) Arabinoxylans and inulin differentially modulate the mucosal and luminal gut microbiota and mucin-degradation in humanized rats. Environ Microbiol 13: 2667–2680.
29. Andoh A, Tsujikawa T, Fujiyama Y (2003) Role of dietary fiber and short-chain fatty acids in the colon. Curr Pharm Des 9: 347–358.
30. Turnbaugh PJ, Hamady M, Yatsunenko T, Cantarel BL, Duncan A, et al. (2009) A core gut microbiome in obese and lean twins. Nature 457: 480–484.
31. Hakansson A, Molin G (2011) Gut microbiota and inflammation. Nutrients 3: 637–682.

32. Bajaj JS, Hylemon PB, Ridlon JM, Heuman DM, Daita K, et al. (2012) Colonic mucosal microbiome differs from stool microbiome in cirrhosis and hepatic encephalopathy and is linked to cognition and inflammation. Am J Physiol Gastrointest Liver Physiol 303: G675–685.

33. Peuhkuri K, Vapaatalo H, Korpela R (2010) Even low-grade inflammation impacts on small intestinal function. World J Gastroenterol 16: 1057–1062.

Embryonic Protein Undernutrition by Albumen Removal Programs the Hepatic Amino Acid and Glucose Metabolism during the Perinatal Period in an Avian Model

Els Willems[1], Tjing-Tjing Hu[2], Laura Soler Vasco[3], Johan Buyse[1*], Eddy Decuypere[1], Lutgarde Arckens[2], Nadia Everaert[1,4]

1 Laboratory of Livestock Physiology, Department of Biosystems, KU Leuven, Leuven, Belgium, **2** Laboratory of Neuroplasticity and Neuroproteomics, KU Leuven, Leuven, Belgium, **3** Division of Livestock-Nutrition-Quality, Department of Biosystems, KU Leuven, Leuven, Belgium, **4** Animal Science Unit, Gembloux Agro-Bio Tech, University of Liège, Gembloux, Belgium

Abstract

Different animal models have been used to study the effects of prenatal protein undernutrition and the mechanisms by which these occur. In mammals, the maternal diet is manipulated, exerting both direct nutritional and indirect hormonal effects. Chicken embryos develop independent from the hen in the egg. Therefore, in the chicken, the direct effects of protein deficiency by albumen removal early during incubation can be examined. Prenatal protein undernutrition was established in layer-type eggs by the partial replacement of albumen by saline at embryonic day 1 (albumen-deprived group), compared to a mock-treated sham and a non-treated control group. At hatch, survival of the albumen-deprived group was lower compared to the control and sham group due to increased early mortality by the manipulation. No treatment differences in yolk-free body weight or yolk weight could be detected. The water content of the yolk was reduced, whereas the water content of the carcass was increased in the albumen-deprived group, compared to the control group, indicating less uptake of nutrients from the yolk. At embryonic day 16, 20 and at hatch, plasma triiodothyronine (T_3), corticosterone, lactate or glucose concentrations and hepatic glycogen content were not affected by treatment. At embryonic day 20, the plasma thyroxine (T_4) concentrations of the albumen-deprived embryos was reduced compared to the control group, indicating a decreased metabolic rate. Screening for differential protein expression in the liver at hatch using two-dimensional difference gel electrophoresis revealed not only changed abundance of proteins important for amino acid metabolism, but also of enzymes related to energy and glucose metabolism. Interestingly, GLUT1, a glucose transporter, and PCK2 and FBP1, two out of three regulatory enzymes of the gluconeogenesis were dysregulated. No parallel differences in gene expressions causing the differences in protein abundance could be detected pointing to post-transcriptional or post-translational regulation of the observed differences.

Editor: Marinus F.W. te Pas, Wageningen UR Livestock Research, Netherlands

Funding: This research was supported by the Fund for Scientific Research Flanders (FWO-Vlaanderen, www.fwo.be) (FWO nr. G.0566.08). The funders had no role in study design, data collection and analysis, decision to publish, or preparation of the manuscript.

Competing Interests: The authors have declared that no competing interests exist.

* E-mail: Johan.buyse@biw.kuleuven.be

Introduction

Studies of the Dutch Hunger Winter (1944–1945) clearly showed that reduced growth *in utero* has detrimental effects on health in later life [1]. An association between a low birth weight and type II diabetes or impaired glucose tolerance has been found in people born around the time of the famine [2]. This means that poor nutrition *in utero* may lead to permanent changes in insulin-glucose metabolism. Indeed, by restricting the nutrient supply during the prenatal period, the fetus adapts to a low nutrient environment and makes metabolic adaptations to survive. However, when nutrition is adequate or overabundant in the postnatal life, a conflict between the programming and the postnatal conditions arises [3,4]. The latter is referred to as the 'fetal origins' hypothesis' [5], which states that it is the conflict between the prenatal metabolic programming and the postnatal conditions that leads to disease and malfunction.

Prenatal protein undernutrition has been studied in several animal models. In these models, the maternal diet is manipulated, exerting direct nutritional effects as well as indirect effects such as hormonal changes on the fetus. As proposed by [6], the approach of albumen removal in avian eggs, as a model of prenatal protein undernutrition, offers a unique avian model to investigate the direct effect of reduced protein availability during embryogenesis on growth and metabolism. Recently, the effect of a low protein diet provided to the hens on metabolic programming of the offspring was investigated in the chicken [7]. Both the investigation of the direct (i.e. chicken embryos) and indirect animals models of prenatal protein deprivation can contribute to unraveling the prenatal programming effects. Several studies have already been conducted examining the effects of albumen removal in chicken for various reasons [6,8,9,10]. A long-term study was previously conducted to examine the importance of albumen as a protein source during embryonic development in the chicken [9]. Before sexual maturation, the body weight and feed intake were reduced. In contrast, during adulthood, an increased body weight was accompanied by reduced reproduction performance (reduced laying rate and egg weight), indicating long-lasting programming effects.

The objective of the present study was to investigate if the chicken model of prenatal protein undernutrition already displays significant differences during the perinatal period, before the conflict between the prenatal and postnatal conditions arises and whether it is possible to detect effects on programming on the protein and gene expression during this period. For this purpose, 3 mL of albumen was removed from layer-type eggs and replaced with saline. During the perinatal period, the present model showed little differences in growth, hormones and metabolites and hepatic glycogen content, supporting the 'fetal origins' hypothesis'. However, metabolic programming caused by prenatal protein undernutrition was revealed by the observed hepatic proteome changes related with amino acids catabolism and glucose metabolism. Interestingly, the differential protein expression of these enzymes was not accompanied by a differential mRNA expression, suggesting that the observed proteome changes are related with post-transcriptional or post-translational events. The present results point to an interesting model, that can be used complementary to mammalian models for the further elucidation of the effects and mechanisms of prenatal protein undernutrition.

Materials and Methods

Ethics statement

All experiments were conducted in strict accordance with the European Communities Council Directive (2003/65/EC) and were approved by the Institutional Ethical Committee of KU Leuven (P132/2008).

Experimental design

Incubation. A total of 528 fertilized Isa Brown layer-type eggs (Vepymo, Poppel, Belgium) from a 48-week-old breeder flock were individually numbered, weighed and randomLy divided over the three treatments. From 19 additional eggs, the albumen and yolk weight were determined. The eggs consisted of 26.6±0.4% yolk, 59.2±0.5% albumen and 14.2±0.3% egg shell. The eggs were incubated with the blunt end up in one forced-draft incubator (PAS Reform, Zeddam, the Netherlands) at a dry bulb temperature of 37.6°C and a wet bulb temperature of 29.0°C and were turned every hour over 90°. On embryonic day (**ED**) 18, all eggs were candled and those with living embryos were transferred from the turning trays to individual hatching baskets. After 22 days of standard incubation, the unhatched eggs were opened and checked for fertility or time of death in order to calculate survival percentage. Infertility was calculated as the number of infertile eggs relative to the total number of set eggs (%). Survival percentage was calculated as the number of hatched chicks relative to the number of fertile eggs (%). Early mortality was defined as dead embryos before ED 10 and mid mortality between ED 10–18. Embryos that died after ED 18 or were ready to hatch and alive in the shell, but had not hatched after 22 days of incubation, were classified as late embryonic mortality. Mortality rates were calculated relative to the number of fertile eggs (%).

Albumen removal. This method was previously described in [9]. Briefly, after one day of incubation (ED 1), albumen removal was established in 240 eggs (albumen-deprived group). After disinfection, a hole was drilled near the sharp end of the egg, 3 mL of albumen was replaced by the same volume of sterile saline, the hole was sealed using a drop of paraffin and the eggs were weighed. Albumen is the main source of protein for the developing embryo [11] and so the net effect is a prenatal protein undernutrition. A sham group of 144 eggs was mock-treated, similar to the albumen-deprived group, except for the actual albumen removal and saline injection. A third group of 144 eggs received no treatment (control group). The difference in the number of eggs for each treatment was based on the higher expected mortality due to albumen removal. To verify that the replacement of the albumen by saline was successful, the mean egg weight before incubation and after manipulation were compared.

Sampling

At embryonic day (ED) 16 and 20 and at hatch, 15 embryos/chicks per group were weighed and killed by decapitation. The residual yolk was dissected and relative weights of both yolk and yolk-free body weight (YFBW) to egg weight at ED 1 were calculated. Weight of liver, heart, digestive tract and carcass was measured and proportional weights relative to YFBW were calculated. The digestive tract was defined as starting from the end of the esophagus, containing the proventriculus, the gizzard, the small and large intestine until the beginning of the cloaca. The carcass was defined as the YFBW minus liver, heart and digestive tract. Water content of yolk and carcass was determined by first drying at 65°C for 48 h and then at 105°C until a constant weight was reached.

At ED 16, blood was taken from the chorioallantoic membrane with a 1-mL syringe and 30 G needle and collected in tubes with heparine (Sigma, Bornem, Belgium). At ED20 and at hatch, blood was taken from the vena jugularis of the embryo or chick with a 1-mL syringe and 27 G needle and collected in tubes with heparine (Sigma, Bornem, Belgium). The blood was centrifuged at 1.500 × g for 10 min at 6°C. The plasma was collected and stored at −20°C for later analyses of triiodothyronine (T_3), thyroxine (T_4), corticosterone, lactate and glucose. Liver samples were taken and snap frozen in liquid nitrogen before storage at −80°C. Frozen liver tissue was homogenized by grinding into powder in liquid nitrogen before use.

Hormones and Metabolites

Plasma analysis was performed on 15 samples per group per sampling day for each measurement. Plasma T_3 and T_4 concentrations were measured by radio-immunoassay (RIA) as described by [12]. The antisera for T_3 and T_4 were purchased from Byk-Belga (Brussels, Belgium). Intra-assay coefficients of variation are 4.5% and 5.4% for T_3 and T_4 respectively. Corticosterone was measured with the Corticosterone Double Antibody – 125I RIA Kit for Animal Testing (07120103, MP Biomedicals, Carlsbad, California, USA). The intra-assay coefficient for corticosterone is 7.1%.

Plasma lactate was measured using a commercially available kit (LAT8840, Ben S.r.l.-Biochemical Enterprise, Milan, Italy) following the manufacturer's instruction. The intra-assay coefficient for lactate is 2.3%. Plasma glucose concentration was determined using a commercially available kit (298–65701, WAKO Pure Chemical Industries Ltd., Osaka, Japan). The absorbance was measured at 490 nm (Victor 1420 Multilabel counter, PerkinElmer, MA, USA). The intra-assay coefficient for glucose is 2.2%.

Glycogen determination

For the determination of the hepatic glycogen content, a method adapted from [13] was used. Tissue was homogenized in exactly the same volume (µL) 7% $HClO_4$ as mg tissue was taken. Homogenates were centrifuged at 4°C at 14,000 g until a clear supernatant was obtained. The supernatant was washed with 1 mL of petroleum ether and stored at −80°C. An iodine color reagent [0.39 mL of an iodine solution (0.104 g I_2, 1.04 g KI_2 in 4 mL of milli-Q water) +30 mL of 10% $CaCl_2$] was added to standards or tissue extracts in a microtiter plate. After mixing and an incubation period of 10 min, the absorbance was measured at 450 nm (Victor 1420 Multilabel counter, PerkinElmer, MA, USA). Tissue glycogen concentration (n = 12) could then be calculated using a standard curve of rabbit liver glycogen (Sigma, Bornem, Belgium). Total glycogen content (ng) was calculated by multiplying the glycogen concentration (ng/mg) with the wet weight of the liver (mg).

Two-dimensional difference gel electrophoresis (2-D DIGE)

The 2-D DIGE was performed as previously described [14]. The fluorescent cyanine dyes (Cy2, propyl-Cy3 and methyl-Cy5) were synthesized as described previously [15,16] according to the method by [17]. All other chemicals were purchased from GE Healthcare, unless mentioned otherwise.

Protein lysates. 100 mg liver tissue taken at hatch (n = 6 per group) was transferred to 500 µL ice-cold lysis buffer, containing 7 M urea, 2 M thiourea, 4% w/v CHAPS (Sigma-Aldrich), 1% w/v DTT (Serva), 40 mM Tris base (ICN; Aurora), pH 8 and Complete Protease Inhibitor Cocktail (Roche Diagnostics, Basel, Switserland). Liver tissue was homogenized on ice, briefly centrifuged at 13,000 rpm, sonicated (3 times 25 sec), followed by a complete solubilization of the proteins for 1 h at room temperature. The proteins were sonicated again briefly and centrifuged for 20 min at 13,000 rpm at 4°C to precipitate cell debris. The supernatant was dialyzed against milli-Q water for 2 h to remove residual salt using a membrane with a 500-Da cutoff (Spectra/Por, Biotech, Omnilabo) and aliquots were stored at −80°C. Protein concentrations were determined with the Quant-iT Protein Assay kit (Q33211, Invitrogen, Carlsbad, CA, USA) using the Qubit Fluorometer 2.0 (Q32866, Invitrogen).

Analytical gels. Pre-cast Immobiline DryStrips (24 cm, pH 3–11 nonlinear) were rehydrated overnight in DeStreak Rehydration Solution containing 0.5% v/v immobilized pH gradient (IPG) buffer in a reswelling tray covered with paraffin oil (Merck). The next day 50 µg protein of each liver samples (n = 6 per group) was randomLy labeled with either propyl-Cy3 (n = 3) or methyl-Cy5 (n = 3) dissolved in dimethylformamide (DMF). The samples were incubated for 30 min on ice in the dark to achieve minimal labeling of proteins with approximately 200 pmol dye and the highest signal-to-noise ratio and maximal number of labeled spots. Labelling was terminated by addition of 1 µL lysine (10 mM; Merck) for 15 min on ice in the dark. Equal fractions of all 18 samples were pooled and per gel 50 µg of this pool was labeled with 200 pmol Cy2 dissolved in DMF to serve as an internal standard. In total, 9 gels were run. The Cy2-, Cy3-, and Cy5-labeled fractions were mixed together, and an equal volume of lysis solution was added. Isoelectric focusing (IEF) was performed in 24-cm long pre-cast Immobiline DryStrips over a pH range of 3–11 (non-linear) on an Ettan IPGphor Cup Loading Manifold system according to manufacturer's instructions. Actual run conditions were 300 V for 3 h, 600 V for 3 h, followed by a 6-h gradient to 1000 V, a 3-h gradient to 8000 V, and 8 h at 8000 V for a total of 75–85 kVh (at 50 µA/strip). After IEF, the strips were reduced with DTT (1% w/v) in equilibration buffer (6 M urea, 34.5% v/v glycerol and 10% w/v SDS in Tris-HCl buffer [1.5 M, pH 8.8]) for 15 min followed by alkylation with 4.5% w/v iodoacetamide (Sigma-Aldrich) in equilibration buffer for 15 min. Electrophoresis of the IPG strips was done on 1.5-mm-thick SDS-polyacrylamide gels (12.5% T; 2.6% C) in the Ettan DALT twelve system for 30 min at 30 mA and 24 h at 15 mA/gel at 13°C. The 2-D DIGE gel plates were rinsed with milli-Q water.

Image analysis. Gels were scanned with the Ettan DIGE Imager (software 1.0; GE Healthcare) and generated gel image triplets (Cy2, Cy3, and Cy5) comprising the CyDye-labeled proteins. Quantitative analysis was carried out with the DeCyder 2D difference analysis software (Version 6.5; GE Healthcare). Spot detection and matching was performed automatically with the DeCyder Batch processor. For spot detection, the estimated number of spots for each co-detection procedure was set to 2500. The best internal standard image (Cy2 labeled samples) based on the number of detected spots and overall similarity of the protein spot pattern with that of other gels was assigned as the "Master" and used as a template. The matching was checked manually in the biological variation analysis (BVA) module to ascertain the accuracy of the match process. Volume ratios were calculated for every spot on every gel by dividing the spot volume (Cy3 or Cy5), by the spot volume of the internal standard (Cy2), thereby correcting for inter-gel variations.

Preparative gels and protein identification. Two preparative gels were run under the same conditions as described above. Each gel was loaded with 1.5 mg of protein from the pool sample, from which only a 50 µg fraction was labeled with Cy3. Glass plates were pretreated with BindSilane, and 2 reference markers were applied to enable automatic spot picking. The preparative gels were scanned in the Ettan DIGE Imager to obtain an image of the Cy3 signal. Subsequently, the total protein load was visualized by fluorescent LavaPurple Total protein stain according to the manufacturer's instructions (GelCompany, San Fransisco, California, USA), and the gels were scanned again. Matching with the analytical gels was carried out automatically with manual correction by the BVA module of the DeCyder software. A pick list of the proteins of interest was generated and imported into the Spot Picker Version 1.20 software that controls the Ettan Spot Picker (GE Healthcare, Little Chalfont, UK) and the relevant spots were excised. All subsequent steps were carried out under a laminar flow hood in dust-free conditions to prevent keratin contamination of the samples. Identical spots from the two preparative gels were pooled. Before tryptic digestion, the gel pieces were thoroughly rinsed with milli-Q water, 50% v/v acetonitrile (ACN) (Biosolve) and again with milli-Q water. After drying in a SpeedVac vacuum centrifuge, they were incubated overnight at 37°C in a 40 µL digestion solution containing 100 ng modified porcine trypsin (sequencing grade, Promega, Fitchburg, Wisconsin, USA), 25 mM NH_4HCO_3, and 5% v/v ACN. Tryptic peptides were extracted from the gel pieces by 2 washing steps of 30 min in a bath sonicator. In the first step, a 100 µL solution of 5% v/v ACN and 0.5% formic acid (FA) (Riedel-de-Haën), and the second step was carried out in a 50 µL solution containing 10% ACN and 0.5% FA. The supernatant was concentrated to a volume of approximately 20 µL using SpeedVac vacuum centrifugation. Automated LC-MS analyses were run on an Ultimate 3000 Nano LC System (Dionex) coupled on-line to a microTOF-Q mass spectrometer (Bruker Daltonics). The total volume of each sample was pipetted in a polypropylene vial (Dionex, LC-Packings) and loaded in the LC autosampler. 5 µL of this peptide solution was transferred to the precolumn (C18 PepMap100 internal diameter (i.d.) 300 lm 3 5 mm; Dionex, LC Packings) and reversed phase eluted over a 75 µm i.d.×15 cm PepMap 100 C18 nanocolumn at a flow rate of 200 nL/min, using a linear gradient from 5% to 40% of ACN/0.5% FA in 25 min. The column outlet was coupled to the Q-TOF through a stainless steel needle at 2000 V. The ionized peptides in the range of 400–1400 m/z were automatically selected and fragmented using predefined collision energy profiles, depending on the detected peptide charge. LC-MS data were processed using the Data Analysis software version 3.4 of Bruker Daltonics and submitted to the Mascot MS/MS ions search engine using the same parameters. For protein identification, the SwissProt 51.6 database (limited to Chordata) was used and a 95% confidence interval threshold ($P<0.05$) was set. The molecular function and subcellular location of these proteins were examined using UNIPROT.

Identification of relevant canonical pathways. The list of differentially expressed proteins was imported into the Ingenuity Pathway Analysis (IPA; Ingenuity Systems, Redwood City, CA, USA) to identify biological interactions between the proteins. The biological interaction scores were defined by the IPA statistical algorithm based on its knowledge base, and the P-value was corrected for multiple comparisons with the Benjamini–Hochberg test.

Quantitative real-time PCR

RNA extraction and reverse transcription. Total RNA was extracted using 750 µL of TRIzol (Invitrogen, Paisley, UK) added to approximately 50 mg of crushed liver sample taken at hatch ($n=8$ per group), and incubated for 5 min at room temperature. 300 µL of chloroform (Sigma Aldrich, Missouri, USA) was added to create a phase separation. After a short vortex step, the samples were centrifuged at 14,000 rpm for 15 min at 4°C. The aqueous phase was transferred to fresh tubes, mixed with 375 µL ice-cold isopropanol (Prolabo, VWR, West Chester, Pennsylvania, USA) and incubated for 10 min at room temperature. After centrifugation (14,000 rpm, 10 min, 4°C), the supernatant was discarded and the remaining RNA pellet was washed with 750 µL ice-cold 70% ethanol (Prolabo, VWR, West Chester, Pennsylvania, USA). After a final centrifugation step (7,500 rpm, 5 min, 4°C), the supernatant was carefully removed and the remaining RNA pellet was dissolved in 1:1000 DEPC-treated water (Fluka). The RNA concentration and quality (260/280 ratio) was measured using UV-spectroscopy (Implen, Westburg, Leusden, The Netherlands). The integrity of the RNA was electrophoretically verified using 2% agarose (Sigma Aldrich, Missouri, USA) gel electrophoresis and Midori Green DNA Stain (MG02, NIPPON Genetics Europe GmbH, Dueren, DE).

The RNA was transcribed into cDNA using the Reverse Transcription system (A3500, Promega, Madison, WI, USA). Denaturation was performed for 3 min at 80°C followed by 45 min at 42°C for the reverse transcription. The reaction was stopped by heating the samples for 5 min at 95°C.

Primer design. The intron-spanning primers for the different genes were designed using Primer Designing Tool (NCBI). The primers were purchased from IDT (Integrated DNA Technologies Inc., Coralville, Iowa, USA). In table 1, all primers are listed, both for reference genes and the genes of interest. For every pair of primers used, standard curves were made and PCR efficiencies were calculated according to the following formula: PCR efficiency $= -1+10^{-1/\text{slope}}$ [18]. A PCR efficiency between 90% and 110% is generally considered acceptable, with correlation coefficient >0.99. Final primer concentration was 0.3 µM for all primer pairs.

qRT-PCR. Quantitative real-time PCR (qRT-PCR) measurements were performed in duplicate using the ABI StepOnePlus (Applied Biosystems, Carlsbad, USA) and Maxima SYBR Green/ROX qPCR Master Mix (2x, Fermentas Life Sciences, St. Leon-Rot, Germany). 1 µL of 1:2 diluted cDNA was used as input in 25 µL reaction. The PCR reaction program began with 10 min heating at 95°C followed by 40 cycles of 15 seconds at 95°C and 60 seconds at 60°C. For the analysis of the qRT-PCR output, the $2^{-\Delta\Delta CT}$ method of relative quantification was used [19]. Expression of genes was normalized to the geometric average of the two references genes: β-actine (ACTB) and peptidylprolylisomerase D (PPID). In addition, a melting curve analysis was performed to check the specificity of the primers (15 seconds at 95°C, 1 minute at 60°C, temperature gradually increased by 0.3°C until 95°C is reached).

Statistical Analysis

All data were processed with the statistical software package SAS version 9.2 (SAS Institute Inc., Cary, NC). A GLM was used to analyse the effect of treatment (control, sham and albumen-deprived group), age (ED 16, ED 20 and at hatch) and their interaction on the measured parameters: absolute and relative YFBW and residual yolk weight, water content of the residual yolk and carcass, absolute and proportional liver, digestive tract and heart weight, plasma T_3, T_4, corticosterone, glucose and lactate concentrations. The liver glycogen content, logarithms of the volume ratios (Cy3/Cy2 or Cy5/Cy2) of the protein spots of 2-D DIGE and the fold change of phosphoenolpyruvate carboxykinase 1 (PCK1) and 2 (PCK2), fructose-1,6-bisphosphatase 1 (FBP1) and 3-hydroxyisobutyrate dehydrogenase (HIBADH) were analysed using the one-way ANOVA with treatment as variable. When there was a significant overall effect of treatment, or interaction with age, the means were further compared by a post-hoc Tukey's test. Survival rate, early, mid and late embryonic mortality, and infertility were analyzed using the logistic regression model with treatment as the classification variable. For all parameters, a degree of significance of 5% was used. All data are shown as mean ± SEM.

Results

Survival and mortality

Survival until hatch (Table 2) differed between all three experimental groups. The albumen-deprived group had a lower survival compared to both the control ($P<0.001$)) and the sham group ($P<0.001$). Furthermore, the survival was also reduced in the sham group compared to the control group ($P=0.001$). The albumen-deprived group had a higher early mortality (Table 2) than the control group ($P<0.001$), with the sham group being intermediate and different from both the control ($P<0.001$) and the albumen-deprived group ($P<0.001$). No differences between treatments were found for the mid or late mortality (Table 2). Infertility was similar in all treatments (Table 2).

Yolk-free body and residual yolk weight

The absolute and relative (to egg weight at ED1) YFBW and residual yolk weight (Table 3) were only affected by age ($P<0.001$) but not by treatment or the interaction. The water content of the yolk (Table 3) however, was affected by treatment ($P=0.016$), but not by age or the interaction. The albumen-deprived group had a lower water content of the yolk compared with the control group ($P=0.012$), whereas the sham group was not different from either the control or the albumen-deprived group.

Table 1. List of primers used for quantification of the genes of interest and reference genes.

Gene	Accession number		5′-primer-3′	Tm (°C)	Size (bp)	Efficiency (%)
PCK2	NM_205470	F	GGCCGAGCACATGCTGATTT	61.7	62	102.7
		R	CCGCCATGTAACGCTTCTCA	60.7		
PCK1	NM_205471	F	GGAAGTAGCCAGCTGGGTCGC	59.5	91	105.1
		R	TTGTGCGTCCTTGCATGCAGC	59.1		
FBP1	NM_001278048	F	TGCTGCGGTCACCGAGTATCTCA	59.8	56	95.6
		R	GCGAACTGCCGTCCTCAGGG	59.8		
HIBADH	NM_001006362	F	CCTGGGTGCTCAGGTAACAG	60.0	84	99.4
		R	TTGGGACTTGAAGGCAGCAT	59.9		
ACTB	NM_205518	F	TCGCCCCAGACATCAGGGTGTGA	61.5	75	103.3
		R	TTGCTCTGGGCTTCATCACCAACGT	60.9		
PPID	XM_426283	F	GTCGCACCCGTCCCCTGTAGA	60.0	93	101.8
		R	ATTCGTCCAACTCGCTCTCCCC	58.4		

For every gene the NCBI accession number, the sequences and the theoretical melting temperature (Tm, °C) of the forward (F) and reverse primer (R), the size of the amplified fragment (bp) and the efficiency of amplification (%) are provided.

Body composition

Only age had an effect on the absolute liver, absolute carcass, absolute and proportional digestive tract and absolute and proportional heart weight (data not shown). The proportional liver (to YFBW) weight, however, was affected by age ($P<0.001$) and almost by treatment ($P=0.057$), but not by the interaction. The albumen-deprived chicks had a numerically lower proportional liver weight (2.00±0.03%) than the control (2.10±0.04%) and the sham group (2.08±0.04%). The proportional carcass weight was affected by treatment ($P=0.024$), age ($P<0.001$) and the interaction ($P=0.026$). At hatch, the albumen-deprived chicks had a higher proportional carcass weight (84.0±0.3 g) than the control (82.1±0.4 g, $P=0.032$) and the sham group (82.1±0.4 g, $P=0.034$). The water content of the carcass was affected both by age ($P<0.001$) and treatment ($P=0.017$). The albumen-deprived chicks had a higher water content of the carcass (82.2±0.3%) than the control chicks (81.3±0.3%, $P=0.014$), whereas the sham group (81.6±0.3%) was not different from both other groups.

Plasma hormones and metabolites and liver glycogen

Only an effect of age ($P<0.001$) was observed on the plasma T_3 concentrations, with concentrations increasing with age (Figure 1A). The plasma T_4 levels (Figure 1B) were affected by treatment ($P=0.033$), age ($P<0.001$) and the interaction ($P=0.001$). On ED20, the albumen-deprived group had lower T_4 levels than the control group ($P<0.001$). Corticosterone levels were not influenced by age, treatment or the interaction (data not shown). Glucose and lactate levels were only affected by age ($P<0.001$, data not shown). The glycogen content of the liver (Figure 2) had an effect of age ($P<0.001$) but not of treatment or the interaction.

Screening for differential proteins in liver samples at hatch using 2-D DIGE

Of the approximately 1400 spots present on the gels (Figure 3), 15 spots were affected by treatment ($P<0.05$). Spots exhibiting differences between the control and the sham group were excluded, as these differences are induced by the manipulation of the egg and not the prenatal undernutrition effect. Only the spots for which the expression in the albumen-deprived group differed from the control group (4 spots), the sham group (1 spot) or both (3 spots) were selected for identification by mass spectrometry. Table 4 shows the proteins that were identified in each of the spots. Four of these protein spots were upregulated,

Table 2. Survival percentage (%), early, mid and late mortality (%) and infertility (%) of the eggs of the control, sham and albumen-deprived group.

Item (%)	control	sham	albumen-deprived	P-value
Survival	87.7[a]	69.3[b]	38.1[c]	<0.001
Early mortality	7.0[a]	25.4[b]	55.7[c]	<0.001
Mid mortality	0.0	0.0	0.5	NS
Late mortality	5.3	5.3	5.7	NS
Infertility	2.6	4.2	2.3	NS

Number of fertile eggs in control (n = 144), sham (n = 144) and albumen-deprived group (n = 240).
[a–c]Within a row, treatment means with different superscript are significantly different ($P<0.001$). P-values of effect of treatment are added in a separate column.
Survival (%) = (number of hatched chicks/number of fertile eggs)*100
Mortality (%) = (number of dead eggs/number of fertile eggs)*100
Infertility (%) = (number of infertile eggs/total number of set eggs) *100

Table 3. Yolk-free body weight (YFWB) (g), relative YFBW to egg weight at embryonic day 1 (ED1) (%), absolute (g) and relative residual yolk to egg weight at ED1 (%) at ED 16, 20 and at hatch of the control, sham, and albumen-deprived group (n = 15 per group per age).

	control		sham		albumen-deprived		P-value treatment	P-value age	P-value interaction
	Mean	SEM	Mean	SEM	Mean	SEM			
YFBW weight (g)	28.7	1.3	29.0	1.3	28.5	1.4	NS	<0.001	NS
Relative YFBW weight (%)	48.3	2.2	47.6	2.2	47.0	2.2	NS	<0.001	NS
Residual yolk weight (g)	9.0	0.5	9.1	0.5	8.8	0.5	NS	<0.001	NS
Relative residual yolk weight (%)	14.9	0.7	14.7	0.7	14.8	0.8	NS	<0.001	NS
Water content residual yolk (%)	52.4[a]	0.5	51.8[ab]	0.4	50.8[b]	0.4	0.016	NS	NS

[a–b]Within a row, treatment means with different superscript are significantly different (P<0.05). P-values of effect of treatment, age and interaction are added in separate columns. Data are shown as mean ± SEM.

while 4 were downregulated in the liver of albumen-deprived chicks. Key metabolic pathways and protein networks affected by the treatment of prenatal protein undernutrion by albumen removal in the chicken were identified by systems biology analysis using Ingenuity Pathways analysis (IPA) software. Relevant pathways are listed in Table 5. Several of these pathways are involved in the degradation of amino acids such as valine, methionine, cysteine and glutamate. Moreover, pathways direct or indirect involved in the glucose metabolism are also apparent: glycolysis/gluconeogenesis, tricarboxylic acid cycle (TCA) and fermentation of pyruvate to lactate. Finally, activation of TR/RXR (thyroid and retinoid X receptor) and FXR/RXR (farnesoid X receptor, retinoid X receptor, cholesterol homeostasis) were detected.

Gene expression of PCK1, PCK2, FBP1 and HIBADH

To investigate if differences in gene expression might cause the difference in protein abundance, several proteins were selected and the mRNA expression was examined. No effect of treatment could be detected on the gene expression of PCK1, PCK2, HIBADH or FBP1 (Table 6), although a trend was observed towards decreased expression of FBP1 ($P = 0.094$). The expression of FBP1 in the liver of albumen-deprived chicks at hatch tended to be reduced compared to the control or sham chicks.

Discussion

Our previous study demonstrated the existence of long-term effects of prenatal protein undernutrition by albumen removal on the body weight and reproduction performance of laying hens [9]. According to the 'fetal origins' hypothesis' [5], it is the conflict between prenatal environment (i.e. reduced protein availability) and the postnatal conditions (i.e. adequate protein levels) that causes disease and malfunction in later life. Indeed, by restricting the nutrient supply during the prenatal period, the fetus adapts to a low nutrient environment and makes metabolic adaptations to survive. However, when nutrition is adequate or overabundant in the postnatal life, a conflict between the programming and the postnatal conditions arises. The objective of the present study was to investigate if the chicken model of prenatal protein undernutrition by albumen removal already displays metabolic programming effects during the late embryonic period until hatch (before access to feed), before the conflict is created.

Effects on YFBW and body composition were examined as phenotypic parameters. In the current study, the equal absolute and relative YFBW and yolk weight together with a lower water content of the yolk (and hence higher weight of dry matter in the yolk) of the albumen-deprived chicks, would suggest a lower utilisation of solids to obtain an equal body weight. In contrast, results from [9] implied a higher consumption of the available yolk by the albumen-deprived group to support an equal embryonic growth until hatch. This discrepancy is remarkable, however, the higher water content of the carcass (and hence less solids in the carcass) is in agreement with increased amount of solids remaining in the yolk, as less were used to synthesize tissue. In addition, no differences in body composition was observed in the albumen-deprived chicks except for a marginally lower proportional liver weight together with an equal YFBW and reduced carcass weight. These results are in agreement with the 'fetal origins' hypothesis' [5]. Since these investigations are focused on the perinatal period, no conflict between the prenatal prenatal (i.e. reduced protein availability) and postnatal environment (i.e. adequate protein levels) has emerged.

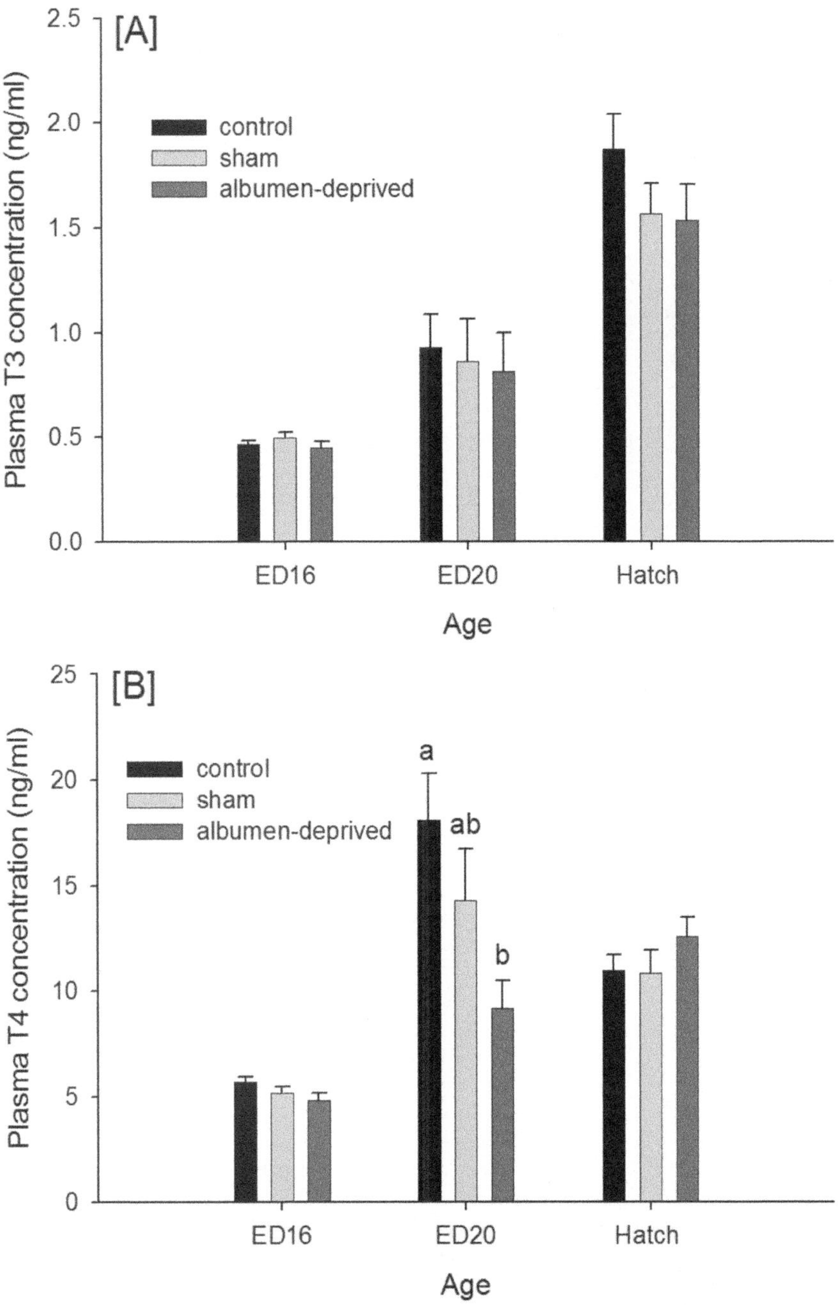

Figure 1. Plasma thyroid hormones. T_3 (A) and T_4 (B) concentrations (ng/mL) of the control, sham and the albumen-deprived chicks at embryonic day (ED) 16, ED 20 and at hatch (n = 15). Data are shown as mean ± SEM.[a–b] Treatment means differ per timepoint (P<0.05).

The metabolic programming effect was examined by screening for differences in hepatic proteome at hatch. Four proteins spots were upregulated, whereas 4 others were downregulated in the albumen-deprived chicks. To investigate the biological significance of these results, the IPA software was implemented to identify key canonical pathways. As expected, several pathways involved in the catabolism of amino acids such as valine, methionine, cysteine and glutamate were enriched in our dataset. Downregulation of mitochondrial 3-hydroxybutyrate dehydrogenase (HIBADH) and upregulation of dihydrolipoyl dehydrogenase (DLD) was detected. These enzymes are involved in the degradation of branched-chain amino acids such as valine, leucine and isoleucine. HIBADH converts 3-hydroxy-2-methylpropanoate to 2-methyl-3-oxopropanoate, whereas DLD is a component of several enzyme complexes such as the branched chain α-keto acid dehydrogenase involved in the catabolism of leucine, isoleucine and valine. Cystathionine gamma-lyase (CTH) was upregulated and is involved in the last step in the trans-sulfuration pathway from methionine to cysteine and can be both involved in the degradation of methionine and cysteine. Finally, upregulated glutamate dehydrogenase 1 (GLUD1) is involved in the biosynthesis or catabolism of glutamate and catalyzes the oxidative deamination of glutamate to 2-ketoglutarate which is an important intermediate in the TCA cycle. The observed increase in amino

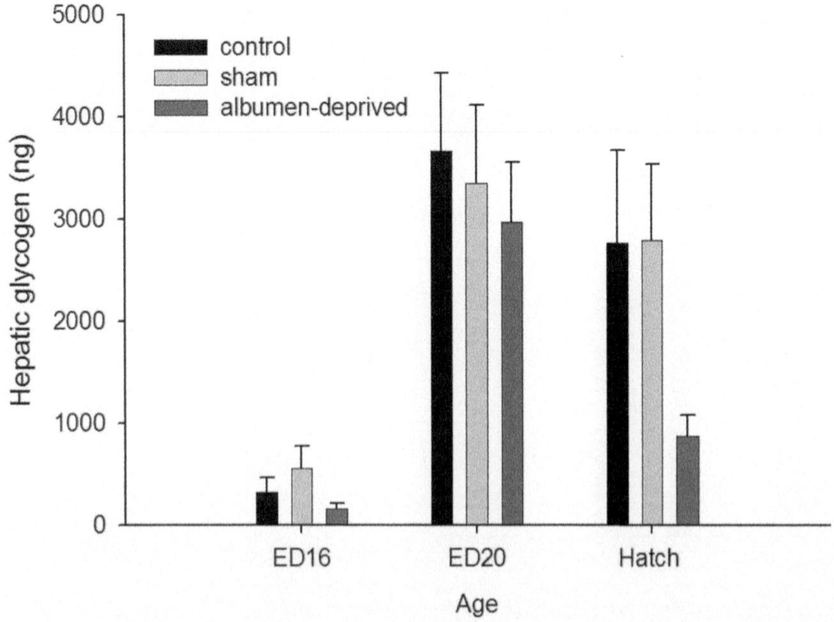

Figure 2. Glycogen in the liver. Hepatic glycogen content (ng) of the control, sham and the albumen-deprived chicks at embryonic day (ED) 16, ED 20 and at hatch (n = 12). Data are shown as mean ± SEM.

acids catabolism may be necessary to compensate for the lack of energy available caused by the embryonic undernutrition. As the albumen removal decreased the protein availability at the end of the incubation, changes in the expression of enzymes involved in amino acid metabolism could be foreseen. Indeed, a previous study also found indications of an altered protein metabolism in broilers treated by albumen removal before incubation, suggesting a transient increase in muscle proteolysis [8].

Metabolic programming caused by prenatal protein undernutrition was revealed by the observed hepatic proteome changes related with glucose metabolism. Upregulation of L-lactate dehydrogenase B chain (LDHB) suggests an increased conversion of pyruvate to lactate in the absence of oxygen in the liver. This lactate can subsequently be converted to glucose by the gluconeogenesis. Two of the regulatory enzymes of the latter pathway were dysregulated in the liver. Fructose-1,6-biphosphatase 1 (FBP1) was downregulated, whereas phosphoenolpyruvate 2 (PCK2) was upregulated. FBP1 catalyzes the conversion of D-fructose-1,6-biphosphate to D-fructose-6-phosphate, whereas PCK2 catalyzes the conversion of oxaloacetate to phosphoenolpyruvate, the rate-limiting step. Upregulated α-enolase (ENO1) is also involved in both the gluconeogenesis and glycolysis and catalyzes the conversion of 2-phospho-D-glycerate to phosphoenolpyruvate. In addition, glucose transporter 1 (GLUT1), a facilitative low capacity/high affinity glucose transporter across the plasma membrane was upregulated. Hepatic GLUT1 is primarily involved in cellular uptake of glucose from the plasma into the hepatocytes when nutrients are in reduced supply [20]. As no differences in plasma glucose or lactate levels were found, it is not clear whether the gluconeogenesis pathway in general is up- or downregulated.

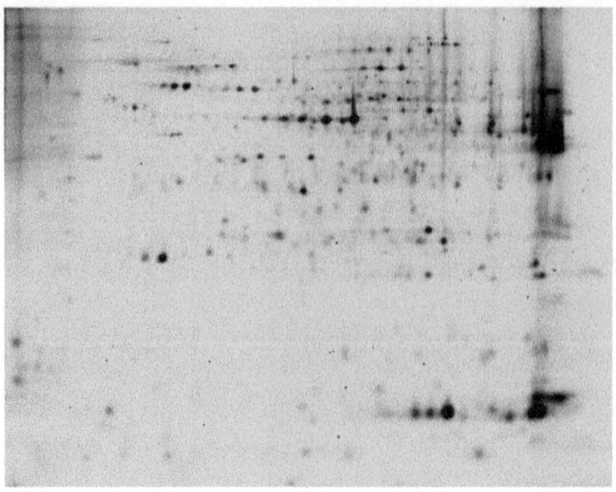

Figure 3. Hepatic proteome of the newly-hatched chick. Visualization of the total number of spots in the hepatic proteome of the newly-hatched chick on a Cy2 image (pooled sample) of an analytic two-dimensional gel electrophoresis (2-D DIGE) gel.

Furthermore, a general upregulation of the TCA pathway was observed, from the upregulation of several enzymes involved such as DLD, aconitate hydratase (ACO2) and malate dehydrogenase 1 (MDH1). DLD is a component of the pyruvate dehydrogenase complex, which converts pyruvate, originating from the breakdown of carbohydrates to acetyl-CoA, the input for the TCA cycle. ACO2 catalyzes the isomerization of citrate to isocitrate via cis-aconitate, and MDH1 the conversion of malate to oxaloacetate. As previously stated, upregulation of GLUD1 leads to increased production of 2-ketoglutarate, an important intermediate of the TCA cycle. Upregulation of the TCA cycle leads to an increase in energy generation from the oxidation of acetate, derived from carbohydrates, fat and proteins.

As synthesis and degradation of **glycogen** are vital for embryonic survival during the last phase of incubation [21], glycogen levels were determined in liver, the most metabolically active tissue of the embryo. Although no significant effects of treatment or an interaction with age could be observed, the albumen-deprived chicks had lower hepatic glycogen content at hatch as compared to both the control and the sham group, suggesting that the released glucose can be distributed to extra-

Table 4. Identification with LC-MS/MS of the proteins present in the 4 upregulated and 4 downregulated spots in the liver of albumen-deprived chicks at hatch compared to either the control chicks or the sham chicks or both (n = 6).

Gene	Full name	Spot	Uniprot ID	pI	Mass (kDa)	Mascot Score	Queries	Coverage (%)	Location	control	sham	albumen-deprived	P-value
UP													
HSPA9	Stress-70 protein, mitochondrial precursor	407	Q5ZM98	6.09	73,2	188	5	10	Mt	1.00 ± 0.09^{b}	1.10 ± 0.07^{ab}	1.44 ± 0.12^{a}	0.010
ALB	Serum albumin		P19121	5.51	69,9	145	16	26	Pl				
HSPA2	Heat shock 70 kDa protein		P08106	5.52	69,8	137	4	9	Cs				
ALB	Serum albumin	439	P19121	5.51	69,9	88	12		Pl	1.00 ± 0.11^{b}	1.04 ± 0.07^{ab}	1.38 ± 0.14^{a}	0.035
PCK2	Phosphoenolpyruvate carboxykinase2	232	P21642	7.56	71,1	364	10	16	Mt	1.00 ± 0.05^{b}	1.12 ± 0.04^{ab}	1.28 ± 0.09^{a}	0.021
LMNA	Lamin-A		P13648	6.50	73,2	113	2	3	Mt, Nu				
ENO1	Alpha-enolase§		P51913	6.17	47,3	112	3	10	Cp				
TUFM	Elongation factor Tu		P84172	8.98	38,3	52	1	3	Mt				
MDH1	Malate dehydrogenase 1		Q5ZME2	6.92	36,5	36	1	3	Cp				
ACO2	Aconitate hydratase§	274	Q8AYI3	8.04	85,8	261	6	9	Mt	1.00 ± 0.03^{b}	1.01 ± 0.02^{b}	1.12 ± 0.04^{a}	0.010
DLD	Dihydrolipoyl dehydrogenase§		Q5ZM32	8.19	54.0	138	6	14	Mt				
GLUD1	Glutamate dehydrogenase 1		P00368	8.48	55,7	65	4	12	Mt				
ALB	Serum albumin§		P19121	5.51	69,9	69	1	3	Pl				
PCK2	Phosphoenolpyruvate carboxykinase		P21642	7.56	71,1	59	1	2	Mt				
CTH	Cystathionine gamma-lyase§		E1BYF1	6.85	43,9	51	1	3	Cp				
GLUT1	Solute carrier family 2, facilitated glucose transporter member 1		P46896	8.82	54,1	42	2	1	Cm				
SMAD3	Mothers against decapentaplegic homolog 3		P84023	6.70	48,3	37	1	3	Cp, Nu				
LDHB	L-lactate dehydrogenase B chain		P00337	7.07	36,3	36	1	3	Cp				
DOWN													
RPLP0	60S acidic ribosomal protein P0§	1033	P47826	5.71	34,3	42	1	3	Rb	1.00 ± 0.07^{ab}	1.04 ± 0.09^{a}	0.78 ± 0.07^{b}	0.050
FBP1	Fructose-1,6-bisphosphatase 1§	1045	Q9I8D4	5.22	18,2	81	3	7	Cp	1.00 ± 0.10^{a}	0.89 ± 0.08^{ab}	0.63 ± 0.12^{b}	0.036
HIBADH	3-hydroxyisobutyrate dehydrogenase §	1126	Q5ZLI9	8.60	35,3	421	10	16	Mt	1.00 ± 0.10^{a}	0.99 ± 0.06^{a}	0.58 ± 0.14^{b}	0.011
TST	Thiosulfate sulfurtransferase	1135	P25324	6.56	32,3	92	7	15	Mt	1.00 ± 0.20^{a}	1.16 ± 0.16^{a}	0.42 ± 0.16^{b}	0.007

The spot number (Spot), Uniprot accession number (Uniprot ID), theoretical iso-electric point (pI), theoretical molecular weight (Mass), Mascot score, number of matched peptides (Queries) and sequence coverage (Coverage) are shown. The cellular localization (Location) is also indicated: Cm = cell membrane, Cp = cytoplasm, Cs = cell surface, Mt = mitochondria, Nu = nucleus, Pl = plasma and Rb = Ribosome. The mean fluorescence (Cy3 or Cy5) of the different spots normalized according to the fluorescence signal of the pooled sample (Cy2) ± SEM are shown in the table for the control, sham and albumen-deprived chicks. [a–b] Within a row, treatment means with different superscript are significantly different ($P<0.05$). P-values of effect of treatment are added in a separate column. Most of the identified spots contained just one protein, but several enclosed multiple proteins. On the other hand, some proteins were present in more than one spot. Porcine trypsine was added for fragmentation before LC-MS/MS and this was consequently identified in the samples but this was omitted for clarity. §Homologous protein was identified in different species, but results are always displayed for the chicken (*Gallus gallus*).

Table 5. Identification of relevant canonical pathways affected by albumen removal by grouping of the differential expressed proteins through the use of Ingenuity Pathway Analysis (IPA).

	Molecules	B-H P-value	Ratio
Ingenuity canonical pathways			
TCA cycle II	ACO2, DLD, MDH1	3.55E-04	3/41
Gluconeogenesis I	ENO1, FBP1, MDH1	3.55E-04	3/48
Glucocorticoid receptor signaling	PCK2, SMAD3, HSPA9, HSPA2	2.57E-03	4/299
Valine Degradation I	HIBADH, DLD	8.13E-03	2/35
Glycolysis I	ENO1, FBP1	8.51E-03	2/41
Superpathway of Methionine Degradation	DLD, CTH	1.82E-02	2/64
TR/RXR Activation	ENO1, GLUT1	2.88E-02	2/109
FXR/RXR Activation	PCK2, FBP1	2.88E-02	2/110
L-cysteine degradation II	CTH	2.88E-02	1/5
Glutamate Biosynthesis/Degradation X	GLUD1	2.95E-02	1/7
Pyruvate Fermentation to Lactate	LDHB	2.95E-02	1/9

IPA-analysis (www.ingenuity.com) was used to identify key biological pathways comprising the differentially identified proteins after prenatal protein undernutrition by albumen removal in chicken. The significance of the canonical pathways was tested by the stringent Benjamini-Hochberg (B-H) multiple testing correction method. The ratio indicates the number of differential proteins in a given pathway divided by the total number of molecules that make up that pathway. The following proteins, annotated with their gene names, are included in the canonical pathways. Abbreviations: ACO2 (Aconitate hydratase); CTH (Cystathionine gamma-lyase); DLD (Dihydrolipoyl dehydrogenase); ENO1 (Alpha-enolase); FBP1 (Fructose-1,6-bisphosphatase 1); GLUD1 (Glutamate dehydrogenase 1); GLUT1 (Solute carrier family 2, facilitated glucose transporter member 1); HIBADH (3-hydroxyisobutyrate dehydrogenase); HSPA2 (Heat shock 70 kDa protein); HSPA9 (Stress-70 protein, mitochondrial precursor); LDHB (L-lactate dehydrogenase B chain); MDH1 (Malate dehydrogenase); PCK2 (Phosphoenolpyruvate carboxykinase); SMAD3 (Mothers against decapentaplegic homolog 3).

hepatic tissue or be used as an energy source in the liver. The variation in glycogen content between individual chicks, however, was very high, but since chicks were randomly selected for sampling, individual chicks may exhibit different hatch times and it is known that time of hatching has an impact on hepatic glycogen content [22]. Reduced liver glycogen content at hatch can be caused by either an increased use of glycogen during the hatching process or a decreased build-up of glycogen before hatch, although the latter is not likely since no differences in glycogen content were detected at ED20. It seems that the albumen-deprived chicks had to degrade more of the hepatic glycogen content, needed as energy source during the energy demanding hatching process [21].

Interestingly, several of the affected proteins are involved in glucocorticoid receptor (GR) signaling. Glucocorticoid hormones have a central role in the regulation of the glucose metabolism and bind to the GR, which is a transcription factor for regulating gene expression. In sheep, glucocorticoid receptor expression is increased in the liver of neonatal offspring born to ewes which were nutrient restricted during early-mid-gestation [23]. Offspring of rat dams that were protein-restricted throughout gestation had increased glucocorticoid receptor protein and mRNA expression in liver during fetal and postnatal life [24,25]. The GR was not identified amongst the upregulated proteins, yet may not appear in a 2-D DIGE gel due to its membrane location. However, several proteins involved in GR signaling were upregulated. The level of plasma corticosterone, an important glucocorticoid in birds, however, was not affected in our model.

An upregulation of ENO1 and GLUT1 can be associated with increased TR/RXR activation. The thyroid hormone receptor (TR) is usually found as a heterodimer with RXR (retinoid X receptor) and regulates gene expression. Thyroid hormones are involved in a range of biological processes such as growth, development and metabolism. Plasma thyroid hormone concentrations, both T_3 and T_4, are reference measurements for evaluating the level of metabolism of the embryos [26]. Plasma T_3 concentrations, the biologically active form of thyroid hormone, however, did not differ between groups, although the T_4 concentrations at ED20 were significantly lower for the albumen-deprived embryos as compared to the control, indicating a decreased metabolism. The sham embryos had an intermediate plasma T_4 value.

Some of the affected proteins (i.e. GLUT1, FBP1 and PCK2) have previously been associated with effects of prenatal protein undernutrition in mammalian models and will be discussed in more detail.

The GLUT proteins are a family of facilitative transport proteins, catalyzing glucose uptake across the plasma membrane, the rate-limiting step in glucose metabolism. In mammals, GLUT1 is expressed ubiquitously and facilitates the basal glucose uptake, which is essential for growth and development in most cells [27]. Expression of GLUT1 has previously been examined in other mammalian models of prenatal undernutrition, but no differences could be detected [28,29]. Chickens exhibit a peculiar glucose transport and glucose homeostasis, since they are lacking GLUT4, the major insulin-responsive transporter [30]. The mechanism for regulation of blood glucose concentration in chickens is not well understood. Furthermore, no information is available on the roles of the chickens GLUT isoforms in relation to glucose metabolism. Most likely, GLUT1 will act in maintaining basal glucose transport in most chicken cell types as in mammals, however the precise function of GLUT1 in the chicken remains to be elucidated [27].

Chickens maintain an elevated level of blood glucose (10 mM), which is supported by high rates of gluconeogenesis. In the present study, prenatal protein undernutrition caused an increase in PCK2 protein abundance, as opposite to the decreased FBP1 protein abundance and the decreased glycogen content. The liver glycogen content has previously been shown to change in a reciprocal way to the cytosolic PCK activity [31]. Indeed, there

Table 6. Gene expression of PCK1, PCK2, HIBADH and FBP1 normalized to the geometric average of expression of ACTB and PPID of the control, sham and the albumen-deprived chicks (n = 8) in the liver of newly-hatched chicks.

	control		sham		albumen-deprived		P-valuetreatment
	Mean	SEM	Mean	SEM	Mean	SEM	
HIBADH	1.00	0.10	0.95	0.06	0.87	0.05	NS
PCK1	1.00	0.50	0.79	0.26	1.08	0.44	NS
PCK2	1.00	0.05	0.96	0.08	0.94	0.07	NS
FBP1	1.00	0.04	0.97	0.06	0.85	0.04	0.094

Data are shown as mean ± SEM.

are two forms of PCK found in most species, differing in their cellular localization: cytosolic PCK1 and mitochondrial PCK2. The relative abundance of both isoforms is dependent on the animal species and the growth stage of the animal (review [32]). In the avian liver, the mitochondrial PCK activity is the most abundant one but during the perinatal period the cytosolic PCK activity increased considerable from a few days before hatching to 4 days after hatching [31]. As PCK1 is the most abundant form in rats and has been linked previously with effects of prenatal protein undernutrition, the expression of both PCK1 and PCK2 was measured. Both genes were present in similar amounts in the liver at hatch, but were not influenced by the applied treatment.

Rats and mice have been used extensively to examine the effects of the maternal diet on the programming of the progeny. In rat dams fed a protein-restricted diet an increase in PCK1 mRNA and increased activity was detected in liver of the progeny until 11 months of age, suggesting that programming of the metabolism also extends to the regulation of gene expression [33]. In the offspring of intrauterine growth retarded rats by uteroplacental insufficiency, the hepatic expression of both PCK1 and FBP1 were increased [34]. A persistent increase in the gene expression of hepatic PCK, catalyzing the first, committed step of gluconeogenesis, leads to reduced ability of insulin to suppress hepatic glucose output, a change which is characteristic of type 2 diabetes [33]. Conversely in mink, it has been shown that feeding a low protein diet to the dam reduced the FBP1 mRNA expression in the liver of the offspring. The expression of PCK1, however, was not affected [35]. The latter is in agreement with the present study where a reduced FBP1 protein level and a trend for decreased FBP1 mRNA level was found.

Since in mammalian models of prenatal protein undernutrition, differences in gene expression are often found, the mRNA expression of the differential proteins was measured to examine if the same might be true for programming effects in the chicken. Expression of PCK2 and HIBADH, however, was not altered between different groups. The gene expression of FBP1 tended to be numerically lower (15% reduction) in the liver of the albumen-deprived chicks, compared to a 40% reduction in protein abundance. Most likely, the different abundance in these proteins are regulated via post-transcriptional or post-translational modifications.

Finally, the lower embryonic survival of the albumen-deprived chicks compared to both the sham and the control group is in agreement with studies in literature after performance of similar egg manipulations [6,36] and with our previous results [8,9]. The reduced survival is the result of an increased early embryonic mortality caused by the manipulation of the egg and inherent to this animal model. Furthermore, if the embryo survived the early stages of the embryonic development, the chance of a successful hatch was the same in the three treatments, as no differences in mid and late death were detected.

Conclusion

Previous results had already demonstrated the existence of both short- and long-term effects of embryonic protein undernutrition by albumen removal in the chicken. This study demonstrates that these zootechnical and physiological differences are not yet present during the perinatal period, before the conflict between the prenatal and postnatal conditions arises. Metabolic programming was revealed by the observed hepatic proteome changes related with amino acid and glucose metabolism.

Acknowledgments

All authors agreed with the final format of the manuscript. We thank all the authors for practical and scientific assistance. In addition, we would like to thank the technical staff Lieve Geenen of the Laboratory of Neuroplasticity and Neuroproteomics of the KU Leuven for the help with 2-D DIGE, Sofia Eleftheriadis for her contribution to the gene expression measurements, Andy Pironet for the glycogen measurements and Inge Vaesen of the Laboratory of Livestock Physiology of the KU Leuven for the plasma analyses.

Author Contributions

Conceived and designed the experiments: EW NE JB ED LA TTH. Performed the experiments: EW TTH. Analyzed the data: EW LSV TTH LA NE. Contributed reagents/materials/analysis tools: JB LA ED. Wrote the paper: EW.

References

1. Roseboom TJ, Painter RC, Van Abeelen AFM, Veenendaal MVE, De Rooij SR (2011) Hungry in the womb: what are the consequences? Lessons from the Dutch famine. Maturitas 70: 141–145.
2. Ravelli ACJ, Van Der Meulen JHP, Michels RPJ, Osmond C, Barker DJP, et al. (1998) Glucose tolerance in adults after prenatal exposure to famine. Lancet 351: 173–177.
3. Hales CN, Barker DJ (2001) The thrifty phenotype hypothesis. Br Med Bull 60: 5–20.
4. Gluckman PG, Hanson MA (2004) Living with the past: evolution, development, and patterns of disease. Science 305: 1733–1736.
5. Barker DJ (1995) The fetal and infant origins of disease. Eur J Clin Invest 25: 457–463.
6. Hill WL (1993) Importance of prenatal nutrition to the development of a precocial chick. Dev Psychobiol 26: 237–249.
7. Rao K, Xie J, Yang X, Chen L, Grossmann R, et al. (2009) Maternal low-protein diet programmes offspring growth in association with alterations in yolk leptin deposition and gene expression in yolk-sac membrane, hypothalamus and muscle of developing Langshan chicken embryos. Br J Nutr 102: 848–857.
8. Everaert N, Métayer-Coustard S, Willemsen H, Han H, Song Z, et al. (2013) The effect of albumen removal before incubation (embryonic protein undernutrition) on the post-hatch performance, regulators of protein translation activation and proteolysis in neonatal broilers. Br J Nutr 110: 265–274.
9. Willems E, Wang Y, Willemsen H, Lesuisse J, Franssens L, et al. (2013) Partial albumen removal early during embryonic development of layer-type chickens has negative consequences on laying performance in adult life. Poult Sci 92: 1905–1915.
10. Willems E, Decuypere E, Buyse J, Everaert N (2014) Importance of albumen during embryonic development in avian species, with emphasis on domestic chicken. WPSJ (*in press*).
11. Freeman BM, Vince MA (1974) Development of the avian embryo: a behavioural and physiological study. London: Chapman And Hall, 362 p.
12. Darras VM, Katonen SP, Geris KL, Bergham LR, Kuhn ER (1996) Plasma thyroid levels and iodothyronine deiodinase activity following an acute glucocorticoid challenge in embryonic compared to posthatch chickens. Gen Comp Endocrinol 104: 203–212.
13. Dreiling CE, Brown DE, Casale L, Kelly L (1987) Musle glycogen: comparison of iodine binding and enzyme digestion assays and application to meat samples. Meat Sci 20: 167–177.
14. Van den Bergh G, Arckens L (2004) Fluorescent two-dimensional difference gel electrophoresis unveils the potential of gel-based proteomics. Curr Opin Biotechnol 15: 38–43.
15. Van den Bergh G, Clerens S, Cnops L, Vandesande F, Arckens L (2003) Fluorescent two-dimensional difference gel electrophoresis and mass spectrometry identify age-related protein expression differences for the primary visual cortex of kitten and adult cat. J Neurochem 85: 193–205.
16. Van den Bergh G, Clerens S, Firestein BL, Burnat K, Arckens L (2006) Development and plasticity-related changes in protein expression patterns in cat visual cortex: a fluorescent two dimensional difference gel electrophoresis approach. Proteomics 6: 3821–3832.
17. Ünlü M, Morgan ME, Minden JS (1997) Difference gel electrophoresis: a single gel method for detecting changes in protein extracts. Electrophoresis 18: 2071–2077.
18. Rasmussen R (2001) Quantification of the LightCycler. In: Meuer S, Wittwer C, Nakagawara K, editors. Rapid cycle real-time PCR, Methods and applications. Heidelberg: Springer Press, pp. 21–34.
19. Livak KJ, Schmittgen TD (2001) Analysis of relative gene expression data using real-time quantitative PCR and the $2^{-\Delta\Delta Ct}$ method. Methods 25: 402–408.
20. Gould GW (1997) Facilitative glucose transporters. Texas: R.G. Landes Company, 237 pp.
21. Christensen VL, Wineland MJ, Fasenko GM, Donaldson WE (2001) Egg storage effects on plasma glucose and supply and demand tissue glycogen concentrations of broiler embryos. Poult Sci 80: 1729–1735.
22. Wang Y, Li Y, Willems E, Willemsen H, Franssens L, et al. (2014) Effects of spread of hatch and delayed feed access on broiler post-hatch performance up to day 5. Animal 8: 610–617.
23. Whorwood CB, Firth KM, Budge H, Symonds ME (2001) Maternal under nutrition during early to mid gestation programs tissuespecific alterations in the expression of the glucocorticoid receptor, 11β-hydroxysteroid dehydrogenase isoforms, and type 1 angiotensin II receptor in neonatal sheep. Endocrinology 142: 2854–2864.
24. Bertram C, Trowern AR, Copin N, Jackson AA, Whorwood CB (2001) The maternal diet during pregnancy programs altered expression of the glucocorticoid receptor and type 2 11β-hydroxysteroid dehydrogenase: potential molecular mechanisms underlying the programming of hypertension in utero. Endocrinology 142: 2841–2853.
25. Lillycrop KA, Phillips ES, Jackson AA, Hanson MA, Burdge GC (2005) Dietary protein restriction of pregnant rats induces and folic acid supplementation prevents epigenetic modification of hepatic gene expression in the offspring. J Nutr 135: 1382–1386.
26. McNabb FMA (2000) Thyroids. In: Whittow GC, editor. Avian Physiology. New York: Academic Press, pp. 461–471.
27. Kono T, Nishida M, Nishiki Y, Seki Y, Sato K, et al. (2005) Characterisation of glucose transporter (GLUT) gene expression in broiler chickens. Br Poult Sci 46: 510–515.
28. Lesage J, Hahn D, Léonhardt M, Blondeau B, Bréant B, et al. (2002) Maternal undernutrition during late gestation-induced intrauterine growth restriction in the rat is associated with impaired placental GLUT3 expression, but does not correlate with endogenous corticosterone levels. J Endocrinol 174: 37–43.
29. Nguyen LT, Muhlhausler BS, Botting KJ, Morrison JL (2010) Maternal undernutrition alters fat cell size distribution, but not lipogenic gene expression in the visceral fat of the late gestation guinea pig fetus. Placenta 31: 902–909.
30. Seki Y, Sato K, Kono T, Abe H, Akiba Y (2003) Broiler chickens (Ross strain) lack insulin-responsive glucose transporter GLUT4 and have GLUT8 cDNA. Gen Comp Endocrinol 133: 80–87.
31. Hamada T, Matsumoto M (1984) Effects of nutrition and ontogeny of liver cytosolic and mitochondrial phosphoenolpyruvate carboxykinase activity of the rat, hamster, guinea-pig, pig, kid, calf and chick. Comp Biochem Physiol B77: 547–550.
32. Hod Y, Cook JS, Weldon SL, Short JM, Wynshaw-Boris A, et al. (1986) Differential expression of the genes for the mitochondrial and cytosolic forms of phosphoenolpyruvate carboxykinase. Ann N Y Acad Sci 478: 31–45.
33. Desai M, Byrne CD, Zhang J, Petry CJ, Lucas A, et al. (1997) Programming of hepatic insulin-sensitive enzymes in offspring of rat dams fed a protein-restricted diet. Am J Physiol Gastrointest Liver Physiol 272: G1083–1090.
34. Lane RH, MacLennan NK, Hsu JL, Janke SM, Pham TD (2002) Increased hepatic peroxisome proliferator-activated receptor-γ coactivator-1 gene expression in a rat model of intrauterine growth retardation and subsequent insulin resistance. Endocrinology 143: 2486–2490.
35. Matthiesen CF, Blache D, Thomsen PD, Hansen NE, Tauson A-H (2010) Effect of late gestation low protein supply to mink (*Mustela vison*) dams on reproductive performance and metabolism of dam and offspring. Arch Anim Nutr 64: 56–76.
36. Finkler MS, Van Orman JB, Sotherland PR (1998) Experimental manipulation of egg quality in chickens: influence of albumen and yolk on the size and body composition of near-term embryos in a precocial bird. J Comp Physiol B168: 17–24.

Effects of HIV Infection on the Metabolic and Hormonal Status of Children with Severe Acute Malnutrition

Aaloke Mody[1*‡], Sarah Bartz[1‡], Christoph P. Hornik[2], Tonny Kiyimba[6], James Bain[3], Michael Muehlbauer[3], Elizabeth Kiboneka[6], Robert Stevens[3], John V. St. Peter[5], Christopher B. Newgard[3], John Bartlett[4], Michael Freemark[1,3,4]

1 Division of Pediatric Endocrinology and Diabetes, Pediatric Division of Quantitative Sciences, Duke University Medical Center, Durham, North Carolina, United States of America, **2** Duke Clinical Research Institute, Duke University Medical Center, Durham, North Carolina, United States of America, **3** Sarah W. Stedman Nutrition and Metabolism Center, Duke University Medical Center, Durham, North Carolina, United States of America, **4** Duke Global Health Institute, Duke University Medical Center, Durham, North Carolina, United States of America, **5** Global Research & Development, Long Term Research, PepsiCo, Inc., Purchase, New York, United States of America, **6** Mwanamugimu Nutrition Unit, Mulago Hospital Complex, Kampala, Uganda

Abstract

Background: HIV infection occurs in 30% of children with severe acute malnutrition in sub-Saharan Africa. Effects of HIV on the pathophysiology and recovery from malnutrition are poorly understood.

Methods: We conducted a prospective cohort study of 75 severely malnourished Ugandan children. HIV status/CD4 counts were assessed at baseline; auxologic data and blood samples were obtained at admission and after 14 days of inpatient treatment. We utilized metabolomic profiling to characterize effects of HIV infection on metabolic status and subsequent responses to nutritional therapy.

Findings: At admission, patients (mean age 16.3 mo) had growth failure (mean W/H z-score −4.27 in non-edematous patients) that improved with formula feeding (mean increase 1.00). 24% (18/75) were HIV-infected. Nine children died within the first 14 days of hospitalization; mortality was higher for HIV-infected patients (33% v. 5%, OR = 8.83). HIV-infected and HIV-negative children presented with elevated NEFA, ketones, and even-numbered acylcarnitines and reductions in albumin and amino acids. Leptin, adiponectin, insulin, and IGF-1 levels were low while growth hormone, cortisol, and ghrelin levels were high. At baseline, HIV-infected patients had higher triglycerides, ketones, and even-chain acylcarnitines and lower leptin and adiponectin levels than HIV-negative patients. Leptin levels rose in all patients following nutritional intervention, but adiponectin levels remained depressed in HIV-infected children. Baseline hypoleptinemia and hypoadiponectinemia were associated with increased mortality.

Conclusions: Our findings suggest a critical interplay between HIV infection and adipose tissue storage and function in the adaptation to malnutrition. Hypoleptinemia and hypoadiponectinemia may contribute to high mortality rates among malnourished, HIV-infected children.

Editor: Geetha P. Bansal, Tulane University, United States of America

Funding: This work was supported by grants from the Genentech Foundation, PepsiCo, Inc., and the Duke Global Health Institute (to SB, MF, and AM). John A. Bartlett is supported by US National Institutes of Health awards P30AI64518, U01AI067854, D43CA153722, and D43TW06732, and HRSA award T84HA21123. Christopher Newgard and the Stedman Metabolomics Center are supported by NIH grant DK58398. The funders had no role in study design, data collection, decision to publish, or preparation of the manuscript. Dr. St. Peter, who is employed by PepsiCo, Inc., assisted with data analysis and approved the final manuscript as submitted.

Competing Interests: The authors have read the journal's policy and have the following conflicts: John V. St. Peter is an author on this study and concurrently employed by PepsiCo, Inc. This does not alter the authors' adherence to PLOS ONE policies on sharing data and materials. The views expressed in this report are those of the authors and do not necessarily reflect the position or policy of PepsiCo, Inc.

* Email: aalokemody@gmail.com

‡ These authors contributed equally to this work.

Introduction

Malnutrition is a major determinant of morbidity and mortality in the developing world and is the underlying cause of 3.5 million child deaths each year [1]. Poor nutrition increases greatly a child's risk of dying from diarrhea, pneumonia, measles, and malaria and is associated with decreased adult height, lower educational achievement, lower socioeconomic status, and a possible increase in chronic diseases during adulthood [2,3]. Worldwide, malnutrition represents 35% of the burden of disease in children less than five years of age and 11% of disability-adjusted life years (DALYs) [1].

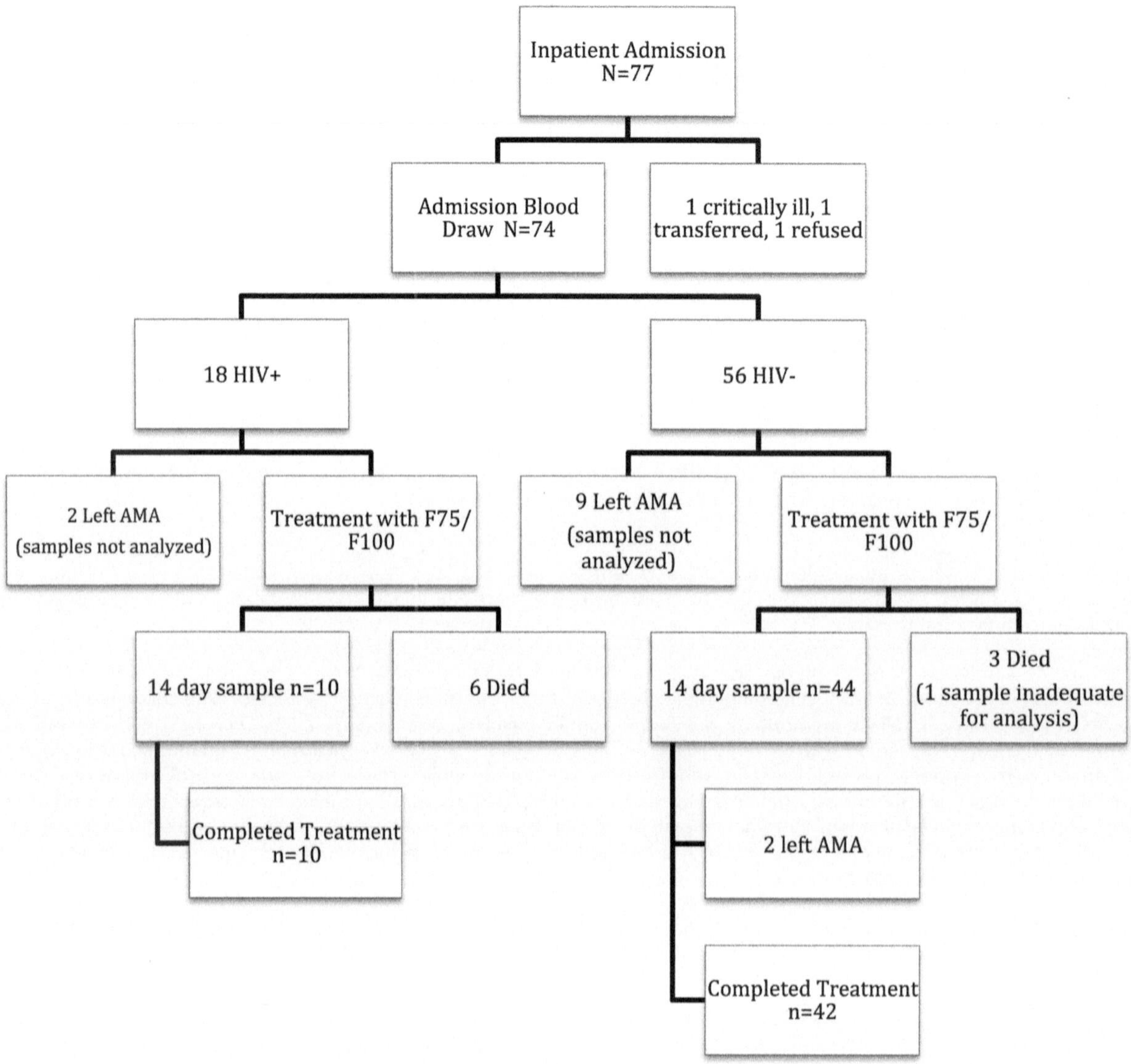

Figure 1. Flowchart of Patient Outcomes.

In sub-Saharan Africa, 30% of children with severe acute malnutrition (SAM) are infected with HIV, which increases mortality rates substantially; those with CD4 count <20% are at greatest risk [4,5]. However, the factors underlying the increased risk of mortality from HIV are poorly understood. Rates of pneumonia (68%), urinary tract infection (26%), and bacteremia (18%) are comparable in severely malnourished HIV-infected and HIV-negative children [6]. Furthermore, among those who survive, the rates of nutritional recovery are similar [7]. There is consequently a critical need to elucidate the pathophysiology of SAM in children with concurrent HIV infection.

In a previous study we used metabolomic profiling to characterize changes in various hormones, growth factors, cytokines, and metabolites during nutritional rehabilitation of severely malnourished Ugandan children [8]. Here we characterized differences in baseline metabolic and hormonal status between HIV-infected and HIV-negative children with SAM and compared their subsequent responses to nutritional therapy. We hypothesized that HIV infection would modify the hormonal and metabolic responses to malnutrition and nutrient therapy and that hormones and metabolites measured at baseline might be associated with mortality in HIV-infected children.

Methods

Study Cohort

The study was conducted at Mwanamugimu Nutrition Unit at Mulago Hospital, in Kampala, Uganda. Children ages six months to five years who met WHO criteria for SAM were eligible for enrollment. SAM was defined as having a weight-for-height z-score (W/H z) <-3, mid-upper arm circumference (MUAC) $<$ 11.5 cm, or bilateral pitting edema. Referrals came from the Mulago pediatric acute care unit (emergency department) and community clinics in and around Kampala.

Study Variables

A complete medical and diet history, sociodemographic profile, and physical exam including anthropometric data were obtained at time of enrollment. Lab studies included CBC and differential, blood smear, and CD4/CD8 counts (FACSCalibur, BD Biosci-

Table 1. Baseline Anthropometric and Hematologic Characteristics of HIV-infected and HIV-negative Patients.

	HIV-infected (n = 18)	HIV-negative (n = 56)	
	Number (%)		**p-value**
Male Sex	10/18 (55.6)	32/56 (57.1)	1.00
Edema Present	9/18 (50)	33/56 (58.9)	0.589
Positive Malaria Smear	1/18 (5.6)	6/56 (10.7))	0.555
Newly Diagnosed HIV infection	12/18 (66.7)	-	-
Current ARV treatment	4/6 (66.7)	-	-
Mortality	6/18 (33.3)	3/56 (5.4)	**0.0051**
	Mean±SEM		
Age	19.2±2.6	15.4±1.1	0.315
Days in Treatment	26.4±3.9	24.9±1.5	0.850
Admission Anthropometry			
W/H % (nonedematous)	70.5±2.4	71.3±1.4	0.571
W/H Z-Score (nonedematous)	−4.44±0.48	−4.20±0.28	0.615
W/A Z-Score (nonedematous)	−5.14±0.61	−4.87±0.33	0.870
MUAC (nonedematous)	9.6±0.5	9.9±0.2	0.599
L/A Z-score (all patients)	−3.17±0.40	−2.90±0.20	0.492
H/C Z-score (all patients)	−0.72±0.32	−1.25±0.21	0.246
Hematology			
Abs CD4 Count	644±103	2734±253	**<0.0001**
CD4%	14.6±2.1	34.8±1.2	**<0.0001**
Abs CD8 Count	1724±387	1610±120	0.638
CD8%	37.3±2.6	21.3±1.0	**<0.0001**
CD4/CD8 Ratio	0.44±0.08	1.83±0.10	**<0.0001**
WBC (10^3/μl)	8.5±1.2	13.2±1.0	**0.0082**
Hemoglobin (g/dL)	7.7±0.4	9.0±0.2	**0.0130**
Platelets (10^3/μl)	267±37	371±24	**0.0231**

ences, USA). HIV status was assessed using an HIV rapid antibody test (Determine, Abbott, USA; STAT-Pak, Chembio Diagnostics, USA; Uni-Gold, Trinity Biotech, Ireland) for patients >18 months of age and HIV DNA PCR (AMPLICOR HIV-1 Monitor Test version 1.5, Roche, USA) for patients <18 months. Children whose mothers had a documented negative HIV test within the previous 30 days were presumed to be HIV negative. Children with known HIV infection did not have repeat HIV testing. Those with malaria were treated with anti-malarials. All patients received counseling from a trained HIV counselor at Mwanamugimu Nutrition Unit before delivering results; HIV-infected patients were referred for appropriate HIV-related care.

Nutritional Interventions

Nutrition rehabilitation and management of medical complications were carried out according to WHO guidelines for inpatient treatment of SAM by medical house officers at Mwanamugimu Nutrition Unit [9]. Inpatient therapy was administered in two phases according to WHO guidelines: an initial stabilization phase during which acute medical conditions were managed; and a longer rehabilitation phase once clinical status improved. Patients were fed F75 mild-based liquid formula (75 kcal and 0.9 g protein/100 mL) during the first phase and F100 (100 kcal and 2.9 g protein/100 mL) during the rehabilitation phase. Micronutrient deficiencies were corrected with vitamin A, folic acid, zinc, and iron. All patients received empiric antibiotics [9]. Patients were followed from time of enrollment until death or discharge from the inpatient unit.

Metabolomic Analysis

Blood samples (maximum 5 mL) were collected at time of enrollment (within 24 h of admission). A second blood sample was collected after 14 days of inpatient treatment or at time of discharge from the inpatient unit, whichever occurred first. Aprotinin (500 KIU/mL of blood; Sigma-Aldrich, USA) was added to prevent protein degradation. Blood samples were collected on ice and processed promptly; EDTA plasma was stored at −70°C and shipped in bulk to the Duke University Stedman Nutrition Center for analysis. Detailed methods of the metabolic and hormonal analyses are described in the **Supporting Information (Methods S1)**.

Statistical Analysis

Sample size was based on commonly reported concentrations and variability of classical hormones (insulin, growth hormone, cortisol) in infants and children. We evaluated pre-treatment anthropometric variables and biomarkers using non-parametric Wilcoxon Rank-Sum and absolute change during treatment using Wilcoxon Signed-Rank based on variables of interest (HIV status, mortality). The association between HIV status and mortality was

Table 2. Baseline Metabolic Profile of HIV-infected and HIV-negative Patients.

	HIV-infected (n = 16)	HIV-negative (n = 46)	
	Mean±SEM		**p-value**
Fatty Acid Metabolites			
NEFA (mmol/L)	0.65±0.10	0.54±0.06	0.285
Total Ketones (μmol/L)	826±259	424±95	**0.0387**
Acylcarnitines			
C2 (μmol/L)	22.3±3.5	14.4±2.4	0.0103
C3 (μmol/L)	0.47±0.07	0.38±0.04	0.179
C2/C3 Ratio	54.3±9.7	44.7±5.7	0.195
Even-Chain Acylcarnitine Molar Sum (μmol/L)	24.0±3.7	16.0±2.6	**0.0108**
Hormones			
Insulin (μIU/ml)	1.81±0.48	2.45±0.45	0.321
Growth Hormone (ng/ml)	12.4±2.7	11.0±1.3	0.380
IGF-1 (ng/ml)	13.3±4.4	9.4±1.7	0.597
Total Ghrelin (pg/ml)	3577±566	4040±320	0.435
GLP-1 (pg/ml)	128.8±21.3	96.0±12.8	0.106
PYY (pg/ml)	1195±160	1202±105	0.866
Cortisol (μg/dl)	54.0±3.2	46.0±2.7	0.106
Adipocytokines*	**n = 13**	**n = 46**	
Leptin (pg/ml)	69.8±26.6	292±52	**0.0163**
Total Adiponectin (ng/ml)	8049±1081	15268±1133	**0.0017**
HMW Adiponectin (ng/ml)	4409±757	9356±761	**0.0014**
Amino Acids			
Amino Acid Molar Sum (μmol/L)	1230±62	1190±51	0.417
Inflammatory Cytokines			
IL-2 (pg/ml)	7.7±2.7	3.6±1.2	**0.0158**
IL-6 (pg/ml)	96.3±58.4	25.6±15.9	0.139
IL-8 (pg/ml)	299.3±191.0	75.2±25.9	0.060
TNF-α (pg/ml)	43.0±5.5	37.4±9.5	**0.0248**
Other			
Glucose (mg/dl)	77.1±7.9	85.9±3.9	0.474
Creatinine (mg/dl)	0.30±0.04	0.27±0.03	0.296
Phosphorus (mg/dl)	2.99±1.40	3.28±1.02	0.390
Albumin (g/dl)	2.0±0.2	2.0±0.1	0.847
CRP (mg/L)	63.7±16.5	26.8±5.3	0.0730
Triglycerides (mg/dl)	177.6±14.0	122.9±12.2	**0.0008**

*Excludes patients on ARVs.

assessed utilizing an odds ratio. We performed multivariable logistic and linear regression to evaluate associations between biomarkers levels, HIV status, and mortality. Analysis of leptin and total and high molecular weight (HMW) adiponectin excluded patients taking antiretroviral drugs (ARVs), given the known effects of these medications on these hormones [10–14]. Edematous children were excluded from analysis of anthropometric variables based on weight. All analyses were conducted using JMP Pro 9.0 (Cary, NC); a two-sided p-value<0.05 was considered statistically significant for all tests.

Ethical considerations

The study protocol was approved by the institutional review boards at Duke University, Makerere University School of Public Health, and the Uganda National Council of Science and Technology. Sponsors of the study assisted with data interpretation but had no role in study design, data collection, or data analysis.

Written informed consent (in English and Luganda) to participate in the study and all its components was obtained from all guardians. Each patient received an insecticide-treated bed net at enrollment and transportation money to return home at the time of discharge as compensation for participation.

Results

Study Population

A total of 77 patients were referred to Mwanamugimu Inpatient Nutrition Unit and screened for study enrollment between

Table 3. Baseline Amino Acid Levels of HIV-infected and HIV-negative patients.

	HIV-infected (n = 16)	HIV-negative (n = 46)	
	Mean±SEM		p-value
Glycine (μmol/L)	235±21.4	237±12.6	0.866
Alanine	153±27.4	217±16.2	**0.0330**
Serine	99.2±99.5	113±5.6	0.464
Proline	152±14.4	153±8.5	0.904
Valine	100±10.7	75.6±6.3	**0.0248**
Leucine/Isoleucine	82.0±8.9	70.5±5.2	0.237
Methionine	16.1±1.7	15.6±1.0	0.742
Histidine	69.1±7.0	53.3±4.1	0.250
Phenylalanine	79.6±7.7	43.0±4.5	**0.0067**
Tyrosine	30.1±4.6	22.6±2.7	0.207
Aspartate	39.2±4.8	36.5±2.8	0.853
Glutamate	111±10.5	91.3±6.2	0.435
Ornithine	27.4±3.5	26.2±2.1	0.381
Citrulline	8.9±1.2	8.2±0.7	0.421
Arginine	28.3±3.3	27.7±1.9	0.323

December 2010 and March 2011. One patient refused to participate, another was deemed clinically unstable by the medical house officer for extra blood draws, and a third was transferred from the ward after only HIV status was assessed. Therefore, 75 patients had known HIV status and 74 had complete admission anthropometry. Analyses of hormones, metabolites, and cytokines were performed on blood samples from 62 patients at admission (16 HIV-infected including three on ARVs and 46 HIV-negative); 54 of these patients had repeat samples analyzed after 14 days of hospitalization and eight patients died before the second sample was obtained. Initial samples were insufficient in one additional patient (who died) and were not analyzed in 11 patients who left the ward prior to completing at least 14 days of treatment (including two HIV-infected patients, one of whom was on ARVs) (**Figure 1**).

The patient population was 57.3% male; mean age was 16.3±1.0 months (mean±SE). 56.8% (42/74) presented with edematous malnutrition. Non-edematous children had an initial W/H z-score −4.27±0.24 and MUAC 9.8±0.2 cm. Mean length-for-age (L/A) z-score was −2.97±0.18; head circumference-for-age (HC/A) z-score was −1.15±0.18. 9.5% (7/74) had malaria; one HIV-infected patient had concurrent malaria (**Table 1**).

As previously reported, overall mortality was 12.2% (9/74). Of those who successfully completed inpatient nutritional rehabilitation, mean length of stay was 25.2 days. During hospitalization, mean W/H z-score increased 1.00±0.18 in non-edematous children. Among surviving patients, 80% (52/65) were followed until discharge and 20% (13/65) left the ward against medical advice before achieving nutritional stability.

Baseline Characteristics of HIV-infected and HIV-negative Patients

HIV prevalence in the study population was 24% (18/75); two-thirds (12/18) of these were newly diagnosed HIV infections. Four of the six previously diagnosed patients were being treated with ARVs upon admission (**Table 1**).

Similar proportions of HIV-infected and HIV-negative patients presented with edematous malnutrition ($p = 0.589$). Non-edematous HIV-infected and HIV-negative patients presented with similar degrees of wasting (W/H z-score −4.44 vs. −4.20, $p = 0.615$). HIV-infected children had lower absolute CD4 counts (644 vs. 2734, $p < 0.0001$), WBC counts, hemoglobin, and platelets (**Table 1**).

HIV-infected patients had increased mortality rates: 33.3% for seropositive children compared with 5.4% for seronegative children (OR = 8.83, CI 1.93–40.43, $p = 0.0051$). Among those who survived, there were similar improvements in W/H z in (non-edematous) HIV-infected and HIV-negative patients after 14 days (0.85 vs. 0.43, $p = 0.412$).

Table 4. Multivariate regression assessing the effect of HIV status on leptin, total adiponectin, and HMW adiponectin when controlling for admission W/H z-score.

	Beta (HIV status)	p-value	Adjusted R^2
Leptin	63.7±44.4	0.1573	0.294
Total Adiponectin	2752±1051	**0.0113**	0.274
HMW Adiponectin	1949±720	**0.0090**	0.253

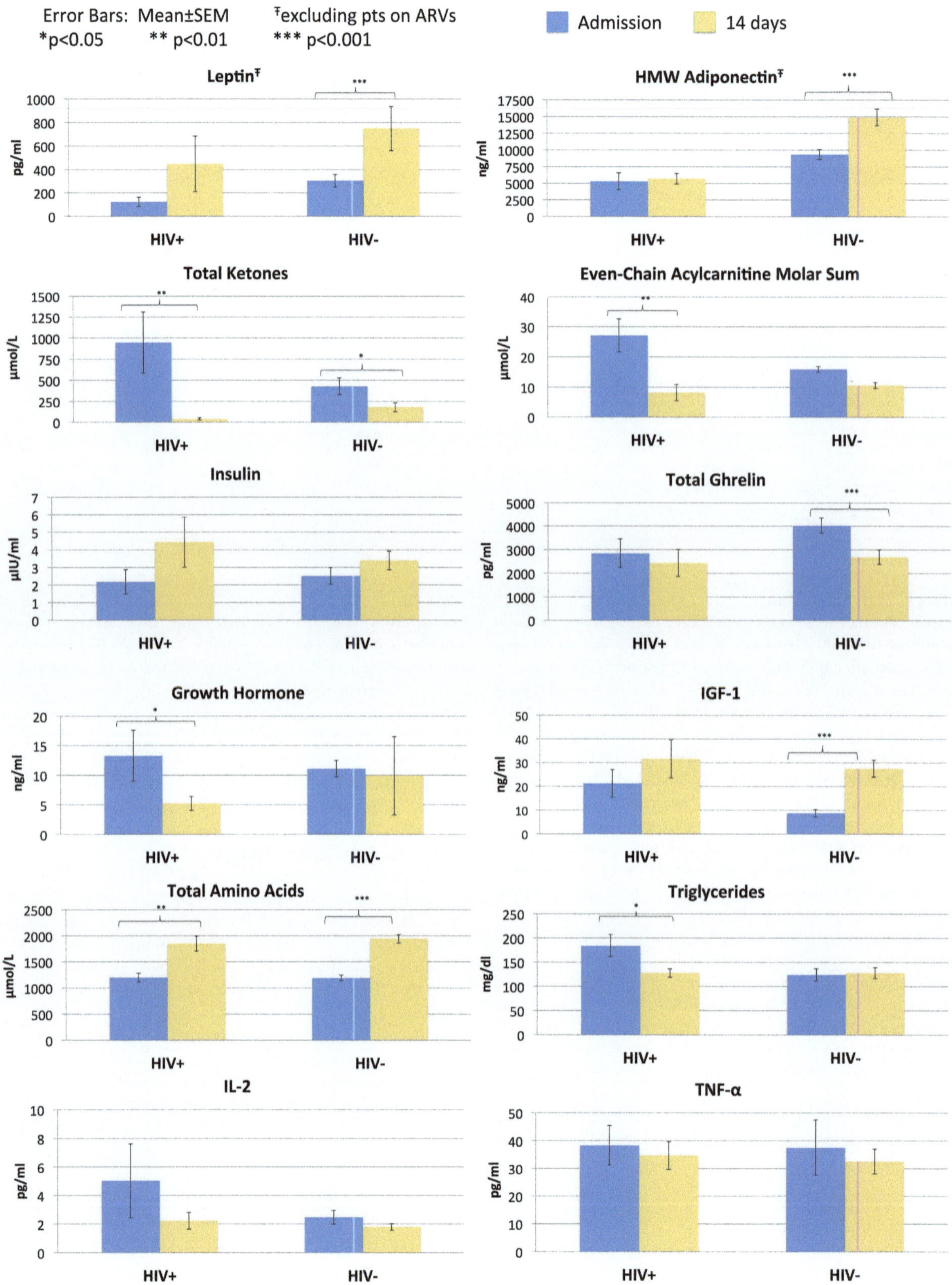

Figure 2. Comparison of metabolic response to inpatient rehabilitation in 54 patients who completed treatment (10 HIV-infected and 44 HIV-negative children). Analysis of leptin and HMW adiponectin excluded those patients taking ARVs. Data are represented as the mean±SEM.

Table 5. Changes in Metabolic Profiles of HIV-infected (surviving) and HIV-negative patients.

	HIV-infected (n = 10)			HIV-negative (n = 44)		
	Mean±SEM		p-value	Mean±SEM		p-value
	Admission	14-day		Admission	14-day	
Fatty Acid Metabolites						
NEFA (mmol/L)	0.72±0.16	0.24±0.06	**0.0020**	0.53±0.06	0.36±0.037	0.0723
Total Ketones (µmol/L)	948±362	39±14	**0.0098**	431±99	179±56	**0.0256**
Acylcarnitines						
C2 (µmol/L)	25.2±5.2	7.2±0.8	**0.0098**	14.5±2.6	9.3±0.94	0.171
C3 (µmol/L)	0.50±0.11	0.65±0.11	0.275	0.36±0.03	0.67±0.06	**<0.0001**
C2/C3 Ratio	60.6±14.7	13.4±2.0	**0.0020**	45.7±5.9	22.5±4.5	**<0.0001**
Even-Chain Acylcarnitine Molar Sum (µmol/L)	27.1±5.5	8.2±0.9	**0.0098**	16±2.7	10.6±1	0.216
Hormones						
Insulin (µIU/ml)	2.18±0.70	4.43±1.42	0.084	2.52±0.47	3.4±0.53	0.108
Growth Hormone (ng/ml	13.3±4.3	5.2±1.2	**0.027**	11.2±1.4	10.1±1.7	0.147
IGF-1 (ng/ml)	21.3±5.8	31.6±8.1	0.250	8.8±1.6	27.6±3.6	**<0.0001**
Total Ghrelin (pg/ml)	2851±603	2439±570	0.084	4029±319	2692±303	**<0.0001**
GLP-1 (pg/ml)	116.7±27.5	86.0±22.1	0.375	93.6±13.0	88.8±12.4	0.863
PYY (pg/ml)	916±118	893±112	1.0	1144±101	1011±78	0.100
Cortisol (µg/dl)	56.6±3.4	41.1±6.7	0.0625	45.3±2.8	38.3±3	**0.0123**
Adipocytokines*	**n = 7**			**n = 44**		
Leptin (pg/ml)	123.1±39.7	446±238	0.128	305±53.5	748.8±188	**0.0011**
Total Adiponectin (ng/ml)	8383±1569	10154±1815	0.297	15115±1093	20792±1329	**<0.0001**
HMW Adiponectin (ng/ml)	5308±1259	5717±795	0.625	9350±748	14895±1245	**<0.0001**
Amino Acids						
Amino Acid Molar Sum (µmol/L)	1198±84.4	1850±145	**0.005**	1192±53.6	1944±80.5	**<0.0001**
Inflammatory Cytokines						
IL-2 (pg/ml)	5.0±2.6	2.2±0.6	0.477	2.5±0.5	1.8±0.2	0.255
IL-6 (pg/ml)	49±32	3.4±0.7	**0.0371**	9.9±1.5	7.8±2.8	**0.0256**
IL-8 (pg/ml)	344±300	29.7±3.4	0.0645	50.6±9.0	41.7±4.4	0.638
TNF-α (pg/ml)	38.3±7.1	34.7±5	0.922	37.5±10	32.5±4.5	1.0
Other						
Glucose (mg/dl)	72.1±9.3	75.4±3.7	0.625	84.2±3.8	77.0±2.2	0.0634
Creatinine (mg/dl)	0.32±0.06	0.36±0.11	0.910	0.25±0.03	0.32±0.07	0.694
Phosphorus (mg/dl)	3.2±0.4	4.2±0.2	0.086	3.4±0.2	4.6±0.1	**<0.0001**
Albumin (g/dl)	2.03±0.32	2.28±0.20	0.219	2.01±0.17	2.51±0.12	**<0.0001**
CRP (mg/L)	70.7±21.1	14.2±7.2	**0.0391**	26.8±5.7	9.9±4.1	**0.0003**
Triglycerides (mg/dl)	184±22.8	127±8.7	**0.0391**	124.3±12.7	127.7±11.2	0.416

*Excludes patients on ARVs.

Effects of HIV Infection on Baseline Metabolic Profile

Both HIV-infected and HIV-negative patients presented in a severe catabolic state with exaggerated lipolysis, fatty acid oxidation, and hypoaminoacidemia (**Table 2 and 3**). Non-esterified fatty acids (NEFA), ketones, C2 acyl (acetyl)carnitine, and even-chained acylcarnitine molar sum were elevated in both groups at presentation, though ketones ($p = 0.039$), acetylcarnitine ($p = 0.0103$), and even-chained acylcarnitine molar sum ($p = 0.0108$) were higher in HIV-infected patients. Levels of albumin, amino acids, and C3 acyl (propionyl)carnitine, a byproduct of branched chain amino acid catabolism, were comparably low in both groups. Yet blood glucose levels were maintained in the normal range. Triglycerides were higher in HIV-infected patients ($p<0.001$). Moreover, a number of inflammatory markers, including CRP, IL-2, IL-6, IL-8, and TNF-α were higher in HIV-infected patients, with IL-2 ($p = 0.016$) and TNF-α ($p = 0.025$) reaching statistical significance (**Table 2**). Edematous patients had higher alanine amino transferase (ALT) and gamma glutamyl transpeptidase (GGT) levels and lower albumin and amino acid levels than non-edematous patients (data not shown); these metrics did not differ among the HIV-infected and HIV-negative groups. Edematous patients also had lower total and HMW adiponectin levels; however, edema did not modify the association between HIV status and hypoadiponectinemia.

Table 6. Changes in Amino Acid Levels of HIV-infected (surviving) and HIV-negative patients.

	HIV-infected (n = 10)			HIV-negative (n = 44)		
	Mean±SEM		p-value	Mean±SEM		p-value
	Admission	14-day		Admission	14-day	
Glycine (μmol/L)	216±16.6	313±28.1	**0.0020**	238±13.7	305±13.4	**<0.0001**
Alanine	150±18.1	409±57.7	**0.0020**	218±18.6	418±27.5	**<0.0001**
Serine	98.8±4.5	125±14.6	**0.0371**	113±6.4	157±6.9	**<0.0001**
Proline	155±14.5	296±42.6	**0.0098**	152±9.4	282±20.3	**<0.0001**
Valine	102±15.8	130±21.3	0.375	76.8±6.2	152±10.2	**<0.0001**
Leucine/Isoleucine	80.1±15.0	112±15.2	0.106	71.0±5.2	132±7.3	**<0.0001**
Methionine	16.8±2.8	19.7±3.3	0.193	15.6±1.0	24.5±1.6	**<0.0001**
Histidine	64.5±12.7	53.9±5.7	0.432	52.8±3.4	50.7±2.7	0.954
Phenylalanine	78.4±18.2	59.8±5.3	0.432	43.3±2.8	53.0±2.5	**0.0184**
Tyrosine	29.8±7.2	45.8±10.6	0.0840	22.6±2.7	52.1±5.0	**<0.0001**
Aspartate	31.3±6.3	50.4±10.5	**0.0039**	35.4±2.7	51.0±5.0	**<0.0001**
Glutamate	109±12.7	135±17.3	0.275	91.3±4.7	152±8.2	**<0.0001**
Ornithine	29.3±3.1	40.2±6.8	**0.0195**	26.7±2.3	47.9±3.3	**<0.0001**
Citrulline	8.9±1.1	16.3±3.4	**0.0098**	8.3±0.7	19.0±1.6	**<0.0001**
Arginine	29.2±2.4	44.5±6.9	**0.0137**	27.8±2.2	49.7±3.3	**<0.0001**

Insulin and IGF-1 levels were low in both HIV-infected and HIV-negative subjects, while growth hormone (GH), ghrelin, cortisol, GLP-1, and peptide YY (PYY) were high (compare levels to those in references [15–18]). Excluding analysis of three patients taking ARVs, which are known to affect adipose tissue function, the levels of leptin ($p = 0.016$), total adiponectin ($p = 0.0017$), and high molecular weight (HMW) adiponectin ($p = 0.0014$) were significantly lower in HIV-infected than in HIV-negative subjects (**Table 2**). Multivariate logistic regression controlling for the degree of wasting (as assessed by W/H z-score) established that HIV infection was associated with lower total adiponectin ($p = 0.0113$) and HMW adiponectin ($p = 0.009$), but not lower leptin ($p = 0.157$) (**Table 4**).

Effects of HIV Infection on Metabolic Response to Nutritional Rehabilitation

54 patients had blood samples drawn both at admission and after 14 days of treatment. We were unable to obtain day-14 samples in any of the patients who died.

HIV-infected and HIV-negative patients demonstrated similar trends in most metabolites, hormones, and cytokines in response to nutritional treatment. NEFA, total ketones, and even-chained acylcarnitines decreased (**Figure 2 and Table 5**), while albumin and the majority of amino acids increased (**Table 6**). There was a rise in the levels of propionylcarnitine (HIV-infected: 0.50 vs. 0.65, $p = 0.2754$; HIV-negative 0.36 vs. 0.67, $p < 0.0001$), likely reflecting the catabolism of (newly available) dietary branched chain amino acids [19]. Plasma insulin, IGF-1, and leptin increased while plasma ghrelin, GH, and cortisol declined. The majority of inflammatory markers decreased in both groups (statistically significant for IL-6 and CRP). After 14 days of nutritional therapy, there were no significant differences among surviving HIV-infected and HIV-negative patients with respect to NEFA, total ketones, insulin, IGF-1, leptin, ghrelin, GH, cortisol, GLP-1, PYY, IL2, IL6, IL8, or TNF-α levels (**Figure 2 and Table 5**).

However, HIV status was associated with differential effects on adiponectin levels during nutritional recovery. Excluding patients on ARVs, HIV-infected patients had no significant changes in total (8383 vs. 10154, $p = 0.2969$) or HMW adiponectin (5308 vs. 5717, $p = 0.625$). In contrast, HIV-negative patients had marked increases in total (15115 vs. 20792, $p < 0.0001$) and HMW adiponectin (9350 vs. 14895, $p < 0.0001$) during recovery. Furthermore, after 14 days of treatment, HIV-infected patients still had significantly lower levels of total ($p = 0.0023$) and HMW adiponectin ($p = 0.0019$) than HIV-negative patients (**Figure 2 and Table 5**).

Predictors of Mortality During Inpatient Treatment

Non-edematous patients who died had more striking manifestations of wasting than those who survived, as reflected in lower W/H z-score (−6.28 vs. −3.98, $p = 0.0244$) and MUAC (7.8 vs. 10.1, $p = 0.0019$). In all patients, there was a greater degree of stunting in those who died (L/A z-score −4.03 vs. −2.82, $p = 0.0454$) (**Table 7**).

In addition to HIV infection, factors at baseline associated with subsequent mortality were hypoleptinemia ($p = 0.0002$), low levels of HMW adiponectin ($p = 0.0149$), and high levels of PYY ($p = 0.0087$), IL2 ($p = 0.0004$), IL6 ($p = 0.004$), and TNF-α ($p = 0.0203$) (**Table 7**) [8]. Multivariate logistic regression analysis controlling for HIV status and admission W/H z showed that hypoleptinemia at baseline remained a significant predictor of mortality (OR 0.906, CI 0.827–0.993, $p = 0.035$) while HMW adiponectin at baseline became insignificant. Mortality did not vary with other baseline measures including presence of edema, hemoglobin, glucose, creatinine, albumin, phosphorus, other hormones and growth factors, fatty acid metabolites, or amino acid or cytokine levels.

Table 7. Baseline Characteristics and Metabolic Profiles associated with Mortality.

	Died (n = 8)	Survived (n = 54)	
	Mean±SEM		p-value
Anthropometry (nonedematous)			
Admission W/H %	61.1±4.6	72.5±1.0	**0.0121**
Admission W/H Z-Score	−6.28±1.05	−3.98±0.19	**0.0244**
Admission W/A Z-Score	−7.01±0.86	−4.63±0.26	**0.0221**
Admission MUAC	7.8±0.3	10.1±0.2	**0.0019**
L/A z-score (all patients)	−4.03±0.58	−2.82±0.18	**0.0454**
Fatty Acid Metabolites			
NEFA (mmol/L)	0.57±0.15	0.56±0.06	0.557
Total Ketones (μmol/L)	539±276	526±106	0.456
Acylcarnitines			
C2 (μmol/L)	16.3±2.2	16.5±2.3	0.139
C3 (μmol/L)	0.51±0.09	0.38±0.03	0.128
C2/C3 Ratio	38.5±7.7	48.4±5.5	0.858
Even-Chain Acylcarnitine Molar Sum (μmol/L)	17.9±2.2	18.1±2.5	0.139
Hormones			
Insulin (μIU/ml)	1.10±0.97	2.46±0.38	0.182
Growth Hormone (ng/ml)	10.5±3.4	11.5±1.3	0.442
IGF-1 (ng/ml)	5.6±4.8	11.1±1.8	0.118
Total Ghrelin (pg/ml)	4660±771	3811±297	0.361
GLP-1 (pg/ml)	149.1±30.3	97.9±11.7	0.080
PYY (pg/ml)	1866±227	1101±87	**0.0089**
Cortisol (μg/dl)	52.2±6.2	47.4±2.4	0.484
Adipocytokines*	**n = 8**	**n = 51**	
Leptin (pg/ml)	7.1±4.4	280±47	**0.0002**
Total Adiponectin (ng/ml)	10403±3360	14191±1017	0.075
HMW Adiponectin (ng/ml)	4894±1922	8795±693	**0.0184**
Amino Acids			
Amino Acid Molar Sum (μmol/L)	1248±70	1193±46	0.319
Inflammatory Cytokines			
IL-2 (pg/ml)	16.2±2.8	2.9±1.1	**0.0004**
IL-6 (pg/ml)	223.6±47.9	17.2±18.4	0.166
IL-8 (pg/ml)	323±147	105±57	**0.0042**
TNF-α (pg/ml)	46.8±20.2	37.6±7.8	**0.0203**

*Excludes patients on ARVs.

Discussion

Malnutrition remains a major cause of morbidity and mortality, with the greatest impact in low-income countries. HIV infection is detected in 30% of children with SAM and is associated with greatly increased mortality rates [4]. The role of HIV in the pathophysiology of malnutrition is poorly understood. Here we characterized differences in baseline metabolic and hormonal status between HIV-infected and HIV-negative children with SAM and compared their subsequent responses to current WHO recommended nutritional therapy. A major finding of this study is that HIV-infected children with SAM present with significant reductions in the adipocytokines leptin and adiponectin that are associated with mortality during inpatient hospitalization.

In our study the prevalence of HIV infection was 24%, with two-thirds of these representing new diagnoses. Mortality in HIV-infected children was very high (33.3%), similar to results from a previous meta-analysis [4]. HIV-infected and HIV-negative patients presented with similar degrees of wasting and edema, and among those who survived, achieved similar rates of growth and recovery. A previous study found HIV-infected patients to be more wasted at baseline; nevertheless that study, like ours, noted that seropositive and seronegative patients achieve similar rates of catch-up growth during nutritional treatment and that increased wasting at presentation is associated with mortality [7].

Both HIV-infected and HIV-negative children presented in a severe catabolic state characterized by elevated NEFA, total ketones, and even-numbered acylcarnitines (derived from fatty acid oxidation) and striking reductions in serum albumin and amino acids. At the same time, blood glucose levels were maintained in the normal range. Leptin, adiponectin, insulin, and IGF-1 levels were low while growth hormone, cortisol, and ghrelin levels were high. [8] This profile suggests a state in which fat catabolism and glucose production are prioritized above energy storage and growth [8,20–25]. At baseline, serum triglycerides, ketones, and even-chain acylcarnitines were higher and leptin and HMW adiponectin lower in HIV-infected patients than in HIV-negative patients. When controlling for W/H z-score, lower HMW adiponectin levels remained significantly associated with HIV infection, though leptin levels did not.

Nutritional treatment reversed the state of lipid mobilization and fatty acid oxidation and increased the levels of amino acids and C3 acyl (propionyl)carnitine. Insulin and IGF-1 rose while GH, cortisol, and ghrelin declined. HIV status did not modify the effect of treatment on most metabolites, hormones, growth factors, and cytokines. However, nutritional intervention increased HMW and total adiponectin levels in HIV-negative patients but not in HIV-infected patients; their levels remained significantly lower despite high calorie feeds. Leptin, on the other hand, increased in both HIV-infected and HIV-negative subjects.

Previous studies have linked decreased levels of leptin and adiponectin to HIV infection, particularly in the context of HIV-associated lipodystrophy, a syndrome characterized by fat redistribution, dyslipidemia, and metabolic syndrome. Many investigations implicate ARVs in the development of this syndrome, citing medication-induced adipose dysregulation and mitochondrial toxicity as potential mechanisms [10–14]. Additional studies, however, in untreated adults and mice have shown that HIV infection itself may be associated with adipose tissue dysfunction and decreased levels of adiponectin and leptin [26–28].

Adiponectin is produced by mature adipocytes; over-expression of adiponectin increases hepatic insulin sensitivity, while low levels of adiponectin are associated with insulin resistance and the metabolic syndrome [29]. Circulating leptin levels rise in proportion to white adipose tissue mass; higher levels are associated with obesity and lower levels with fasting and malnutrition [22]. The severe hypoadiponectinemia and hypoleptinemia in our HIV-infected children suggest a state of insulin resistance associated with depletion of white adipose tissue reserves.

The pre-existing mass and function of white adipose tissue appear to play roles in the adaptation to, and recovery from, malnutrition because low levels of leptin and adiponectin at baseline were associated with subsequent mortality. Indeed, baseline hypoleptinemia remained a strong predictor of mortality when controlling for HIV infection and W/H z-score in a multivariate analysis. While these findings do not prove that mortality is caused by hypoadiponectinemia and/or hypoleptinemia, there are potential mechanisms by which hypoadiponectinemia and hypoleptinemia might contribute to mortality risk. For example, a lack of pre-existing adipose tissue stores, suggested by hypoleptinemia at presentation, may limit a child's ability to sustain energy production for critical cardiorespiratory function during the initial phases of acute severe malnutrition. Moreover, leptin and adiponectin have immunoregulatory properties that may modulate the response to infectious pathogens. Leptin activates NK cells, induces neutrophil chemotaxis, enhances secretion of pro-inflammatory cytokines, and induces activation and proliferation of T-cells, while adiponectin promotes production of numerous anti-inflammatory cytokines [30,31]. It is possible that the combined effects of HIV infection and malnutrition on adipose tissue and immune function may increase mortality risk.

There were several limitations to our study. Blood samples were not obtained after fasting, as this could not be justified in critically ill patients. Our small sample size prevented us from conducting potentially important analyses of subgroups including HIV-infected patients who died ($n = 6$) and those already taking ARVs. Additionally, 17.6% ($n = 13$) of the original patient population left the ward prior to completing nutritional rehabilitation.

Nevertheless, this study provides a comprehensive analysis of the effects of HIV on the pathophysiology and recovery from SAM in childhood. Our findings suggest a critical interplay between HIV infection and adipose tissue storage and function in the adaptation to malnutrition.

Mortality in malnutrition is predicted by low W/H z and low MUAC. However, these can be difficult or impossible to interpret in infants and children with nutritional edema. Currently, all patients with nutritional edema are categorized as having SAM and treated accordingly. Our finding that hypoleptinemia predicts mortality in edematous as well as non-edematous subjects suggests that leptin assays might in the future be used to identify and target malnourished children at highest risk of death [8].

Finally, it should be noted that the optimal timing for initiating ARV treatment in HIV-infected children with SAM is currently unknown. In some cases, early initiation of therapy may increase the risk of clinical deterioration; in clinically stable children, however, it appears to improve outcomes [12,32–35]. Future studies should determine if the effects of ARVs on adipose tissue metabolism and function influence the clinical response to treatment of severely malnourished children.

Supporting Information

Methods S1 Detailed methods on the assays used for the metabolic and hormonal analyses.
(DOC)

Acknowledgments

The authors gratefully acknowledge the hard work and dedication of the staff of Mwanamugimu Nutrition Unit, particularly Esther, Jane Buyonjo, Justine Nalwadda, and Vicki Nabunnya for their help in completing this study. The authors also thank the staff of the Mulago University-Johns Hopkins University (MU-JHU) Core Lab at the Infectious Disease Institute (IDI).

Author Contributions

Conceived and designed the experiments: AM SB MF. Performed the experiments: AM SB TK EK. Analyzed the data: AM SB MF CH JVP CN. Contributed reagents/materials/analysis tools: J. Bain MM RS CN J. Bartlett. Wrote the paper: AM SB MF. Facilitated site coordination: J. Bartlett.

References

1. Black RE, Allen LH, Bhutta ZA, Caulfield LE, de Onis M, et al. (2008) Maternal and child undernutrition: global and regional exposures and health consequences. Lancet 371: 243–260.
2. Caulfield LE, de Onis M, Blossner M, Black RE (2004) Undernutrition as an underlying cause of child deaths associated with diarrhea, pneumonia, malaria, and measles. Am J Clin Nutr 80: 193–198.
3. Victora CG, Adair L, Fall C, Hallal PC, Martorell R, et al. (2008) Maternal and child undernutrition: consequences for adult health and human capital. Lancet 371: 340–357.
4. Fergusson P, Tomkins A (2009) HIV prevalence and mortality among children undergoing treatment for severe acute malnutrition in sub-Saharan Africa: a

systematic review and meta-analysis. Transactions of the Royal Society of Tropical Medicine and Hygiene 103: 541–548.

5. Chinkhumba J, Tomkins A, Banda T, Mkangama C, Fergusson P (2008) The impact of HIV on mortality during in-patient rehabilitation of severely malnourished children in Malawi. Transactions of the Royal Society of Tropical Medicine and Hygiene 102: 639–644.
6. Bachou H, Tylleskar T, Downing R, Tumwine JK (2006) Severe malnutrition with and without HIV-1 infection in hospitalised children in Kampala, Uganda: differences in clinical features, haematological findings and CD4+ cell counts. Nutrition journal 5: 27.
7. Fergusson P, Chinkhumba J, Grijalva-Eternod C, Banda T, Mkangama C, et al. (2009) Nutritional recovery in HIV-infected and HIV-uninfected children with severe acute malnutrition. Archives of disease in childhood 94: 512–516.
8. Bartz S, Mody A, Hornik C, Bain J, Muehlbauer M, et al. (2014) Severe acute malnutrition in childhood: hormonal and metabolic status at presentation, response to treatment, and predictors of mortality. J Clin Endocrinol Metab: Epub Feb 27 2014.
9. Ashworth A, Khanum S, Jackson A, Schofield C (2003) Guidelines for the inpatient treatment of severely malnourisehd children. Geneva: World Health Organization.
10. Verkauskiene R, Dollfus C, Levine M, Faye A, Deghmoun S, et al. (2006) Serum adiponectin and leptin concentrations in HIV-infected children with fat redistribution syndrome. Pediatr Res 60: 225–230.
11. Hammond E, McKinnon E, Nolan D (2010) Human immunodeficiency virus treatment-induced adipose tissue pathology and lipoatrophy: prevalence and metabolic consequences. Clin Infect Dis 51: 591–599.
12. Musoke PM, Fergusson P (2011) Severe malnutrition and metabolic complications of HIV-infected children in the antiretroviral era: clinical care and management in resource-limited settings. Am J Clin Nutr 94: 1716S–1720S.
13. Sweeney LL, Brennan AM, Mantzoros CS (2007) The role of adipokines in relation to HIV lipodystrophy. AIDS 21: 895–904.
14. Tsiodras S, Mantzoros C (2006) Leptin and Adiponectin in the HIV Associated Metabolic Syndrome: Physiologic and Therapeutic Implications. Am J Infect Dis 2: 141–152.
15. Feigerlova E, Diene G, Conte-Auriol F, Molinas C, Gennero I, et al. (2008) Hyperghrelinemia precedes obesity in Prader-Willi syndrome. J Clin Endocrinol Metab 93: 2800–2805.
16. Higgins PB, Fernandez JR, Garvey WT, Granger WM, Gower BA (2008) Entero-insular axis and postprandial insulin differences in African American and European American children. Am J Clin Nutr 88: 1277–1283.
17. Lomenick JP, Melguizo MS, Mitchell SL, Summar ML, Anderson JW (2009) Effects of meals high in carbohydrate, protein, and fat on ghrelin and peptide YY secretion in prepubertal children. J Clin Endocrinol Metab 94: 4463–4471.
18. Lomenick JP, Clasey JL, Anderson JW (2008) Meal-related changes in ghrelin, peptide YY, and appetite in normal weight and overweight children. Obesity (Silver Spring) 16: 547–552.
19. Batch BC, Shah SH, Newgard CB, Turer CB, Haynes C, et al. (2013) Branched chain amino acids are novel biomarkers for discrimination of metabolic wellness. Metabolism 62: 961–969.
20. Warren MP (2011) Endocrine manifestations of eating disorders. The Journal of clinical endocrinology and metabolism 96: 333–343.
21. Norrelund H (2005) The metabolic role of growth hormone in humans with particular reference to fasting. Growth hormone & IGF research: official journal of the Growth Hormone Research Society and the International IGF Research Society 15: 95–122.
22. Ahima RS (2006) Adipose tissue as an endocrine organ. Obesity 14 Suppl 5: 242S–249S.
23. Nonogaki K (2008) Ghrelin and feedback systems. Vitamins and hormones 77: 149–170.
24. Soliman AT, ElZalabany MM, Salama M, Ansari BM (2000) Serum leptin concentrations during severe protein-energy malnutrition: correlation with growth parameters and endocrine function. Metabolism: clinical and experimental 49: 819–825.
25. Manary MJ, Muglia LJ, Vogt SK, Yarasheski KE (2006) Cortisol and its action on the glucocorticoid receptor in malnutrition and acute infection. Metabolism: clinical and experimental 55: 550–554.
26. Villarroya J, Diaz-Delfin J, Hyink D, Domingo P, Giralt M, et al. (2010) HIV type-1 transgene expression in mice alters adipose tissue and adipokine levels: towards a rodent model of HIV type-1 lipodystrophy. Antivir Ther 15: 1021–1028.
27. Giralt M, Domingo P, Guallar JP, Rodriguez de la Concepcion ML, Alegre M, et al. (2006) HIV-1 infection alters gene expression in adipose tissue, which contributes to HIV- 1/HAART-associated lipodystrophy. Antivir Ther 11: 729–740.
28. Azzoni L, Crowther NJ, Firnhaber C, Foulkes AS, Yin X, et al. (2010) Association between HIV replication and serum leptin levels: an observational study of a cohort of HIV-1-infected South African women. J Int AIDS Soc 13: 33.
29. Turer AT, Scherer PE (2012) Adiponectin: mechanistic insights and clinical implications. Diabetologia 55: 2319–2326.
30. Carbone F, La Rocca C, Matarese G (2012) Immunological functions of leptin and adiponectin. Biochimie 94: 2082–2088.
31. Procaccini C, Jirillo E, Matarese G (2012) Leptin as an immunomodulator. Mol Aspects Med 33: 35–45.
32. Liu E, Spiegelman D, Semu H, Hawkins C, Chalamilla G, et al. (2011) Nutritional status and mortality among HIV-infected patients receiving antiretroviral therapy in Tanzania. The Journal of infectious diseases 204: 282–290.
33. Prendergast A, Bwakura-Dangarembizi MF, Cook AD, Bakeera-Kitaka S, Natukunda E, et al. (2011) Hospitalization for severe malnutrition among HIV-infected children starting antiretroviral therapy. AIDS 25: 951–956.
34. Heikens GT, Bunn J, Amadi B, Manary M, Chhagan M, et al. (2008) Case management of HIV-infected severely malnourished children: challenges in the area of highest prevalence. Lancet 371: 1305–1307.
35. Kim MH, Cox C, Dave A, Draper HR, Kabue M, et al. (2012) Prompt initiation of ART With therapeutic food is associated with improved outcomes in HIV-infected Malawian children with malnutrition. J Acquir Immune Defic Syndr 59: 173–176.

Poor Nutrition Status and Associated Feeding Practices among HIV-Positive Children in a Food Secure Region in Tanzania: A Call for Tailored Nutrition Training

Bruno F. Sunguya[1], Krishna C. Poudel[2], Linda B. Mlunde[1], David P. Urassa[3], Junko Yasuoka[1]*, Masamine Jimba[1]

1 Department of Community and Global Health, Graduate School of Medicine, The University of Tokyo, Tokyo, Japan, **2** Department of Public Health, School of Public Health and Health Sciences, University of Massachusetts Amherst, Amherst, Massachusetts, United States of America, **3** School of Public Health and Social Sciences, Muhimbili University of Health and Allied Sciences, Dar es Salaam, Tanzania

Abstract

Undernutrition among HIV-positive children can be ameliorated if they are given adequate foods in the right frequency and diversity. Food insecurity is known to undermine such efforts, but even in food rich areas, people have undernutrition. As yet no study has examined feeding practices and their associations with nutrition status among as HIV-positive children in regions with high food production. We therefore examined the magnitude of undernutrition and its association with feeding practices among HIV-positive children in a high food production region in Tanzania.

Methods: We conducted this mixed-method study among 748 children aged 6 months-14 years attending 9 of a total of 32 care and treatment centers in Tanga region, Tanzania. We collected quantitative data using a standard questionnaire and qualitative data through seven focus group discussions (FGDs).

Results: HIV-positive children had high magnitudes of undernutrition. Stunting, underweight, wasting, and thinness were prevalent among 61.9%, 38.7%, 26.0%, and 21.1% of HIV-positive children, respectively. They also had poor feeding practices: 88.1% were fed at a frequency below the recommendations, and 62.3% had a low level of dietary diversity. Lower feeding frequency was associated with stunting ($\beta = 0.11$, $p = 0.016$); underweight ($\beta = 0.12$, $p = 0.029$); and thinness ($\beta = 0.11$, $p = 0.026$). Lower feeding frequency was associated with low wealth index ($\beta = 0.06$, $p < 0.001$), food insecurity ($\beta = -0.05$, $p < 0.001$), and caregiver's education. In the FGDs, participants discussed the causal relationships among the key associations; undernutrition was mainly due to low feeding frequency and dietary diversity. Such poor feeding practices resulted from poor nutrition knowledge, food insecurity, low income, and poverty.

Conclusion: Feeding practices and nutrition status were poor among HIV-positive children even in food rich areas. Improving feeding frequency may help to ameliorate undernutrition. To improve it, tailored interventions should target children of poor households, the food insecure, and caregivers who have received only a low level of education.

Editor: Grace C. John-Stewart, University of Washington, United States of America

Funding: This study is funded by a grant from the Directorate of Research and Publication of the Muhimbili University of Health and Allied Sciences (Ref. No: MU/01/1022/0130/21), and the Ministry of Health, Labor and Welfare of Japan (Research Grant No: H24-Chikyukibo-Ippan-008). Funders did not have influence on the results or conduct of this study. The funders had no role in study design, data collection and analysis, decision to publish, or preparation of the manuscript.

Competing Interests: The authors have declared that no competing interests exist.

* E-mail: jyasuoka@post.harvard.edu

Background

Poor feeding practices undermine efforts to combat unacceptably high rates of undernutrition among children in developing countries [1,2]. Such practices include low feeding frequency, low dietary diversity, inadequate quantity, and diets with poor quality [1,3]. Efforts to improve feeding practices can also improve undernutrition among children in developing countries [4–7].

Poverty and other socio-demographic disadvantages can limit adequate feeding practices [8,9]. Households in low economic strata are prone to food insecurity [10–12]. Under such circumstance, poor households have limited choices for food with adequate nutritional values [10,12]. They usually adapt themselves to this situation by cutting down the number of basic meals or reducing the amount in each meal [13,14]. In a typical household affected by food insecurity, children are usually less afflicted during its early stage. At this stage, other members of the household tend to reduce amount and frequency of food for themselves for the sake of children. However, children are more likely to be affected by extreme forms of food insecurity and later, hunger. Socio-economic disadvantages and the cycle of poverty are also associated with poor education. Children of poorly educated caregivers succumb to various forms of undernutrition [15]. The possible link could be through poor feeding practices [16].

Through high agricultural yield or high purchasing power, food availability can reduce a household's food insecurity [17].

However, even when sufficient food is available, its consumption may not be adequate. This is because the consumption of diverse types of foods in adequate quality, quantity, and frequency may depend on nutrition knowledge of caregivers [3,18]. This may also be a reason behind the high rates of undernutrition among children in the general populations of many developing countries, including Tanzania, even where food productivity is high [19,20].

In developing countries, if children are affected by HIV/AIDS in a household, such household is more likely to have lower potential to provide them with food of adequate quality, quantity, and in the required frequency [14–16,21]. Furthermore, HIV-positive children have special nutritional needs, different from their HIV-negative counterparts [22]. The World Health Organization (WHO) recommends a 10% increase in energy intake for the HIV-positive child growing well on antiretroviral therapy (ART) above the normal requirement of an otherwise HIV-negative child of the same age [22]. A 20–30% increase in energy intake is required to sustain an HIV-positive child with HIV-related symptoms including TB, chronic lung infections, or persistent diarrhea [22]. HIV-positive children need an extra 50–100% of energy intake compared to an otherwise normal child if they have severe malnutrition or severe failure to thrive, regardless of their ART status [22]. These energy requirements are supposed to be met from the foods consumed daily. To achieve adequate nutrition, an HIV-positive child is supposed to eat at least five times a day [22]. Such meals have to be balanced, diverse, and adequate in amount.

Food insecurity and poor feeding practices can also affect the effectiveness of ART and drive the HIV-positive children further into undernutrition. Appropriate use of ART should reduce the risk of a child succumbing to opportunistic infections that can affect his/her nutrition status [23–25]. However, its use comes with its own risks especially in the context of food insecurity and hunger [26]. Food insecurity is known to intensify ART's side effects to the extent of intolerability [21]. To avoid symptoms of ART's side effects, caregivers in some areas give their children ART when they are sure of accessing food to accompany it [27]. This results in poor adherence and sometimes pushing the children further into advanced stages of HIV and undernutrition [21,26]. In Tanzania, too, households with HIV-positive children had a lower dietary diversity score, feeding frequency, and a higher proportion of food insecurity compared to households with HIV-negative children [28].

To decrease undernutrition among HIV-positive children in Tanzania and in other similar areas, feeding practices should be improved [28]. However, to provide culturally appropriate interventions, it is important to understand the local determinants of poor feeding practices among such children. So far, little has been examined about the determinants of poor feeding practices among HIV-positive children in areas where food production is high. In this study, we therefore first examined the magnitude of undernutrition and poor feeding practices. Next, we examined local determinants of undernutrition including its association with feeding practices. Third, we examined the local factors associated with poor feeding practices, in particular, low feeding frequency, among children living with HIV/AIDS in Tanga, Tanzania. Finally, we further explored the key associations by conducting a qualitative inquiry.

Methods

Study design and area

We employed a mixed method design for this study. First, we conducted a cross-sectional quantitative study to examine the magnitude and determinants of undernutrition and poor feeding practices among HIV-positive children in Tanga, Tanzania. Results of this study guided a qualitative study. Through seven focus group discussions (FGDs), we explored possible explanations of the findings and the key associations between various determinants and undernutrition among HIV-positive children. Finally, we triangulated results from both methods to help explain the causal relations of the associations between feeding practices and nutrition statuses among HIV-positive children in this food rich region. This study seeks to contribute to the operational research [29], aiming to improve feeding practices and thus nutritional status of such vulnerable children.

In the Tanga region, a vast diversity of food is available and grown. It is the leading region in fruit and vegetable production in the country and supplies other regions with cereal, fruits, marine, and diary products. The presence of such quantity and diversity of foods is not correlated with consumption and nutrition statuses. Only 59.4% of 292 sampled under-five children in Tanga consumed foods rich in Vitamin A [19]. Tanga has the worst nutrition outcomes in the country despite the foods available. For example, stunting prevalence was the highest in the country with about 49% of 315 under-five sampled children, 12% were underweight, and 5.5% had wasting. Poor feeding practices could also be behind poor micronutrient markers among children. In the same population, 38.9% of children had Vitamin A deficiency, 36.5% had iron deficiency, and 52.2% had iron deficiency anemia [19].

A total of 20,773 people living with HIV/AIDS were enrolled in care and treatment centers (CTCs) in the Tanga region in 2009. Although the magnitude of HIV/AIDS among children has not been reported for Tanga, about 1,800 HIV-positive children have been enrolled in the CTCs for care and treatment. The current study was a hospital-based study and conducted among participants who were attending CTCs in the region. We described the CTCs' organization and distribution in a separate article [29].

After obtaining confirmatory test results using the standard algorithm [30], HIV-positive children are usually enrolled in the CTCs to receive care. Such care includes treatment with Highly Active Antiretroviral Therapy (HAART), follow up, adherence counseling, and treatment of other associated opportunistic infections [30]. They are also supposed to receive nutrition care and monitoring. However, during this study period, no specific nutrition intervention was carried out targeting HIV-positive children attending these CTCs. Health workers attending these children also were not equipped with any inservice nutrition training to improve their management skills, and the new WHO *Guidelines for an integrated approach to the nutritional care of HIV-infected children (6 months – 14 years)* [22] had not yet been locally adapted.

Participants

We recruited pairs of HIV-positive children and their caregivers who were attending the CTCs for the child to receive care and/or treatment. Inclusion criteria were children aged between six months and fourteen years, who are registered at or have been transferred to the CTC, who have ART records, and whose caregiver gave consent to participate in the study. We excluded children with missing medical records.

We selected a convenience sample of nine out of 32 CTCs that give care to such patients. The selected health facilities represented most districts of the Tanga region and have at least 20 children registered. Out of 32 CTCs, 15 fulfilled this criterion. We selected the CTC with the highest number of children if the district had two or more CTCs with at least 20 children. Because of its size and high number of patients, we selected three CTCs from the Tanga municipality. This process resulted in a final selection of nine CTCs for this study which, according to medical records, had a total of 1,248 children registered. We recruited a total of 797 pairs of children and their caregivers for this study, who attended the clinic on the day of data collection, and fulfilled the criteria. We excluded the data of 49 children after data collection. Among them, 41 had missing variables or erroneous entries for the outcome variable, and eight had not met the selection criteria.

We also conducted seven FGD sessions with the caregivers of HIV-positive children attending CTCs in Tanga region. The initial plan was to conduct nine focus group discussions; one from each CTC selected for the quantitative survey. However, we had reached the saturation point at the seventh group and no new information was emerging. We conducted each FGD in a separate district to reach participants in different geographic areas within the region. We conveniently selected participants who agreed to participate and who had time for the discussions when they were done with care and treatment or an ART refill for their HIV-positive children. We invited eight participants for each group, for a total of 56 caregivers.

Measurements

The outcome variables of interest were measures of nutrition status including stunting, underweight, thinness, and wasting. A low height for age, below or equal to −2 SD of the reference population, signifies moderate stunting while below or equal to −3 SD signifies severe stunting [31–33]. To measure height, we used a standard measuring board calibrated in centimeters and converted it to height-for-age z-scores (HAZ).

Wasting is measured by weight for height of children aged 6–60 months. A low weight for height, below or equal to −2 SD of the reference population, signifies acute moderate wasting, while below or equal to −3 SD signifies severe wasting [31–33]. We measured weight in grams using a standard Salter scale with minimal clothing and converted them into weight-for-height z-scores.

We also used underweight as a measure of weight for age of children up to 10 years of age [34]. A child with a weight-for-age z score below or equal to −2 SD of the reference population is moderately underweight while a child below or equal to −3 SD is severely underweight. Finally, we used BMI-z scores as a measure of thinness among children aged above five years. A BMI-z score below or equal to −2SD was considered moderate thinness, while below or equal to −3SD is severe thinness. All anthropometric calculations used WHO Anthro version 3.22 [34].

To measure feeding practices, we assessed the most common measures, which are feeding frequency and dietary diversity. In this study, we assessed feeding frequency and dietary diversity separately.

We assessed feeding frequency by asking the caregivers to recall the number of times they fed their children in the previous 24 hours. This measurement was also used in previous studies in Tanzania among HIV-positive children [35,36]. We considered a feeding frequency below five to be a low feeding frequency. The WHO recommends a feeding frequency of at least five times a day for HIV-positive children [22,37].

We measured dietary diversity using the dietary diversity scale (DDS) [38]. The scale is made of common food items usually found in the area of interest. We extracted a list of twelve food items from the Tanzania Demographic and Health Survey [20,39]. In our questionnaire, we asked caregivers about the food items they had given to their children in the previous 24 hours and summed them to make the total dietary diversity score. To establish the cutoff point for low dietary diversity, we used the median value, which was three. This value also coincided with the mean DDS of the lowest two terciles of the DDS score as recommended by the developer [38]. Therefore, a DDS score of three or below was considered low DDS. The DDS scale was also used in previous studies of HIV-positive children in Tanzania [28,36].

We assessed food insecurity using the household food insecurity access scale (HFIAS) [40]. HFIAS is a nine-item questionnaire used to measure the severity of food insecurity and household access to food according to a Likert scale. Options in this scale are 0 = 'no', 1 = 'rarely', 2 = 'sometimes', and 3 = 'often'. The lowest total score is 0 and the highest is 27. The scale can be used as a continuous variable or categorized into four groups: food secure, mildly insecure, moderately insecure, and severely insecure. HFIAS uses a recall period of 30 days and has been used in several studies within the region [2,41–45]. In this study, HFIAS had a Cronbach's alpha of 0.96, an item-rest correlation ranging from 0.63 to 0.89, and an average variance of 0.36.

To determine HIV/AIDS progression, we used the WHO clinical staging system, a four-stage classification system. We classified the first two stages as "early stages" and clinical HIV stages 3 and 4 as "advanced stages" [46]. We retrieved the data on HIV stage from the medical files of each patient. The health workers update the clinical stage on a routine basis with each patient visit to the CTC.

We measured adherence to ART using a four-day recall. We asked patients whether they took their medications, when during the day, how many times each day, and how many pills each time. Based on the HAART regimen, doctors can prescribe a once or twice a day dosage. For the twice a day dosage regimen, we considered missing one dose in four days as low adherence. For the once a day dosage regimen, we considered missing one in four day regimen as low adherence.

To assess the burden of common opportunistic infections, we asked the caregivers whether their children had been affected by tuberculosis (TB), malaria, acute respiratory infections, or diarrhea in the past six months. As in previous studies [28,47], we defined diarrhea as the presence of three or more watery stools during the previous 24 hours. We defined malaria as a febrile illness with symptoms such as fever, chills and sweating, confirmed with laboratory investigation [48].

As in previous studies [28,36] and other population surveys in Tanzania [20,39,49], we used a weighted wealth index to assess the economic status of households with HIV-positive children. The wealth index was calculated based on ownership of household durable assets. Factor analysis was used to reduce the constructed dichotomous variables from 59 to 22, which loaded as factor 1. We treated the factor loadings as item weights summed to give the wealth index for each household like in the previous studies [50–52].

We adopted other socio-demographic variables from the women and household questionnaires of the TDHS [20,39]. The population surveys tested and used such variables in both 2005 and 2010 in Tanzania. Such variables included caregivers' education level, child's orphanhood state, sex, and age. We defined a caregiver as being a child's parent, relative, guardian, or anyone else above 18 years old who takes care of the child and supervises their treatment or accompanies them to the CTCs [28]. We measured education level according to the education levels in Tanzania and divided them into three levels: no formal education, having a primary level education, and above primary level, including secondary, college, and others. A child who lost one or both parents was regarded as an orphan [20,39].

Data collection

We collected data using a pre-tested questionnaire. We conducted a one-day training of two research assistants from each CTC on interview techniques, questionnaire content, and ethics in data collection. We collected data through face-to-face interviews and retrieved medical data from medical records from April to May 2013.

For the focus group discussions, we used an IC recorder to record the participants' discussions. Before each discussion, participants introduced their age, occupation, marital status, and number of children they care for. The moderator, who is the first author, introduced the study, explained its aims, and set ground rules. The stem questions asked by the moderator sought to find the local factors associated with undernutrition in the region despite its known vast food production, participants' feeding practices, food access, the role of nutrition education, occurrence of opportunistic infections, and local challenges encountered when feeding HIV-positive children in each district. Finally, participants were given opportunities to suggest their local solutions and what they needed from the health workers to combat poor feeding practices and undernutrition among HIV-positive children and those of the general population. All discussions were conducted in Swahili language. The conduct and reporting of the FGDs was in accordance with the consolidated criteria for reporting qualitative research (COREQ) [53].

Data analysis

We conducted analysis using both descriptive and regression methods. For descriptive analyses, we used Chi-square tests to compare the characteristics of participants. A similar method was used to examine the magnitude of undernutrition and feeding characteristics presented in categorical variables while comparing them between males and females. We conducted bivariate linear regression to examine association between independent variables and dependent variables. In this case, we examined factors associated with each type of undernutrition. Statistical associations with p-values below or equal to 0.2 were entered into a multivariate regression to find factors associated with undernutrition after adjusting for confounders and important covariates [54].

Feeding frequency was low and associated with most of the nutrition status measures. Therefore a separate model was built to examine factors associated with feeding frequency among HIV-positive children attending CTCs in Tanga region. For this model, independent variables included sex; household wealth index; caregivers' education level; orphanhood; household food insecurity access score; acute respiratory infection or diarrhea in the past six months; and HAART adherence.

In both models, we examined multicollinearity using variance-inflating factors. None of the independent variables had a VIF value above 10 or below 0.1. We set the statistical significance at *p-value*<0.05. We conducted all analyses using STATA version 12.

A research assistant transcribed the recorded focus group discussions into Swahili scripts. A separate research assistant then translated each of the Swahili scripts into English. A local expert on qualitative research checked for quality of each step. We analyzed the transcribed text based on the themes that emerged from the discussion [55].

When the main study and all publications are completed, the data collected in this study will be made available to other researchers upon request. Data will be coded to ensure confidentiality and anonymity.

Ethics statement

We obtained written consent from participants before the interviews and focus group discussion. Participants were assured of confidentiality and anonymity throughout the process and for all reports and publications generated. Participation was voluntary and there were no implications for care at the CTC upon refusal to participate. This study was approved by the Research Ethics Committee of the University of Tokyo, and the Expedited Review Sub-committee of the Senate Research and Publication Directorate of the Muhimbili University of Health and Allied Sciences.

Results

Quantitative study

General characteristics. We recruited 63.8% of all HIV-positive children attending the nine selected CTCs in Tanga region. Data were available for analyses from 748 pairs of HIV-positive children and their caregivers who were attending CTCs. Of the 748 HIV-positive children in this study, 666 (89.0%) were on HAART. Of those on treatment, 85.3% had high adherence to the treatment. Of all children included in this study, 69.6% were in the advanced HIV clinical stage. Among the 666 HIV-positive children on HAART, 75.7% were in the advanced HIV clinical stage. In this respect, no differences were observed between male and female participants. Table 1 shows that two thirds (66.7%) of the children had lost at least one parent. A high proportion of their caregivers (22.1%) had no formal education while only 7.6% of all caregivers had at least secondary education.

Feeding practices and nutrition status of HIV-positive children in Tanga. HIV-positive children in this study had a mean dietary diversity score of 3.3 (SD 1.3) and a mean feeding frequency of 3.2 (SD 1.0). The WHO's standard recommended feeding frequency for this population is ideally five times a day. As shown in Table 2, a high proportion of HIV-positive children (88.1%) were fed at a low frequency. Feeding frequency did not differ between male and female participants. A high proportion of HIV-positive children (62.3%) had a low dietary diversity score.

HIV-positive children also presented with a high burden of undernutrition. A high magnitude (61.9%) of HIV-positive children attending CTCs had moderate to severe stunting. Moderate to severe underweight was also prevalent among 38.7% of children below ten years of age. More than one quarter (26.0%) of HIV-positive children aged between six months and five years presented with moderate to severe wasting. Moderate to severe thinness was prevalent among 21.1% of HIV-positive children aged six years and above. For all types of undernutrition, there were no statistical differences between male and female children.

Determinants of undernutrition among HIV-positive children attending CTCs in Tanga. Table 3 shows the results of regression analysis on the factors associated with undernutrition among HIV-positive children attending CTCs with their caregivers. After adjusting for covariates and confounders, a unit increase in age of HIV-positive children (in months) was more likely to be associated with poor linear growth ($\beta = -0.35$, $p<0.001$). Compared to uneducated caregivers, caregivers with at least primary education had a lower chance of having stunted children ($\beta = 0.87$, $p = 0.035$). Household food insecurity was also associated with children's poor linear growth ($\beta = -0.01$, $p = 0.027$). Low feeding frequency was also associated with poor linear growth among HIV-positive children ($\beta = 0.11$, $p = 0.016$). Malaria episodes in the past six months and advanced HIV clinical stage were also associated with poor linear growth among HIV-positive children.

Table 1. Descriptive characteristics of HIV-positive children attending CTCs in Tanga.

Variable	Total		Male		Female		p-value
	n	%	n	%	n	%	
Age (months)							
6–59	152	20.3	81	23.7	71	17.5	0.105
60–143	422	56.4	183	53.5	239	58.9	
144–168	174	23.3	78	22.8	96	23.6	
Parental status							
Non-orphan	249	33.3	122	35.7	127	31.3	0.204
Orphan	499	66.7	220	64.3	279	68.7	
Caregiver education							
None	165	22.1	73	21.3	92	22.7	0.852
Primary	526	70.3	244	71.4	282	69.4	
>Primary	57	7.6	25	7.3	32	7.9	
Wealth index							
High	251	33.6	123	36.0	128	31.5	0.327
Middle	248	33.2	105	30.7	143	35.2	
Low	249	33.2	114	33.3	135	33.3	
ART status							
Yes	666	89.0	303	88.6	363	89.4	0.490
No	82	11.0	39	11.4	43	10.6	
HIV stage							
Early	227	30.4	101	29.5	126	31.0	0.656
Advanced	521	69.6	241	70.5	280	69.0	
ART adherence							
Low	98	14.7	49	16.1	49	13.5	0.349
High	568	85.3	255	83.9	313	86.5	
Household food security							
Food secure	146	19.6	70	20.5	76	18.8	0.899
Mild insecure	46	6.2	22	6.5	24	5.9	
Moderate insecure	112	15.0	49	14.4	63	15.6	
Severe insecure	442	59.2	200	58.6	242	59.7	

CTC- Care and treatment center; ART- Antiretroviral therapy; HIV- Human immunodeficiency virus.

Table 2. Magnitude of poor feeding practices and nutrition status.

Nutrition status	Male		Female		Total		p-value
	n	%	n	%	N	%	
Feeding Frequency							
Low	298	87.1	361	88.9	659	88.1	0.454
High	44	12.9	45	11.1	89	11.9	
Dietary Diversity Score							
Low	220	64.3	246	60.6	466	62.3	0.293
High	122	39.7	160	39.4	282	37.7	
Wasting (≤ 60 months)							
Wasted (WHZ ≤−2SD)	29	30.2	18	21.2	47	26.0	0.167
Normal (WHZ>−2SD)	67	69.8	67	78.8	134	74.0	
Thinness (>60 months)							
Thin (BMIZ ≤−2SD)	56	23.1	62	19.6	118	21.1	0.316
Normal (BMIZ>−2SD)	187	76.9	255	80.4	442	78.9	
Underweight (≤120 months)							
Underweight (WAZ≤−2SD)	95	40.6	103	37.1	198	38.7	0.412
Normal (WAZ>−2SD)	139	59.4	175	62.9	314	61.3	
Stunting (6 months-14 years)							
Stunted (HAZ≤−2SD)	208	60.8	255	62.8	463	61.9	0.577
Normal (HAZ>−2SD)	134	39.2	151	37.2	285	38.1	

WHZ- Weight-for-height z-score; BMIZ- Body Mass Index-for-age z-score; WAZ- Weight-for-age z-score; HAZ- Height-for-age z-score.

Table 3. Regression analyses of factors associated with undernutrition (stunting, wasting, underweight, and thinness) among HIV-positive children.

Variable	Stunting (HAZ-score)				Wasting (WHZ-score)				Underweight (WAZ-score)				Thinness (BMIZ-score)			
	Bivariate		Multivariate		Bivariate		Multivariate		Bivariate		Multivariate		Bivariate		Multivariate	
	Beta	p-value	Beta	p-value	Beta	p-value	Beta	p-value	Beta	p-value	Beta	p-value	Beta	p-value	Beta	p-value
Age	−0.32	<0.001	−0.35	<0.001	0.17	0.024	0.20	0.009	−0.04	0.363	−0.06	0.180	−0.27	<0.001	−0.28	<0.001
Sex	−0.07	0.071	−0.06	0.076	0.06	0.413	0.06	0.411	0.05	0.308	0.31	0.484	0.06	0.182	0.04	0.353
Education																
None	1.00												1.00			
Primary	0.15	<0.001	0.87	0.035	0.16	0.841	0.02	0.808	0.09	0.095	−0.01	0.942	−0.01	0.950	−0.05	0.273
>Primary	0.10	0.011	0.36	0.395	0.11	0.195	0.07	0.451	0.18	0.001	0.07	0.196	0.13	0.008	0.06	0.186
Wealth index	0.11	0.002	−0.02	0.606	0.15	0.036	0.09	0.294	0.17	<0.001	−0.01	0.790	0.08	0.053	0.01	0.876
Food insecurity	−0.20	<0.001	−0.01	0.027	−0.15	0.038	0.06	0.541	−0.29	<0.001	−0.17	0.003	−0.13	0.002	−0.08	0.134
Food frequency	0.18	<0.001	0.11	0.016	0.14	0.054	0.05	0.601	0.25	<0.001	0.12	0.029	0.14	0.001	0.11	0.026
Dietary diversity	0.17	<0.001	0.08	0.050	0.08	0.305			0.20	<0.001	0.07	0.165	0.08	0.074	−0.01	0.972
TB	−0.07	0.070	−0.06	0.096	−0.04	0.579			−0.09	0.053	−0.07	0.111	−0.07	−0.103	−0.07	0.066
Diarrhea	−0.04	0.261			−0.08	0.267			−0.07	0.160	−0.04	0.452	−0.04	0.365		
Malaria	−0.71	0.051	−0.09	0.013	−0.17	0.020	−0.12	0.119	−0.16	0.001	−0.14	0.002	0.03	0.438		
ARI	−0.05	0.163	0.03	0.350	−0.15	0.051	−0.13	0.120	−0.12	0.008	−0.01	0.826	0.01	0.840		
HIV stage	−0.12	0.001	−0.12	0.001	−0.25	0.001	−0.25	0.001	−0.18	<0.001	−0.14	0.001	−0.03	0.461		
HAART	0.03	0.479			0.09	0.227			0.03	0.565			−0.11	0.011	−0.12	0.002
Adherence	0.05	0.177	0.03	0.423	0.02	0.849			−0.03	0.501			−0.05	0.276		

WHZ- Weight-for-height z-score; BMIZ- Body Mass Index-for-age z-score; WAZ- Weight-for-age z-score; HAZ- Height-for-age z-score; TB- Tuberculosis; ARI- Acute respiratory infection; ART- Antiretroviral therapy.

Wasting was associated with age and HIV clinical stage (Table 3). Younger children were more likely to experience wasting ($\beta = 0.20$, $p = 0.009$), and an increase child's HIV clinical stage from early to advanced was more likely to be associated with severity of wasting ($\beta = -0.25$, $p = 0.001$). Feeding practices were not significantly associated with wasting among children of this population.

Food insecurity, feeding frequency, malaria, and HIV clinical stage were associated with poor weight gain for age after controlling for covariates and confounders (Table 3). HIV-positive children residing in households with food insecurity were more likely to be underweight ($\beta = -0.17$, $p = 0.003$). Low feeding frequency was also associated with poor weight gain for age among HIV-positive children ($\beta = 0.12$, $p = 0.029$). Having malaria in the past six months ($\beta = -0.14$, $p = 0.002$) and advanced HIV clinical stage ($\beta = -0.14$, $p = 0.001$) were associated with poor weight gain among children in this population.

Factors associated with thinness included age in months, feeding frequency, and ART use (Table 3). After adjusting for covariates and confounders, a unit increase in age of HIV-positive children (in months) was more likely to be associated with poor body mass index for age ($\beta = -0.28$, $p < 0.001$). Feeding frequency was also more likely to be associated with poor body mass index for age among HIV-positive children ($\beta = 0.11$, $p = 0.026$). HIV-positive children on ART were more likely to have poor body mass index for age ($\beta = -0.12$, $p = 0.002$).

Factors associated with feeding frequency. Table 4 shows the results of bivariate and multivariate regression analysis for the factors associated with feeding frequency among the HIV-positive children attending CTCs. Children residing in households with a low wealth index were less likely to have a high feeding frequency ($\beta = 0.06$, $p < 0.001$) so were children whose households had high levels of food insecurity ($\beta = -0.05$, $p < 0.001$). HIV-positive children whose caregivers had higher than primary school education were more likely to have higher feeding frequency ($\beta = 0.34$, $p = 0.015$), Finally, having acute respiratory tract infections in the previous six months was associated with low feeding frequency among HIV-positive children ($\beta = -0.23$, $p = 0.001$).

Results of the focus group discussions

We identified seven major themes from the seven focus group discussions that were conducted. The themes evolved from the locally identified determinants of undernutrition and poor feeding practices. They included low feeding frequency and dietary diversity, food insecurity, poverty and low income, and opportunistic infections. These four themes were related to the factors associated with undernutrition in the quantitative survey. Three other themes emerged that were unrelated to the quantitative survey: stigma, lack of nutrition education or misconceptions, and traditions and ways of life.

Feeding frequency and dietary diversity. In this study, low feeding frequency was a common practice among participants. Caregivers fed their children twice a day or at the same frequency as adults or otherwise normal children.

> "...my children eat only twice a day although I am a food vendor. In the morning I give them porridge until at 4 PM, when they eat the last meal of a day. We skip lunch because we cannot afford it. I prefer giving the last meal closer to night just to make them survive." (A 26-year-old food vendor and mother of two HIV-positive children)

Participants explained that when they increased their children's feeding frequency, their nutrition statuses improved.

> "My child's hair was so weak, so thin, and she had a large abdomen and thin legs. I was told that she had kwashiorkor. This was when her biological mother had just died. She was checked for worms, and treated for it, also given Septrin (an antibiotic given routinely for HIV-positive children). I

Table 4. Factors associated with feeding frequency.

Variable	Bivariate regression			Multivariate regression		
	Coefficient	Beta	P-value	Coefficient	Beta	p-value
Age (months)	−0.01	−0.05	0.160	−0.01	−0.04	0.201
Sex	−0.06	−0.03	0.401	−0.10	−0.05	0.138
Education						
None	1.00					
Primary	0.43	0.20	<0.001	0.07	0.03	0.420
>Primary	0.93	0.26	<0.001	0.34	0.09	0.015
Wealth index	0.17	0.38	<0.001	0.06	0.14	<0.001
Food insecurity	−0.06	−0.49	<0.001	−0.05	−0.39	<0.001
TB	0.13	0.03	0.344			
Diarrhea	−0.26	−0.13	<0.001	−0.04	−0.02	0.563
Malaria	−0.01	−0.01	0.982			
ARI	−0.53	−0.26	<0.001	−0.23	−0.11	0.001
HIV stage	−0.02	−0.01	0.811			
HAART	0.08	0.03	0.459			
ART adherence	0.15	0.13	0.001	0.04	0.04	0.286

TB- Tuberculosis; ARI- Acute respiratory infection; ART- Antiretroviral therapy.

started to give her more food, many times a day. As a result, she started to thrive. She was later started on ARV, and now she looks healthy, all symptoms of kwashiorkor are gone." (A 28-year-old caregiver and mother of four children)

Increasing feeding frequency also showed improvements in micronutrients profiles. It happens when the quality of diets is improved among children living with HIV/AIDS.

"I did not feed my child five times a day. Instead, I gave her three times just like the rest of the family including adults. When I came to hospital, she was found to have low weight, failed to grow, and had low blood contents. I then started to feed actively, especially fruits, vegetables, mixing porridge with peanuts.... she started to grow healthy, her blood contents increased, and weight too, even other diseases had stopped." (A 28-year-old married woman, mother of three children, one of whom is HIV-positive)

HIV-positive children in Tanga are fed with fewer food types. Caregivers pointed to a lack of money to buy other types of food although such foods are available in the markets.

"...nowadays, we cook only once a day, either plain corn porridge or stiff porridge, so the child eats only what is available in the morning until evening. If we are lucky to have something to eat at night, we give her otherwise we sleep hungry. We are taught to give them mixture of eggs, meat, milk, and vegetables. Although these foods are available, we can not afford them." (A 50-year-old caregiver, mother of four children and a small-scale farmer)

Caregivers may be given nutrition education on how to mix foods for their children. But many of them still consume a mixture of similar types of foods unknowingly. These foods have similar nutrition contents and might not provide added benefits, no matter the number of items included or frequency at which they are fed.

"...in her porridge, I mix flour from corn, millet, sorghum, rice, and other cereals. I was advised to mix a variety of foods to improve nutrition. This porridge I give many times in a day." (A 24-year-old mother of two who is also an entrepreneur, selling a similar mixture to her peers)

When asked who taught her this mixture, she said, "This is what I was taught by my nurses here."

Giving high dietary diversity can improve nutrition status and even physical body functions. Several caregivers explained that their children had improved after they received nutrition advice to increase diversity.

"My child had poor health, weak, and very thin when I started her in this clinic. She could not stand up by herself or play, although she had the age of a child who could walk and run. She started ARV, and I was given nutrition advice, which I followed, I started to give milk, adequate volumes of various foods, and fruits everyday. Her health status improved, and gained weight. She could then play and walk." She went on and say, "I have stopped giving that quality foods now because, now I can not afford it... we cook only once for what we have...I cannot give milk, I can't even cook with cooking oil...as a result, she is falling back so fast." (A 30-year-old farmer and caregiver of seven children)

Food insecurity and hunger. The HIV-positive participants mentioned that low food availability in their households is common because they cannot do manual farm work due to their health condition. They have low purchasing power for foods despite being available in the markets. As a result, they cannot have the recommended feeding frequency and dietary diversity. Ultimately, their children suffer from undernutrition.

"I am a farmer, and depend on agriculture. Last year for example, it did not rain enough. We did not get harvests, especially corn. Foods were little and less diverse...we did not have income, and could not even buy enough foods from markets. This child ate less and lost weight. When this child is sick with fever, he wants to eat some good foods; it was impossible for him to get it. He did not want to eat stiff porridge available all day, everyday." (A 56-year-old grandmother of an HIV-positive child)

"For farmers like me, sometimes, we do not harvest enough because we depend on rain and can do it manually with hand hoe, so we cannot cultivate enough because of our health. Our yields are low and we are in a constant food shortage." (A 59-year-old widow and farmer)

Poverty and low income. Participants pointed to poverty and low income as an underlying cause of poor feeding practices and undernutrition among HIV-positive children in this region.

"..now life has become so difficult. I am sick, and cannot do hard work, especially farming. It causes children to lose weight because good food requires a lot of money. I do not have income. I know that milk is important especially when you use strong medications like ARVs, but, I can stay one year before I or my child could drink it. Sometimes in my family we sleep without eating anything... my child goes to school without breakfast. When I am well I go to work, and get paid 2000 shillings for example, I can only afford to buy basic cheap food. That is why children are undernourished." (A 50-year-old mother of four children)

"...low income is the reason for undernutrition. I struggle to look for money, the child eat only twice, in the morning and then at evening even when I myself sell food and fruits...when my husband died, he left us a little money. My family income suddenly dropped. I am the only person who has to provide for my family and it is not enough." (A 37-year-old mother of two)

Opportunistic infections. HIV/AIDS suppresses immunity leading to opportunistic infections. Participants in this study gave examples where undernutrition of their children resulted from such infections.

"My child had swellings on his neck. During the time of this illness, he was not eating well, and complained of painful swallowing. He became wasted, like those people who are real sick of AIDS. But after medication (not ARVs), he improved; now he eats well and his weight gained." (A 31-year-old mother of two children)

Tanga is also an endemic area for malaria transmission. Participants also explained how malaria contributed to their children's poor nutrition status.

"This week, my child was sick of malaria, she could not hold food, she has fever, and she also has oral curd-like condition they say is fungus. She has pain when eating and has lost too much weight... her suffering gives me depression." (A 32-year-old mother of two HIV-positive children)

Stigma related to HIV status and child undernutrition. Participants indicated that stigma against people living with HIV/AIDS can lead to a child's poor health including undernutrition. For example:

"Another problem is stigma. Colleague of my child tells her at school that she has AIDS... this created stigma. As a result, she lost hope at first then refused to eat; at the end she lost weight. She told me that her friends did not want to play with her. People in our society stigmatize our children and us. Even if we feed them with whatever food available, the stigma they face weakens them physically and psychologically." (A 24-year-old entrepreneur and mother of two HIV-positive children)

"...another reason is stigma especially for those who are older children attending schools. They are isolated and mocked. They feel weak and lose hope. Their feeding deteriorates even in the presence of enough food as well." (A 20-year-old mother of one HIV-positive child)

Stigma also exists within families. A 30-year-old housewife and mother to two while caring for her late sister's HIV-positive child said:

"My husband leaves money for his children's food only, not for this HIV-positive one. Even when I leave some for this affected child, he does not like it, and get mad at me."

Lack of nutrition education or misconceptions, and traditional beliefs. In the current study, caregivers had low levels of nutrition knowledge especially of adequate feeding frequency, proper dietary diversity, and mixing of foods for young HIV-positive children.

"Majority of us do not understand what is a good quality food. Education on nutrition is lacking...we have our myths from our traditions. We thought that artificial juice had equal nutrition values as natural juice based on fruits available in our environment, such as pawpaw, mangoes, oranges, banana, etc. I would like to know how to make them. With such knowledge, I believe, I will be able to make right decisions on foods. All quality food substances are available I believe, I just need to understand how to combine them in to a quality diet. For example, if I cannot afford meat, what else should I replace with? What cheap options can I substitute with?" (A 33-year-old father of four children)

A 19-year-old participant thinks that vegetables are not 'good food' as it is the food of poor, and said "I eat vegetables a few days only when I do not have money for alternatives like red meat." She added, "Good food is anything other than green vegetables. Vegetables are not considered as good food here. In our normal diet we do not eat them, even when available."

Discussion

HIV-positive children attending CTCs had poor nutrition status despite vast food availability in the Tanga region. For example, 61.9% of all recruited HIV-positive children were stunted; 38.7% of HIV-positive children below ten years were underweight; 26.0% of HIV-positive children between six months and five years had wasting; and 21.1% of HIV-positive children above five years were thin. Feeding practices of HIV-positive children attending HIV care and treatment centers were poor. Among the children recruited to participate in this study, 88.1% had a feeding frequency below the recommended value of five times a day. About two thirds of the children had dietary diversity scores of three or below. Triangulated evidence of the quantitative and qualitative studies showed that the poor feeding practices in Tanga region were associated with undernutrition in this region. Regression analyses of factors associated with different types of undernutrition pointed to feeding frequency as a common risk factor for stunting, underweight, and thinness. This is the first study to demonstrate the high magnitudes of poor feeding practices among HIV-positive children in areas known to have adequate food production and its association with undernutrition.

Magnitudes of poor nutrition status in this food rich region among HIV-positive children was higher compared to the general population [19]. For example, while 49.0% of children in the general population were stunted, 61.9% of the HIV-positive children in this study were stunted. Similarly, for all other types of undernutrition, magnitudes were higher in this study than in the general population. Contrary to our prior thoughts, magnitudes of undernutrition among HIV-positive children in this food secure region were also higher compared to those of ART-treated HIV-positive children in another city in Tanzania [28]. As in our previous study [28], ART did not have a statistically significant influence over nutrition status of most types of undernutrition.

This study found an inverse association between age in months and linear growth. Stunting is a chronic form of undernutrition resulting from the cumulative effects of food shortages and poor feeding practices [56]. Compared to other forms of undernutrition, stunting is an irreversible condition. Its effects are long term and can result in poor brain and intellectual development. Our results are different from another study we conducted in another city in Tanzania [28]. Results of the qualitative study showed that low feeding frequency, low amounts, and limited variety of feeding were also common and contributed to poor nutrition statuses.

Low feeding frequency was associated with stunting, underweight, and thinness among HIV-positive children in this study. Similar conclusions were made for stunting, wasting, and underweight in our previous study among HIV-positive children in a different city in Tanzania [28]. WHO recommends a feeding frequency of at least five times a day to provide for the high energy and nutrients demand among HIV-positive children [22]. Improvement in feeding frequency and other feeding practices can bring about positive changes in nutrition status among children in the general population [4]. Our study strengthens the need for improvement in feeding practices, particularly feeding frequency, in the fight against undernutrition.

In this study, overall feeding practices of HIV-positive children were poor, despite food production being high in the region. Households of HIV-positive children also had high levels of food insecurity; about three quarters of the children resided in households with moderate to severe food insecurity. Caregivers of HIV-positive children, in particular, may therefore not be able to provide enough food for their families even if general food availability in the area is good [21]. As in other regions in Tanzania [28], such caregivers may succumb to socio-economic disadvantages and are also prone to a high burden of opportunistic infections as they are also more likely to be HIV-positive. The main sources of food in this region are small-scale farming and animal husbandry. Therefore, poor families with no or small farmlands, or HIV-positive people who are not strong enough to do the manual labor required on a farm, may have less food for their households. This in turn may lead to a chronic shortage of food and may bring about low dietary diversity and inadequate intake of nutrients [10,11].

Feeding frequency might also be affected in a similar way. In this study, an independent association was detected between feeding frequency among households affected by food insecurity and poverty. Results from focus group discussions among caregivers of HIV-positive children also showed that households with food insecurity were more prone to low feeding frequency of their children. Because of the lack of food, children ate twice a day on most occasions. Similar results were observed in Ethiopia among adolescents with unknown serostatus [57] and HIV-positive adults.[58] However, these areas have been known to have long periods of hunger and food insecurity, characteristics that differ from our study.

Feeding practices, and in particular feeding frequency, were also associated with the caregiver's education level. In this case, even when food is available at the household level and other factors are controlled for; caregivers with low education levels may not provide foods to their children at the recommended frequency. More than one fifth of the caregivers of HIV-positive children in this population were not educated. In the qualitative study, too, caregivers had little knowledge of nutrition and how to feed their children. There were many misconceptions based on local beliefs and traditions that also led to wrong choices of foods. The level of education may determine nutrition knowledge [59]. When caregivers are given such knowledge, they improve feeding practices, including feeding frequency and dietary diversity, of their children [3,58,60,61].

Poor feeding practices were associated with a burden of other diseases. For example, low feeding frequency was associated with the chance of having had acute respiratory tract infections at the same time. Such acute diseases are especially common among children with HIV/AIDS and undernutrition [25]. Results from our qualitative study may help to explain this phenomenon. Because of low immunity, HIV-positive children who are also affected by undernutrition are prone to other infections including upper respiratory tract infections. Children with these conditions improved upon proper feeding in adequate amount and frequency.

The results of this study should be interpreted with care owing to the following limitations. First, the nature of our cross-sectional design limits our conclusions on causality. For example, the direction of associations between feeding practices and infections such as respiratory tract infections cannot be ascertained. However, triangulation of the quantitative and the qualitative study can help further explore such associations, though it is not sufficient to ascertain causality. Previous models have also suggested the association between diseases such as malaria and respiratory tract infections with undernutrition is possibly through poor feeding practices among HIV-positive children [62]. Second, this study may be subjected to recall bias based on self-reporting by caregivers of HIV-positive children on items such as feeding practices, food insecurity, and other demographic characteristics. Third, our findings may not be generalizable beyond the settings of high food productivity. Evidence already exists on the high magnitude of poor feeding practices among HIV-positive children in general settings [15] and in food insecure areas among HIV-negative [57] and HIV-positive adults [58]. Fourth, the reliability of our measurement for ART adherence may be questionable, as it was not validated in scientific articles from the settings of this study. However similar method is being used in CTC clinics to monitor ART adherence and conduct adherence counseling. Fifth, we did not translate the translated script from Swahili to English, to the original Swahili language to compare with the original script. This could have lead to the unintended translation. However, the first author who supervised the overall translation process is fluent both in English and Swahili language and tried to avoid the fatal misunderstandings.

Conclusion

In conclusion, HIV-positive children attending care and treatment centers in Tanga, a region with adequate food production, had poor nutrition statuses and low feeding frequency and dietary diversity scores. Low feeding frequency was associated with stunting, underweight, and thinness. Factors associated with low feeding frequency included low wealth index, low maternal or caregiver education, household food insecurity, and acute respiratory tract infections in the past six months.

To ameliorate the high burden of undernutrition among HIV-positive children, feeding practices, in particular feeding frequency, should be improved even in areas where food production is high and food is available at low cost. To achieve this, more focused interventions may be necessary to help HIV-positive children in those households that face high food insecurity, poverty, and low education of caregivers. Nutrition training of health workers can help provide this support, reduce misconceptions regarding healthy foods [63], and help caregivers utilize efficiently and well the vast food availability in the region [3]. Nutrition counseling may also teach methods of food storage households who are affected by food insecurity but live in food rich regions [22]. Frequent nutrition counseling can help to guide such families into proper use of available resources including foods and give priorities to children with high nutritional demand.

Acknowledgments

The authors would like to thank Prof. William Urassa (World Health Organization), Dr. Honorath Massanja (Ifakara Health Institute), and Dr. Adelheid Onyango (World Health Organization) for their invaluable inputs that helped to revise the initial protocol. Heartfelt regards also goes to the Tanga regional administrators including Dr. Selemani Msangi (RACC), Dr.Uredi Ally (RMO), all DMOs and CTC in-charges who agreed and helped to facilitate this study. Last but not least, we would like to thank Dr. Robert Kissanga (AIDS Relief), Dr. Omary Ubuguyu (MNH), Dr. Namala Mkopi (MNH/ChT), and Dr. Joseph Mihayo (AIDS Relief) for their invaluable technical and logistical support in this study.

Author Contributions

Conceived and designed the experiments: BFS KCP DPU MJ. Performed the experiments: BFS DPU MJ. Analyzed the data: BFS LBM JY MJ. Contributed reagents/materials/analysis tools: DPU MJ. Wrote the paper: BFS LBM JY MJ.

References

1. Lutter CK, Daelmans BM, de Onis M, Kothari MT, Ruel MT, et al. (2011) Undernutrition, poor feeding practices, and low coverage of key nutrition interventions. Pediatrics 128: e1418–1427.
2. Kadiyala S, Rawat R (2012) Food access and diet quality independently predict nutritional status among people living with HIV in Uganda. Public Health Nutr: 1–7.
3. Sunguya BF, Poudel KC, Mlunde LB, Shakya P, Urassa DP, et al. (2013) Effectiveness of nutrition training of health workers toward improving caregivers' feeding practices for children aged six months to two years: a systematic review. Nutr J 12: 66.
4. Imdad A, Yakoob MY, Bhutta ZA (2011) Impact of maternal education about complementary feeding and provision of complementary foods on child growth in developing countries. BMC Public Health 11 Suppl 3: S25.
5. Vitolo MR, Rauber F, Campagnolo PD, Feldens CA, Hoffman DJ (2010) Maternal dietary counseling in the first year of life is associated with a higher healthy eating index in childhood. J Nutr 140: 2002–2007.
6. Shi L, Zhang J, Wang Y, Caulfield LE, Guyer B (2010) Effectiveness of an educational intervention on complementary feeding practices and growth in rural China: a cluster randomised controlled trial. Public Health Nutr 13: 556–565.
7. Shi L, Zhang J (2011) Recent Evidence of the Effectiveness of Educational Interventions for Improving Complementary Feeding Practices in Developing Countries. Journal of Tropical Pediatrics 57: 91–98.
8. Mullie P, Clarys P, Hulens M, Vansant G (2010) Dietary patterns and socioeconomic position. Eur J Clin Nutr 64: 231–238.
9. Aggarwal A, Monsivais P, Cook AJ, Drewnowski A (2011) Does diet cost mediate the relation between socioeconomic position and diet quality? Eur J Clin Nutr 65: 1059–1066.
10. Ivers LC, Cullen KA (2011) Food insecurity: special considerations for women. Am J Clin Nutr 94: 1740S–1744S.
11. Ivers LC, Cullen KA, Freedberg KA, Block S, Coates J, et al. (2009) HIV/AIDS, undernutrition, and food insecurity. Clin Infect Dis 49: 1096–1102.
12. Saaka M, Shaibu M (2013) Does Household Food Insecurity Affect the Nutritional Status of Preschool Children Aged 6–36 Months? International Journal of Population Research 2013.
13. Keenan DP, Olson C, Hersey JC, Parmer SM (2001) Measures of food insecurity/security. J Nutr Educ 33 Suppl 1: S49–58.
14. Anema A, Vogenthaler N, Frongillo EA, Kadiyala S, Weiser SD (2009) Food insecurity and HIV/AIDS: current knowledge, gaps, and research priorities. Curr HIV/AIDS Rep 6: 224–231.
15. Saloojee H, De Maayer T, Garenne M, Kahn K (2007) What's new? Investigating risk factors for severe childhood malnutrition in a high HIV prevalence South African setting. Scand J Public Health Suppl 69: 96–106.
16. Mpontshane N, Van den Broeck J, Chhagan M, Luabeya KK, Johnson A, et al. (2008) HIV infection is associated with decreased dietary diversity in South African children. J Nutr 138: 1705–1711.
17. FAO (2010) The State of Food Insecurity in the World. Rome, Italy: Food and Agriculture Program.
18. Choi ES, Shin NR, Jung EI, Park HR, Lee HM, et al. (2008) A study on nutrition knowledge and dietary behavior of elementary school children in Seoul. Nutr Res Pract 2: 308–316.
19. ICF Macro, NBS (2011) Micronutrients: Results of the 2010 Tanzania Demographic and Health Survey Dar es Salaam, Tanzania NBS and ICF Macro
20. NBS, ORC-Macro (2010) Tanzania Demographic and Health Survey 2009–2010. Dar es Salaam, Tanzania: National Bureau of Statistics and ORC Macro.
21. Weiser SD, Young SL, Cohen CR, Kushel MB, Tsai AC, et al. (2011) Conceptual framework for understanding the bidirectional links between food insecurity and HIV/AIDS. Am J Clin Nutr 94: 1729S–1739S.
22. WHO (2009) Guidelines for an integrated approach to the nutritional care of HIV-infected children (6months to 14 years). Geneva, Switzerland: World Health Organization.
23. Yeung S, Wilkinson D, Escott S, Gilks C (2000) Paediatric HIV infection in a rural South African district hospital. J Trop Pediatr 46: 107–110.
24. Bachou H, Tylleskär T, Downing R, Tumwine J (2006) Severe malnutrition with and without HIV-1 infection in hospitalised children in Kampala, Uganda: differences in clinical features, haematological findings and CD4+ cell counts. Nutr J 5: 27.
25. Berkley J, Bejon P, Mwangi T, Gwer S, Maitland K, et al. (2009) HIV infection, malnutrition, and invasive bacterial infection among children with severe malaria. Clin Infect Dis 49: 336–343.
26. Weiser SD, Tuller DM, Frongillo EA, Senkungu J, Mukiibi N, et al. (2010) Food insecurity as a barrier to sustained antiretroviral therapy adherence in Uganda. PLoS One 5: e10340.
27. Nagata JM, Magerenge RO, Young SL, Oguta JO, Weiser SD, et al. (2012) Social determinants, lived experiences, and consequences of household food insecurity among persons living with HIV/AIDS on the shore of Lake Victoria, Kenya. AIDS Care 24: 728–736.
28. Sunguya BF, Poudel KC, Otsuka K, Yasuoka J, Mlunde LB, et al. (2011) Undernutrition among HIV-positive children in Dar es Salaam, Tanzania: antiretroviral therapy alone is not enough. BMC Public Health 11: 869.
29. Sunguya BF, Poudel KC, Mlunde LB, Urassa DP, Jimba M, et al. (2013) Efficacy of in-service nutrition training for mid-level providers to improve feeding practices among HIV-positive children in Tanga, Tanzania: study protocol for a cluster randomized controlled trial. Trials 14: 352.
30. NACP, Tanzania TURo, Health Mo, Programme NAC, Health Mo, Programme NAC (2009) National guideline for management of HIV/AIDS. 3 ed. Dar es Salaam, Tanzania.
31. WHO (1978) A growth chart for international use in maternal and child health care. Geneva, Switzerland: World Health Organization.
32. WHO (1995) Physical Status: The Use and Interpretation of Anthropometry. Report of a WHO Expert Committee. WHO Technical Report Series no. 854. Geneva, Switzerland: World Health Organization.
33. Van den Broeck J, Willie D, Younger N (2009) The World Health Organization child growth standards: expected implications for clinical and epidemiological research. Eur J Pediatr 168: 247–251.
34. WHO (2009) WHO AnthroPlus for personal computers Manual: Software for assessing growth of the world's children and adolescents. Geneva: World Health Organization.
35. Sunguya BF, Poudel KC, Otsuka K, Yasuoka J, Mlunde LB, et al. (2011) Undernutrition among HIV-positive children in Dar es Salaam, Tanzania: antiretroviral therapy alone is not enough. BMC Public Health 11: 869.
36. Sunguya BF, Poudel KC, Mlunde LB, Otsuka K, Yasuoka J, et al. (2012) Ready to Use Therapeutic Foods (RUTF) improves undernutrition among ART-treated, HIV-positive children in Dar es Salaam, Tanzania. Nutr J 11: 60.
37. WHO (2003) Nutrient requirements for people living with HIV/AIDS: report of a technical consultation. Geneva, Switzerland: World Health Organization.
38. Swindale A, Bilinsky P (2006) Household Dietary Diversity Score Household Food Access: Indicator Guide. Washington, D.C: Food and Nutrition Technical Assistance Project, Academy for Educational Development.
39. NBS, ORC-Macro (2005) Tanzania Demographic and Health Survey 2004–2005. Dar es Salaam, Tanzania: National Bureau of Statistics(Tanzania) and ORC Macro.
40. Coates J, Swindale A, Bilinsky P (2007) *Household Food Insecurity Access Scale (HFIAS) for Measurement of Household Food Access: Indicator Guide (v. 3)*. Washington, D.C: Food and Nutrition Technical Assistance Project, Academy for Educational Development.
41. Nagata JM, Magerenge RO, Young SL, Oguta JO, Weiser SD, et al. (2012) Social determinants, lived experiences, and consequences of household food insecurity among persons living with HIV/AIDS on the shore of Lake Victoria, Kenya. AIDS Care 24: 728–736.
42. Tsai AC, Bangsberg DR, Emenyonu N, Senkungu JK, Martin JN, et al. (2011) The social context of food insecurity among persons living with HIV/AIDS in rural Uganda. Soc Sci Med 73: 1717–1724.
43. Tsai AC, Bangsberg DR, Frongillo EA, Hunt PW, Muzoora C, et al. (2012) Food insecurity, depression and the modifying role of social support among people living with HIV/AIDS in rural Uganda. Soc Sci Med 74: 2012–2019.
44. Weiser SD, Young SL, Cohen CR, Kushel MB, Tsai AC, et al. (2011) Conceptual framework for understanding the bidirectional links between food insecurity and HIV/AIDS. Am J Clin Nutr 94: 1729S–1739S.
45. Weiser SD, Gupta R, Tsai AC, Frongillo EA, Grede N, et al. (2012) Changes in food insecurity, nutritional status, and physical health status after antiretroviral therapy initiation in rural Uganda. J Acquir Immune Defic Syndr.
46. WHO (2006) WHO Case Definitions of HIV for Surveillance and Revised Clinical Staging and Immunological Classification of HIV-Related Disease in Adults and Children. Geneva, Switzerland: World Health Organization.
47. Sunguya B, Koola J, Atkinson S (2006) Infections associated with severe malnutrition among hospitalised children in East Africa. Tanzan Health Res Bull 8: 189–192.
48. Nyarango PM, Gebremeskel T, Mebrahtu G, Mufunda J, Abdulmumini U, et al. (2006) A steep decline of malaria morbidity and mortality trends in Eritrea between 2000 and 2004: the effect of combination of control methods. Malar J 5: 33.
49. TACAIDS ZAC, NBS OCGS, ICF (2013) Tanzania HIV/AIDS and Malaria Indicator Survey 2011–12. Dar es Salaam, Tanzania. Dar es Salaam, Tanzania: Tanzania Commission for AIDS (TACAIDS), Zanzibar AIDS Commission (ZAC), National Bureau of Statistics (NBS), Office of the Chief Government Statistician (OCGS), and ICF International.
50. Howe DL, Hargreaves RJ, Huttly RS (2008) Issues in the construction of wealth indices for the measurement of socio-economic position in low-income countries. Emerging Themes in Epidemiology 5: 3.

51. Gwatkin DR, Rutstein S, Johnson K, Pande RP, Wagstaff A (2000) Socio-economic difference in health, nutrition and population in Ghana. HNP/Poverty Thematic Group of the World Bank. Washington, D.C: World Bank.
52. Vyas S, Kumaranayake L (2006) Constructing socio-economic status indices: how to use principal components analysis. Health Policy Plan 21: 459–468.
53. Tong A, Sainsbury P, Craig J (2007) Consolidated criteria for reporting qualitative research (COREQ): a 32-item checklist for interviews and focus groups. Int J Qual Health Care 19: 349–357.
54. Katz M (1999) Multivariable Analysis: A Practical Guide for Clinicians. Cambridge, UK: Cambridge University Press.
55. Patton M (2001) Qualitative research and evaluation methods. Thousands Oaks, USA: Sage.
56. WHO (2005) Nutrition and HIV/AIDS. Geneva, Switzerland: World Health Organization.
57. Belachew T, Lindstrom D, Gebremariam A, Hogan D, Lachat C, et al. (2013) Food insecurity, food based coping strategies and suboptimal dietary practices of adolescents in Jimma zone Southwest Ethiopia. PLoS One 8.
58. Tiyou A, Belachew T, Alemseged F, Biadgilign S (2012) Food insecurity and associated factors among HIV-infected individuals receiving highly active antiretroviral therapy in Jimma zone Southwest Ethiopia. Nutr J 11: 51.
59. Paul K, Muti M, Khalfan S, Humphrey J, Caffarella R, et al. (2011) Beyond food insecurity: how context can improve complementary feeding interventions. Food Nutr Bull 32: 244–253.
60. Palwala M, Sharma S, Udipi SA, Ghugre PS, Kothari G, et al. (2009) Nutritional quality of diets fed to young children in urban slums can be improved by intensive nutrition education. Food Nutr Bull 30: 317–326.
61. Paul KH, Muti M, Chasekwa B, Mbuya MN, Madzima RC, et al. (2012) Complementary feeding messages that target cultural barriers enhance both the use of lipid-based nutrient supplements and underlying feeding practices to improve infant diets in rural Zimbabwe. Matern Child Nutr 8: 225–238.
62. Buonomo E, de Luca S, Tembo D, Scarcella P, Germano P, et al. (2012) Nutritional rehabilitation of HIV-exposed infants in Malawi: results from the drug resources enhancement against AIDS and malnutrition program. Int J Environ Res Public Health 9: 421–434.
63. Sunguya B, Poudel K, Mlunde L, Urassa D, Yasuoka J, et al. (2013) Nutrition training improves health workers' nutrition knowledge and competence to manage child undernutrition: a systematic review. Front Public Health 1:37.

17

Phylogenetic Analyses and Characterization of RNase X25 from *Drosophila melanogaster* Suggest a Conserved Housekeeping Role and Additional Functions for RNase T2 Enzymes in Protostomes

Linda Ambrosio[1]*, Stephanie Morriss[1]⁹, Ayesha Riaz[2]⁹, Ryan Bailey[1], Jian Ding[3], Gustavo C. MacIntosh[1]*

1 Roy J. Carver Department of Biochemistry, Biophysics and Molecular Biology, Iowa State University, Ames, Iowa, United States of America, **2** Interdepartmental Genetics Graduate Program, Iowa State University, Ames, Iowa, United States of America, **3** Children's Hospital Boston, Harvard Medical School, Boston, Massachusetts, United States of America

Abstract

Ribonucleases belonging to the RNase T2 family are enzymes associated with the secretory pathway that are almost absolutely conserved in all eukaryotes. Studies in plants and vertebrates suggest they have an important housekeeping function in rRNA recycling. However, little is known about this family of enzymes in protostomes. We characterized RNase X25, the only RNase T2 enzyme in *Drosophila melanogaster*. We found that RNase X25 is the major contributor of ribonuclease activity in flies as detected by *in gel* assays, and has an acidic pH preference. Gene expression analyses showed that the *RNase X25* transcript is present in all adult tissues and developmental stages. *RNase X25* expression is elevated in response to nutritional stresses; consistent with the hypothesis that this enzyme has a housekeeping role in recycling RNA. A correlation between induction of *RNase X25* expression and autophagy was observed. Moreover, induction of gene expression was triggered by oxidative stress suggesting that RNase X25 may have additional roles in stress responses. Phylogenetic analyses of this family in protostomes showed that RNase T2 genes have undergone duplication events followed by divergence in several phyla, including the loss of catalytic residues, and suggest that RNase T2 proteins have acquired novel functions. Among those, it is likely that a role in host immunosuppression evolved independently in several groups, including parasitic Platyhelminthes and parasitoid wasps. The presence of only one RNase T2 gene in the *D. melanogaster* genome, without any other evident secretory RNase activity detected, makes this organism an ideal system to study the cellular functions of RNase T2 proteins associated with RNA recycling and maintenance of cellular homeostasis. On the other hand, the discovery of gene duplications in several protostome genomes also presents interesting new avenues to study additional biological functions of this ancient family of proteins.

Editor: Dmitri Boudko, Rosalind Franklin University, United States of America

Funding: A.R. is the recipient of a Fulbright Fellowship. This work was supported by grant No. MBC-1051818 from the United States National Science Foundation to G.C.M. The funders had no role in study design, data collection and analysis, decision to publish, or preparation of the manuscript.

Competing Interests: The authors have declared that no competing interests exist.

* Email: lima@iastate.edu (LA); gustavo@iastate.edu (GCM)

⁹ These authors contributed equally to this work.

Introduction

Members of the RNase T2 family of enzymes catalyze endonucleolytic RNA cleavage via a 2′-3′-cyclic phosphate intermediate [1]. These ribonucleases (RNases) are found ubiquitously, with RNase T2 genes in genomes of most eukaryotes, many bacteria, as well as some viruses [1,2]. Although primary sequence identity between eukaryotic and prokaryotic enzymes is low, there are conserved secondary structures that contain key core hydrophobic residues associated with the RNase T2 active site [2,3]. All characterized RNase T2 family members consist of a central four-stranded antiparallel β-sheet (strands β1, β2, β4 and β5), a small two-stranded antiparallel β-sheet (β3 and β7), and three α-helices (αB, αC, αD), with the catalytic site of the enzyme residing mainly within strands β2 and β5 and helix αC (Kurihara et al. 1996; Tanaka et al. 2000; Rodriguez et al. 2008). Two histidine residues within β2 and αC, together with surrounding residues form the conserved active site (CAS) motifs CAS I and CAS II [2]. Importantly, each histidine is a direct participant in the acid-base catalysis mechanism that enables the transphosphorylation and hydrolysis reactions of RNase T2 enzymes [1,4].

These ancient ribonucleases are secreted or targeted to membrane-bound intracellular compartments (lysosomes and vacuoles) where they degrade single stranded RNAs. Long known for their function in gametophytic self-incompatibility, and as part of the response to phosphate starvation in plants [2,5], the RNase T2 family has been recently shown to play distinctly different developmental and physiological roles in plants and animals. Recent insights from *Arabidopsis thaliana* and zebrafish indicate that conservation of the RNase T2 family in all eukaryotes may be related to an important housekeeping function carried out by these enzymes, which includes recycling of ribosomal RNAs [6,7]. A ribophagy-like pathway is thought to mediate this turnover of rRNAs in normal, non-stressed cells [8], which is essential to maintain cellular homeostasis. Additionally, in *Saccharomyces cerevisiae* and *Tetrahymena thermophila*, the enzymatic activities of RNase T2 proteins have been associated with cleavage of mature tRNAs to produce tRNA halves in response to starvation and oxidative stress [9,10]. The significance of the accumulation of these degradation intermediates is unknown, although it has been suggested that they may play a signaling role in the maintenance of cellular homeostasis [5]. Alternatively, they may accumulate as a consequence of targeted degradation of the translation machinery during stress conditions that leads to suppression of cell division [10]. Interestingly, a different ribonuclease carries out tRNA cleavage function in response to stress in vertebrate cells. In this case angiogenin, a member of the vertebrate-specific RNase A family, is responsible for the accumulation of tRNA fragments [11].

At least one member of the RNase T2 family has been found in every eukaryotic genome that has been sequenced, with Trypanosomatids as the only exception [2]. High frequency of gene duplication and extensive divergence of the T2 RNases has occurred in plants [12,13]. On the other hand, only one, well-conserved gene, is found in most vertebrate genomes [14]; and it has been proposed that RNase A members have replaced RNase T2 in several biological roles in these organisms [2,14]. Thus, characterization of the biological role played by RNase T2 enzymes in multicellular organisms is complicated in plants and vertebrates due to the presence of potentially redundant enzymatic activities. In contrast, the *Drosophila melanogaster* genome contains only one RNase T2 gene, *RNase X25* (also known as *DmRNase-66B*), and no RNase A homolog; thus, this organism could be used as a simpler system to demonstrate the conserved function(s) of this enzyme family in animals. *RNase X25* (CG8194), located at 66A21 on chromosome 3, is 1658 nucleotides in length and encodes a single form of mRNA transcript with a 325 amino acid open reading frame [15]. A signal peptide cleavage site is anticipated between residues 21 and 22 suggesting transport of the predicted polypeptide chain to the secretory pathway. In addition, two asparagine residues (positions 214 and 231) and a threonine (residue 34) may serve as N- and O-glycosylation sites, respectively. N-glycosylation is the most common modification found for the RNase T2 family, while a few cases of O-glycosylation have been observed for fungal enzymes (reviewed in [2]).

As a first step towards understanding the role of RNases T2 in animals, biochemical analyses and gene expression studies were initiated in the fruit fly *D. melanogaster*. RNase T2 activity was detected in all *Drosophila* life cycle stages examined, and this correlated well with *RNase X25* gene expression patterns. Furthermore, *RNase X25* gene expression levels were responsive to nutritional and oxidative stress as determined by the accumulation of *RNase X25* mRNAs in larvae starved for nutrients or exposed to wheat germ agglutinin (WGA), or hydrogen peroxide. A correlation between induction of autophagy and increased RNase X25 expression and activity was also observed in response to starvation. Finally, we used phylogenetic analyses to shed light on the evolution of the RNase T2 family of ribonucleases in protostomes and found evidence for gene duplications followed by divergence and the potential acquisition of new functions in several phyla, in contrast to the pattern observed in most deuterostomes. Together, these analyses suggest that RNase X25 carries out a conserved housekeeping function as proposed for other RNases T2 in plants and animals, and that *Drosophila*, with a single RNase T2 gene, is a good eukaryotic model system in which to investigate the role of RNases T2 in the process of ribophagy. The discovery of gene duplications in several protostome genomes also presents interesting new avenues to study additional roles of this ancient family of proteins.

Material and Methods

D. melanogaster strains, and tissue preparations

In this study the *Drosophila melanogaster* strain w^{1118}/w^{1118} with two wild type *RNase X25* genes and w^{1118}/w^{1118}; *Df(3L)Excel6279/+* (denoted *Df(3L)Excel6279/+* in the text), with one wild type *RNase X25* gene were raised at 25°C on standard cornmeal media.

For staged embryo collections, females were placed in collecting bottles and eggs were gathered after aging from molasses-agar plates dusted with yeast.

Stress treatments

To provide standardized non-crowded growing conditions prior to stress treatments, 43 w^{1118}/w^{1118} embryos (0–2 hrs) were gently transferred onto Formula 4–24 instant blue *D. melanogaster* diet (363.6 mg/1.625 µl H_2O; Carolina Biological Supply, Burlington, NC, USA), that had been placed into a small petri dish (60×15 mm). Baker's yeast was not sprinkled on this medium. Petri plates were placed in an incubator at 22°C and 80% humidity for 128 hours. Then 25 young, newly molted third instar larvae were gently transferred from each plate to either control *D. melanogaster* diet, or experimental media consisting of *D. melanogaster* diet containing 1% unconjugated wheat germ agglutinin (Vector Laboratories, Burlingame, CA, USA), or hydrogen peroxide at 0.1% [w/w] or 0.5% [w/w]. For starvation conditions larvae were placed onto PBS-saturated Whatman 1 filter paper. After 14 hours, larvae were collected, frozen at −80°C and stored for further processing. For detection of autophagy in fat body cells of starved and fed control larvae, embryos were placed onto Bloomington's Drosophila Stock Center cornmeal/molasses/yeast soft media, sprinkled with Baker's yeast, and subsequently processed as described above. LysoTracker Red DND-99 (Life Technologies, Carlsbad, CA, USA) staining of lysosomes and autolysosomes, and Hoescհst 33342 (Thermo Fisher Scientific Inc, Rockford, IL, USA) staining of DNA was performed as described by Scott et al. [16] and Juhasz and Neufeld [17]. Stained fat body lobes were imaged in PBS using a Zeiss Axio Imager.Z2 microscope equipped with AxioCam HR digital camera using a LD Plan-Neofluar 40x/0.6 objective lens and ZEN imaging software.

Protein extracts and RNase activity assays

Protein was prepared from flies at different stages or collected from stress experiments, using approximately 100 mg of each sample. The material was homogenized in 1.5 ml eppendorf tubes and protein extractions were performed as described by Hillwig et al [14], using the protease inhibitor cocktail Complete Mini EDTA Free (Roche Diagnostics, Indianapolis, IN, USA) or Protease Inhibitor Cocktail P8340 (Sigma-Aldrich, St. Louis, MO, USA). *In gel* RNase activity assays were performed following the protocol used by Yen and Green [18] using high molecular weight Torula Yeast RNA (Sigma-Aldrich) as substrate, loading 20–80 µg of protein per lane. After running and washes, gels were incubated at pH 6.0 or 7.0, as indicated in the figures. SDS-PAGE was run in parallel for each sample as loading and quality control, also using 20 µg of protein per lane, and then stained with Coomassie Brilliant Blue. Experiments were repeated at least 3 times. A representative gel is shown.

qPCR analysis

RNA was extracted from 100 mg of sample using Trizol (Fisher) according to manufacturers' instructions. RNA was DNase-treated using Turbo DNA-free (Ambion), and cDNA was synthesized using the iScript Select cDNA Synthesis kit (Bio-Rad), also following manufacturers' instructions for each procedure. qPCR was completed on a Stratagene MX4000 using the Absolute qPCR with SYBR Green + Rox kit (Fisher Scientific) according to manufacturers' instructions. The transcript of ribosomal protein L32 gene (*RPL-32)* was used as the control for data normalization, using the Pfaffl method [19]. Primers used for *RNase X25* were: Forward (5′-3′): TCCACGCCCCTCAGCGACATA, and Reverse (5′-3′): ACGCCAAGTGAGCCCCTGCT; for *RPL-32*: Forward (5′-3′): TGGGACACCTTCTTCAAGAT, and Reverse (5′-3′): CAGGCGACCGTTGGGGTTG; for *Atg5*: Forward (5′-3′): ATCTGGGAGGGCCAGATAGG, and Reverse (5′-3′): TAGCTCCTTGGAGTTGAGCTTG; for *Amyrel*: Forward (5′-3′): GATCTAGAGTACATCTACAGCAGCC, and Reverse (5′-3′): ACTTGTAGTTCAGCACGGCA; and for *Lip3*: Forward (5′-3′): GCCTATTTCTGATTGCGGTGAG, and Reverse (5′-3′): AGTACTTGTGCGCCTTGGAG.

Experiments were performed using triplicates, and repeated 3 times using independent samples. Statistical significance of the differences between treatments was determined using *t*-test. Graphs show averages of each sample normalized using the average value of the control sample. One star = $P<0.05$, two stars = $P<0.01$.

Phylogenetic analysis

Identification of protostome RNase T2 genes or proteins was done by BLAST searches [20] using Ensembl Genomes [21], VectorBase [22], the Genome Portal of the Department of Energy Joint Genome Institute [23], the *Clonorchis sinensis* Genome Database [24], SmedGD [25], the Hymenoptera Genome Database [26], SilkDB [27], Beetle Base [28], GeneDB [29], AphidBase [30], and the National Center for Biotechnology Information Map Viewer (http://www.ncbi.nlm.nih.gov/projects/mapview/).

Protein sequences were aligned using ClustalW2 [31] followed by manual adjustments. PAUP 4.0 software [32] was used for neighbor-joining (1,000 bootstrap replications) and parsimony analyses, using default parameters.

Results

Characterization of RNase activity in Drosophila development

The activity of the RNases with characteristics similar to the RNase T2 family, i.e. endonucleases with no sequence/base specificity, has not been characterized in *Drosophila*. To detect RNase activities in extracts from different *Drosophila* developmental stages we used a standard *in gel* activity assay that allows size separation of different proteins with RNase activity. Embryos at 0–2, 2–6, and 0–16 hr after egg deposition, as well as wandering third instar larvae, white prepupae, pupae, adult males, females, and isolated ovaries were collected. Protein extracts were prepared and analyzed for RNase activities (Figure 1, top panel). At all developmental stages, RNase activities in the apparent 25–30 kDa range, which correspond to the predicted size range of RNase T2 enzymes, were observed. It is important to note that the PAGE method used for this assay is semi-denaturing, since it includes SDS but not reducing agents, and the apparent molecular weight observed for each protein band does not necessarily correspond to the predicted mass. Detection of RNase activities with distinct molecular weights in this range may be indicative of posttranslational processing, including N- and O-glycosylation, a common posttranslational modification of RNase T2 proteins. While most stages showed a similar level of RNase activity, samples collected from early 0–2 hr embryos and third instar larvae showed lower RNase activity. This result was not due to general protein degradation since protein integrity seems evident in a Coomassie stained SDS-PAGE (Figure 1, bottom panel). In addition, a band of RNase activity at a very large apparent molecular weight (~200 kDa) was observed primarily in third instar larvae, white prepupae, and pupae (Figure 1, top panel, arrow).

We undertook a combined biochemical-genetics strategy to more definitely assign the RNase activity observed on our activity gels to the *RNase X25* gene product. One important defining characteristic of the T2 family of RNases in animals is their pH sensitivity and acidic preference [1,2,3]. Thus, we compared RNase activities in *Drosophila* ovarian and embryonic extracts using *in gel* activity assays at different pH conditions (Figure 2). At pH 7, little to no RNase activity was observed at the 25-30 kDa range, while robust activity was evident in samples from ovary and embryos at acidic pH. A large number of endo and exoribonuclease activities are predicted based on sequence analysis of the *Drosophila* genome. Classical genetic mutations in *RNase X25* are currently unavailable and RNA interference stocks without off-target effects have not been produced. Therefore, we employed a chromosomal deletion approach to determine whether a decrease in gene dose could affect the relative amount of RNase activity detected in our assays.

The *Df(3L)Excel6279* chromosome was chosen, with deficiency break points mapped to 66A17 and 66B5. This is the smallest known deletion that removes the *RNase X25* gene located at position 66A21. Importantly, *RNase X25* is the only RNase encoding gene that lies between the breakpoints of the *Df(3L)Excel6279* chromosome. RNA and protein extracts were produced from ovarian tissue from either a wild type (+/+) genetic background with two *RNase X25* gene copies or the *Df(3L)Excel6279/+* background with one *RNase X25* gene copy. A homozygous mutant line could not be obtained, since homozygous deletions of this region are lethal. Quantitative RT-PCR analysis indicated approximately one-half of wild-type *RNase X25* mRNA levels were detected for the *Df(3L)Excel6279/+* ovaries (Figure 3C). Furthermore, a corresponding decrease in RNase activity was observed for the 25–30 kDa bands in *Df(3L)Excel6279/+* extracts (Figure 3A), when similar amounts of protein were examined for wild-type and heterozygous deletion mutants (Figure 3B). These results strongly suggested that the enzymatic activity observed by our *in gel* analysis was, in fact, RNase T2 activity, encoded by the *Drosophila RNase X25* gene.

Total RNA was also isolated from developmental samples, and *RNase X25* expression was analyzed using quantitative real time PCR (qRT-PCR) studies (Figure 4). This analysis indicated that *RNase X25* transcripts are present in all the stages analyzed, showing constitutive expression throughout *Drosophila* development. No significant stage-specific differences in mRNA accumulation were apparent in this experiment. Our gene expression analyses correspond well with expression data obtained from genome-wide transcriptome analyses deposited in FlyBase (http://flybase.org). Moreover, data obtained from the modENCODE [33] and FlyAtlas [34] databases indicated that *RNase X25* expression is constitutive for all tissues of the fly at the 3rd instar larva and adult developmental stages with tissue specific expression ranging from very low to high levels (Figures S1 and S2). It is intriguing that early embryos and third instar larvae, the two samples with low RNase activity, had at least as much expression of *RNase X25* as samples with high activity. The discrepancy between enzymatic activity and mRNA accumu-

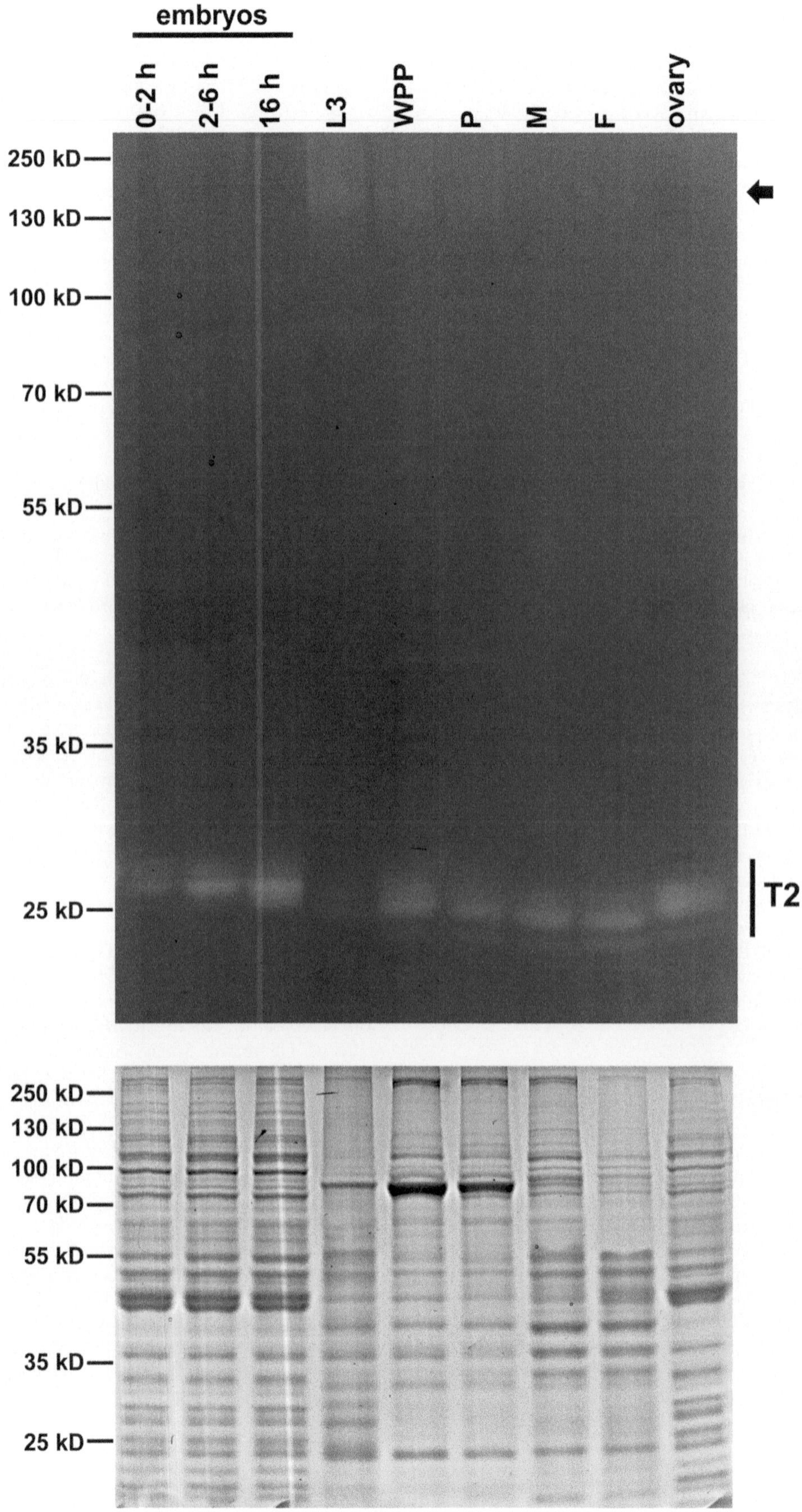
embryos
0-2 h
2-6 h
16 h
L3
WPP
P
M
F
ovary
250 kD
130 kD
100 kD
70 kD
55 kD
35 kD
25 kD
T2

Figure 1. Developmental profile of *Drosophila* RNase activities. Protein extracts were produced from embryos at 0–2 hours (h), 2–6 h, and 0–16 h after egg deposition and from animals at 3rd instar larval (L3), white prepupal (WPP), pupal (P), and adult male (M) or female (F) stages of development. Ovarian tissue (ovary) was prepared from 3–5 day old females. (Upper panel) Protein was fractionated by electrophoresis through a 12% polyacrylamide gel containing 3 mg/ml Torula yeast RNA, washed to remove SDS, incubated in 100 mM Tris-HCl at pH 6.0 and stained with toluidine blue to visualize regions of nuclease activity. Low molecular weight (~25–30 kD) activities in the size range of the RNase T2 family were detected at all developmental stages assayed. High molecular weight (~200 kD) activities were also apparent (arrow), but absent from embryos. (Lower panel) Protein extracts were analyzed by SDS/PAGE and stained with Coomassie Blue R-250 to control for equal loading and protein integrity. Each lane in both gels contains 20 μg of protein.

lation could suggest that RNase X25 is postrancriptionally or posttranslationally regulated.

RNase X25 expression is altered by stress

In addition to a general housekeeping function in rRNA recycling, the RNase T2 family of enzymes is thought to play specialized roles in unicellular and multicellular eukaryotes. In yeast and *Tetrahymena*, RNase T2 activity is responsible for the cleavage of mature tRNAs to produce tRNA halves [9,10] during the response to oxidative stress or amino acid starvation. Several microarray and RNAseq reports on the fly's transcriptional response to a variety of stresses are available in the literature and public databases. However, results related to the effect of starvation on *RNase X25* are not clear (Table S1). To begin exploring the possibility that RNase T2 may play a role in the fruit fly's response to nutritional and oxidative stress, we determined whether *RNase X25* gene expression levels were altered after exposure to these pressures. It was also reported by Li *et al.* [35] that accumulation of *RNase X25* mRNAs was altered in *Drosophila* larval midgut tissue after animals were fed a diet supplemented with wheat germ agglutinin (WGA). Thus, we also

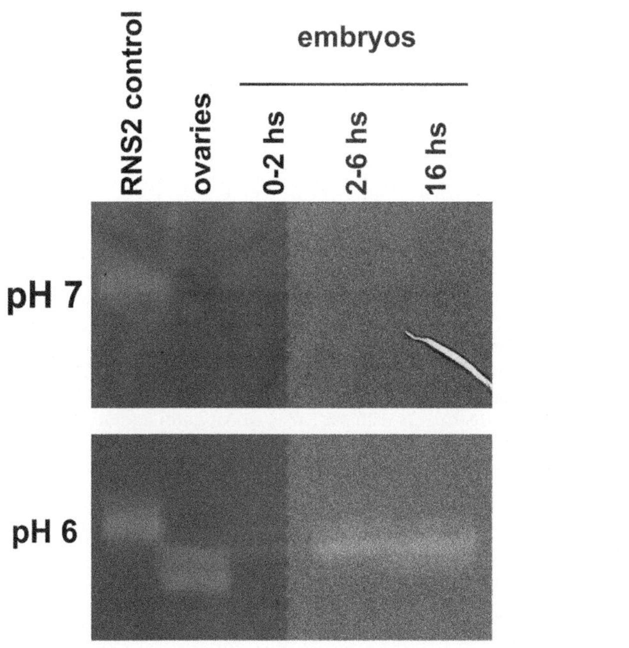

Figure 2. Effect of pH on *Drosophila* RNase activities. Protein extracts from ovaries and embryos were analyzed using RNase *in gel* activity assays as described in Figure 1, with incubations at neutral (pH 7.0; upper panel) and acidic (pH 6.0; lower panel) conditions. RNase activity in the size range corresponding to RNase T2 enzymes was abundant after incubation at pH 6, while almost no activity was observed at neutral pH. Each lane in both gels contains 20 μg of protein. A plant protein that is active at the two pH conditions, *Arabidopsis thaliana* RNS2 [7], was used as control.

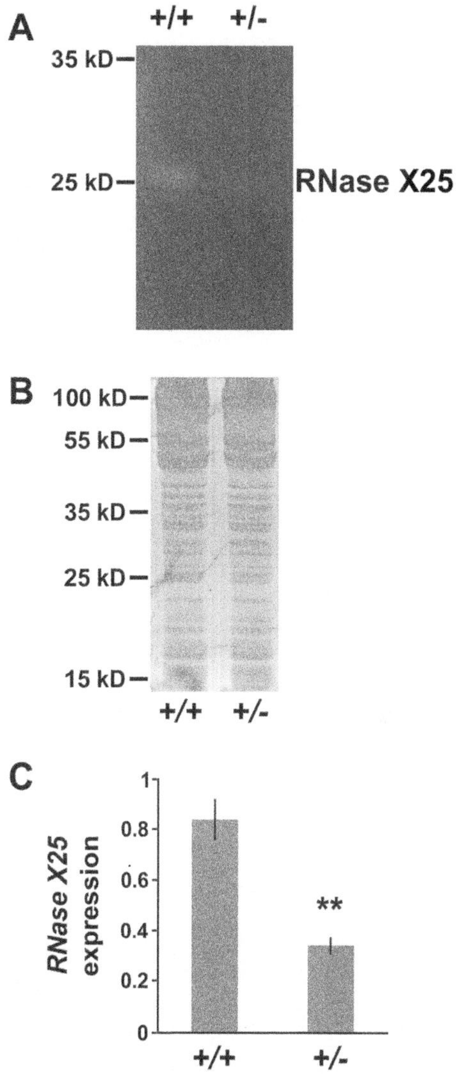

Figure 3. Reduced RNase activity and expression correlates with reduced *RNase X25* gene dose. Ovarian extracts were prepared from wild type control (+/+), or deletion mutant *Df(3L)Excel6279/+* females (+/−), carrying two or one copy of the *RNase X25* gene, respectively. Protein samples were analyzed using (A) *in gel* RNase activity assay, or (B) standard SDS/PAGE analysis. Compared to the control (+/+), RNase activity was reduced in ovaries dissected from females with one copy of the *RNase X25* gene (+/−). Each lane in both gels contains 20 μg of protein. (C) RNA was isolated from ovaries and qPCR quantification of the relative level of *RNase X25* mRNAs in these samples was carried out using the ribosomal protein L3 (*RpL3*) transcript as internal standard control for normalization. *RNase X25* expression levels were reduced in tissue samples from mutant *Df(3L)Excel6279/+* females (+/−), compared to control females (+/+). Data are representative of 3 independent experiments and are means and S.E. of triplicates. **, $P<0.01$ (*t*-test).

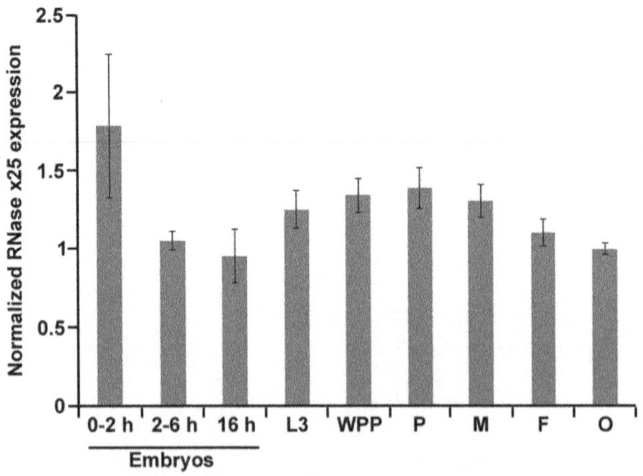

Figure 4. Developmental profile of *RNase X25* transcript accumulation. RNA was isolated from embryos at 0–2 h, 2–6 h, and 0–16 h after egg deposition and from animals at 3rd instar larval (L3), white prepupal (WPP), pupal (P), and adult male (M) or female (F) stages of development. Ovarian tissue (O) was prepared from 3–5 day old females. qPCR quantification of the relative level of *RNase X25* mRNAs in these samples was carried out using the ribosomal protein L3 (*RpL3*) transcript as internal standard control for normalization. *RNase X25* expression was detected at all stages analyzed. Data are representative of 3 independent experiments and are means and S.E. of triplicates.

determined if a change in *RNase X25* expression levels could be detected in whole animal extracts after larval ingestion of WGA (1% w/w).

Whole animal extracts were prepared for molecular analysis from third instar larvae fed a control diet or subjected to starvation for 14 h (see Materials and Methods). As shown in Figure 5A, the accumulation of *RNase X25* mRNA transcripts increased approximately 80% for animals starved for nutrients ($P<0.05$) when compared to fed control larvae. It has been proposed that diets containing WGA produce a starvation-like effect on flies [35]; thus, a WGA-containing diet was also used to feed *D. melanogaster* larvae. Consistent with a starvation-like effect, a WGA diet resulted in a significant increase in *RNase X25* expression ($P<0.01$), similar to that observed in starved flies (Figure 5A).

We also observed an increase in *RNase X25* mRNA when larvae were fed a diet containing the oxidative stressor hydrogen peroxide (Figure 5B). In this set of experiments, the normalized *RNase X25* expression levels for whole animals exposed to 0.5% hydrogen peroxide were 50% higher ($P<0.05$) than observed for control animals. At a lower dosage, 0.1 %, a 20% increase in *RNase X25* mRNA was observed, although this change was not statistically significant. Thus, analysis of whole larval extracts indicated that the *RNase X25* gene was responsive to various stressors including starvation, and treatments with 1% WGA or 0.5% hydrogen peroxide. Data from microarray experiments performed by other laboratories suggest that a few other stress conditions and chemical treatments can also alter the expression of *RNase X25* (Table S1).

Starvation, *RNase X25* Expression and Autophagy

Since starvation induces autophagy and autophagy mediated RNA degradation, we also tested whether expression of *Atg5*, which encodes a protein that participates in an ubiquitin-like protein conjugation system essential for autophagy[36], was altered in our starved larvae. We found a small but significant ($P<0.05$) increase in the expression of this autophagy marker in

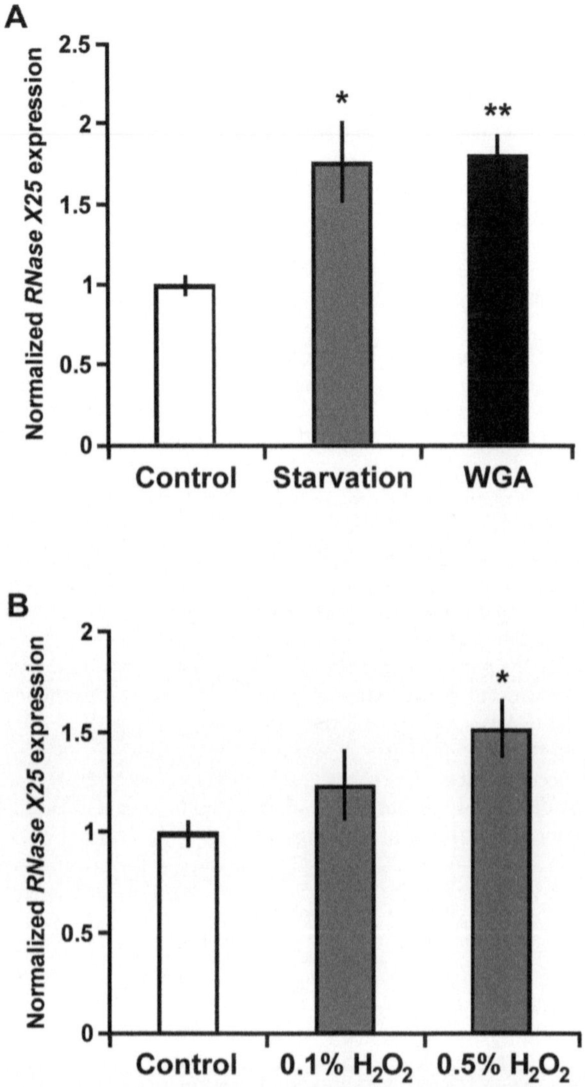

Figure 5. *RNase X25* gene expression is regulated by nutritional and oxidative stress. RNA was isolated from whole 3rd instar larvae, 14 h after transfer to control or experimental media (see Materials and methods). qPCR quantification of the relative level of *RNase X25* mRNAs in these samples was carried out using the ribosomal protein L3 (*RpL3*) transcript as internal standard control for normalization. Increased levels of *RNase X25* transcripts were apparent in samples after (A) starvation and treatments with 1% [w/w] wheat germ agglutinin (WGA), and (B) 0.1% [w/w] or 0.5% [w/w] hydrogen peroxide. Data are representative of 3 independent experiments and are means and S.E. of triplicates. *, $P<0.05$; **, $P<0.01$ (*t*-test).

starved, as compared with fed control larval samples (Figure 6A left F 4–24 panel). Since only a low level of induced *Atg5* expression was detected in our starved samples, we used two gene markers, *Amyrel* (α-amylase related) [35] and *Lip3* (lipase) [37] to monitor the starvation response for these animals grown on Formula 4-24 instant blue *D. melanogaster* diet. As shown in Figure 6B (F 4–24 panels) significant ($P<0.01$) increases in the level of *Amyrel* (2.5 fold) and *Lip3* (14 fold) were apparent, indicating that the starved animals were indeed nutritionally stressed.

Next, we followed autophagy by examining the formation of Lysotracker-positive vesicles in larval fat body, as previously

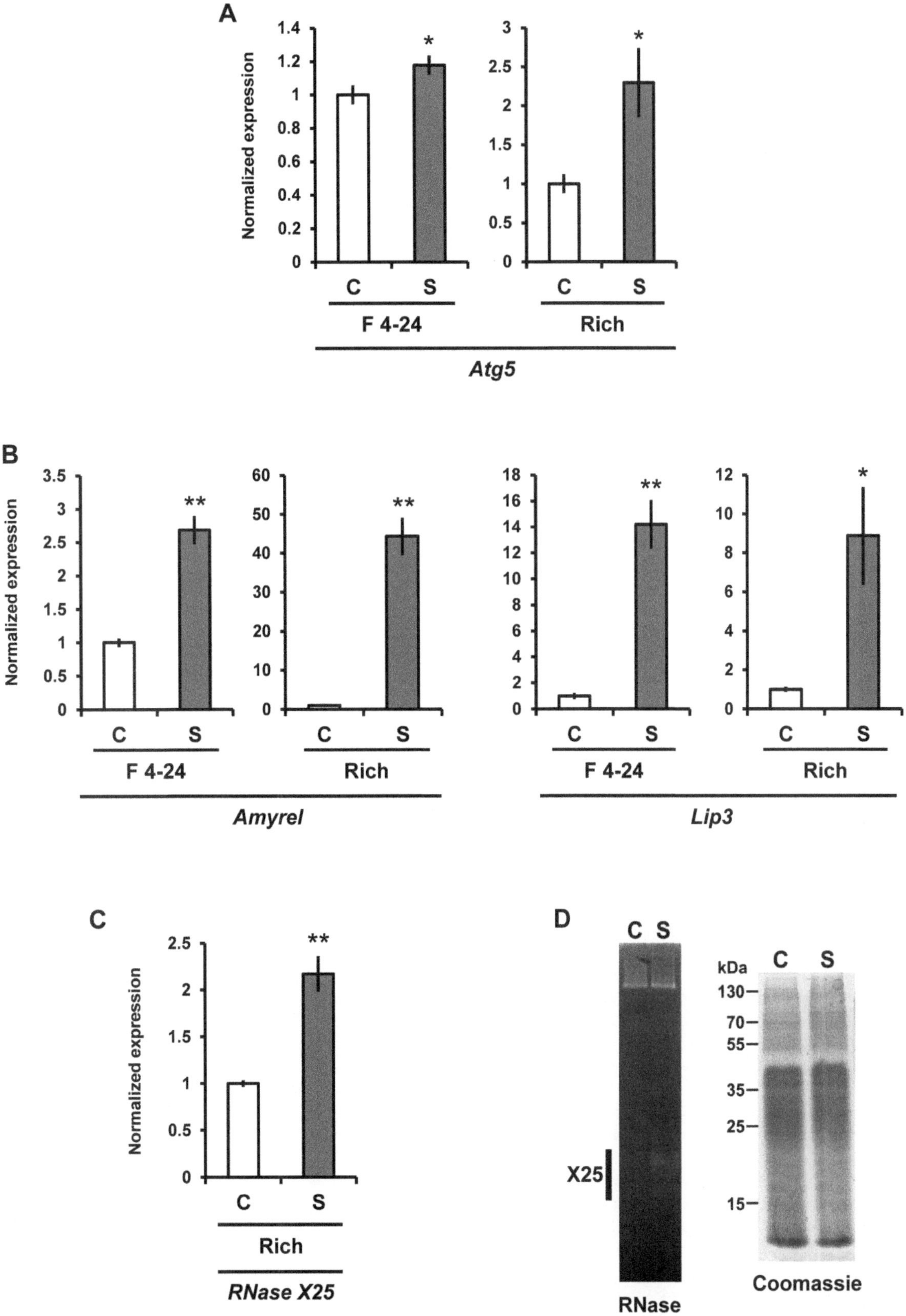

Figure 6. Starvation induces expression of the autophagy marker, *Atg 5* and *Amyrel, Lip3* and *RNase X25* in larvae. RNA was isolated from whole 3rd instar larvae, 14 h after transfer to control (C) or starvation (S) conditions (see Materials and methods). qPCR quantification of the relative level of (A) autophagy marker *Atg5,* (B) starvation markers *Amyrel*, and *Lip3*, and (C) *RNase X25* mRNAs in these samples was carried out using the ribosomal protein L3 (*RpL3*) transcript as internal standard control for normalization. Increased levels of *Atg5, Amyrel, Lip3*, and *RNase X25* transcripts were apparent in samples after starvation as compared with fed-control animals. Data are representative of 3 independent experiments

and are means and S.E. of triplicates. *, $P<0.05$; **, $P<0.01$ (*t*-test). (D) Protein extracts from 14 h starved (S) and fed-control (C) whole 3rd instar larvae were analyzed using RNase *in gel* activity assays as described in Figure 1. RNase activity in the size range corresponding to RNase T2 enzymes was evident in starved as compared with fed-control animals. Each lane in both gels contains 80 µg of protein. "F 4–24" denotes extracts from animals nourished with Formula 4–24 instant *D. melanogaster* diet without yeast; "Rich" denotes extracts from animals fed a yeast rich diet (see Materials and methods).

described by Jimenez-Sanchez et al. [38]. For animals nourished with Formula 4–24 instant *D. melanogaster* diet, very high, but diffuse accumulation of Lysotracker was found for both fed control and starved larval fat body, complicating the interpretation of results (data not shown). The diet of these animals was not supplemented with Baker's yeast, an important and major source of nutrients for Drosophila larvae [39]. However, for 3rd instar larvae growing on rich media containing yeast (see Materials and Methods), after a 14-hour starvation period, characteristic Lysotracker-positive vesicles were observed in fat body cells (Figure 7B, D and F), with little to no puncta visible for fed control animals (Figure 7A, C and E). Importantly, quantitative RT-PCR analysis demonstrated that a significantly ($P<0.01$) higher level of *Atg5* mRNA transcripts was present after 14 hours of starvation, as compared with those from non-starved control animals in rich media-fed larval samples (Figure 6A), confirming the induction of autophagy in these nutritionally stressed animals. The starved state of these animals was verified by the presence of significantly ($P<0.01$) higher levels of both *Amyrel* and *Lip3* mRNA transcripts, as compared with fed-control larvae (Figure 6B). Finally, the level of *RNase X25* gene expression and enzymatic activity were probed and found to be at higher levels for starved compared with fed-control animals (Figure 6C and D). Together, these results suggest that the autophagy process is concomitantly induced with an increase in *RNase X25* mRNA expression and enzymatic activity after starvation.

Phylogenetic analysis of T2 RNase genes in protostomes

Phylogenetic analyses of deuterostomes and plants suggested that RNase T2 enzymes carry out an essential housekeeping role that justifies their presence in all eukaryotic genomes [2]. In addition, the RNase T2 family in plants has undergone many gene duplication events followed by gene sorting and diversification, which led to the acquisition of new biological roles [13], but this diversification was not been observed in the animal genomes so far analyzed [14], which did not include almost any protostome. The presence of only one *RNase T2* gene in the *Drosophila* genome also seemed to confirm that only one gene is present in animal genomes; nevertheless, the recent availability of a large number of fully sequenced protostome genomes led us to perform a search for members of the RNase T2 family in those genomes, followed by phylogenetic analyses.

Extensive searches in all the available Drosophilidae genomes (Table S2) confirmed that this family possesses only one *RNase T2* gene. A similar result was obtained in extensive searches of other fully sequenced insect genomes, including seven species of ants, two bees, two bumblebees, red flour beetle, silkworm, and pea aphid (Table S2). Surprisingly, the analysis of parasitoid wasp genomes provided a different result. We identified eight *RNase T2* genes in the *Nasonia vitripennis* genome (Table S2 and Figure 8), seven that encoded for potential full-length proteins (RNase Nvi1 - RNase Nvi7) and one pseudogene (RNase Nvi8, sequence not shown). Analysis of expressed sequence tag (EST) databases indicated that at least two of these genes are expressed in *N. vitripennis* (not shown). Protein database searches also revealed that another parasitoid wasp species, *Glyptapanteles flavicoxis*, contained more than one *RNase T2* gene in its genome (Table S2).

Extending the search to other fully sequenced protostome genomes and EST databases produced similar results (Table S2). RNase T2 was absolutely conserved in all the genomes analyzed, supporting the hypothesis that these enzymes carry out an important housekeeping function. Additionally, different phyla or subgroups varied on whether a single or multiple genes were present in their genomes. Among Arthropoda, only one gene was found on most Hexapoda genomes except parasitic wasp, and only one full RNase T2 gene seems to be present in the only Crustacean genome (*Daphnia pulex*) available; however, Arachnids genomes have multiple expressed genes corresponding to this family. Nematoda and Annelida have only one T2 gene, based on the analysis of three and two full genome sequences, respectively. On the other hand, Mollusca and Platyhelminthes have multiple copies of RNase T2 genes in their genomes.

Neighbor-joining analysis was used to create a phylogenetic tree (Figure 9) of the protostome RNase T2 proteins extracted from full genomes and protein and EST databases. The tree showed a well-defined clade for most individual phyla, but overall it did not have good definition. This could be due to significant divergence for proteins in each phylum clade, or it could also indicate that more sequences are needed for a better resolution. A parsimony analysis showed similar results (not shown). In any case, several inferences can be made with respect to the evolution of RNase T2 proteins in protostomes. Gene duplication events seem to have happened independently in each phylum. Moreover, in some cases we found species-specific clades, in particular the one corresponding to *Nasonia vitripennis* (parasitic wasp, see below) or *Lottia gigantea* (Mollusca) that suggest that gene duplication occurred after speciation. In contrast, gene duplications in Platyhelminthes may have occurred before speciation in some cases, since it is possible to find conserved ortholog pairs for *Schistosoma japonicum* and *Schistosoma mansoni*; however proteins from *Schmidtea mediterranea* do not cluster with those from *Schistosoma* spp, suggesting either duplication after speciation or rapid divergence.

The parasitic wasp RNases are an interesting case. In our analysis, parasitic wasps were the only insects with multiple T2 genes in their genome. Remarkably, wasps from the Braconidae family form a symbiosis with polydnaviruses that help the insect parasitize its host [40]. Bracovirus in the Braconidae contain an RNase T2 gene in their genome, which has a role in immunosuppression of the wasp's host [41]. The RNase T2 protein predictions derived from ESTs from *Glyptapanteles flavicoxis*, a wasp from the Braconidae family, cluster with bracovirus RNases included in our phylogenetic analysis (Figure 7), indicating that these RNases are expressed from the symbiotic viral genome. However, the RNases in *N. vitripennis*, which belongs to the Pteromalidae family and does not form a symbiotic relation with polydnaviruses, form an independent clade. One *N. vitripennis* gene, *RNase Nvi1*, is included in the clade that includes the RNases from all other Hymenoptera. This gene is located in chromosome 4 in this wasp (Figure 8). The other six full-length genes (*RNase Nvi2 - RNase Nvi7*) and a pseudogene (*RNase Nvi8*) are located in tandem in chromosome 3, and are likely the result of later gene duplications. We searched for any potential viral gene that could be linked to the RNases in chromosome 3 without success, suggesting that these RNases do

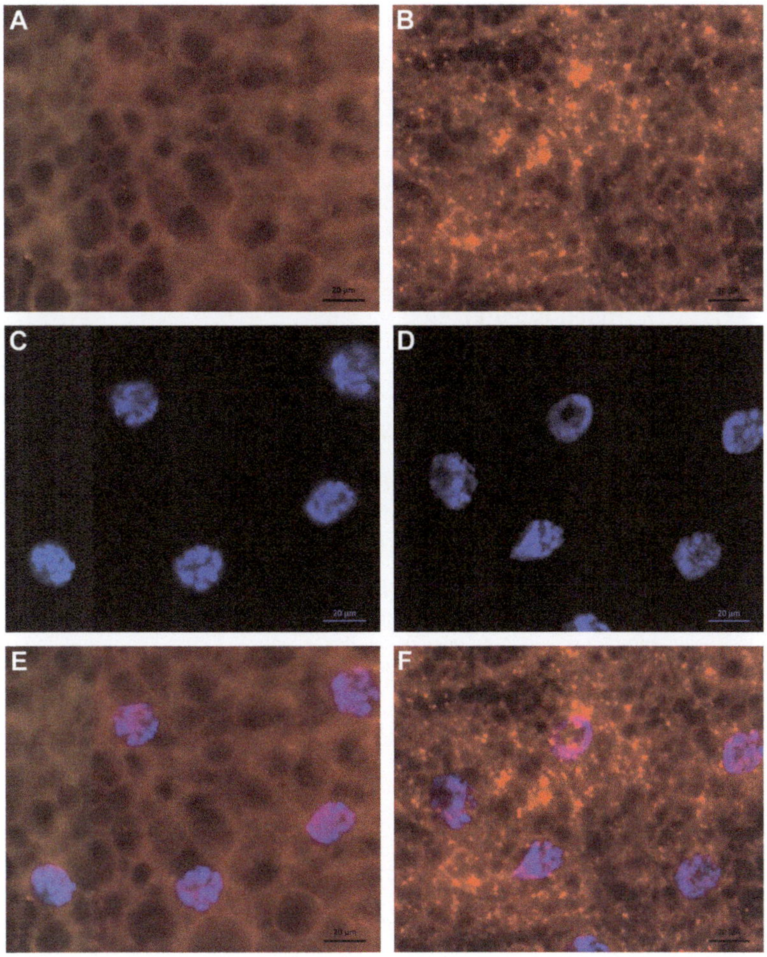

Figure 7. Effect of starvation on the accumulation of Lysotracker-positive vesicles in larval fat body. (A and B) A high level of bright red Lysotracker-positive vesicles accumulate in fat body cells isolated from (B) 14 h starved 3rd instar larvae, with few observed for (A) fed-control larvae. (C and D) Hoescht 33342 staining of DNA, and (E and F) merged images. Scale bar = 20 μm.

not have a viral origin. The fact that these RNases form an independent cluster with strong bootstrap support suggests that these proteins diverged quickly after the initial gene duplication event. Identification of an EST from *Nasonia giraulti* (GeneBank Accession number ES622650) with 97% identity at the nucleotide level with *RNase Nvi2* indicated that this duplication event(s) should have occurred before speciation in the genus *Nasonia*. Analysis of protein sequences indicated that all the RNases from chromosome 3 have an H to Y amino acid substitution in the conserved active site II (CAS II, Figure 10) that may lead to an attenuation of enzymatic activity, as has been previously observed in other animal and plant RNase T2 proteins [2]. Substitutions in this position were also observed in some Platyhelminthes and mollusk RNases (Figure 10). Moreover, some flatworm RNases (RNase Sja2, RNase Sja3, and RNase Sja6) may have lost enzymatic activity completely, since they also have a substitution in a CAS I histidine that is essential for RNase activity [1].

Discussion

In this work we performed an initial characterization of *Drosophila* RNase X25, the only member of the RNase T2 family present in this insect. We found constitutive expression of *RNase X25* mRNA during *Drosophila* development, and we were able to show a correlation between the main RNase activity detected in zymograms and expression of this gene in wild-type and deletion mutants, indicating that RNase X25 is a major contributor of endonuclease activity in *Drosophila* extracts. This activity has a pH optimum in the acidic range, a common characteristic of animal RNase T2 enzymes, which indicates that the active enzyme may normally be sequestered in an acidic compartment within cells to carry out its function. Animal RNase T2 proteins have been localized to lysosomes in zebrafish and humans [6,42], and prediction of subcellular localization for RNase X25 indicated that this protein is also targeted to the secretory pathway [15].

Based on our results and data extracted from databases, RNase X25 seems to be active at all stages of development and in all larval and adult tissues investigated. This result is in agreement with those studies that have characterized the RNase T2 family in other eukaryotes [2], and suggest that, as it has been proposed for other eukaryotic RNase T2 enzymes constitutively expressed, RNase X25 may perform a housekeeping function. Absence of this constitutive RNase activity in *Arabidopsis thaliana* and zebrafish leads to accumulation of rRNA in vacuoles or lysosomes [6,7]. Additionally, Arabidopsis plants lacking expression of *RNS2*, the housekeeping RNase T2 in this organism, show constitutive autophagy [7]. Thus, it has been proposed that the role of these

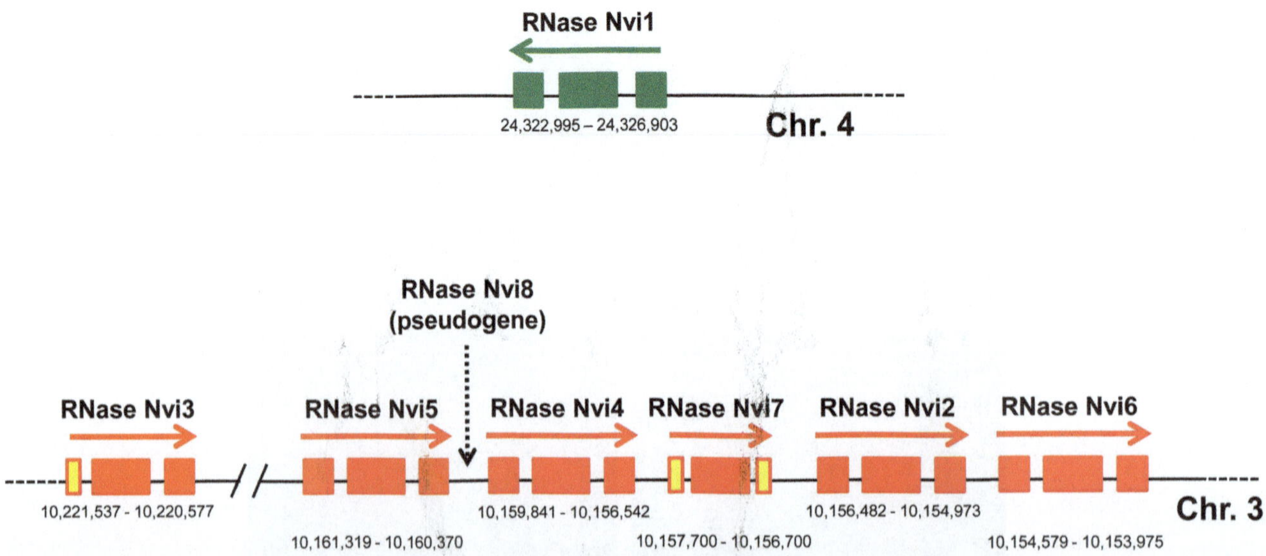

Figure 8. Genomic organization of the *RNase T2* genes found in the *Nasonia vitripennis* genome. Genes belonging to the RNase T2 family were identified by homology searches of the wasp genome. Boxes represent exons. The gene more closely related to other insect RNase T2 genes is shown in green. Genes with more divergence are shown in orange. Yellow boxes indicate exons with uncertain boundaries. Numbers below each gene are the coordinates of each gene based on the *Nasonia vitripennis* genome assembly Nvit_2.0. The location of the pseudogene is indicated but the gene is not depicted.

RNases is to maintain normal cellular homeostasis by recycling rRNA.

A role in rRNA recycling and cellular homeostasis may also be carried out by RNase T2 enzymes in cells under nutritional stress conditions, likely through a specialized autophagy process known as ribophagy. Ribophagy, the targeted degradation of ribosomes through a mechanism that uses the autophagy machinery, has been described for yeast cells undergoing starvation [43]; and Rny1, the only RNase T2 enzyme in yeast [44], may mediate rRNA degradation under stress conditions [9]. While a direct role for RNase T2 enzymes in ribophagy has not been established, their participation in this process has been suggested for plants, animals, and unicellular eukaryotes [6,8,10]. Moreover, several plant *RNase T2* genes are induced under conditions of phosphate starvation, probably as a mechanism to scavenge nutrients [2], and at least two *Tetrahymena RNase T2* genes are also induced by starvation conditions [45]. We observed that expression of *RNase X25* is significantly induced in fly larvae subjected to starvation or fed WGA. Concomitant with this response we could also observe an increase in the expression of *Atg5*, which encodes one of the core components of the autophagy machinery that has been previously shown to be induced by starvation in *Drosophila* ovaries [46], and the robust appearance of Lysotracker-positive vesicles in larval fat body cells, marking lysosomes and autolysosomes participating in the autophagy process [16,38]. Induction of *RNase X25* by nutritional stresses and evidence of autophagy may indicate that this enzyme also has a role in cellular homeostasis through recycling of cellular RNAs.

Data from a genome-wide microarray analysis of mRNA expression had previously identified *RNase X25* as one of 61 transcripts differentially expressed when animals were fed a 1% WGA diet [35]. In that study, a 9-fold increase in *RNase X25* transcript levels was observed for midgut tissue dissected from third instar larvae. Since whole animals were harvested for our analysis, it is conceivable that the modest ~2 fold increase in *RNase X25* mRNA levels we observed reflects a tissue specific differential response to WGA. Higher levels of *RNase X25* mRNAs may accumulate in tissues of the gut, with stable expression levels in remaining tissues. This effect could also explain the discrepancies in results observed in several high throughput analyses of starved *Drosophila* larvae or adults (see Table S1). This "dilution effect" may also explain the difference between the *Atg5* levels of expression observed in our experiment and the experiments of Barth et al. [46], who isolated ovaries for their analyses.

In addition to the housekeeping role, RNase T2 enzymes have acquired novel functions during eukaryote evolution. In some cases, novel functions appeared after gene duplications. This seems to be the case for plant RNase T2 enzymes that participate in defense mechanisms, and also for S-RNases, specialized T2 enzymes that determine gametophytic self-incompatibility in several plant species [12,13]. In other cases, a single protein can have multiple roles. For example, both RNase activity-dependent and -independent functions have been proposed for human RNASET2. Lack of RNASET2 causes cystic leukoencephalopathy in humans and a similar phenotype in zebrafish [6,47]. This neurological disorder is likely caused by lysosomal malfunction due to the high levels of rRNA that accumulate in these organelles when the enzyme is absent [6]. In addition, human RNASET2 has been shown to have anti-metastatic properties independent of its catalytic activity [48]. Another enzyme with more than one function is yeast Rny1. This protein may work in rRNA recycling during ribophagy-like processes, given its localization in vacuoles in normal growth conditions [9]. Additionally, Rny1 is responsible for tRNA cleavage during the cell's response to oxidative stress, after the enzyme is likely released from the vacuole into the cytoplasm. The accumulation of stable tRNA halves is thought to act as a signal during the stress response [9,10]. Moreover, during the oxidative stress response, Rny1 is able to promote cell death through an unknown mechanism that is independent of its RNase activity [9]. Cleavage of tRNAs in stress conditions that inhibit cell growth is a response conserved in plants and animals [10,49], and there is some evidence that tRNA fragments also accumulate in *Drosophila* [50,51]. We showed here that *RNase X25* expression is

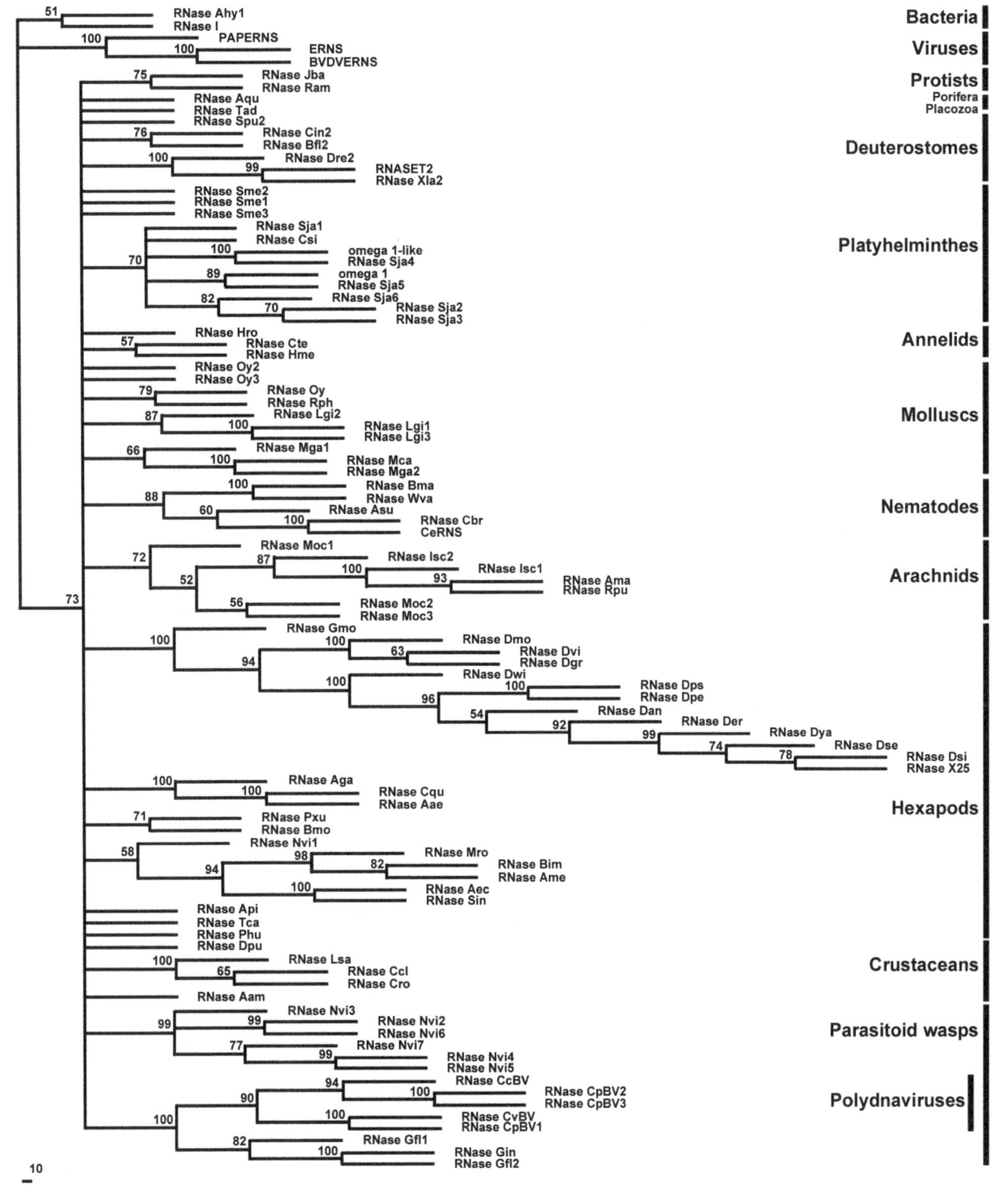

Figure 9. Phylogenetic tree of protostome RNase T2 proteins. Tree was obtained by the Neighbor-Joining method using only conserved regions. Bootstrap percentages (for 1,000 replications) greater than 50 are shown on interior branches. The tree was rooted using bacteria sequences. Groups discussed in the text are labeled on the right.

increased in flies subjected to oxidative stress, making this enzyme the logical candidate for a role in tRNA cleavage in these insects, and suggesting that RNase X25 may have dual function, as shown for other members of the RNase T2 family.

Our phylogenetic analyses showed that most insects have only one gene belonging to the RNase T2 family in their genomes. However, parasitoid wasps of the genus *Nasonia* seem to be the exception. In these insects, several gene duplications have

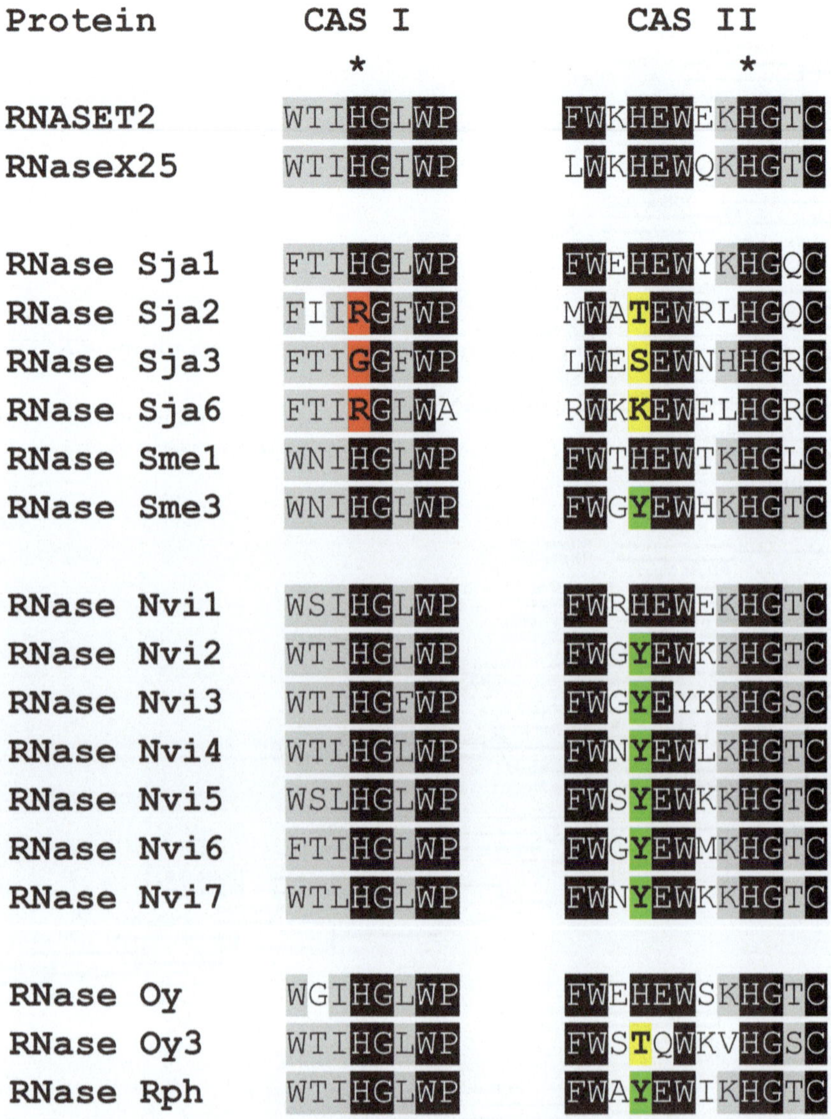
Protein
CAS I
CAS II
*
*
RNASET2 WTIHGLWP FWKHEWEKHGTC
RNaseX25 WTIHGIWP LWKHEWQKHGTC
RNase Sja1 FTIHGLWP FWEHEWYKHGQC
RNase Sja2 FIIRGFWP MWATEWRLHGQC
RNase Sja3 FTIGGFWP LWESEWNHHGRC
RNase Sja6 FTIRGLWA RWKKEWELHGRC
RNase Sme1 WNIHGLWP FWTHEWTKHGLC
RNase Sme3 WNIHGLWP FWGYEWHKHGTC
RNase Nvi1 WSIHGLWP FWRHEWEKHGTC
RNase Nvi2 WTIHGLWP FWGYEWKKHGTC
RNase Nvi3 WTIHGFWP FWGYEYKKHGSC
RNase Nvi4 WTLHGLWP FWNYEWLKHGTC
RNase Nvi5 WSLHGLWP FWSYEWKKHGTC
RNase Nvi6 FTIHGLWP FWGYEWMKHGTC
RNase Nvi7 WTLHGLWP FWNYEWKKHGTC
RNase Oy WGIHGLWP FWEHEWSKHGTC
RNase Oy3 WTIHGLWP FWSTQWKVHGSC
RNase Rph WTIHGLWP FWAYEWIKHGTC

Figure 10. Identification of mutations in conserved active site residues in protostome RNase T2 proteins. The alignment shows the conserved CAS I and CAS II regions characteristic of RNase T2 enzymes. The catalytic histidines are marked with asterisks. Mutations in the catalytic histidine in CAS I should result in complete loss of activity (shown in red). Mutations in the additional histidine in CAS II, implicated in binding to the substrate or stabilization of the pentacovalent intermediate [2], should result in enzymes with reduced activity (shown in green or yellow). The active sites of human RNASET2 and RNase X25, two active RNases, are shown for comparison.

occurred, and there is EST evidence indicating that the duplicated genes are expressed. In addition, mutations in the conserved active site of these proteins suggest that the duplicated enzymes have attenuated activity. Interestingly, parasitoid wasps from other families have a symbiotic relationship with polydnaviruses that provide protein factors essential for parasitism [40], including proteins belonging to the RNase T2 family [52]. These virus-encoded RNase T2 proteins are expressed in the parasitoid larva and likely delivered into the host during the parasitization process [52]. Expression of the viral RNase alone in the host larva resulted in reduction in hemocyte populations and increase in susceptibility of the larva to bacterial and baculovirus infections, indicating that these RNases have an important immunosuppressive function during parasitism [41,53]. *Nasonia* wasps do not have a polydnavirus symbiont. It is possible, then, that upon duplication of the conserved housekeeping *RNase T2* gene, the new proteins diverged and were recruited for a novel function in immunosuppression during parasitism, in a case of convergent evolution.

It is intriguing that the duplicated *Nasonia* RNases have mutations in the enzymes' active site. These changes have been previously reported in other proteins of the RNase T2 family, and it has been speculated that they may result in attenuated yet active enzymes [13,14]. However, the biological significance of this mutation is not yet understood. Other RNase T2 proteins are also able to modulate immune responses. E^{rns}, a Bovine Viral Diarrhea Virus RNase T2 protein, can inhibit the host beta interferon response potentially by interfering with the dsRNA signal [54], or through an intracellular mechanism involving cell-to-cell signaling even in the absence of virion particles [55]. This inhibitory effect on the beta interferon response depends on the RNase activity of E^{rns} [54,55]. However, a catalysis-independent cytotoxic effect for this protein has also been proposed based on the ability of mutant proteins without RNase activity to induce cell death in swine kidney cells [56]. Omega-1, a secreted RNase T2 protein from *Schistosoma mansoni*, also has a cytotoxic effect on its host hepatic cells [57]. This protein is also able to induce a strong Th2-polarized immune response in the host, which is necessary for the efficient passage of parasite eggs from the intravascular sites of deposition to the intestinal or bladder lumen [58]. In this case, modulation of the immune response seems to be caused by suppression of protein synthesis after internalization by dendritic cells following recognition of the glycosylation signature of omega-1 [59]. The RNase activity of omega-1 is necessary for this immunomodulating role. However, other *Schistosoma* species appear to have inactive RNase T2 proteins in addition to enzymes with conserved active sites. It is possible that these proteins could also play a role in immunoregulation, although these inactive proteins are present also in free living planarians.

Recent insights from *Arabidopsis thaliana*, zebrafish, and human indicate that the RNase T2 enzymes carry out an important housekeeping function in normal cells [6,7]. Arabidopsis mutants lacking this conserved RNase T2 activity accumulate RNA, mainly in the vacuole, have an increased rRNA half-life, and exhibit constitutive autophagy [7]; while *rnaset2* mutant zebrafish show aberrant accumulation of undigested rRNA in neuronal lysosomes and present brain lesions similar to those observed in leukocephalopathies associated with deficiencies in RNASET2 in humans [6,47]. Thus, RNase T2 enzymes participate in the normal recycling of rRNA, and this housekeeping function seems to be essential for cellular homeostasis. Duplication and divergence of the RNase T2 gene family has occurred in the evolution of plants and fishes. Secreted RNases of the RNase A family seem to have acquired in vertebrates, including humans, some of the biological roles carried out by RNase T2 enzymes in other systems (reviewed by MacIntosh [2]). Use of the *Drosophila* model, whose genome encodes only one *RNase T2* gene and lacks RNase A homologs or other evident secretory RNases with similar activity, is likely to provide insight into the ancestral physiological function of this gene family in multicellular animals during normal growth and development, and also under stress conditions. Analyses of *Drosophila* mutants with reduced RNase X25 activity may lead to identification of phenotypic characteristics that could be the basis of genetic modifier screens to identify other key genes that participate in RNase T2 function. These may also prove important to understand how RNA degradation systems interface with other cellular processes.

Supporting Information

Figure S1 Expression profile of *RNase X25* in different adult tissues from the modENCODE database.
(PDF)

Figure S2 Expression profile of *RNase X25* in different adult and larval tissues from the FlyAtlas database.
(PDF)

Table S1 Regulation of RNase X25 expression under nutritional stress or other conditions, obtained from public databases or the literature.
(PDF)

Table S2 Proteins belonging to the RNase T2 family used for phylogenetic analyses.
(XLSX)

Acknowledgments

The authors would like to thank Shelby Gosa, Amanda Haffarnan, and Joanne Tran for their help collecting fly samples.

Author Contributions

Conceived and designed the experiments: GCM LA SM AR. Performed the experiments: LA SM AR RB JD. Analyzed the data: GCM LA SM AR RB JD. Contributed reagents/materials/analysis tools: GCM LA. Wrote the paper: GCM LA.

References

1. Irie M (1999) Structure-function relationships of acid ribonucleases: lysosomal, vacuolar, and periplasmic enzymes. Pharmacol Ther 81: 77–89.
2. MacIntosh GC (2011) RNase T2 Family: Enzymatic Properties, Functional Diversity, and Evolution of Ancient Ribonucleases. In: Nicholson AWW, editor. Ribonucleases: Springer Berlin Heidelberg. pp. 89–114.
3. Deshpande RA, Shankar V (2002) Ribonucleases from T2 family. Crit Rev Microbiol 28: 79–122.
4. Tanaka N, Arai J, Inokuchi N, Koyama T, Ohgi K, et al. (2000) Crystal structure of a plant ribonuclease, RNase LE. J Mol Biol 298: 859–873.
5. Luhtala N, Parker R (2010) T2 Family ribonucleases: ancient enzymes with diverse roles. Trends Biochem Sci 35: 253–259.
6. Haud N, Kara F, Diekmann S, Henneke M, Willer JR, et al. (2011) *rnaset2* mutant zebrafish model familial cystic leukoencephalopathy and reveal a role for RNase T2 in degrading ribosomal RNA. Proc Natl Acad Sci U S A 108: 1099–1103.
7. Hillwig MS, Contento AL, Meyer A, Ebany D, Bassham DC, et al. (2011) RNS2, a conserved member of the RNase T2 family, is necessary for ribosomal RNA decay in plants. Proc Natl Acad Sci U S A 108: 1093–1098.
8. MacIntosh GC, Bassham DC (2011) The connection between ribophagy, autophagy and ribosomal RNA decay. Autophagy 7: 662–663.
9. Thompson DM, Parker R (2009) The RNase Rny1p cleaves tRNAs and promotes cell death during oxidative stress in *Saccharomyces cerevisiae*. J Cell Biol 185: 43–50.
10. Andersen KL, Collins K (2012) Several RNase T2 enzymes function in induced tRNA and rRNA turnover in the ciliate *Tetrahymena*. Mol Biol Cell 23: 36–44.
11. Yamasaki S, Ivanov P, Hu GF, Anderson P (2009) Angiogenin cleaves tRNA and promotes stress-induced translational repression. J Cell Biol 185: 35–42.
12. Igic B, Kohn JR (2001) Evolutionary relationships among self-incompatibility RNases. Proc Natl Acad Sci U S A 98: 13167–13171.
13. MacIntosh GC, Hillwig MS, Meyer A, Flagel L (2010) RNase T2 genes from rice and the evolution of secretory ribonucleases in plants. Mol Genet Genomics 283: 381–396.
14. Hillwig MS, Rizhsky L, Wang Y, Umanskaya A, Essner JJ, et al. (2009) Zebrafish RNase T2 genes and the evolution of secretory ribonucleases in animals. BMC Evol Biol 9: 170.
15. Hime G, Prior L, Saint R (1995) The *Drosophila melanogaster* genome contains a member of the Rh/T2/S-glycoprotein family of ribonuclease-encoding genes. Gene 158: 203–207.
16. Scott RC, Schuldiner O, Neufeld TP (2004) Role and Regulation of Starvation-Induced Autophagy in the Drosophila Fat Body. Dev Cell 7: 167–178.
17. Juhasz G, Neufeld T (2008) Experimental Control and Characterization of Autophagy in Drosophila. Methods in Molecular Biology 445: 125–133.
18. Yen Y, Green PJ (1991) Identification and Properties of the Major Ribonucleases of *Arabidopsis thaliana*. Plant Physiol 97: 1487–1493.
19. Pfaffl MW (2001) A new mathematical model for relative quantification in real-time RT–PCR. Nucleic Acids Res 29: e45.
20. Altschul SF, Gish W, Miller W, Myers EW, Lipman DJ (1990) Basic Local Alignment Search Tool. J Mol Biol 215: 403–410.
21. Kersey PJ, Staines DM, Lawson D, Kulesha E, Derwent P, et al. (2012) Ensembl Genomes: an integrative resource for genome-scale data from non-vertebrate species. Nucleic Acids Res 40: D91–D97.
22. Megy K, Emrich SJ, Lawson D, Campbell D, Dialynas E, et al. (2012) VectorBase: improvements to a bioinformatics resource for invertebrate vector genomics. Nucleic Acids Res 40: D729–D734.
23. Grigoriev IV, Nordberg H, Shabalov I, Aerts A, Cantor M, et al. (2012) The Genome Portal of the Department of Energy Joint Genome Institute. Nucleic Acids Res 40: D26–D32.
24. Wang X, Chen W, Huang Y, Sun J, Men J, et al. (2011) The draft genome of the carcinogenic human liver fluke *Clonorchis sinensis*. Genome Biol 12: R107.
25. Robb SMC, Ross E, Sánchez Alvarado A (2008) SmedGD: the *Schmidtea mediterranea* genome database. Nucleic Acids Res 36: D599–D606.
26. Munoz-Torres MC, Reese JT, Childers CP, Bennett AK, Sundaram JP, et al. (2011) Hymenoptera Genome Database: integrated community resources for insect species of the order Hymenoptera. Nucleic Acids Res 39: D658–D662.

27. Wang J, Xia Q, He X, Dai M, Ruan J, et al. (2005) SilkDB: a knowledgebase for silkworm biology and genomics. Nucleic Acids Res 33: D399–D402.
28. Kim HS, Murphy T, Xia J, Caragea D, Park Y, et al. (2010) BeetleBase in 2010: revisions to provide comprehensive genomic information for *Tribolium castaneum*. Nucleic Acids Res 38: D437–D442.
29. Logan-Klumpler FJ, De Silva N, Boehme U, Rogers MB, Velarde G, et al. (2012) GeneDB—an annotation database for pathogens. Nucleic Acids Res 40: D98–D108.
30. Legeai F, Shigenobu S, Gauthier JP, Colbourne J, Rispe C, et al. (2010) AphidBase: a centralized bioinformatic resource for annotation of the pea aphid genome. Insect Mol Biol 19: 5–12.
31. Larkin MA, Blackshields G, Brown NP, Chenna R, McGettigan PA, et al. (2007) Clustal W and Clustal X version 2.0. Bioinformatics 23: 2947–2948.
32. Swofford DL (2002) PAUP*. Phylogenetic analysis using parsimony (*and other methods). Version 4.0b10. Sunderland, Massachusetts: Sinauer Associates.
33. Celniker SE, Dillon LAL, Gerstein MB, Gunsalus KC, Henikoff S, et al. (2009) Unlocking the secrets of the genome. Nature 459: 927–930.
34. Robinson SW, Herzyk P, Dow JAT, Leader DP (2013) FlyAtlas: database of gene expression in the tissues of *Drosophila melanogaster*. Nucleic Acids Res 41: D744–D750.
35. Li HM, Sun L, Mittapalli O, Muir WM, Xie J, et al. (2009) Transcriptional signatures in response to wheat germ agglutinin and starvation in *Drosophila melanogaster* larval midgut. Insect Mol Biol 18: 21–31.
36. Chang YY, Neufeld TP (2010) Autophagy takes flight in *Drosophila*. Febs Lett 584: 1342–1349.
37. Zinke I, Schütz CS, Katzenberger JD, Bauer M, Pankratz MJ (2002) Nutrient control of gene expression in *Drosophila*: microarray analysis of starvation and sugar-dependent response. EMBO J 21: 6162–6173.
38. Jimenez-Sanchez M, Menzies FM, Chang YY, Simecek N, Neufeld TP, et al. (2012) The Hedgehog signalling pathway regulates autophagy. Nat Commun 3: 1200.
39. Ashburner M, Golic KG, Hawley RS (2005) *Drosophila*: A Laboratory Handbook: Cold Spring Harbor Laboratory Press.
40. Burke GR, Strand MR (2012) Polydnaviruses of Parasitic Wasps: Domestication of Viruses To Act as Gene Delivery Vectors. Insects 3: 91–119.
41. Park B, Kim Y (2010) Transient transcription of a putative RNase containing BEN domain encoded in *Cotesia plutellae* bracovirus induces an immunosuppression of the diamondback moth, *Plutella xylostella*. J Invertebr Pathol 105: 156–163.
42. Campomenosi P, Salis S, Lindqvist C, Mariani D, Nordstrom T, et al. (2006) Characterization of RNASET2, the first human member of the Rh/T2/S family of glycoproteins. Arch Biochem Biophys 449: 17–26.
43. Kraft C, Deplazes A, Sohrmann M, Peter M (2008) Mature ribosomes are selectively degraded upon starvation by an autophagy pathway requiring the Ubp3p/Bre5p ubiquitin protease. Nat Cell Biol 10: 602–610.
44. MacIntosh GC, Bariola PA, Newbigin E, Green PJ (2001) Characterization of Rny1, the *Saccharomyces cerevisiae* member of the T_2 RNase family of RNases: Unexpected functions for ancient enzymes? Proc Natl Acad Sci U S A 98: 1018–1023.
45. Miao W, Xiong J, Bowen J, Wang W, Liu Y, et al. (2009) Microarray Analyses of Gene Expression during the *Tetrahymena thermophila* Life Cycle. PLoS One 4: e4429.
46. Barth JMI, Szabad J, Hafen E, Kohler K (2011) Autophagy in *Drosophila* ovaries is induced by starvation and is required for oogenesis. Cell Death Differ 18: 915–924.
47. Henneke M, Diekmann S, Ohlenbusch A, Kaiser J, Engelbrecht V, et al. (2009) RNASET2-deficient cystic leukoencephalopathy resembles congenital cytomegalovirus brain infection. Nat Genet 41: 773–775.
48. Acquati F, Possati L, Ferrante L, Campomenosi P, Talevi S, et al. (2005) Tumor and metastasis suppression by the human RNASET2 gene. Int J Oncol 26: 1159–1168.
49. Thompson DM, Lu C, Green PJ, Parker R (2008) tRNA cleavage is a conserved response to oxidative stress in eukaryotes. RNA 14: 2095–2103.
50. Brennecke J, Aravin AA, Stark A, Dus M, Kellis M, et al. (2007) Discrete Small RNA-Generating Loci as Master Regulators of Transposon Activity in *Drosophila*. Cell 128: 1089–1103.
51. Aravin AA, Lagos-Quintana M, Yalcin A, Zavolan M, Marks D, et al. (2003) The Small RNA Profile during *Drosophila melanogaster* Development. Dev Cell 5: 337–350.
52. Ramjan Ali M, Kim Y (2012) A novel polydnaviral gene family, BEN, and its immunosuppressive function in larvae of *Plutella xylostella* parasitized by *Cotesia plutellae*. J Invertebr Pathol 110: 389–397.
53. Park B, Kim Y (2012) Immunosuppression induced by expression of a viral RNase enhances susceptibility of *Plutella xylostella* to microbial pesticides. Insect Sci 19: 47–54.
54. Iqbal M, Poole E, Goodbourn S, McCauley JW (2004) Role for Bovine Viral Diarrhea Virus E^{rns} Glycoprotein in the Control of Activation of Beta Interferon by Double-Stranded RNA. J Virol 78: 136–145.
55. Python S, Gerber M, Suter R, Ruggli N, Summerfield A (2013) Efficient Sensing of Infected Cells in Absence of Virus Particles by Blasmacytoid Dendritic Cells Is Blocked by the Viral Ribonuclease E^{rns}. PLoS Pathog 9: e1003412.
56. Hulst MM, Panoto FE, Hoekman A, van Gennip HGP, Moormann RJM (1998) Inactivation of the RNase Activity of Glycoprotein E^{rns} of Classical Swine Fever Virus Results in a Cytopathogenic Virus. J Virol 72: 151–157.
57. Fitzsimmons CM, Schramm G, Jones FM, Chalmers IW, Hoffmann KF, et al. (2005) Molecular characterization of omega-1: a hepatotoxic ribonuclease from *Schistosoma mansoni* eggs. Mol Biochem Parasitol 144: 123–127.
58. Pearce EJ (2005) Priming of the immune response by schistosome eggs. Parasite Immunol 27: 265–270.
59. Everts B, Hussaarts L, Driessen NN, Meevissen MHJ, Schramm G, et al. (2012) Schistosome-derived omega-1 drives Th2 polarization by suppressing protein synthesis following internalization by the mannose receptor. J Exp Med 209: 1753–1767.

18

Protein-Energy Malnutrition Developing after Global Brain Ischemia Induces an Atypical Acute-Phase Response and Hinders Expression of GAP-43

Shari E. Smith[1,3], Sarah A. Figley[1,3], David J. Schreyer[2,3], Phyllis G. Paterson[1,3]*

1 College of Pharmacy and Nutrition, University of Saskatchewan, Saskatoon, Saskatchewan, Canada, **2** Department of Anatomy and Cell Biology, University of Saskatchewan, Saskatoon, Saskatchewan, Canada, **3** Cameco MS Neuroscience Research Center, Saskatoon City Hospital, Saskatoon, Saskatchewan, Canada

Abstract

Protein-energy malnutrition (PEM) is a common post-stroke problem. PEM can independently induce a systemic acute-phase response, and pre-existing malnutrition can exacerbate neuroinflammation induced by brain ischemia. In contrast, the effects of PEM developing in the post-ischemic period have not been studied. Since excessive inflammation can impede brain remodeling, we investigated the effects of post-ischemic malnutrition on neuroinflammation, the acute-phase reaction, and neuroplasticity-related proteins. Male, Sprague-Dawley rats were exposed to global forebrain ischemia using the 2-vessel occlusion model or sham surgery. The sham rats were assigned to control diet (18% protein) on day 3 after surgery, whereas the rats exposed to global ischemia were assigned to either control diet or a low protein (PEM, 2% protein) diet. Post-ischemic PEM decreased growth associated protein-43, synaptophysin and synaptosomal-associated protein-25 immunofluorescence within the hippocampal CA3 mossy fiber terminals on day 21, whereas the glial response in the hippocampal CA1 and CA3 subregions was unaltered by PEM. No systemic acute-phase reaction attributable to global ischemia was detected in control diet-fed rats, as reflected by serum concentrations of alpha-2-macroglobulin, alpha-1-acid glycoprotein, haptoglobin, and albumin. Acute exposure to the PEM regimen after global brain ischemia caused an atypical acute-phase response. PEM decreased the serum concentrations of albumin and haptoglobin on day 5, with the decreases sustained to day 21. Serum alpha-2-macroglobulin concentrations were significantly higher in malnourished rats on day 21. This provides the first direct evidence that PEM developing after brain ischemia exerts wide-ranging effects on mechanisms important to stroke recovery.

Editor: Muzamil Ahmad, Indian Institute of Integrative Medicine, India

Funding: P. Paterson gratefully acknowledges funding support from the Heart and Stroke Foundation of Saskatchewan and the Canadian Institutes of Health Research (Operating Grant 111124). S. Smith was supported by a University Graduate Scholarship from the University of Saskatchewan. The funders had no role in study design, data collection and analysis, decision to publish, or preparation of the manuscript.

Competing Interests: The authors have declared that no competing interests exist.

* Email: phyllis.paterson@usask.ca

Introduction

Protein-energy malnutrition (PEM) is commonly associated with stroke. Pre-existing PEM is present in 12–19% of patients admitted to hospital with a diagnosis of stroke [1,2,3]. With post-stroke feeding challenges, PEM prevalence rises to 20–35% after one week [2,4] and 35–49% by admission to a rehabilitation unit [5,6]. These unfortunate statistics were first documented more than two decades ago and span many countries [7,8].

In clinical studies, PEM is associated with poorer functional outcome following stroke [1,2,9], implicating malnutrition as an important stroke co-morbidity factor. Using a preclinical model, we found pre-existing PEM to be a direct cause of impaired short-term cognitive function after global brain ischemia [10]. While clinical studies have focused on the relationship between nutritional status and infection rates, length of hospital stay [8], and muscle strength [11], we identified direct effects on the ischemic brain. In rodent models of global brain ischemia mimicking the clinical scenario of PEM pre-existing at the time of ischemia and continuing untreated, PEM appeared to lower the set-point for the inflammatory response in the vulnerable hippocampal CA1 subregion [10,12]. This was evident as an increase in activation of the predominant pro-inflammatory transcription factor, nuclear factor kappa B [12], and, in a subset of malnourished rodents, an augmented glial response to global brain ischemia [10]. While pre-existing PEM did not exacerbate neuronal death, neuroplasticity-related proteins were altered [10,13]. The latter might be due to an increase in glial cell activation and neuroinflammation, which can modulate post-stroke neuroplasticity [14]. Whereas glial cells activated by brain ischemia can secrete growth factors [15,16] that promote neuroplasticity, over-expression of pro-inflammatory cytokines and neuroinflammation can inhibit synaptic plasticity [17,18].

No studies have addressed the response of the brain to the more common clinical problem of PEM developing after stroke. Thus, the first aim of the current study was to investigate the effects of post-ischemic PEM on glial activation, neuronal growth state, and synaptic organization. Since inflammation can persist for weeks to months after brain ischemia [19] when the brain is receptive to remodeling [20], we hypothesized that PEM would intensify the neuroinflammatory response, thus inhibiting the expression of growth associated protein-43 (GAP-43), synaptophysin and synaptosomal-associated protein-25 (SNAP-25).

PEM may also influence post-stroke recovery by altering the acute-phase reaction triggered by brain ischemia [21]. Although PEM can independently stimulate systemic inflammation [22,23] and an atypical acute-phase response [24], malnutrition can also blunt such a response to injury or infection [25,26]. Thus, the second objective was to investigate whether post-ischemic malnutrition would alter an acute-phase response induced by global ischemia. This was assessed by examining serum concentrations of the rat acute-phase proteins, albumin [27], alpha-2-macroglobulin (A2M), haptoglobin, and alpha-1-acid glycoprotein (AGP) [28].

Materials and Methods

Animals

Sixty-nine male Sprague-Dawley rats (52–55 day old) (Charles River Canada, QC, Canada) were acclimatized on rat chow for 2 days before placement on a protein adequate control diet (CON, 18% protein) [24]. Rats were housed in groups of 2–4 and maintained on a 12 hour light/dark cycle in a temperature controlled room with free access to food and water. This work was approved by the University of Saskatchewan's Animal Research Ethics Board and adhered to the Canadian Council on Animal Care guidelines for humane animal use.

Global brain ischemia

Following a 4–6 day acclimation period on CON diet, rats were randomly allocated to undergo either sham surgery (Sham) or transient forebrain ischemia via the 2-vessel occlusion (2-VO) model (ISC), as previously described [29] and modified from Smith *et al.* [30]. Surgical procedures were performed aseptically under isoflurane anaesthesia (1.75–4% in 70% N_2O and 30% O_2). Before surgery, rats were fasted for ~16 hours to achieve consistent blood glucose levels. Following anaesthesia induction, animals were placed on a heated water blanket and a tympanic probe was inserted to estimate brain temperature (IT-18 flexible probe; Physitemp Instruments Inc. NJ, USA). Tympanic temperature was maintained close to 37.5°C with the use of an overhead infrared lamp (250W) controlled by an automated feedback temperature controller (CN9500; Omega Engineering Inc., CT, USA). Tail artery cannulation allowed for continuous measurement of mean arterial blood pressure (PressureMAT PDKTP4-PCS; PendoTech, NJ, USA) and collection of arterial blood samples (100 μL) for measurement of blood gases, hematocrit, and glucose concentration. Samples for the latter were taken prior to and after the period of ischemia. Both common carotid arteries were isolated and the right jugular vein was cannulated. Blood was withdrawn via the jugular vein into a warmed heparinized syringe until blood pressure reached ~35 mmHg. At this time, micro-aneurysm clips (S&T Vascular Clamps HD-S; Fine Science Tools, BC, Canada) were applied to both carotid arteries for 10 minutes. Blood pressure was recorded at 1 minute intervals and maintained at 35–40 mmHg throughout the occlusion period by withdrawing or infusing blood as needed. After releasing the clamps, blood was slowly re-infused and incisions were sutured. A dose of bupivacaine (2 mg/kg) was divided equally for injection around the 2 incision sites. Sham rats were treated identically except that carotid arteries were not occluded and hypotension was not induced. Post-surgical care included monitoring recovery from anaesthesia in the acute period as well as monitoring and documenting healing of incisions, physical appearance, grooming, and body weight for the entire experimental period. During the first 3 days of the post-surgical recovery period, food was available in the cages for ease of access. Rats were singly housed until post-surgical day 3, at which time the rats were placed back with their original cage mates.

Diet assignment

At 3 days following surgery, rats previously exposed to global ischemia were randomly assigned to either a protein-deficient diet (PEM, 2% protein) or to continue on the CON diet (18% protein) (Dyets, Inc., PA, USA). All rats exposed to sham surgery were provided with CON diet. Diets were modified from the American Institute of Nutrition-93G diet [31]; the diet composition was previously described in detail [24]. Rats of this age fed a 2% protein diet voluntarily reduce food consumption, thereby causing a decrease in both energy and protein intake [24,32]. Body weight and food intake were recorded on the day of surgery (day 0) and post-surgical days 1 and 2. Following diet assignment (day 3), food intake was recorded daily, and body weight was recorded weekly and on the final day of the experiment. The sample sizes for the six experimental groups generated were: CON-Sham5d (n = 9), CON-ISC5d (n = 13), PEM-ISC5d (n = 12), CON-Sham21d (n = 8), CON-ISC21d (n = 11), and PEM-ISC21d (n = 11).

Histology and immunofluorescence

At 5 or 21 days post-surgery, rats were anaesthetized under isoflurane (5% in 100% O_2) and blood samples were collected via cardiac puncture prior to euthanasia. Rats were then perfused transcardially with 0.9% saline followed by 4% paraformaldehyde. Intact heads were submerged into 4% paraformaldehyde and stored overnight at 4°C. Brains were removed and post-fixed in paraformaldehyde for an additional 24 hours. Following fixation, brains were submerged into a 20% sucrose solution and stored at 4°C for 3 days to prevent ice crystal formation and tissue cracking. Fixed brains were placed in plastic cryomolds and embedded in Optimal Cutting Temperature (OCT) compound. Samples were flash frozen using dry ice-cooled isopentane and stored at −80°C until sectioning. For each rat, the coronal section (14 μm) corresponding to −3.8 mm from Bregma was stained with cresyl violet, while adjacent sections were used for immunofluorescence. Viable CA1 and CA3 pyramidal neurons were counted at 400× magnification in cresyl violet stained sections. Using a 200 μm square (10×10) microscope grid, neurons with intact nucleus and cellular membrane were counted bilaterally in medial, middle, and lateral sectors of the CA1 region and the medial sector of the CA3 bend. Cell counts from the right and left hemisphere were summed to generate the total neuron count for each rat. Assessment of neuronal counts and semi-quantification of immunofluorescence were blinded.

Identical protocols were followed, using Shandon Sequenza Immunostaining Racks (Thermo Scientific, CHS, UK), to immuno-label coronal sections for astrocytes (GFAP), activated microglia (Iba-1), and the axon terminal proteins synaptophysin, SNAP-25, and GAP-43. Sections were blocked with normal goat serum (5%; Sigma-Aldrich, ON, Canada) and incubated at 4°C overnight in a primary antibody either for astrocytes (Rabbit anti-GFAP, 1:400; Z0334, DakoCytomation, ON, Canada), microglia (Rabbit anti-Iba-1, 1:1000; 019–19741, Wako Chemicals, VA, USA), synaptophysin (Mouse anti-synaptophysin, 1:200; clone SY38, Millipore, MA, USA), SNAP-25 (Mouse anti-SNAP-25, 1:500; Millipore, clone SP12, MA, USA) or GAP-43 (Mouse anti-GAP-43, 1:2500; clone 9-1E12 Ascites fluid [33]). Following a wash step with PBS, slides were incubated in a secondary fluorescent antibody (Goat-anti-mouse AlexaFluor488, 1:200 [115-545-166, Jackson Laboratories, PA, USA] or Goat-anti-rabbit AlexaFluor 594, 1:500 [A11012, Molecular Probes, Invitrogen]) in the dark for 2 hours. Slides were washed with PBS and cover slipped with ProLong Gold Antifade Reagent with DAPI (P36931, Molecular Probes, Invitrogen) in order to visualize cell nuclei. Negative control sections were treated identically, except that the sections were not incubated in the primary antibody.

Semi-quantification of the immuno-labeling obtained for each marker was completed using one section per hemisphere from every rat (ImageJ, U.S. National Institutes of Health, MD, USA). The integrated density value (IDV), the sum of the pixel values in the region of interest, was measured using high magnification photographs captured from a fluorescence microscope. All densitometry measurements were adjusted for background staining, as calculated from negative control sections. GFAP and Iba-1 expression was measured by placing a box (pixel area = 265,816) that included the CA1 pyramidal layer, stratum oriens and stratum radiatum. A second box was placed in the CA3 mossy fiber terminals (pixel area = 265,816). Immuno-staining of axon terminal markers was found predominantly within the CA3 region, and therefore semi-quantification was performed in the mossy fiber terminals for synaptophysin (pixel area = 78,402), SNAP-25 (pixel area = 101,936), and GAP-43 (pixel area = 141,778). Values from the right and left hemispheres were averaged.

Serum acute-phase proteins

Blood samples collected at the time of euthanasia were allowed to clot for 30 minutes at room temperature and then centrifuged at 1,500×g for 10 minutes. Following centrifugation, serum was collected and stored at −80°C. Enzyme-linked immunosorbent assay (ELISA) kits were used to measure the serum concentrations of A2M, AGP, and haptoglobin (Immunology Consultants Laboratory, Inc., OR, USA), which are positive acute-phase proteins in the rat [28]. Serum concentrations of the negative acute-phase protein, albumin [27], was measured using the bromocresol green method [34]. A volume of 25 μL of blank, serum sample, or standard solution was added to 5.0 mL bromocresol green reagent (0.15 mmol/L bromocresol green, 0.075 mol/L succinate buffer, 30% Brij-35). After 30 minutes, absorbance was measured spectrophotometrically at 628 nm (Biochrom Ultrospec 3100 Pro). Linear regression was used to determine the albumin concentration of the samples.

Statistical analyses

Statistical analyses were conducted using SPSS 20.0 for Windows. All data are presented as mean ± SEM, and the significance level was set at $p<0.05$. Body weight and food intake differences between rats exposed to sham surgery or global ischemia were analyzed on post-surgical days 0, 1, 2, and 3 using an independent-sample Student's t-test. Following assignment to experimental diet on day 3, food intake was analyzed for rats fed the low protein diet or CON diet for each day until it reached significance using an independent-sample Student's t-test. Significant differences in body weight were determined using a 1-factor ANOVA and Tukey's test. Differences in neuronal cell counts, serum acute-phase protein concentrations, and immunofluorescence among the three treatment groups at each time-point were determined using a 1-factor ANOVA and Tukey's test for two *posthoc* comparisons only; comparing the CON-Sham and the CON-ISC groups identified an ischemia effect, whereas the CON-ISC versus PEM-ISC comparison detected an effect of diet on ischemic outcome. Selected unadjusted pair-wise comparisons were also made for the immunofluorescence data.

Results

Exclusion from the study

Five rats were excluded from the study due to blood pressure readings not meeting criteria, unsuccessful tail artery cannulation, or poor recovery demonstrated by severe weight loss. These rats were humanely euthanized with isoflurane (5% in 100% O_2).

Physiological parameters measured during surgery

A summary of the physiological parameters measured during 2-VO and sham surgeries in the remaining rats is shown in **Table S1**. Although all rats were still on CON diet at the time of surgery, the table separates the CON-ISC and PEM-ISC groups to illustrate baseline comparison prior to dietary assignment. Mean pre- and post-ischemic values for all physiological parameters were within the target range. Tympanic temperature was tightly regulated throughout the 10 minute occlusion period, and thus the resulting tympanic temperature values fell within the desired range for the three experimental groups. Blood pressure was carefully manipulated in the two groups exposed to global ischemia, resulting in values within the desired range.

Impact of surgery on food intake and body weight prior to diet assignment

Mean initial body weight on the day of surgery was not significantly different between sham and ischemic treatment groups, at which time all rats were on CON diet ($t(62) = -0.38$, $p = 0.71$; Sham, $n = 17$; ISC, $n = 47$). A significant decrease in body weight was reported on post-surgical days 1, 2 and 3 in the group exposed to the 2-VO surgery, relative to that of sham animals (day 1, $t(62) = 5.23$, $p<0.001$; data not shown). Individual rat food intake was monitored on post-surgical days 1, 2, and 3, which was possible due to individual rat housing (Sham, $n = 17$; ISC, $n = 47$). Daily food intake was significantly decreased in the ischemia treatment group compared to sham-operated rats on days 1, 2 and 3 (day 1, $t(62) = 13.29$, $p<0.001$; data not shown).

Indices of PEM

Fig. 1A shows the pattern of body weight change for the day 21 treatment groups resulting from experimental diet assignment initiated on post-surgical day 3. On day 7 post-surgery (4 days after diet assignment), there was a significant difference in body weight ($F_{2,27} = 31.74$, $p<0.001$), with PEM-ISC rats weighing significantly less than CON-Sham (Tukey's test; $p<0.001$) and CON-ISC ($p<0.001$) rats; this pattern continued throughout the post-surgical period ($p<0.001$). Malnourished rats gained 6% of their initial body weight by day 21, compared to a 59% increase observed in both the CON-ISC and CON-Sham groups. This resulted in a mean difference in final body weight of 33% between the PEM-ISC group and both CON-fed groups.

Fig. 1B shows mean (± SEM) daily food intake starting on post-surgical day 4 (1 day after diet assignment) for rats fed the low protein (PEM-ISC21d, $n = 5$ cages [2–3 rats/cage]) or CON diet (CON-Sham21d + CON-ISC21d, $n = 8$ cages [2–3 rats/cage]). Mean food intake was calculated based on cage data (daily cage food intake/number of rats per cage). Since CON-ISC and CON-Sham rats were sometimes housed in the same cages, differences between these groups could not be analyzed. A significant decrease in food intake in the PEM-ISC group was first observed on post-surgical day 7 (4 days after diet assignment), as compared to the other two CON groups combined ($t(11) = 2.57$, $p = 0.026$). Total

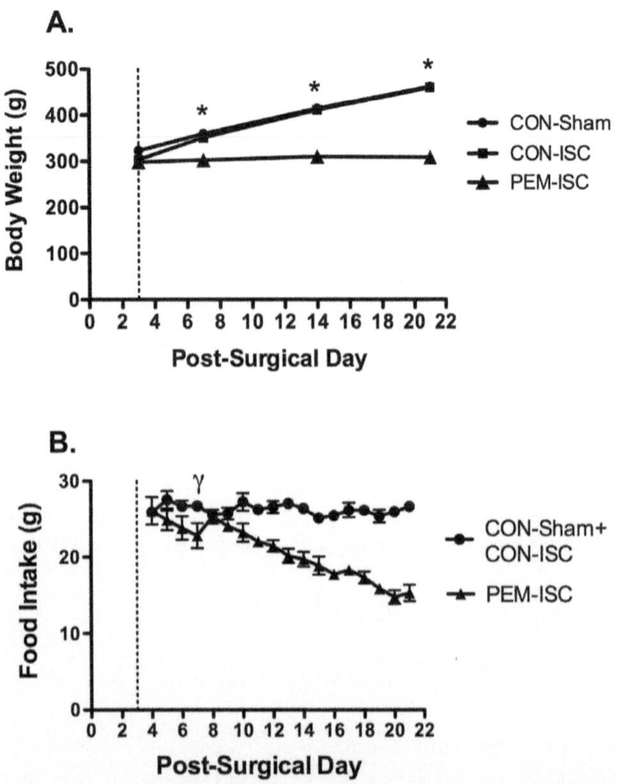

Figure 1. The PEM regimen introduced on day 3 after global brain ischemia depressed body weight and food intake. Data are shown as mean ± SEM for the day 21 treatment groups. The dashed vertical line illustrates the day on which rats were assigned to experimental diet. (**A**) Body weights are shown for days 3, 7, 14 and 21 (CON-Sham21d, n = 8; CON-ISC21d, n = 11; PEM-ISC21d, n = 11).*Indicates a significant effect of experimental diet on body weight (PEM-ISC compared to CON-Sham and CON-ISC groups) by Tukey's Test ($p < 0.05$). (**B**) Food intake was collected daily on a cage basis (CON-Sham21d + CON-ISC21d, n = 8 cages [2–3 rats/cage]; PEM-ISC21d, n = 5 cages [2–3 rats/cage]) and calculated as daily cage food intake/number of rats per cage. γ Indicates the first day on which PEM-ISC rats experienced a significant reduction in food intake, when compared to that for the combined CON groups, as detected by an independent-sample Student's t-test ($p < 0.05$).

food intake over the 18 days on experimental diet was depressed by 21% in PEM-ISC rats. Rats in the day 5 treatment groups had similar body weight and food intake patterns to the day 21 groups (data not shown).

CA1 and CA3 neuronal death

Hippocampal CA1 neuronal counts are shown in **Table 1**. On both days 5 and 21 post-ischemia, there was a significant group effect (5 day, $F_{2,24} = 217.41$, $p < 0.001$; 21 day, $F_{2,22} = 296.29$, $p < 0.001$). There was extensive CA1 neuronal death in the CON-ISC rats compared to CON-Sham rats (Tukey's test; $p < 0.001$), but no significant difference between the PEM-ISC and CON-ISC groups ($p > 0.87$). Hippocampal CA3 neuronal counts did not differ among treatment groups at post-surgery day 21 ($F_{2,21} = 2.41$, $p = 0.114$). Mean (± SEM) counts were 77±3 (CON-Sham; n = 8), 72±3 (CON-ISC; n = 10), and 81±2 (PEM-ISC; n = 8). CA3 neurons were counted to verify that the differences in axon terminal marker proteins within the CA3 mossy fibers between PEM-ISC and CON-ISC groups on day 21 were not related to CA3 neuronal loss.

The 2-VO model of global brain ischemia yields some variability in CA1 neuronal death, and thus the statistical analyses for the neuron counts in Table 1 excluded those rats exposed to 2-VO surgery that showed CA1 neuronal death that was unilateral or minimal (<50% reduction in CA1 neurons in either hemisphere). This was done only after first verifying that there were no significant differences in neuronal loss between the PEM-ISC and CON-ISC groups. That is, it was first demonstrated that excluding rats with incomplete forebrain ischemia did not bias the results by masking an effect of PEM on neuronal death at either time-point (day 5, t (23) = −1.35, $p = 0.16$).

Analyses of the other endpoints (below) were conducted only on rats with extensive bilateral hippocampal damage on day 5 (CON-Sham, n = 8; CON-ISC, n = 11; PEM-ISC, n = 8) and day 21 (CON-Sham, n = 8; CON-ISC, n = 7; PEM-ISC, n = 10). Exceptions to this sample size were related to instances in which blood samples were unattainable or tissue quality prevented immunofluorescence analysis (Iba-1, CON-ISC21d, n = 6; GAP-43, PEM-ISC21d, n = 9; SNAP-25, CON-ISC5d, n = 9).

Glial response to global brain ischemia

Semi-quantification of Iba-1 immunofluorescence is shown for the CA1 (**Fig. 2A**) and CA3 (**Fig. 2B**) hippocampal subregions. Within the CA1 subregion at both time-points, there was a significant group effect on Iba-1 levels (day 5, $F_{2,24} = 4.55$, $p = 0.021$; day 21, $F_{2,24} = 12.85$, $p < 0.001$). Iba-1 staining was significantly increased by ischemia in the control-fed rats (CON-Sham vs CON-ISC by Tukey's test; day 5, $p = 0.040$; day 21, $p = 0.001$), but this was not influenced by post-ischemic PEM at either time-point (CON-ISC vs PEM-ISC; day 5, $p = 0.957$; day 21, $p = 0.997$). A representative photograph of Iba-1 staining in the CA1 subregion on day 21 is shown in **Fig. 3A** for each experimental group. Within the CA3 subregion, Iba-1 staining was not as pronounced, and there was no significant effect of experimental group at either time-point (day 5, $F_{2,23} = 0.26$, $p = 0.771$; day 21, $F_{2,21} = 1.30$, $p = 0.294$).

GFAP expression analysis is also presented for the hippocampal CA1 (**Fig. 2C**) and CA3 (**Fig. 2D**) subregions. There were no group effects on the GFAP signal that reached statistical significance for either time-point within the CA1 (day 5, $F_{2,24} = 2.61$, $p = 0.095$; day 21, $F_{2,22} = 1.79$, $p = 0.191$) or CA3 (day 5, $F_{2,24} = 1.35$, $p = 0.278$; day 21, $F_{2,22} = 0.27$, $p = 0.769$) subregions. A representative photograph of GFAP staining in the CA1 subregion on day 21 is shown in **Fig. 3B**.

Axon terminal markers following global brain ischemia

Semi-quantification of GAP-43, synaptophysin, and SNAP-25 within the CA3 mossy fiber terminals is shown in **Fig. 4A, 4B, and 4C**, respectively. There was no effect of treatment on GAP-43 expression at day 5 ($F_{2,24} = 1.13$, $p = 0.339$). On post-ischemic day 21, the group effect was significant ($F_{2,21} = 4.23$, $p = 0.029$), with GAP-43 decreased in the PEM-ISC group as compared to that in the CON-ISC rats (Tukey's test; $p = 0.030$). A trend was present for GAP-43 immuno-staining to increase in the CON-ISC group at post-ischemic day 21 as compared to that in the CON-Sham rats (Tukey's test; $p = 0.082$).

For synaptophysin expression, there was no significant effect of treatment on post-ischemic day 5 ($F_{2,24} = 0.62$, $p = 0.548$). On day 21, the group effect was not statistically significant although a trend was evident ($F_{2,22} = 2.91$, $p = 0.076$). An unadjusted pairwise comparison demonstrated a significant depression in the synaptophysin signal in the PEM-ISC group as compared to that in the CON-ISC rats (t (15) = 2.23, $p = 0.041$).

Table 1. PEM initiated at 3 days after global brain ischemia did not exacerbate hippocampal CA1 neuronal death.

	CON-Sham	CON-ISC	PEM-ISC
Day 5	258±10 (n = 8)	46±7 (n = 11)*	41±7 (n = 8)
Day 21	241±10 (n = 8)	27±7 (n = 7)*	22±4 (n = 10)

Data are presented as mean ± SEM. *CA1 neuronal counts were significantly decreased in the CON-ISC group, as compared to the CON-Sham group by 1- factor ANOVA and Tukey's test (p<0.001), but the CON-ISC and PEM-ISC groups did not differ (p>0.87).

There was a significant group effect on SNAP-25 expression on day 5 ($F_{2,22} = 4.36$, $p = 0.025$), with a marked increase due to ischemia in the control-fed rats (CON-Sham vs CON-ISC by Tukey's test; $p = 0.022$). PEM had no effect on the ischemic response at day 5 (CON-ISC vs PEM-ISC; $p = 0.169$). Although the 1-factor ANOVA did not reveal a significant group effect at post-ischemic day 21 ($F_{2,22} = 2.17$, $p = 0.138$), an unadjusted pairwise comparison demonstrated a significant decrease in SNAP-25 in the PEM-ISC group as compared to that in the CON-ISC rats ($t(15) = 3.38$, $p = 0.004$).

Representative photographs of the CA3 mossy fiber region for GAP-43 (**Fig. 5A**), synaptophysin (**Fig. 5B**) and SNAP-25 (**Fig. 5C**) are shown for post-ischemic day 21.

Acute-phase response after global brain ischemia

Fig. 6 shows the serum concentrations of positive (A2M, AGP, and haptoglobin) and negative (albumin) acute-phase proteins for post-surgery days 5 and 21. Serum A2M concentrations were not significantly different among the three treatment groups on day 5 ($F_{2,22} = 1.96$, $p = 0.165$). A significant group effect was evident by day 21 ($F_{2,21} = 9.27$, $p = 0.001$), with significantly higher circulating levels of A2M in the PEM-ISC group as compared to those of CON-ISC rats (Tukey's test; $p = 0.005$). Serum haptoglobin concentrations were significantly different among treatment groups at both time-points (day 5, $F_{2,22} = 8.00$, $p = 0.002$; day 21, $F_{2,21} = 4.67$, $p = 0.021$). The PEM-ISC group had a decrease in haptoglobin levels, relative to CON-ISC rats, that was statistically significant on day 5 (Tukey's test; $p = 0.011$), but not day 21 ($p = 0.353$). Serum albumin showed a significant group

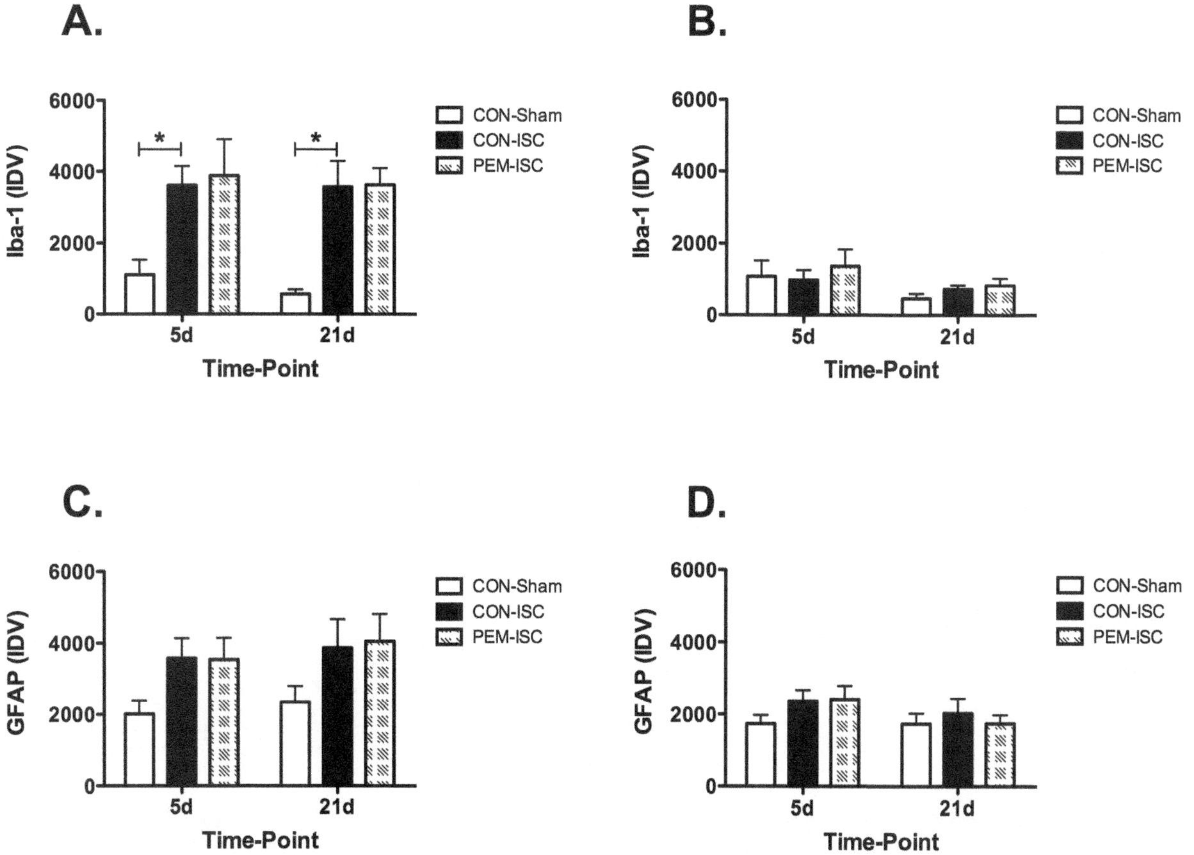

Figure 2. PEM introduced on day 3 after global ischemia did not alter the hippocampal glial response on either day 5 or 21. Immuno-labeling results are shown for Iba-1 in the CA1 (A) and CA3 (B) and for GFAP in the CA1 (C) and CA3 (D) hippocampal subregions.*Indicates a significant difference for the *posthoc* comparisons made by Tukey's Test (CON-Sham versus CON-ISC) within the specific time-point (p<0.05). Results are shown as mean ± SEM integrated density value (IDV).

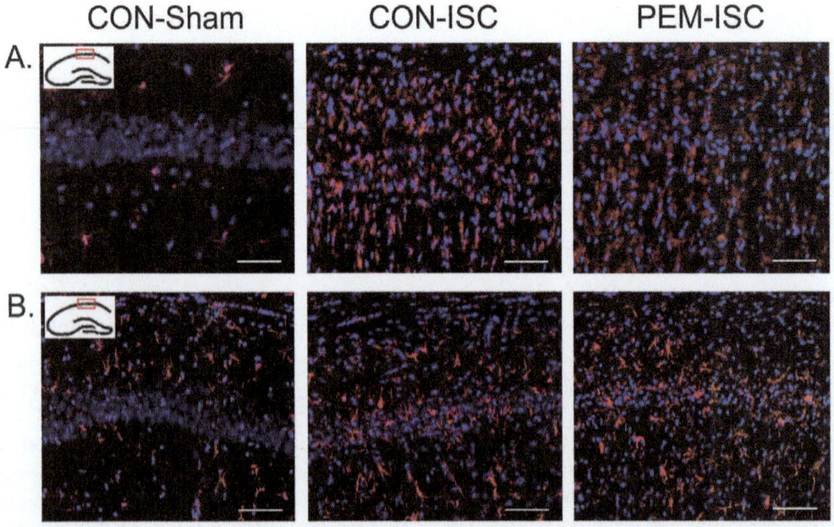

Figure 3. Representative photographs of the Iba-1 (A) and GFAP (B) immunofluorescence in the CA1 hippocampal subregion on day 21 after global brain ischemia. Blue = DAPI (cell nuclei). Red = Iba-1 (activated microglia marker; A) or GFAP (astrocytic marker; B).

effect at both day 5 ($F_{2,22} = 15.49$, $p < 0.001$) and day 21 ($F_{2,21} = 12.38$, $p < 0.001$), with concentrations decreased in the PEM-ISC group as compared to the CON-ISC group (Tukey's test; day 5, $p < 0.001$; day 21, $p = 0.001$). There was no effect of treatment on serum AGP concentrations at either time-point (day 5, $F_{2,22} = 0.13$, $p = 0.88$; day 21, $F_{2,21} = 0.64$, $p = 0.54$).

There were no significant differences between the CON-ISC and CON-Sham groups for any acute-phase protein at either time-point (Tukey's test; $p > 0.40$).

Discussion

Suboptimal protein and energy status is a common problem arising in patients after and because of a stroke. Here, we report on the first study to utilize a well-controlled experimental model to isolate the direct effects of this compromised nutritional state on the post-ischemic brain. Specifically, we found that PEM developing after global brain ischemia inhibits the expression of axon terminal proteins that serve as markers for synaptic remodeling in the hippocampal CA3 mossy fibers. In addition, the induction of PEM elicited a strong systemic response characterized by an immediate and sustained atypical acute-phase reaction. These findings highlight important mechanisms by which malnutrition developing in the post-stroke period could hamper recovery and suggest that treating this co-morbidity factor may be essential for patients to benefit fully from rehabilitation therapy.

To address the specific effects of post-ischemic PEM on the brain, we utilized a well-controlled and previously characterized nutritional regimen in which a low protein diet causes a voluntary reduction in food intake and induces mixed PEM [24]. Introducing this regimen on the third post-ischemic day provided evidence that PEM could interfere with axonal sprouting elicited by brain ischemia. We semi-quantified the SNAP-25, GAP-43 and synaptophysin immunofluorescence since these indicators of synaptic structure have previously been used to evaluate neuroplasticity in other models of cerebral ischemia [13,35,36,37]. Synaptophysin and SNAP-25 are pre-axonal synaptic proteins that are often used to identify functional synaptic connections [38,39]. GAP-43 is expressed in actively sprouting neurons, and specifically in the growth cones of axons [40,41]. The GAP-43 expression showed clearly that by day 21, PEM can significantly hinder the potential for synaptic remodeling that is induced by global ischemia. Although less studied in global brain ischemia, focal (cortical) ischemia induces GAP-43 as part of its program to reactivate the growth potential of neurons in the region of axonal sprouting in the peri-infarct cortex [42]. We acknowledge that further studies are required to provide definitive

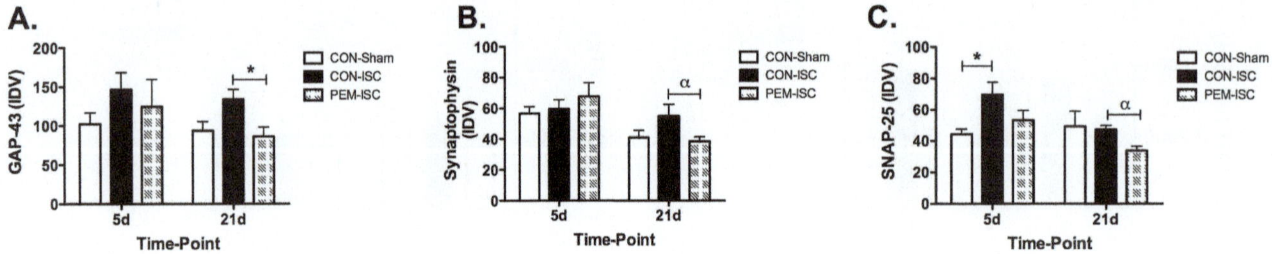

Figure 4. The influence of post-ischemic PEM on expression of GAP-43 (A), synaptophysin (B) and SNAP-25 (C) within the CA3 mossy fibers on days 5 and 21 following global brain ischemia. *Indicates a significant difference for either of the 2 *posthoc* comparisons made by Tukey's Test (CON-Sham versus CON-ISC and CON-ISC versus PEM-ISC) within the specific time-point ($p < 0.05$). α Indicates a significant difference between CON-ISC and PEM-ISC groups detected by unadjusted pairwise comparison ($p < 0.05$). Results are shown as mean ± SEM integrated density value (IDV).

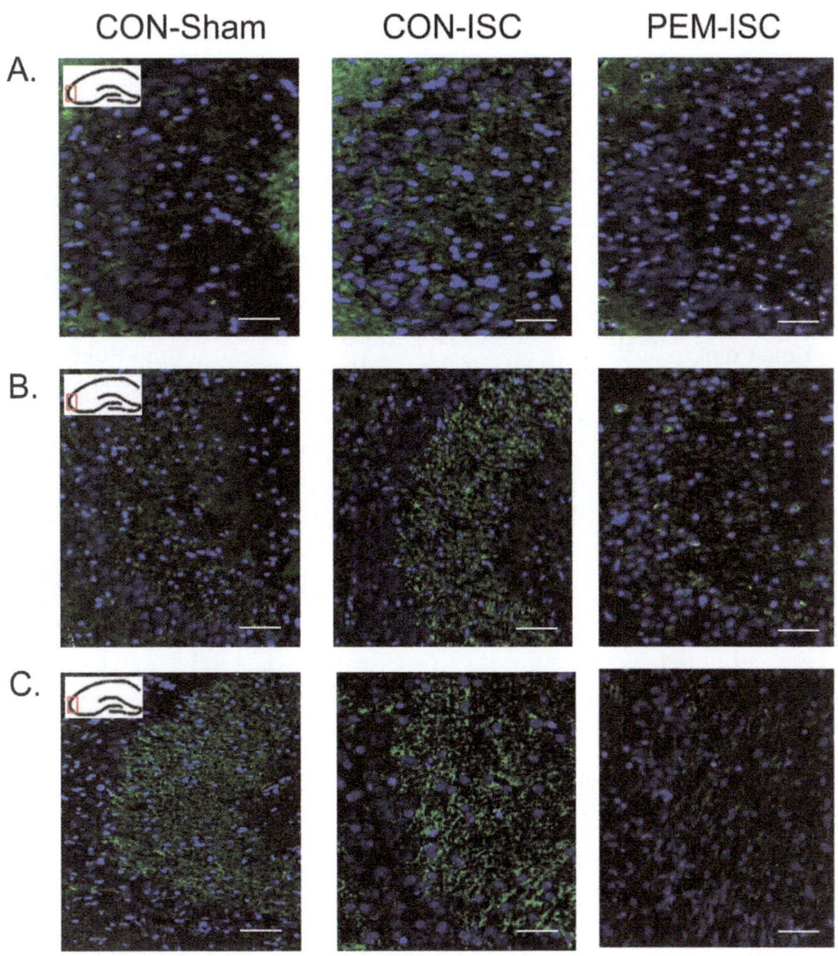

Figure 5. Representative photographs of GAP-43 (A), synaptophysin (B) and SNAP-25 (C) immunofluorescence in the CA3 mossy fibers on day 21 after global brain ischemia. Blue = DAPI (cell nuclei). Green = GAP-43 (A), synaptophysin (B), or SNAP-25 (C).

evidence that PEM inhibits mossy fiber sprouting, since the decreases in synaptophysin and SNAP-25 on day 21 in the PEM-ISC group relative to the CON-ISC rats were not statistically significant by 1-factor ANOVA. Nonetheless, it is important to highlight the significant depression in the signals for these molecules detected by the unadjusted pairwise comparisons between the PEM-ISC and CON-ISC rats, particularly because semi-quantitative densitometry limits statistical power for detecting differences. The consistent inhibitory effect of post-ischemic PEM on all three synaptic markers on day 21 is evident in Fig. 4 and 5. Future studies with Golgi-Cox staining and electrophysiology to examine dendritic morphology and synaptic strength, respectively, will also be needed to reinforce the study results. Our findings are reminiscent of the extensive literature on the adverse effects of perinatal malnutrition on synaptic plasticity in the hippocampal formation [43,44], although some of these studies are limited by flaws in the methodology for the nutritional regimens (reviewed in [45]).

Depending on stroke severity, some spontaneous neurological recovery can occur that can be further enhanced by rehabilitation [46,47]. Because of the link between increased plasticity and improved function after stroke [20], our results suggest that preventing or reversing the common post-stroke problem of PEM [2,4,6] could directly enhance spontaneous recovery and facilitate rehabilitation efforts aimed at enhancing plasticity [48]. While the global brain ischemia model mimicking cardiac arrest has been a valuable way to examine effects of post-ischemic PEM, these findings should be extended to establish functional relevance in an experimental model of focal ischemia mimicking the ischemic stroke patient.

The malnutrition-induced decrease in hippocampal synaptic remodeling is not caused by a different degree of brain injury, since the extent of neuronal death in the vulnerable hippocampal CA1 subregion did not differ between CON-ISC and PEM-ISC groups. Neither did PEM extend neuronal death into the more resistant CA3 subregion. These findings were expected, since the malnutrition was introduced after the period of major CA1 neuronal death [49]. The trigger for the reduced receptivity to brain remodeling also does not appear to be increased neuroinflammation. Microglia and astrocytes are predominant responders and the major inflammatory cells elicited by global brain ischemia [50]. Since the hippocampal CA1 glial response observed at post-ischemic days 5 and 21 in our study was unaffected by nutritional status, we found no evidence that PEM arising after global brain ischemia exacerbates brain inflammation. Future investigation of the balance between specific pro- and anti-inflammatory mediators would further strengthen this conclusion.

The second major finding of our study was that post-ischemic PEM triggered an atypical acute-phase response characterized by immediate and prolonged changes to specific circulating acute-phase

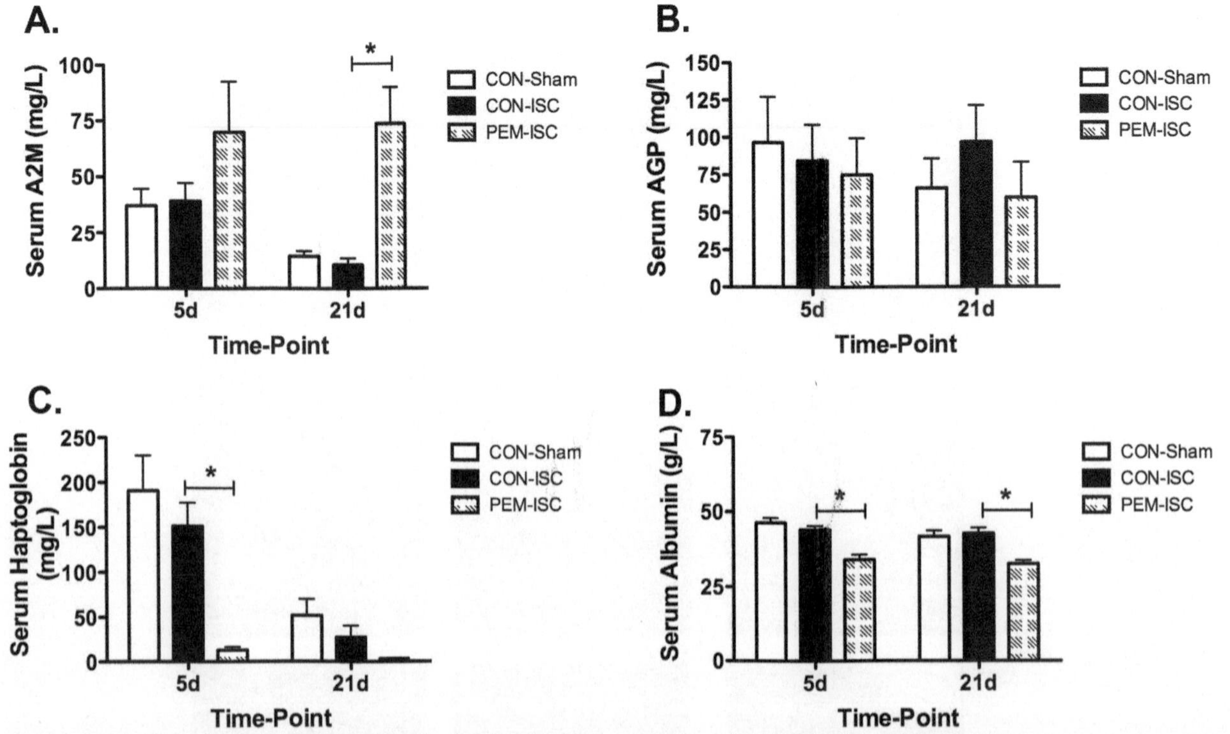

Figure 6. PEM introduced on day 3 following global brain ischemia elicits an atypical acute-phase response. Alpha-2-macroglobulin (A2M) (**A**), alpha-1-acid glycoprotein (AGP) (**B**), and haptoglobin (**C**) are positive acute-phase proteins, and albumin (**D**) is a negative acute-phase protein. *Indicates a significant difference for the 2 *posthoc* comparison made by Tukey's Test (CON-ISC versus PEM-ISC) within the specific time-point ($p<0.05$). Data are shown as mean ± SEM for each experimental group on day 5 (CON-Sham, n = 8; CON-ISC, n = 11; PEM-ISC, n = 6) and day 21 (CON-Sham, n = 8; CON-ISC, n = 6; PEM-ISC, n = 10).

proteins relative to the CON-ISC group. The decrease in the negative acute-phase protein, albumin, on day 2 after nutritional intervention (5 days following global ischemia) was sustained at day 21, at which time the rise in the class 2 positive acute-phase protein, A2M, also became significant. Our previous findings suggest that this reaction exists without a febrile response [24,29]. The acute-phase response was selective, however, as the class 1 acute-phase protein, AGP, was unchanged, and haptoglobin was decreased after 2 days of exposure to the PEM regimen and barely detectable by day 21. The decrease in haptoglobin, a positive acute-phase protein, suggests that post-ischemic PEM induces an aberrant acute-phase reaction.

The implications to stroke recovery of an incomplete acute-phase reaction accompanying post-ischemic PEM should be further explored. A heightened acute-phase response in stroke patients is associated with worse outcome, although it is unclear whether it plays a direct detrimental role [21,51,52]. Prolonged systemic inflammation after focal ischemia can increase brain injury and be more detrimental than pre-existing inflammation [53]. Although PEM did not increase neuronal death, the malnutrition-induced decrease in expression of axon terminal proteins could be related to increased susceptibility of the malnourished, injured post-stroke brain to the systemic inflammation. Decreased long-term potentiation in the hippocampus occurs with systemic inflammation [54,55], although it is of note that the systemic inflammation caused by PEM did not increase microglial activation as was previously reported [54]. Cognitive testing and serum cytokine measurements in future studies will help to address this hypothesis. Individual differences in nutritional status should also be investigated as a possible contributor to the considerable variability in the acute-phase response observed among stroke patients [21,51].

Unfortunately, we were unable to completely unravel the potentially complex interactions among brain ischemia, acute-phase response, and PEM, since no acute-phase reaction was detected after global ischemia in the control diet-fed rats. That is, no differences existed between the CON-ISC and CON-Sham groups for any acute-phase protein at either time-point. Global brain ischemia, unlike focal ischemia, may not trigger an acute-phase reaction. Alternatively, the latter may not have been detectable above the much larger response typically elicited by surgery [56]. The relatively higher serum A2M and haptoglobin concentrations in both CON-Sham and CON-ISC rats on day 5 relative to day 21 is suggestive of a surgery-induced acute-phase response that subsides over time. This raises a potential limitation in using the currently available rat models of brain ischemia to study the role of the acute-phase response as a determinant of stroke outcome, since the major models rely on surgery to generate reproducible brain ischemia. The least surgically invasive model should be chosen if the goal is to study the systemic reaction to brain ischemia.

In summary, the initiation of PEM within days of global brain ischemia triggers an immediate aberrant acute-phase response that is sustained. Post-ischemic PEM also hinders neuroplasticity mechanisms, which do not appear to be triggered by an increase in neuroinflammation. This is the first well-controlled study to demonstrate that post-ischemic PEM exerts direct and wide-ranging effects on mechanisms important to stroke recovery.

Supporting Information

Table S1 Physiological parameters measured during 2-VO and sham surgeries.
(DOC)

Acknowledgments

We thank Angela Cooper for technical assistance.

Author Contributions

Conceived and designed the experiments: SES PGP. Performed the experiments: SES SAF. Analyzed the data: SES SAF DJS PGP. Contributed reagents/materials/analysis tools: DJS PGP. Wrote the paper: SES SAF DJS PGP.

References

1. Davis JP, Wong AA, Schluter PJ, Henderson RD, O'Sullivan JD, et al. (2004) Impact of premorbid undernutrition on outcome in stroke patients. Stroke 35: 1930–1934.
2. Yoo S, Kim JS, Kwon SU, Yun S, Koh J, et al. (2008) Undernutrition as a predictor of poor clinical outcomes in acute ischemic stroke patients. Arch Neurol 65: 39–43.
3. Martineau J, Bauer JD, Isenring E, Cohen S (2005) Malnutrition determined by the patient-generated subjective global assessment is associated with poor outcomes in acute stroke patients. Clin Nutr 24: 1073–1077.
4. Brynningsen PK, Damsgaard EM, Husted SE (2007) Improved nutritional status in elderly patients 6 months after stroke. J Nutr Health Aging 11: 75–79.
5. Finestone HM, Greene-Finestone LS, Wilson ES, Teasell RW (1995) Malnutrition in stroke patients on the rehabilitation service and at follow-up: Prevalence and predictors. Arch Phys Med Rehabil 76: 310–316.
6. Poels BJ, Brinkman-Zijlker HG, Dijkstra PU, Postema K (2006) Malnutrition, eating difficulties and feeding dependence in a stroke rehabilitation centre. Disabil Rehabil 28: 637–643.
7. Paterson PG, Juurlink BHJ (1999) Nutritional regulation of glutathione in stroke. Neurotox Res 1: 99–112.
8. Foley N, Teasell R, Richardson M, Bhogal S, Speechley M (August 2013) Nutritional interventions following stroke. The evidence-based review of stroke rehabilitation (EBRSR). 16th Edition. Available: http://www.ebrsr.com/reviews_details.php?Nutritional-Interventions-Following-Stroke-10). Accessed 2014 March 16.
9. FOOD Trial Collaboration (2003) Poor nutritional status on admission predicts poor outcomes after stroke: Observational data from the FOOD trial. Stroke 34: 1450–1456.
10. Bobyn PJ, Corbett D, Saucier DM, Noyan-Ashraf MH, Juurlink BHJ, et al. (2005) Protein-energy malnutrition impairs functional outcome in global ischemia. Exp Neurol 196: 308–315.
11. Ha L, Hauge T, Spenning AB, Iversen PO (2010) Individual, nutritional support prevents undernutrition, increases muscle strength and improves QoL among elderly at nutritional risk hospitalized for acute stroke: A randomized, controlled trial. Clin Nutr 29: 567–573.
12. Ji L, Nazarali AJ, Paterson PG (2008) Protein–energy malnutrition increases activation of the transcription factor, nuclear factor κB, in the gerbil hippocampus following global ischemia. J Nutr Biochem 19: 770–777.
13. Prosser-Loose EJ, Verge VM, Cayabyab FS, Paterson PG (2010) Protein-energy malnutrition alters hippocampal plasticity-associated protein expression following global ischemia in the gerbil. Curr Neurovasc Res 7: 341–360.
14. Kriz J, Lalancette-Hébert M (2009) Inflammation, plasticity and real-time imaging after cerebral ischemia. Acta Neuropathol 117: 497–509.
15. Imai F, Suzuki H, Oda J, Ninomiya T, Ono K, et al. (2007) Neuroprotective effect of exogenous microglia in global brain ischemia. J Cereb Blood Flow Metab 27: 488–500.
16. Hébert-Lalancette M, Gowing G, Simard A, Weng YC, Kriz J (2007) Selective ablation of proliferating microglial cells exacerbates ischemic injury in the brain. J Neurosci 27: 2596–2605.
17. Jablonka JA, Kossut M, Witte OW, Liguz-Lecznar M (2012) Experience-dependent brain plasticity after stroke: effect of ibuprofen and poststroke delay. Eur J Neurosci 36: 2632–2639.
18. Bellinger FP, Madamba SG, Campbell IL, Siggins GR (1995) Reduced long-term potentiation in the dentate gyrus of transgenic mice with cerebral overexpression of interleukin-6. Neurosci Lett 198: 95–98.
19. Langdon KD, Granter-Button S, Corbett D (2008) Persistent behavioral impairments and neuroinflammation following global ischemia in the rat. Eur J Neurosci 28: 2310–2318.
20. Murphy TH, Corbett D (2009) Plasticity during stroke recovery: from synapse to behaviour. Nat Rev Neurosci 10: 861–872.
21. Dziedzic T (2008) Clinical significance of acute phase reaction in stroke patients. Front Biosci 13: 2922–2927.
22. Ling P-R, Smith RJ, Kie S, Boyce P, Bistrian BR (2004) Effects of protein malnutrition on IL-6-mediated signaling in the liver and the systemic acute-phase response in rats. Am J Physiol Regul Integr Comp Physiol 287: R801–R808.
23. Dülger H, Arik M, Şekeroğlu MR, Tarakçioğlu M, Noyan T, et al. (2002) Pro-inflammatory cytokines in Turkish children with protein-energy malnutrition. Mediators Inflamm 11: 363–365.
24. Smith SE, Andrade Ramos R, Refinetti R, Farthing JP, Paterson PG (2013) Protein-energy malnutrition induces an aberrant acute-phase response and modifies the circadian rhythm of core temperature. Appl Physiol Nutr Metab 38: 844–853.
25. Reid M, Badaloo A, Forrester T, Morlese JF, Heird WC, et al. (2002) The acute-phase protein response to infection in edematous and nonedematous protein-energy malnutrition. Am J Clin Nutr 76: 1409–1415.
26. Jennings G, Bourgeois C, Elia M (1992) The magnitude of the acute phase protein response is attenuated by protein deficiency in rats. J Nutr 122: 1325–1331.
27. Qu Z, Ling P-R, Chow JC, Burke PA, Smith RJ, et al. (1996) Determinants of plasma concentrations of insulin-like growth factor-I and albumin and their hepatic mRNAs: The role of dietary protein content and tumor necrosis factor in malnourished rats. Metabolism 45: 1273–1278.
28. Cray C, Zaias J, Altman NH (2009) Acute phase response in animals: A review. Comp Med 59: 517–526.
29. Smith SE, Prosser-Loose EJ, Colbourne F, Paterson PG (2011) Protein-energy malnutrition alters thermoregulatory homeostasis and the response to brain ischemia. Curr Neurovasc Res 8: 64–74.
30. Smith ML, Bendek G, Dahlgren N, Rosen I, Wieloch T, et al. (1984) Models for studying long-term recovery following forebrain ischemia in the rat. 2. A 2-vessel occlusion model. Acta Neurol Scand 69: 385–401.
31. Reeves PG, Nielsen FH, Fahey GC (1993) AIN-93 purified diets for laboratory rodents: Final report of the American Institute of Nutrition ad hoc writing committee on the reformulation of the AIN-76A rodent diet. J Nutr 123: 1939–1951.
32. Prosser-Loose EJ, Smith SE, Paterson PG (2011) Experimental model considerations for the study of protein-energy malnutrition co-existing with ischemic brain injury. Curr Neurovasc Res 8: 170–182.
33. Schreyer DJ, Skene JHP (1991) Fate of GAP-43 in ascending spinal axons of DRG neurons after peripheral nerve injury: delayed accumulation and correlation with regenerative potential. J Neurosci 11: 3738–3751.
34. Doumas BT, Watson WA, Biggs HG (1971) Albumin standards and the measurement of serum albumin with bromcresol green. Clin Chim Acta 31: 87–96.
35. Schmidt-Kastner R, Bedard A, Hakim A (1997) Transient expression of GAP-43 within the hippocampus after global brain ischemia in rat. Cell Tissue Res 288: 225–238.
36. Silasi G, Klahr AC, Hackett MJ, Auriat AM, Nichol H, et al. (2012) Prolonged therapeutic hypothermia does not adversely impact neuroplasticity after global ischemia in rats. J Cereb Blood Flow Metab 32: 1525–1534.
37. Martí E, Ferrer I, Ballabriga J, Blasi J (1998) Increase in SNAP-25 immunoreactivity in the mossy fibers following transient forebrain ischemia in the gerbil. Acta Neuropathol 95: 254–260.
38. Li S, Reinprecht I, Fahnestock M, Racine RJ (2002) Activity-dependent changes in synaptophysin immunoreactivity in hippocampus, piriform cortex, and entorhinal cortex of the rat. Neuroscience 115: 1221–1229.
39. Oyler GA, Higgins GA, Hart RA, Battenberg E, Billingsley M, et al. (1989) The identification of a novel synaptosomal-associated protein, SNAP-25, differentially expressed by neuronal subpopulations. J Cell Biol 109: 3039–3052.
40. Goslin K, Schreyer DJ, Skene JHP, Banker G (1988) Development of neuronal polarity: GAP-43 distinguishes axonal from dendritic growth cones. Nature 336: 672–674.
41. Benowitz LI, Routtenberg A (1997) GAP-43: an intrinsic determinant of neuronal development and plasticity. Trends Neurosci 20: 84–91.
42. Carmichael ST, Archibeque I, Luke, Nolan T, Momiy J, et al. (2005) Growth-associated gene expression after stroke: Evidence for a growth-promoting region in peri-infarct cortex. Exp Neurol 193: 291–311.
43. Cintra L, Granados L, Aguilar A, Kemper T, DeBassio W, et al. (1997) Effects of prenatal protein malnutrition on mossy fibers of the hippocampal formation in rats of four age groups. Hippocampus 7: 184–191.
44. Morgane PJ, Mokler DJ, Galler JR (2002) Effects of prenatal protein malnutrition on the hippocampal formation. Neurosci Biobehav Rev 26: 471–483.
45. Prosser-Loose EJ, Saucier DM, Paterson PG (2007) Can a reward-based behavioural test be used to investigate the effect of protein-energy malnutrition on hippocampal function? Nutr Neurosci 10: 145–150.
46. Cramer SC (2008) Repairing the human brain after stroke: I. Mechanisms of spontaneous recovery. Ann Neurol 63: 272–287.
47. Kwakkel G, Kollen B, Lindeman E (2004) Understanding the pattern of functional recovery after stroke: facts and theories. Restor Neurol Neurosci 22: 281–299.

48. Krakauer JW, Carmichael ST, Corbett D, Wittenberg GF (2012) Getting neurorehabilitation right: What can be Learned from animal models? Neurorehabil Neural Repair 26: 923–931.
49. Pulsinelli WA, Brierley JB, Plum F (1981) Temporal profile of neuronal damage in a model of transient forebrain ischemia. Ann Neurol 11: 491–498.
50. Stoll G, Jander S, Schroeter M (1998) Inflammation and glial responses in ischemic brain lesions. Prog Neurobiol 56: 149–171.
51. Smith CJ, Emsley HCA, Vail A, Georgiou RF, Rothwell NJ, et al. (2006) Variability of the systemic acute phase response after ischemic stroke. J Neurol Sci 251: 77–81.
52. Idicula T, Brogger J, Naess H, Waje-Andreassen U, Thomassen L (2009) Admission C - reactive protein after acute ischemic stroke is associated with stroke severity and mortality: The 'Bergen stroke study'. BMC Neurol 9: 18. Available: http://www.biomedcentral.com/1471-2377/9/18. Accessed 2014 April 7.
53. Langdon KD, MacLellan CL, Corbett D (2010) Prolonged, 24-h delayed peripheral inflammation increases short- and long-term functional impairment and histopathological damage after focal ischemia in the rat. J Cereb Blood Flow Metab 30: 1450–1459.
54. Di Filippo M, Chiasserini D, Gardoni F, Viviani B, Tozzi A, et al. (2013) Effects of central and peripheral inflammation on hippocampal synaptic plasticity. Neurobiol Dis 52: 229–236.
55. Maggio N, Shavit-Stein E, Dori A, Blatt I, Chapman J (2013) Prolonged systemic inflammation persistently modifies synaptic plasticity in the hippocampus: modulation by the stress hormones. Front Mol Neurosci 6: 46. Available: http://www.ncbi.nlm.nih.gov/pmc/articles/PMC3850065/pdf/fnmol-06-00046.pdf. Accessed 2014 April 7.
56. Lowry SF, Coyle SM (2014) Hypercatabolic states. In: Ross AC, Caballero B, Cousins RJ, Tucker KL, Ziegler TR, editors. Modern Nutrition in Health and Disease. Philadelphia: Wolters Kluwer Health/Lippincott Williams and Wilkins. pp.1261–1272.

19

Protein Aggregation in *E. coli*: Short Term and Long Term Effects of Nutrient Density

Ulfat I. Baig[1,2], **Bharati J. Bhadbhade**[1], **Dincy Mariyam**[2], **Milind G. Watve**[2]*

1 Department of Microbiology, Abasaheb Garware College, Pune, Maharashtra, India, **2** Department of Biology, Indian Institute of Science Education and Research, Pune, Maharashtra, India

Abstract

During exponential growth some cells of *E. coli* undergo senescence mediated by asymmetric segregation of damaged components, particularly protein aggregates. We showed previously that functional cell division asymmetry in *E. coli* was responsive to the nutritional environment. Short term exposure as well as long term selection in low calorie environments led to greater cell division symmetry and decreased frequency of senescent cells as compared to high calorie environments. We show here that long term selection in low nutrient environment decreased protein aggregation as revealed by fluorescence microscopy and proportion of insoluble proteins. Across selection lines protein aggregation was correlated significantly positively with the RNA content, presumably indicating metabolic rate. This suggests that the effects of caloric restriction on cell division symmetry and aging in *E. coli* may work via altered protein handling mechanisms. The demonstrable effects of long term selection on protein aggregation suggest that protein aggregation is an evolvable phenomenon rather than being a passive inevitable process. The aggregated proteins progressively disappeared on facing starvation indicating degradation and recycling demonstrating that protein aggregation is a reversible process in *E. coli.*

Editor: Aamir Nazir, CSIR-Central Drug Research Institute, India

Funding: The authors would like to thank Rajiv Gandhi Science and Technology Commission's Maharashtra Gene Bank Project for the partial funding. The funders had no role in study design, data collection and analysis, decision to publish, or preparation of the manuscript.

Competing Interests: The authors have declared that no competing interests exist.

* Email: milind@iiserpune.ac.in

Introduction

Senescence in bacteria in spite of conditions favoring growth became a focus of active interest only recently. In *Caulobacter* [1], [2] there is a clear distinction between mother cell and daughter cell and the mother cell has been shown to slow down and stop reproducing after a certain number of division cycles. The division in such a species is morphologically and functionally asymmetric. For some time it was thought that there is no senescence or natural death in bacteria that undergo a morphologically symmetric division. On this background the demonstration by Stewart *et al* [3] that even in *E. coli* the cell division was functionally asymmetric and that the "old pole" cell gradually slowed down its growth and stopped dividing came as a surprise. This finding triggered both theoretical and empirical work and gave rise to many new possibilities.

Aging in *E. coli* is thought to happen because of asymmetric segregation of damaged components to the daughter cells. The damaged components were later shown to be mainly, if not exclusively, protein aggregates (PAs) [4], [5], [6]. There appear to be two possible alternative evolutionary interpretations of the asymmetric segregation phenomenon. According to one senescence is inevitable and cellular polarization is suggested to have evolved to restrict senescence to one daughter lineage [7], [8]. According to the other, there are two possible ways of handling damaged proteins. One is to repair or recycle the damaged components and the other is to dump them asymmetrically in one cell to leave the other free of damage. Mathematical models show that repair or recycle could be a better strategy in severely nutrient limited environments and asymmetric dumping may work better in rich nutrient environments [9]. These models expect that the extent of protein aggregation and/or the asymmetry of segregation would be responsive to different nutritional environments.

In the initial concept of bacterial aging the distinction of old pole and new pole was thought to be critical, with the old pole cell always retaining the aggregate and senescing [3], [4], [8]. However there is a possibility that there can be pole flipping, i. e. the damaged components may drift away from the morphologically old pole with some probability. Even if the probability is small the old pole cell may rejuvenate and maintain its growth rate over a long time [10]. Some studies have indicated that the old pole cell is not always the slower of the two in terms of growth and next division [11]. Therefore the role of morphologically old and new poles may be less important than assumed earlier, nevertheless the importance of asymmetric segregation of protein aggregates remains more robust theoretically as well as empirically.

Protein aggregation is associated with aging and related disorders across wide diversity of taxa including humans [12], [13], [14]. Because all organisms face the important challenges of protein misfolding and aggregation, strategies to cope with the problem are expected to have evolved and be conserved [15], [16]. However our understanding of the evolution of protein handling

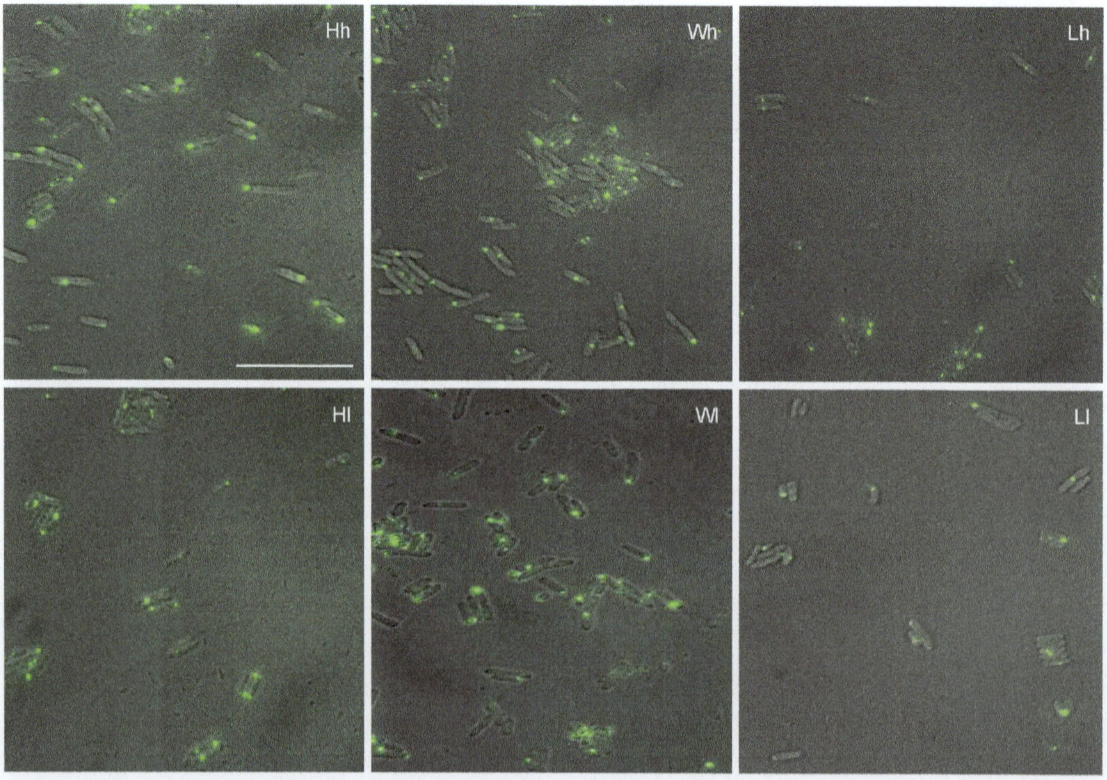

Figure 1. Superimposed DIC and fluorescence images of the three selection lines generated from MGAY in two current nutrient conditions. *W* stands for the wild type or ancestral strain. Selection was carried out for an estimated 1800 generation under constant low (*L*) and high (*H*) nutrient environments. Before microscopy all the three lines were grown in high (*h*) or low (*l*) glucose concentration for 16 hours. (e.g. *Hl:* a lineage selected under high nutrient concentration but currently being grown in low concentration). The same notation is used in all figures. All lineages showed visible protein aggregates under stress free conditions but the proportion of cells with aggregates and mean intensities differed across selection and current nutrient conditions. The scale bar represents 10 μ.

mechanisms is as yet very poor. It is interesting to ask why components of proteostasis machinery are not constitutively expressed at high levels, or why it did not evolve to perfection; whether an efficient proteostasis is impossible or whether the cost benefits of a highly efficient system are not favorable. This question cannot be context independent and it is likely that the cost-benefits of efficient protein handling systems are more beneficial under certain conditions and costly under others. One of the suggested costs in multicellular organisms is the increased potentiation of cancerous growth [17]. Alternatively a trade-off between somatic maintenance and reproduction may decide an optimum level of investment in proteostasis mechanisms in somatic cells [18]. This optimum could be much short of perfection and therefore protein aggregation is commonly observed. Understanding protein folding and mechanisms of PA formation in bacteria can serve as a simpler model for the mechanics as well as the evolutionary dynamics of proteostasis mechanisms which can ultimately help us understand how and why human conformational diseases progress.

In bacteria aggregate formation and features are influenced by various growth conditions such as temperature, pH [19], culture phase [5] and glucose/oxygen availability [20]. All proteins in inclusion bodies were initially considered as misfolded, but it has been shown that some active polypeptides are present inside aggregates [21] presumably due to accidental trapping. Misfolded proteins are presumably deposited in the nucleoid free space because of molecular crowding and these aggregates get deposited more frequently at poles [4], [6]. This leads to asymmetric inheritance of denatured proteins which are a burden for old pole cell. Cells that are less burdened with aggregates divide faster as compared to the ones with a greater burden [16].

Since the association of protein aggregates with asymmetric damage segregation, asymmetry in cell growth and division time and aging has been shown by many studies, we take these associations for granted and investigate,

i. Whether protein aggregation is an inevitable phenomenon or the cell has some control over it. Is it possible to avoid or minimize protein aggregation and whether the cell executes these mechanisms all the time or strategically under certain conditions?
ii. Whether asymmetric segregation of protein aggregation is an inevitable phenomenon or is a strategic behaviour subject to differential natural selection under different environments?
iii. Whether protein aggregates are outright waste products or whether they have any beneficial role under some conditions?

A common approach to study protein aggregation in the context of aging is to follow individual cells and their subsequent daughters for a few generations [3], [4], [6], [10]. This is done using fluorescence microscopy to reveal the protein aggregates. A possible objection to this approach is that the cells under observation are continuously or repeatedly exposed to UV light during imaging which might alter the fate of proteins [22], [23]. Since the extent of alteration in protein handling during fluorescence microscopy has not been estimated we use a cross

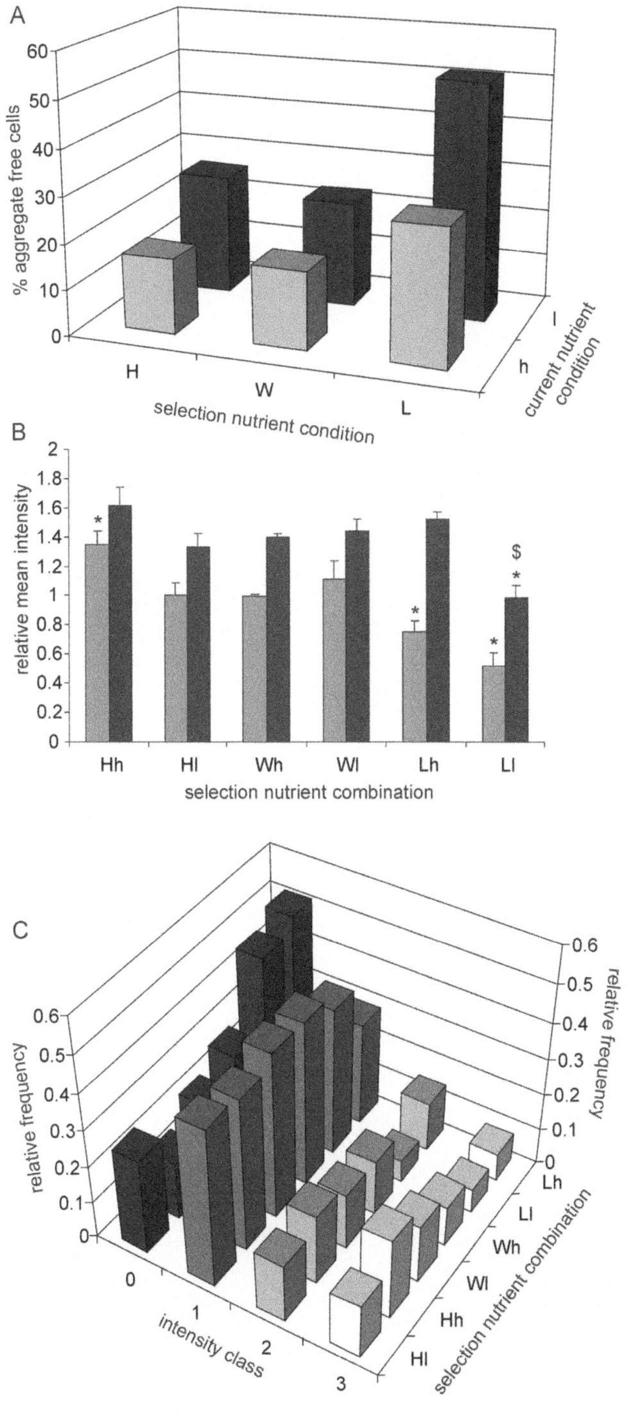

Figure 2. Effect of selection and current nutrient concentration on protein aggregation. (n = 200±20 each for data in Fig. 2A to C). A: The proportion of aggregate free cells: Both short term exposure and long term selection in low nutrient concentrations increased the proportion of aggregate free cells. (chi sq = 38.15, $p<0.0001$). B: The mean fluorescence intensities of cells (expressed relative to mean *Wh* including aggregate free cells) under the 6 selection nutrition combinations: The grey columns denote the average including cells without visible aggregates. The black columns denote average calculated by excluding the aggregate free cells. *denotes significant difference from Wh. $ denotes significant difference between corresponding *h* and *l* conditions (at $p<0.05$). C: Frequency distribution of cells with fluorescence intensity classes of aggregates: The modal class is 1 except in *Lh* and *Ll* where the modal class is 0. The proportion of cells in different intensity classes across the three selection lines differed significantly at high nutrient concentration (for *Wh, Hh* and *Lh* Chi square = 57.157, df = 6, $P<0.0001$) as well as low nutrient concentration (For *Wl, Hl* and *Ll* Chi square = 35.317, df = 6, $P<0.0001$). The effect of current nutrient concentration was not significant for *W* (Chi square = 2.35, df = 3, P = 0.503) but was significant for *H* (Chi square = 7.138, df = 3, P = 0.0676) and *L* (Chi square = 9.415, df = 3, P = 0.0243).

sectional approach where cells are not observed longitudinally but a growing population is sampled at a cross section in time. This does not reveal information of old or new poles and mother or daughter cells but inferences based on the statistical distribution of aggregates are nevertheless possible. The cross sectional data can therefore be cleaner and important despite the limitation that the inferences are necessarily statistical and indirect.

Materials and Methods

Strains used: We studied MGAY, obtained from A. Lindner (INSERM, France) which constitutively expresses yellow fluorescent protein (YFP) fused to the C terminus of Inclusion body protein (Ibp) A under the control of the endogenous chromosomal IbpA promoter. This allows visualization of protein aggregates in the cells under fluorescence microscopy [4] [24].

Selection regime

Similar to Lele *et al* [11] we grew the above strain continuously under two concentrations of glucose in a mineral medium. On agar media with high (10 mg/ml) or low (0.1 mg/ml) concentrations of glucose as the sole source of carbon and energy, cultures were serially transferred up to an estimated 1800 generations so that at the end of the prolonged sub-culturing we had three cell lineages, one each selected for either of the nutritional environments and one wild type. We denote the strain selected under high caloric environment as *H* and the one selected under low caloric environment as *L*. The current medium condition for the experiment is denoted by small letters *h* and *l* for high and low caloric conditions respectively (e.g. a lineage selected under high concentration but currently being grown in low concentration is denoted as *Hl*).

In addition we also used the lines selected by Lele *et al* [11] originating from *E. coli* KL16 and 2563 with an identical protocol for an estimated 3000 generations. These lines did not have the fluorescent tag and therefore could not be used for microscopic observation of protein aggregates but were subject to differential estimation of soluble and insoluble protein contents (see below) which is thought to be a surrogate of protein aggregation. Lele *et al* [11] used three ancestral strains of *E. coli*, but since some of the selected lines from one of them lost viability only two of the three were used for this study.

Growth conditions

All the selection lines were maintained on agar media with the respective nutrient concentration (*h* or *l*). Before preparing for microscopy or cell composition studies they were grown in respective liquid media on shake flask at 180 rpm for 16–18 hours at 37°C.

The starvation experiment was performed with two alternative starvation conditions. In one the cells were continued to be incubated in the same medium after entering the stationary phase and were observed with fluorescence microscopy at every 12 hours up to 48 hours. Alternatively the cells in early stationary phase were harvested, washed in distilled water three times and then suspended in distilled water again and incubated at 37°C.

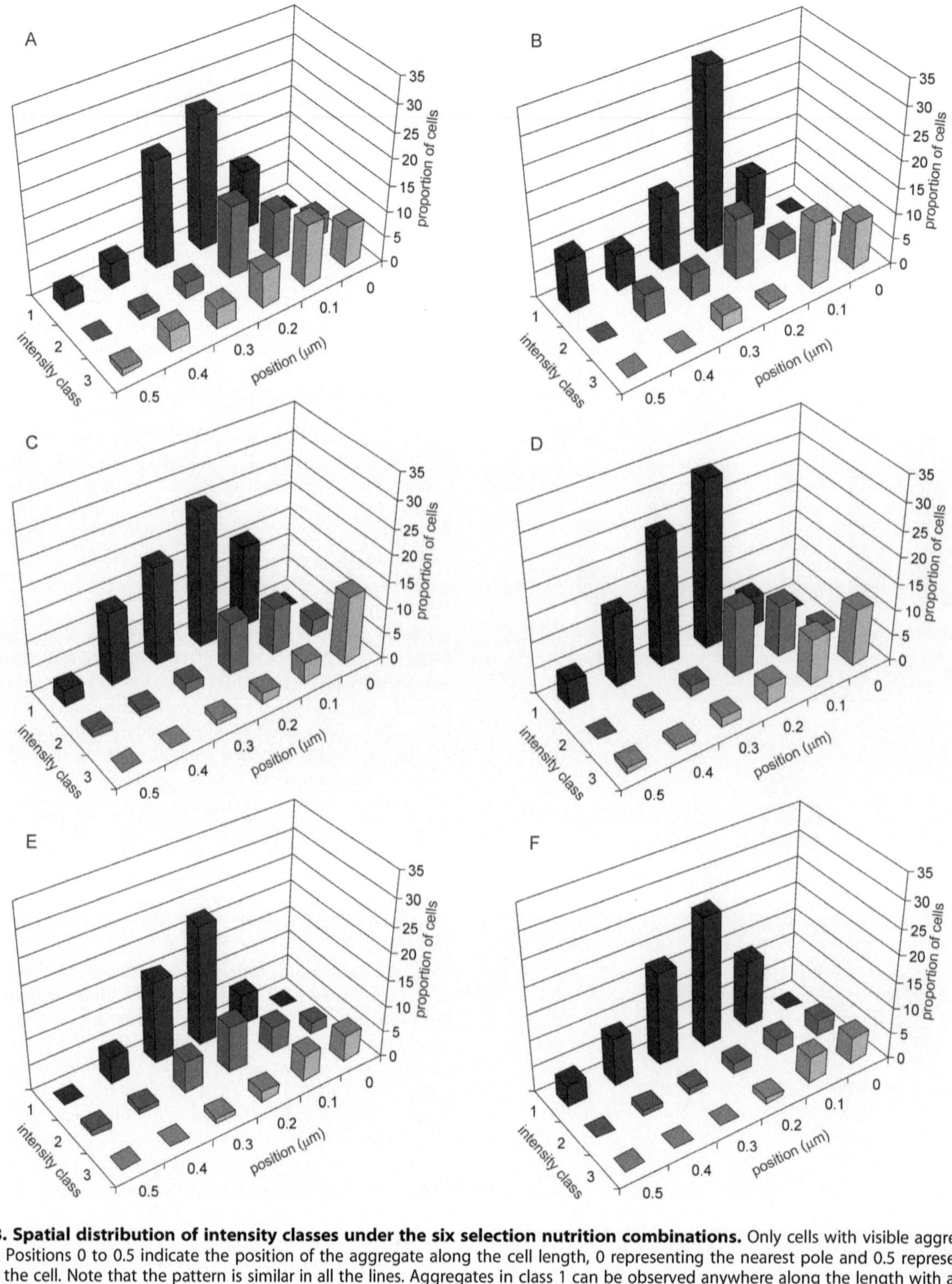

Figure 3. Spatial distribution of intensity classes under the six selection nutrition combinations. Only cells with visible aggregates are included. Positions 0 to 0.5 indicate the position of the aggregate along the cell length, 0 representing the nearest pole and 0.5 representing the centre of the cell. Note that the pattern is similar in all the lines. Aggregates in class 1 can be observed anywhere along the length with a subpolar peak. Older aggregates are more frequently polar. Similarity across selection demonstrates that although there is a difference in the rate of formation of the aggregates, once formed their further fate and spatial dynamics may be unaffected by selection or standing nutrient concentration. A–F represents *Hh, Hl, Wh, Wl, Lh* and *Ll* respectively.

Observations with fluorescence microscopy were made after every 12 hours up to 48 hours.

Fluorescence microscopy

For the selection lines derived from *E. coli* MGAY, when the cells reached an absorbance 0.2 (600 nm), they were placed on a slide that was layered with a 1.5% agarose pad and covered with a cover slip to immobilize the cells. Observations were made using

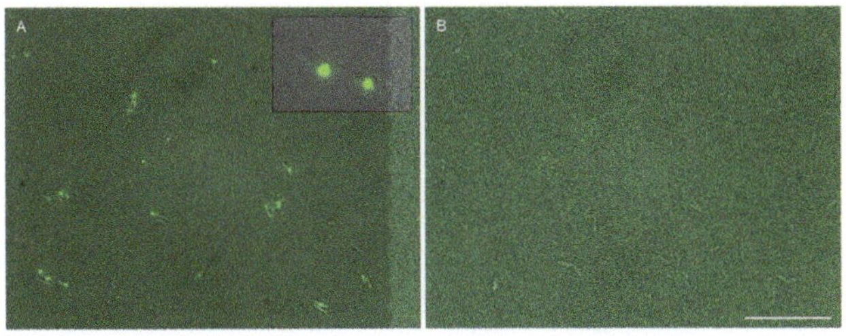

Figure 4. Comparative superimposed DIC and fluorescence images of protein aggregates in cells immediately after entering the stationary phase. (A) and after starvation for 4 days (B). The scale bar represents 20 μ. Inset: some of the larger aggregates did not disappear after prolonged starvation (30 days) but altered the morphology showing diffused fluorescence sometimes even exceeding the cell boundary.

differential interference contrast (DIC) and fluorescence imaging on Zeiss Axioimager M-1 upright microscope (100X/1.40 Oil DIC M27) with a color digital camera controlled by Axio software 4.8. Images both DIC/fluorescence were taken using exposure time of 30 millisecond illumination. The resulting images were processed and analyzed using Image J 1.44c software [25]. The fluorescence image alone was used for quantification of fluorescence intensity reflecting aggregate size whereas composite image formed by merging DIC and fluorescence was used to determine the location of protein aggregates in a cell.

Fluorescence intensity classification

Fluorescence given by the protein aggregates was quantified in arbitrary units using integrated fluorescence intensity corrected for the background. The aggregates were classified into four intensity classes namely 0 (cells with no visible aggregates), 1 with intensity <1500 units, 2 with intensities between 1500 and 3000 and 3 with intensities greater than 3000 units. In an experiment pertaining to the effect of starvation on PAs, classes were resolved at finer intervals with a larger sample size (500 to 800 cells per observation).

To characterize the position of protein aggregates in *E. coli* cells, we measured the distances of an aggregate from the nearest pole. The distance was normalized by the cell length. As a result the normalized positions range from 0 to 0.5 which were divided in to 5 classes. The class 0 to 0.1 represents the polar location and 0.4 to 0.5 represents central position.

Estimation of RNA and protein content of cells

The RNA and soluble and insoluble protein concentrations of cells were determined. A density of 10^7–10^8 cells/ml was used for the studies in which RNA extraction was done by hot phenol method [25], [26]. RNA quality was further checked by Agilent 2100 bioanalyzer and the RIN number for the same was 8 or above. Estimation of nucleic acids was done by Thermo scientific Nano drop 2000 [27]. For the quantification of soluble and insoluble proteins exponentially growing cells were harvested from 10-liter cultures and then soluble and insoluble fractions were extracted by Maisonneuve *et al* method [5] and estimated by bichinconic acid method [28].

Results

Low nutrient concentration reduces protein aggregation

In selection lines derived from MGAY strain fluorescent protein aggregates were visible and quantifiable in all cell lineages under both *h* and *l* conditions in the absence of heat or any other external stress (Fig. 1). The proportion of aggregate free cells showed a gradient along both current nutrient concentration and selection axes. The maximum proportion of aggregate free cells was found in *Ll* whereas the minimum was in *Hh* (Fig. 2A). The mean fluorescence intensities of the aggregates calculated including zero intensity cells (aggregate free cells) showed a similar trend where both the effects of current concentrations and selection could be seen (Fig. 2B). After removing zero intensity cells from the average calculation both the effects remained in the same direction but were weaker (Fig. 2B). When the aggregates were categorized in 4 intensity classes, the frequency distribution was positively skewed in all the lines at both nutrient concentrations with the modal frequency being at zero for *Lh* and *Ll* and at intensity class 1 for all others (Fig. 2C). The decreasing frequency of larger aggregates is expected by the dynamics of cell division and asymmetric segregation. This distribution is similar to the one expected by a Leslie matrix model of stable age structure [9]. Since in an exponentially growing population with stable age class distribution the largest frequency is that of the youngest class, maximum frequency would be in the aggregate free or smaller aggregate class. The frequency of zero aggregate class will be determined by the relative rates of cell growth and division versus protein aggregation. It appears from the frequencies (>50%) that in *W* and *H* lineages under both *h* and *l* conditions, a visible aggregate appears in a cell in the first generation itself whereas in *Lh* and *Ll* since the frequency of cells showing aggregates is less than 50%, the first generation cells are presumably all free of visible aggregates.

Separating the effects of current nutrient concentration and selection, we compared the selection lines at a given nutrient concentration and nutrient concentrations for a given selection. It can be seen (Fig. 2C) that both current nutrient concentration and long term selection altered the distribution of intensity classes significantly. The main difference was in the zero intensity class, i.e. aggregate free cells. Among the cells with aggregates the differences between selection and current nutrition conditions were marginal. This indicates that the main difference caused by nutrient concentration and selection is likely to be in the rate of formation or early development of the aggregates and the difference in the later development could be smaller or absent.

Apart from the rates of aggregate formation and growth, the fate and spatial dynamics of the aggregates does not appear to be affected by the different selection and current conditions. This is apparent in the spatial distribution of the intensity classes in cells having aggregates (Fig. 3). The patterns in this distribution are remarkably similar across groups with the possible exception of *Ll* which has very few aggregates in class 2 and 3. Because of their smaller number it is difficult to decide whether their spatial distribution is significantly different from other lineages. The picture generalizable across selection and treatments is that smaller aggregates may originate anywhere in the cell with a higher probability at sub central or sub polar region. Larger aggregates tend to be polar more frequently, but they can be seen at other positions occasionally.

With a low frequency, cells with more than one aggregate at a time could be observed. Since there is only one aggregate in majority of the cells, it is obvious that this aggregate will go to only one of the daughter cells so that the distribution of aggregated proteins will be asymmetric. Since theoretical models [9] expect more symmetric division in *l* type of environment, it may be expected that cells with more than one aggregates and distribution of these aggregates to both the daughter cells would be more common in *L* and/or *l*. However the total frequency of this

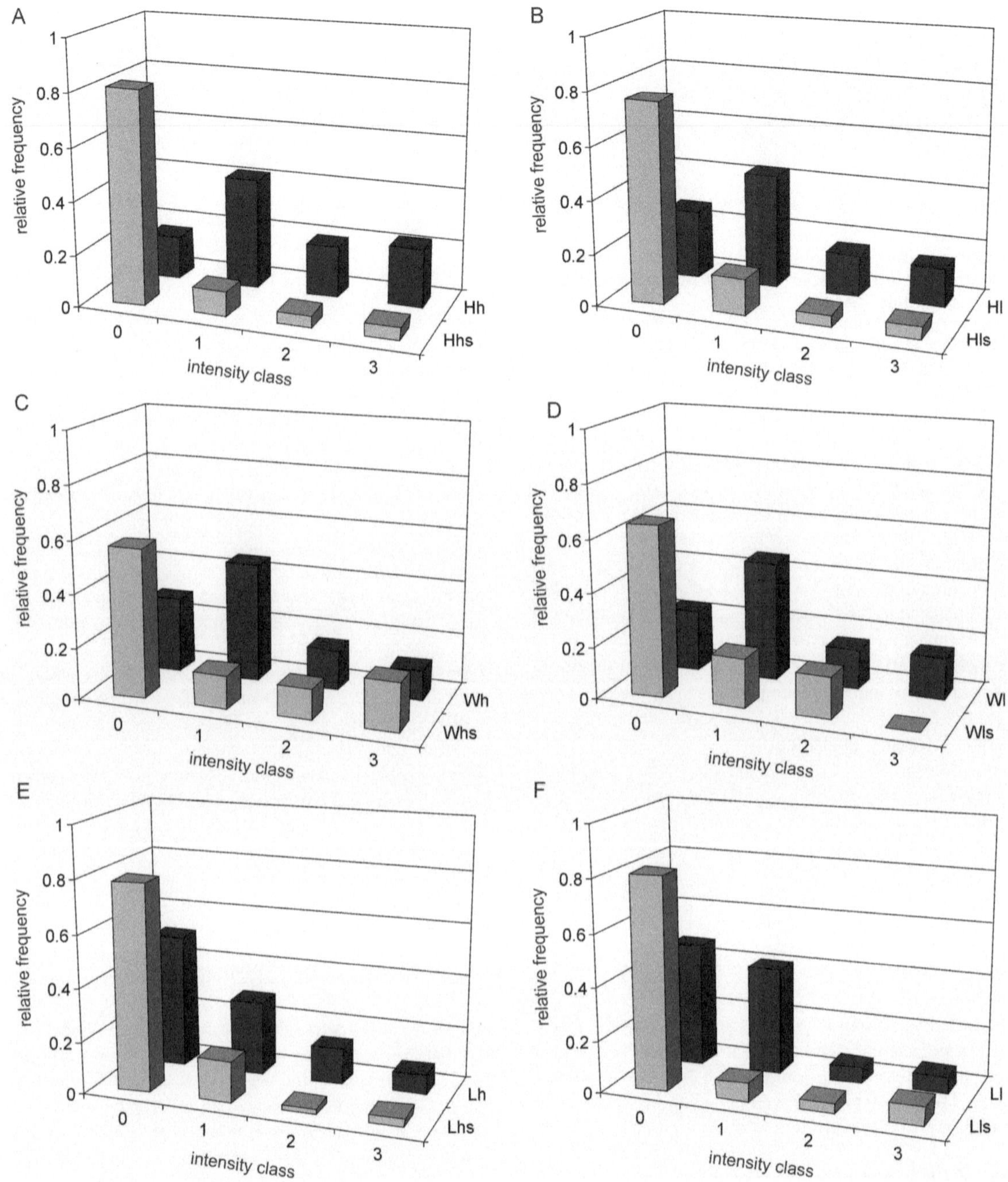

Figure 5. The distribution of intensity classes before and after starvation for 4 days. A–F represents *Hh, Hl, Wh, Wl, Lh* and *Ll* respectively. The suffix *s* stands for starvation. Although the distribution before starvation was different in all selection-concentration combinations, the distribution after starvation is similar. In all lines the aggregate free class increased significantly and class 1 reduced consistently. The trend in class 2 and 3 was less consistent.

phenomenon was so small that this could not be tested. Also at such a low frequency it is unlikely to make a difference to the population.

Protein aggregates progressively disappear on starvation

In order to test whether the aggregated proteins are degraded and recycled on facing starvation we compared aggregate distribution in cells at the end of exponential phase with the same culture continued in the stationary phase for 4, 8, 15 and 30 days. By the 4th day itself the proportion of aggregate free cells had increased in all lineages (Fig. 4). In the 8th, 15th and 30th day pictures, smaller aggregate classes were not observed, some large aggregates were still seen but with an altered morphology and diffused fluorescence around them, the fluorescence occasionally diffusing out of the cell (Fig. 4 inset). The distribution of intensity classes was substantially altered by 4 day starvation (Fig. 5) in all selection lines. The proportion of no aggregate cells increased and that in intensity class 1 decreased consistently. In *Hh* there was a 5 fold rise in the proportion of aggregate free cells and 80% decline in class 1. On the other hand since *Lh* already had over 50% cells in the aggregate free class there was a 1.54 fold rise and class 1

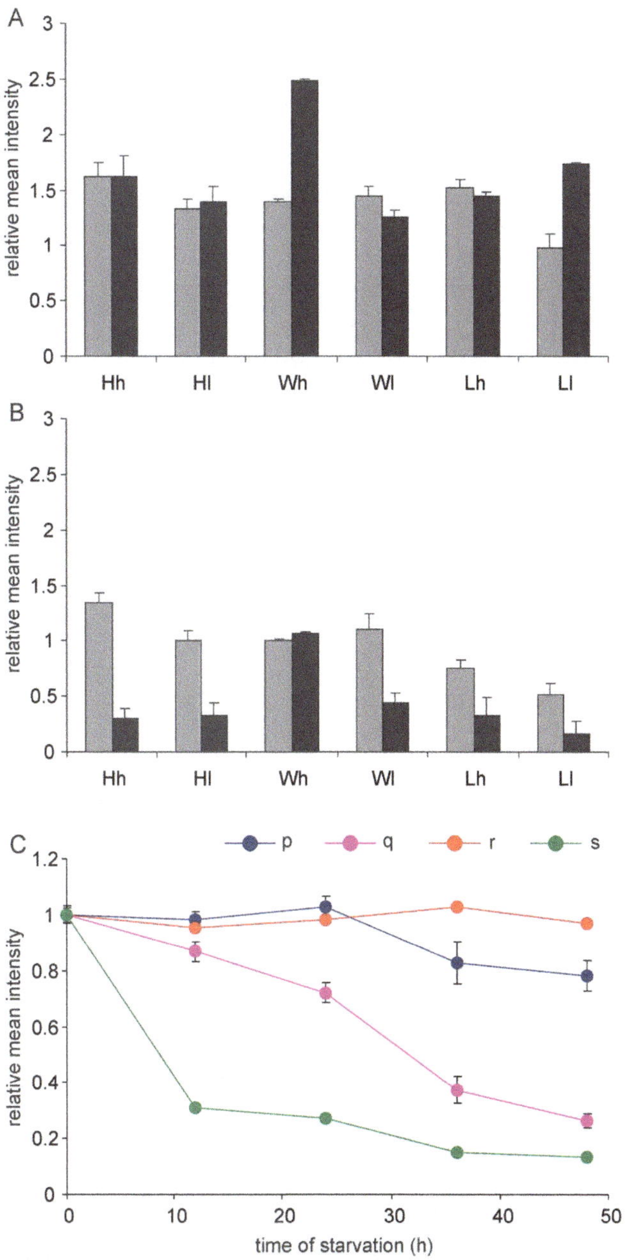

Figure 6. The effect of 4 day's starvation on visible protein aggregates. (n = 100±20 each for data in Fig. 2A to C). A and B: The mean fluorescence intensities before (grey bars) and after (black bars) starvation for 4 days. Means calculated excluding (A) and including (B) aggregate free cells. All columns are significantly reduced in B but not reduced or significantly increased in A. This suggests that all aggregate classes are not degraded proportionately. Many of the larger ones could be relatively resistant to degradation while the smaller ones degrade fast, thereby increasing the mean excluding aggregate free cells after degradation. *denotes significant difference from Wh. $ denotes significance between corresponding starved and unstarved populations (at $p<0.05$). C: The time course of decrease in the mean fluorescence intensity with starvation: The intensities are expressed relative to the mean intensity at zero hours. p: represents mean excluding aggregate free cells and q: represents including them in continued stationary phase. r: represents averages excluding aggregate free cells and s: represents including aggregate free cells in distilled water. Error bars show standard error of the mean.

declined by 46%. There was no consistent trend in classes 2 and 3. Although the trends in classes 2 and 3 are difficult to infer because of smaller frequencies, it is possible that the frequency in these classes does not decline as rapidly as class 1. The mean fluorescence intensity was reduced substantially on starvation when the aggregate free cells were included in the average calculation. However, when these cells were excluded the mean intensity did not decrease significantly or actually increased in some groups (Fig. 6). This indicates that the aggregates were not being degraded proportionately. The smaller aggregates were more likely to be degraded rapidly the larger ones being relatively resistant to degradation. The occasional appearance of large aggregates in 8, 15 and 30 day starved cells with diffusing fluorescence suggests that at least some of the large aggregates may not be degraded at all. This could be either because above a critical size aggregation might become irreversible, or cells containing very large aggregates may be dead. The dynamics of large aggregate degradation, if any, could be qualitatively different than the smaller ones.

In order to get a finer time as well size resolution we studied the fate of protein aggregates during stationary phase of *Wh* at every 12 hours using a larger sample size (500 to 800 cells each). The cells were either incubated in the same medium or washed and transferred to distilled water and both were observed under fluorescence microscopy after every 12 hours up to 48 hours. In the continued stationary phase experiment there was no significant reduction in the viable count whereas during and after washing and incubation in distilled water the viable count decreased by approximately one third. The pattern of change in the frequency distribution of fluorescence intensities with time can help us resolve between alternative hypotheses for the reduction in the mean intensities with time. Apart from the hypothesis of interest that the protein aggregates are degraded and recycled during starvation, the other possible explanations for the reduction in mean intensity and increase in the proportion of aggregate free cells are (i) the fluorescent protein has a short half life compared to the duration of the experiment and therefore fluorescence decreases with time (ii) senescent cells with large PAs die and disintegrate thereby reducing the mean fluorescence in the surviving population (iii) some replication continues in the stationary phase but there is little protein aggregation owing to low nutrient availability and therefore the proportion of aggregate free cells increases. The three alternative explanations make differential predictions that are testable by observing the changes in mean intensities and the frequency distribution of intensities with time. (i) GFP and YFP are known to be stable proteins [29] and therefore are unlikely to have disintegrated during the experimental period. We observed some large PAs retaining fluorescence up to 30 days (Fig. 4) indicating that fluorescence could remain substantially longer. Exponential reduction in fluorescence should give rise to a greater reduction in the high intensity classes than in the low intensity classes on a linear scale. This does not match with the observed pattern of decrease in the mean (Fig. 6 C) as well as frequency distributions (Fig. 7). Also we observed a significant decrease in the insoluble protein fraction (IPF) of the cells which reduced from 0.613 at the beginning of starvation to 0.267 at the end of 72 hours supporting the hypothesis that the aggregates actually degraded and half life of fluorescence is not an adequate explanation of the observed decline. (ii) If the reduction in mean is brought about by the death of cells with large PAs the right hand tail of the distribution would be curtailed first and the reduction in the mean excluding zero class should be comparable or faster than the reduction in the mean including zero class. This did not match with the observed

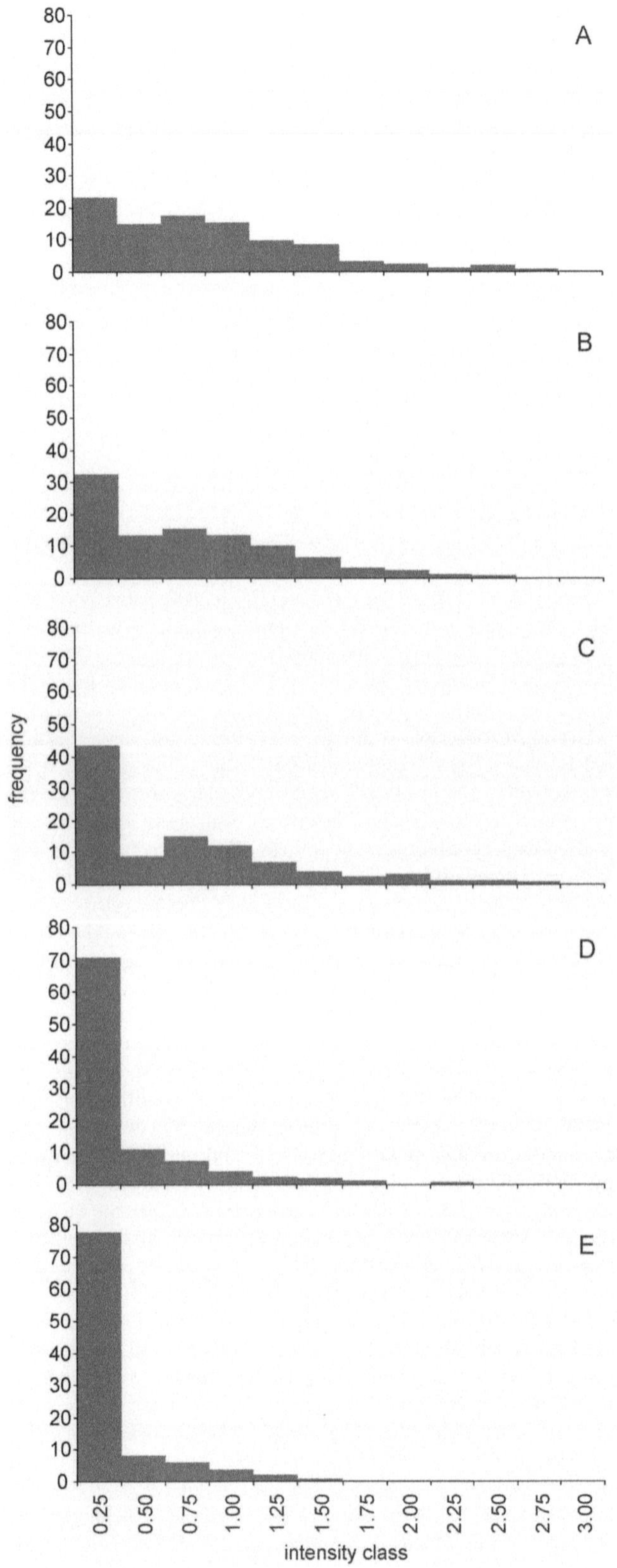

Figure 7. The progressively changing frequency distribution of fluorescence intensities on exposure to starvation. A: at the beginning of stationary phase B to E: 12, 24, 36, and 48 hours of starvation respectively. The intensities are classified at a higher resolution but the scale is matched with that in other figures. Note the transient bimodality created presumably due to faster degradation of smaller aggregate classes. Trends were similar but somewhat slower (not shown here) when cells were followed in the same medium after reaching stationary phase. The transient bimodality was consistently seen across both the conditions.

pattern (Fig. 7). Also when the cells were incubated in continued stationary phase we did not observe a decrease in the total viable count of cells in early stationary phase which makes this explanation unlikely. (iii) If new cells are born without aggregates, the frequency of zero class would increase but there would be no change in the mean calculated excluding zero class. The mean excluding aggregate free cells did not decrease in some and decreased marginally in other sets in this study which is compatible with this hypothesis. However, in order to explain the observed pattern in the decline of mean and the frequency distribution, the population should have increased between 1.5 to 1.8 fold. This is unlikely for a starving population. Also the total viable count did not increase either in continued stationary phase or in distilled water. In distilled water the viable count decreased whereas in continued stationary phase it did not. However, in spite of this difference the percent reduction in fluorescence in the two was not significantly different. Therefore we do not consider selective growth or death as adequate explanations of the observed decline.

A closer look at the pattern of change in the frequency distribution (Fig. 7) reveals that there appears a transient bimodality during early (12 and 24 hours) starvation. This is compatible with our earlier suggestion that the smaller aggregates disappeared at a faster rate than the rate at which the larger ones reduced their size.

Correlation between visible protein aggregates, estimates of insoluble protein fraction and RNA content of cells

The standing RNA content (Fig. 8A) of a cell is a direct indication of metabolic activity and therefore we expect the RNA levels to be different under different nutritional conditions and under differential selection. For all the three strains and in each of the three replicates we use the *Wh* as a reference and express the chemistry of all other lineages relative to it. Therefore throughout the results *Wh* has a mean of unity and variance of zero. Results show that the total RNA content of cells was substantially different. The RNA content of *l* was lower than that of *h* in 8 out of the 9 pairs. Selection had larger and significant effects. In all the three strains *L* selected lines had significantly lower RNA content under both *h* and *l* conditions as compared to *W* and *H* lines. The RNA contents were not consistently affected by *H* selection across all the three strains.

The total protein contents (Fig. 8B) of the cells also followed a similar pattern. In 7 out of the 9 pairs *l* conditions showed lower cell protein content than *h* conditions. Selection played a greater role, particularly *L* having a substantial reduction effect in all the three strains. More dramatic were the differences in soluble versus insoluble fractions in cell proteins (Fig. 8C). There was no consistent pattern across *l* and *h* conditions but *L* selection altered the ratio of insoluble to soluble proteins by almost an order of magnitude. Protein aggregates contribute to the insoluble fraction and therefore the two findings that *L* selection reduces visible protein aggregates and also reduces the fraction of insoluble proteins are mutually supportive. In MGAY there was good correlation between the mean fluorescence intensity of protein aggregates and IPF (Fig. 9). Therefore we can justifiably use IPF as a surrogate for protein aggregation in the other selection lines too. The total protein as well as insoluble protein fraction correlated

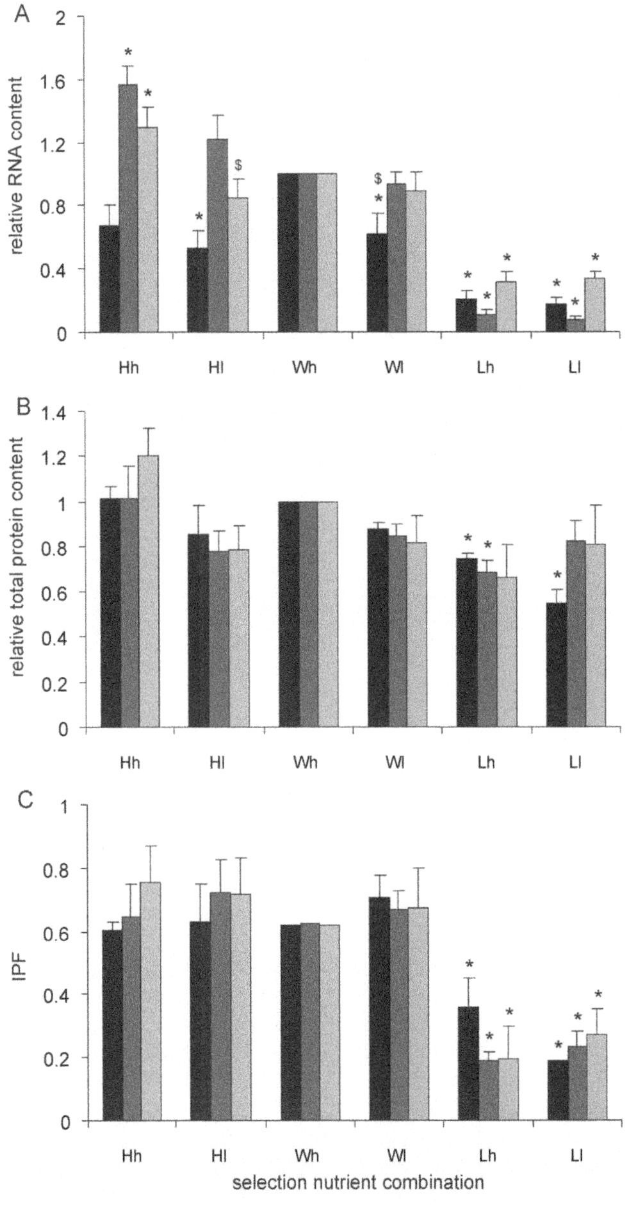

Figure 8. RNA and protein contents of cells. (A) Total RNA (ng/µl) (B) Total protein (µg/ml) and (C) The fraction of insoluble protein (IPF) content of the selection lines under high and low current nutrition. All are expressed relative to Wh. Black columns stand for KL16, dark grey for 2563 and light grey for MGAY. RNA contents differed over an order of magnitude in the *L* selected lines. *denote significant difference from *Wh*. $ denote significant difference between corresponding *h* and *l* conditions.

significantly positively with total RNA content in the pooled data over all the strains and their selection lines (Fig. 10).

The relation between nutritional environment and functional cell division time asymmetry has been shown earlier [11]. If protein aggregates are responsible for cell division asymmetry, we expect our data to correlate with earlier results. Correlations of the insoluble fraction with cell division time asymmetry, frequency of senescent cells, growth rates and growth yields of selection lines derived from KL16 and 2563 (obtained from Lele *et al.* 2011) [11] were not significant parametrically. However when separately ranked for the two strains under the two growth conditions, ranked correlations across the three selection regimes were significantly positive between IPF and asymmetry index ($r = 0.625$, $n = 12$, $p < 0.005$) and significantly negative between IPF and growth rate ($r = -0.625$, $n = 12$, $p < 0.05$). The proportion of senescent cells in the three selection regimes pooled over *h* and *l* and ranked separately for the two strains correlated positively with IPF ($r = 0.875$, $n = 6$, $p < 0.05$). This indicates that the two strains differ substantially in the pattern of quantitative response to *h* and *l* but the direction of response to selection is similar and therefore after correcting for the strain difference and current nutritional environment, protein aggregation is significantly positively correlated with cell division asymmetry and the frequency of senescent cells and negatively with growth rate in a non-parametric correlation. The correlation with growth yield nevertheless remained insignificant even after the correction. It is observed from the combined results of Lele *et al* [11] and this work that growth yield is affected significantly by *h* and *l* conditions whereas protein aggregation and cell division symmetry by *H* and *L* selection.

Discussion

Protein aggregation has an evolvable component

We showed previously that caloric restriction in short as well as long term reduces asymmetry in cell division time in *E. coli* and thereby the frequency of cells showing the signs of aging [11]. This study primarily demonstrates a relationship between caloric restriction and protein aggregation in the species supporting the hypothesis that the effect of caloric restriction on cell division symmetry and aging might be mediated through altered proteostasis. In all the three strains studied, in the lines selected under low nutrient environments there was less protein aggregation as compared to those selected in nutrient rich environments. The effect of nutrients on protein aggregation can potentially be a direct effect of nutrient concentration on the metabolic dynamics or it could be an evolved strategy of the cell to handle proteins differently under different nutrient conditions. The long term selection experiment gives support to the latter although the former is not eliminated. The quantitative effects of selection on protein aggregation suggest that there is some evolvable genetic control over protein aggregation although chemically and thermodynamically protein misfolding and aggregation may be an inevitable process. The possible cellular control over protein aggregation appears to operate more effectively at an early stage before visible protein aggregates appear since the different selection lines differ substantially in the proportion of visibly aggregate free cells but within cells showing aggregates, the frequency distribution of intensity or the spatial distribution along the cell length is only marginally different (Fig. 3). This has important implications for the inevitability versus evolved strategy debate. There appears to be substantial strategic control on protein aggregation, but the asymmetric distribution of the aggregates to the daughter cells is invariant and not responsive to nutrient based selection.

Lele *et al.* [11] demonstrated selection for symmetry in different strains of *E. coli* independently subject to the same selection regime. Protein aggregation could not be demonstrated in these strains by using fluorescence, but we showed here that the insoluble protein fraction showed response to selection in the same direction. Further in MGAY in which both IPF and visible aggregates can be monitored, there was a good correlation between fluorescence intensity of visible aggregates and IPF. Therefore IPF can be used as a reliable surrogate for protein aggregation. This allows us to test the generality of the results

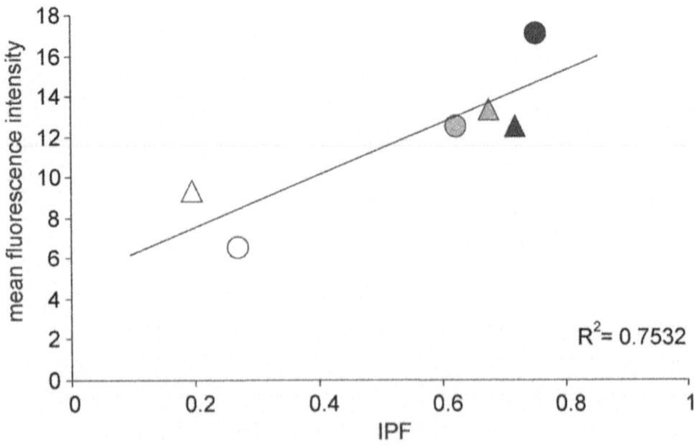

Figure 9. Correlation between mean fluorescence intensity and insoluble protein fraction in MGAY. The circles denote *h* and triangles denote *l* conditions (r = 0.868, n = 6, $p<0.05$). Open circles and triangles stand for *L* selection, grey for *W* and black for *H*. The correlation validates the use of IPF as a surrogate for protein aggregation in strains without a fluorescent marker.

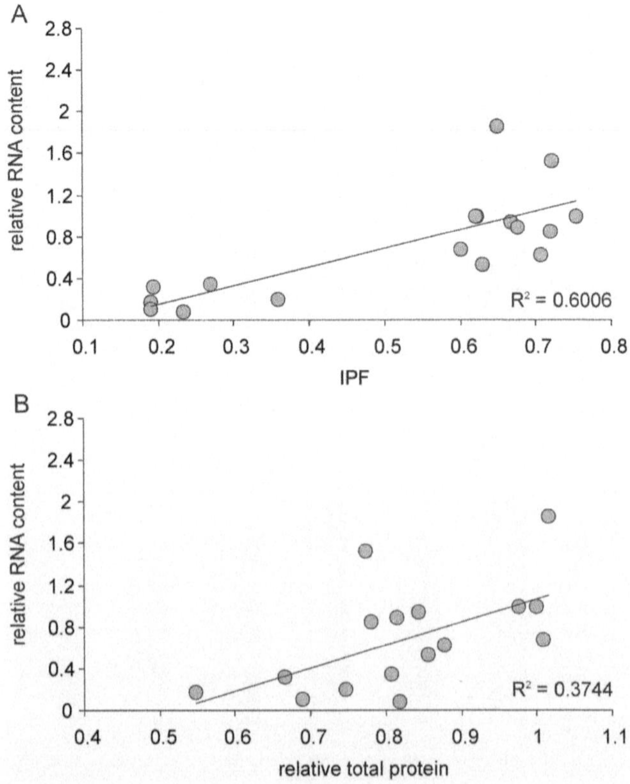

Figure 10. Correlation with total RNA content of insoluble protein fraction (r = 0.7749, n = 18, $p<0.05$) and the total protein (r = .612, n = 18, $p<0.05$) in the pooled data over all the strains and their selection lines.

across different strains. In all the three strains selection in low nutrient environment reduced the tendency to aggregate proteins and selection in high nutrient concentration increased it independent of the effects of standing nutrient concentration. This illustrates the generality and reproducibility of the phenomenon. Unlike some of the earlier studies that used heat or some other stress to induce protein aggregation [24], [30], [31] we observed the phenomenon here with no such external inducer of protein denaturation. Also we made a onetime cross sectional observation without repeatedly exposing the organisms to fluorescence. This is important in the light of the objection raised on the earlier studies that the observed protein aggregation and aging may be a response to the stress rather than being a natural phenomenon [23].

Selection on protein handling?

Since protein aggregation is related to aging in *E. coli* [4], [6], [32], [33], the demonstration that caloric restriction reduces protein aggregates has relevance to aging. It appears that the phenomenon of caloric restriction increasing the lifespan begins with bacteria along the hierarchy of life and here the mechanism is likely to be much simpler as compared to multicellular organisms. In bacteria this phenomenon can perhaps be more easily interpreted simultaneously at proximate and ultimate levels. Although many gaps in data still remain, it appears that when nutrient availability is good, the cells may adopt a use and throw strategy in handling proteins because it allows rapid growth [9] albeit with reduced energy efficiency. On the other hand in nutrient poor environments, energy efficiency could be more important for survival and therefore recycling of proteins is more adaptive than dumping them in the form of aggregates. It is easy to understand why such a strategy would be adaptive in a resource poor environment.

Is there any advantage of protein aggregates?

Our findings point to another dimension of protein aggregation that aggregation is not the end point. The aggregated proteins can be and seem to be reutilized when the cells face starvation. Within four days of starvation the proportion of aggregate free cells increases significantly in all selection lines. But interestingly within the cells that retain aggregates, the mean aggregate intensity is only marginally decreased in some, not significantly decreased, or in fact increased in some cases. If all aggregates degraded with some rate, both the number of aggregate free cells and mean intensity of aggregates should have decreased proportionately. The more sluggish change in the later indicates that the larger aggregates do not degrade as efficiently. Some of them remain undegraded till 30 days. The rate of reutilization of aggregates is likely to be negatively associated with the size of protein aggregates. The smaller aggregates disappear faster on facing starvation and the larger ones appear to linger on disproportionately. This could be simply an effect of decrease in surface to volume ratio of the aggregates or aggregates above a threshold may interfere with some metabolic functions of the cell directly or indirectly making the cell non-viable. This has implications for the biology of aging. If protein aggregation is a mechanism of aging, the reutilization of aggregates points to the possibility of reversibility of aging. Not only that, the aggregated proteins may facilitate survival during starvation. These possibilities need to be tapped in near future.

Implications for the evolution of aging

Many issues in the evolution of aging are debated over a long time and bacterial aging is likely to provide some new insights into it [34]. The demonstration of aging in *E. coli* was taken as a convincing evidence for the universality and therefore inevitability of aging for the living world. Although many of the mechanisms leading to aging including oxidative damages, protein aggregation, telomere shortening, glycosylation etc are inevitable, the patterns of aging are not universal across species [35]. The probability of death and reproductive potential does not necessarily decrease with age in all life forms. The reutilization of protein aggregates raises a possibility that a senescent bacterial cell with a protein aggregate may have better chances of surviving starvation although this has not yet been directly demonstrated.

The reutilization of protein aggregates has a few other possible implications too. *E. coli* is not known to store fat as energy reserve which most multicellular animals do. In humans the tendency to store fat has been popularly known as "thrift" and is said to have evolved as a result of repeated exposure to starvation [36], [37], [38]. There are three close parallels between fat storage in higher animals and protein aggregates in *E. coli*. In both the cases high energy intake increases the storage of fat/proteins, under starvation both can be reutilized and excessive adiposity as well as protein aggregates appear to negatively affect at least some of the normal metabolic processes. This suggests that *E. coli* can be a good model to study the evolution of thrift. Although this was not the objective of the present study, it makes certain suggestions in this context. Continued exposure to low nutrient availability appears to increase the metabolic efficiency, compatible with the thrift hypothesis, but it does not result into excessive storage/aggregation. Instead growth at low nutrients increases growth yield and the efficiency of reutilization rather than the efficiency of storage. Thus there are similarities as well as differences with the prevalent concept of thrift in humans. This warrants further evolutionary experiments specifically designed to probe the evolution of thrift in a bacterial model.

The correlation of protein aggregates with metabolic rate is consistent with the Watve *et al.* [9] hypothesis prediction that asymmetric segregation should increase the net metabolic rate of the population although the cells with aggregates would slow down. Although we did not directly measure metabolic rate, the order of magnitude difference in the standing RNA content probably reflects the increased rate of transcription and thereby metabolism in general. It is important to realize that although we showed that the growth rate is negatively correlated with protein aggregation, this correlation is done after correcting for the main growth rate determining factor that is the currently available nutrient concentration. Without this correction the correlation was positive but non-significant. More surprising is the order of magnitude difference in the total DNA content which most probably reflects the standing chromosomal copy number and simultaneous replication forks [39]. This difference has many implications for the mutation dynamics, mutation tolerance, neutral space and evolvability of the organism. This is an intricate mathematical problem which we do not want to explore here. It is interesting to note that there is a substantial change in the overall cell chemistry indicating some fundamental alterations in metabolic regulation as a result of selection. The cells evolve to become more dilute in terms of protein and nucleic acid concentrations when they evolve in dilute environments.

There are likely to be other direct or indirect benefits of aging like processes in bacteria. Growth arrest accompanying protein aggregation is suggested to give temporary resistance to antibiotics [40]. For accruing this benefit too, the aging process needs to be reversible in bacteria. If such cells have a greater probability of surviving antibiosis or prokaryotic predation [41] and they can reutilize the protein aggregates, the population has a better chance of rejuvenating. Even if a senescent cell with large protein aggregate may have lost its ability to rejuvenate, the stored proteins may be available as a nutrient source to neighboring cells after the death and degeneration of the senescent cell. Thus there can be multiple possible advantages of senescence in bacteria which makes a good case for senescence being an adaptively evolved phenomenon rather than being an inevitable fate. Also since some of the advantages such as better chances of surviving starvation are possible individual advantages and others such as better growth rate are population advantages, both programmed and non-programmed aging are likely to be operative in bacteria. Alternatively the programmed versus non-programmed aging debate may in fact be irrelevant to bacteria [34].

Acknowledgments

The authors would like to extend their most sincere appreciation to Dr. Neelesh Dahanukar who worked with us for final set up of figures. Special mention ought to be made of Mr. Vijay Vital for helping with imaging and Ms. Uttara Lele for sharing the data.

Author Contributions

Conceived and designed the experiments: UB MW. Performed the experiments: UB DM. Analyzed the data: UB DM MW BB. Contributed to the writing of the manuscript: UB MW.

References

1. Ackermann M, Stearns S, Jenal U (2003) Senescence in a bacterium with asymmetric division. Science 300(5627): 1920–1920. doi:10.1126/science.1083532.
2. Ackermann M, Chao L, Bergstrom C, Doebeli M (2007) On the evolutionary origin of aging. Aging Cell 6(2): 235–244. doi:10.1111/j.1474-9726.2007.00281.x.
3. Stewart E, Madden R, Gregory P, Taddei F (2005) Aging and death in an organism that reproduces by morphologically symmetric division. PLoS Biol 3(2): 295–300. doi:10.1371/journal.pbio.0030045.
4. Linder A, Madden R, Demarez A, Stewart E, Taddei F (2008) Asymmetric segregation of proteins aggregates associated with cellular aging and rejuvenation. Proc Natl Acad Sci USA 105(8): 3076–3081. doi:10.1073/pnas.0708931105.
5. Maisonneuve E, Ezraty B, Dukan S (2008) Protein aggregates: an aging factor involved in cell death. Jour of Bact 190(18): 6070–6075. doi:10.1128/JB.00736-08.
6. Coquel A, Jacob J, Primet M, Demarez A, Dimiccoli M, et al. (2013) Localization of protein aggregation in *Escherichia coli* is governed by diffusion and nucleoid macromolecular crowding effect. PLoS Comp Biol 9(4): e1003038. doi:10.1371/journal.pcbi.1003038.
7. Macara I, Mili S (2008) Polarity and differential inheritance–universal attributes of life? Cell 135(5): 801–812. doi:10.1016/j.cell.2008.11.006.
8. Liu B, Larsson L, Caballero A, Hao X, Öling D, et al. (2010) The polarisome is required for segregation and retrograde transport of protein aggregates. Cell 140(2): 257–267. doi:10.1016/j.cell.2009.12.031.
9. Watve M, Parab S, Jogdand P, Keni S (2006) Aging may be a conditional strategic choice and not an inevitable outcome for bacteria. Proc Natl Acad Sci USA 103(40): 14831–14835. doi:10.1073/pnas.0606499103.
10. Wang P, Robert L, Pelletier J, Dang W, Taddei F, et al. (2010) Robust growth of *Escherichia coli*. Curr Biol 20(12): 1099–1103. doi:10.1016/j.cub.2010.04.045.
11. Lele U, Baig U, Watve M (2011) Phenotypic plasticity and effects of selection on cell division symmetry in *Escherichia coli*. PLoS ONE 6(1): e14516. doi:10.1371/journal.pone.0014516.
12. Mullins R, Russell S, Anderson D, Hageman G (2000) Drusen associated with aging and age-related macular degeneration contain proteins common to extracellular deposits associated with atherosclerosis, elastosis, amyloidosis, and dense deposit disease. The FASEB Journal 14(7): 835–846.
13. Butterfield D, Kanski J (2001) Brain protein oxidation in age-related neurodegenerative disorders that are associated with aggregated proteins. Mech Ageing Dev 122(9): 945–962. doi:10.1016/S0047-6374(01)00249-4.
14. Ballatore C, Lee V, Trojanowski J (2007) Tau-mediated neurodegeneration in Alzheimer's disease and related disorders. Nature Rev Neurosci 8(9): 663–672. doi:10.1038/nrn2194.
15. De Groot N, Ventura S (2010) Protein aggregation profile of the bacterial cytosol. PLoS ONE 5(2): e9383. doi:10.1371/journal.pone.0009383.
16. Bukau B, Weissman J, Horwich A (2006) Molecular chaperones and protein quality control. Cell 125(3): 443–451. doi:10.1016/j.cell.2006.04.014.
17. Whitesell L, Lindquist S (2005) HSP90 and the chaperoning of cancer. Nat Rev Cancer 5(10): 761–772. doi:10.1038/nrc1716.
18. Kirkwood T (1977) Evolution of ageing. Nature 270(5635): 301–304. doi:10.1038/270301a0.

19. Strandberg L, Enfors S (1991) Factors influencing inclusion body formation in the production of a fused protein in *Escherichia coli*. Appl Environ Microbiol 57(6): 1669–1674.
20. Kwiatkowska J, Matuszewska E, Kuczyńska-Wiśnik D, Laskowska E (2008) Aggregation of *Escherichia coli* proteins during stationary phase depends on glucose and oxygen availability. Res Microbiol 159: 651–657. doi:10.1016/j.resmic.2008.09.008.
21. Carrio M, Villaverde A (2005) Localization of chaperones DnaK and GroEL in bacterial inclusion bodies. J Bacteriol 187(10): 3599–3601. doi:10.1128/JB.187.10.3599-3601.2005.
22. Neumann M, Gabel D (2002) Simple method for reduction of autofluorescence in fluorescence microscopy. Journal of Histochem Cytochem 50(3): 437–439. doi:10.1177/002215540205000315.
23. Rang C, Peng A, Poon A, Chao L (2012) Ageing in *Escherichia coli* requires damage by an extrinsic agent. Microbiol 158(6): 1553–1559. doi:10.1099/mic.0.057240-0.
24. Laskowska E, Bohdanowicz J, Kuczyńska-Wiśnik D, Matuszewska E, Kędzierska S, et al (2004) Aggregation of heat-shock-denatured, endogenous proteins and distribution of the IbpA/B and Fda marker-proteins in *Escherichia coli* WT and grpE280 cells. Microbiol 150(1): 247–259. doi:10.1099/mic.0.26470-0.
25. Chomczynski P, Sacchi N (1987) Single-step method of RNA isolation by acid guanidinium thiocyanate-phenol-chloroform extraction. Anal Biochem 162(1): 156–159. doi:10.1016/0003-2697(87)90021-2.
26. Ares M (2012) Bacterial RNA isolation. Cold Spring Harbor Protocols 2012(9): 1024–1027. doi:10.1101/pdb.prot071068.
27. Gallagher S, Desjardins P (2001) Quantitation of DNA and RNA with absorption and fluorescence spectroscopy. Current Protocols in Human Genetics, A-3D. doi/10.1002/0471142727.mba03ds76/abstract.
28. Olson B, Markwell J (2007) Assays for Determination of Protein Concentration. Current Protocols in Protein Science. 48: 3.4: 3.4.1–3.4.29. doi:10.1002/0471140864.ps0304s48.
29. Lowder M, Unge A, Maraha N, Jansson J, Swiggett J, et al. (2000) Effect of starvation and the viable-but-nonculturable state on green fluorescent protein (GFP) fluorescence in GFP-tagged *Pseudomonas fluorescens* A506. Appl Environ Microb 66(8): 3160–3165. doi:10.1128/AEM.66.8.3160-3165.2000.
30. Zeng X, Bhasin S, Wu X, Lee J, Maffi S, et al. (2004) Hsp70 dynamics in vivo: effect of heat shock and protein aggregation. J Cell Sci 117(21): 4991–5000. doi:10.1242/jcs.01373.
31. Tyedmers J, Mogk A, Bukau B (2010) Cellular strategies for controlling protein aggregation. Nat Rev Mol Cell Biol 11(11): 777–788. doi:10.1038/nrm2993.
32. Winkler J, Seybert A, König L, Pruggnaller S, Haselmann U, et al. (2010) Quantitative and spatio-temporal features of protein aggregation in *Escherichia coli* and consequences on protein quality control and cellular ageing. The EMBO Journal 29(5): 910–923. doi:10.1038/emboj.2009.412.
33. Lloyd-Price J, Hakkinen A, Kandhavelu M, Marques I, Chowdhury S, et al. (2012) Asymmetric disposal of individual protein aggregates in *Escherichia coli*, One Aggregate at a Time. J of Bacteriol 194(7): 1747–1752. doi:10.1128/JB.06500-11.
34. Baig U, Bhadbhade B, Watve M (2014) Evolution of aging and death: what insights bacteria can give. Quart Rev Biol 89(3): 209–223.
35. Jones O, Scheuerlein A, Salguero-Gómez R, Camarda CG, Schaible R, et al. (2013) Diversity of ageing across the tree of life. Nature 505: 169–173. doi:10.1038/nature12789.
36. Neel J (1962) Diabetes mellitus: a "thrifty" genotype rendered detrimental by "progress"? Am J Hum Genet 14(4): 353–362.
37. Baig U, Belsare P, Watve M, Jog M (2011) Can thrifty gene (s) or predictive fetal programming for thriftiness lead to obesity? 2011:861049 J of Obes doi:10.1155/2011/861049.
38. Watve M (2013) Doves, Diplomats, and Diabetes: A Darwinian Interpretation of Type 2 Diabetes and Related Disorders. Springer. doi:10.1007/978-01-4614-4409-1_1.
39. Fossum S, Crooke E, Skarstad K (2007) Organization of sister origins and replisomes during multifork DNA replication in *Escherichia coli*. The EMBO Journal 26(21): 4514–4522. doi:10.1038/sj.emboj.7601871.
40. Leszczynska D, Matuszewska E, Kuczynska-Wisnik D, Furmanek-Blaszk B, Laskowska E (2013) The formation of persister cells in stationary-phase cultures of *Escherichia Coli* is associated with the aggregation of endogenous proteins. PLoS ONE 8(1): e54737. doi:10.1371/journal.pone.0054737.
41. Kumbhar C, Watve M (2013) Why antibiotics: A comparative evaluation of different hypotheses for the natural role of antibiotics and an evolutionary synthesis. Nat Sci 05(04): 26–40. doi:10.4236/ns.2013.54A005.

Cross-Sectional Study of Malnutrition and Associated Factors among School Aged Children in Rural and Urban Settings of Fogera and Libo Kemkem Districts, Ethiopia

Zaida Herrador[1,2], Luis Sordo[3,4,5], Endalamaw Gadisa[6], Javier Moreno[7], Javier Nieto[7], Agustín Benito[1,2], Abraham Aseffa[6], Carmen Cañavate[7], Estefania Custodio[1,2]*

1 National Centre of Tropical Medicine, Instituto de Salud Carlos III (ISCIII), Madrid, Spain, **2** Tropical Diseases Research Network (RICET in Spanish), Madrid, Spain, **3** National Centre of Epidemiology, ISCIII, Madrid, Spain, **4** Department of Preventive Medicine and Public Health, Faculty of Medicine, Complutense University, Madrid, Spain, **5** Network Biomedical Research Centers, Epidemiology and Public Health (CIBERESP in Spanish), Madrid, Spain, **6** Armauer Hansen Research Institute, Addis Ababa, Ethiopia, **7** National Centre of Microbiology, ISCIII, Madrid, Spain

Abstract

Introduction: Little information is available on malnutrition-related factors among school-aged children ≥5 years in Ethiopia. This study describes the prevalence of stunting and thinness and their related factors in Libo Kemkem and Fogera, Amhara Regional State and assesses differences between urban and rural areas.

Methods: In this cross-sectional study, anthropometrics and individual and household characteristics data were collected from 886 children. Height-for-age z-score for stunting and body-mass-index-for-age z-score for thinness were computed. Dietary data were collected through a 24-hour recall. Bivariate and backward stepwise multivariable statistical methods were employed to assess malnutrition-associated factors in rural and urban communities.

Results: The prevalence of stunting among school-aged children was 42.7% in rural areas and 29.2% in urban areas, while the corresponding figures for thinness were 21.6% and 20.8%. Age differences were significant in both strata. In the rural setting, fever in the previous 2 weeks (OR: 1.62; 95% CI: 1.23–2.32), consumption of food from animal sources (OR: 0.51; 95% CI: 0.29–0.91) and consumption of the family's own cattle products (OR: 0.50; 95% CI: 0.27–0.93), among others factors were significantly associated with stunting, while in the urban setting, only age (OR: 4.62; 95% CI: 2.09–10.21) and years of schooling of the person in charge of food preparation were significant (OR: 0.88; 95% CI: 0.79–0.97). Thinness was statistically associated with number of children living in the house (OR: 1.28; 95% CI: 1.03–1.60) and family rice cultivation (OR: 0.64; 95% CI: 0.41–0.99) in the rural setting, and with consumption of food from animal sources (OR: 0.26; 95% CI: 0.10–0.67) and literacy of head of household (OR: 0.24; 95% CI: 0.09–0.65) in the urban setting.

Conclusion: The prevalence of stunting was significantly higher in rural areas, whereas no significant differences were observed for thinness. Various factors were associated with one or both types of malnutrition, and varied by type of setting. To effectively tackle malnutrition, nutritional programs should be oriented to local needs.

Editor: Heather B. Jaspan, University of Cape Town, South Africa

Funding: The authors gratefully acknowledge the financial support of the UBS-Optimus Foundation in Switzerland, (www.ubs.com/global/en/wealth_management/optimusfoundation.html), via the Visceral Leishmaniasis and Malnutrition in Amhara State, Ethiopia project, and the Tropical Diseases Research Network in Spain (www.ricet.es/es/) via the VI PN de I+D+I 2008–2011, ISCIII -Subdirección General de Redes y Centros de Investigación Cooperativa RD12/0018/0001 and RD12/0018/0003. The funders had no role in study design, data collection and analysis, decision to publish, or preparation of the manuscript.

Competing Interests: The authors have declared that no competing interests exist.

* Email: ecustodio2014@gmail.com

Introduction

Adequate nutrition is essential during childhood to ensure healthy growth, proper organ formation and function, a strong immune system, and neurological and cognitive development [1]. Nutritional status has a major impact on children's survival mainly due to the synergistic relationships between malnutrition and diseases [2,3]. In Eastern and Southern Africa, malnutrition is a major underlying cause of the persistently high child mortality, contributing to more than a third of all deaths among children under age 5 [4].

The two main anthropometric indicators used to define malnutrition– stunting, and wasting or thinness– represent different histories of nutritional insult to the child. Linear growth retardation (chronic malnutrition or stunting) is frequently associated with repeated exposure to adverse economic conditions, poor sanitation, and the interactive effects of poor nutrient intakes and infection. Low weight-for-height or low body mass index (BMI) for age (acute malnutrition, wasting or thinness) is generally associated with recent illness and/or food deprivation [5].

The causes of childhood malnutrition are diverse, multidimensional, and interrelated. An analytical framework suggested by the

United Nations Children's Fund (UNICEF) categorizes the causes into (a) immediate causes: inadequate dietary intake and illness, (b) underlying causes: insufficient access to food in a household; inadequate health services and unhealthy environment; and inadequate care for children and women at the household level, and (c) basic causes: insufficient current and potential resources at societal level [6]. In Sub-Saharan Africa, various indicators of social economic status have been associated with children's nutritional status, such as maternal and paternal educational level, parental income, and family assets [7–9]. In addition, child nutrition outcomes in developing countries have been characterized by large rural-urban disparities over the last few decades [10].

In Ethiopia, child malnutrition continues to be a major public health problem. According to the Ethiopian National Demographic Health Survey (2011), the prevalence of both wasting and stunting in children under 5 years is very high (10% and 44% respectively) [11], while the situation in older children is not so well known [12,13]. Furthermore, rural-urban disparities in child nutrition, as well as growing urbanization that results in increasing inequalities in urban areas, underlines the need to improve our knowledge of the main drivers of urban-rural differences [14].

The Amhara Region is one of the four primary agricultural regions in Ethiopia [15], and most households rely upon livestock and crop sales to generate cash income. This region, and especially the Tana Zuria Zone, has a moderate population density, fertile soils and good rainfall. For this reason, it is amongst the most food self-sufficient regions in the country [16]. Despite this good regional profile, other factors may be determining the high prevalence of infant malnutrition in this area [17]. According to the Food and Agriculture Organization of the United Nations (FAO), the four pillars of food security are food availability, stability of the food supply, food access and the utilization of food by the body [18]. In our context, availability is strongly affected by seasonality; many households are only able to produce sufficient food to meet their food requirements for less than six months of the year [19]. Food access may be affected by market conditions, but also by cultural and religious practices. For example, the high number of fasting days commemorated by the Ethiopian Orthodox Church, the main religion in the country, may have repercussions on the nutritional status of the community, particularly in rural Ethiopia [20].

Even if people get enough to eat, good nutrition requires access to a sufficient, supply of varied, safe and nutritious food to meet daily nutritional requirements [21]. Although diet diversity questionnaires are extensively used in Ethiopia to investigate relationships between food intake and nutritional status, there is limited knowledge of nutrition outcomes, dietary practices and socioeconomic factors among school-aged children in this specific context [17].

The present study aimed to [22] describe the prevalence of stunting and thinness, and their related factors, including dietary habits, and [23] document the differences in nutritional status across urban and rural areas accounting for household and individual characteristics in school-aged children in Libo Kemkem and Fogera, Amhara regional State, Ethiopia.

Material and Methods

Study area and population

The study was carried out during May–June 2009 in the districts (*woredas*) of Libo Kemkem and Fogera (Amhara regional state, Ethiopia). Libo Kemkem and Fogera woredas are located in the Tana Zuria Livelihood Zone, within the Amhara Regional State, northwestern Ethiopia at an altitude of 2,000 m above sea level. According to the 2009 census, the population was 198,374 and 226,595 for Libo Kemkem and Fogera, respectively.

These two districts are located in a black cotton clay soil flat plain. Temperatures are relatively high, but rainfall is unusually abundant, with a mean of 1173 mm per annum. Agricultural activities are dependent on a single rainy season (from June to September). Maize, barley and millet are the main food crops, while rice, vetch and chickpea are the main cash crops. Livestock holdings in sheep and cattle are relatively modest, but livestock and butter sales make a substantial complement to the predominant crop sales. The major hazards to crop production and livestock are pests, occasional flooding, and zoonosis such as anthrax, trypanosomiasis, pasteurellosis and black leg [16].

Study design

This cross-sectional survey was part of a UBS Optimus Foundation funded project called Visceral Leishmaniasis (VL) and Malnutrition in Amhara State, Ethiopia. Among its specific objectives, the project aimed to characterize nutritional, immunological, and parasitological factors in school-aged children in the districts of Fogera and Libo Kemkem. Other methodological aspects have previously been published [24–26].

Sampling was carried out by multistage cluster survey. A total of 886 children aged 4 to 15 years were recruited. Primary sampling units were sub-districts (*kebeles*) with a high incidence of VL according to the 2008 register of the Addis Zemen VL Treatment Centre: one urban (Addis Zemen) and the rest rural: Bura, Yifag Akababi and Agita from Libo Kemkem, and Sifatra and Rib Gebriel from Fogera. Secondary sampling units were randomly selected villages (*gotts*) in each of the selected sub-districts. Third-stage sampling units were randomly selected households in each of the villages. All children with reported age between 4 and 15 years living in the household at the time of the survey were recruited. Sample size was calculated according to previous estimates of malnutrition for children under age 5 in the area and taking into account a design effect of 2, corresponding to the complex design.

Data collection

All children were measured and weighed according to standard WHO procedures [27]. Weight was measured to the nearest 0.1 kg on a battery-powered digital scale (SECA 881©). Standing height was measured to the nearest 0.1 cm using a portable adult/infant measuring unit (PE-AIM-101©).

A pre-tested questionnaire translated into Amharic, the local language, was administered to the caretaker/head of household (HH) of each child in the study by trained medical personnel (nurses and health officers).

We asked about individual demographic characteristics, health status and behavior determinants. The following household variables were also recorded: household socio-demographic characteristics, person in charge of food preparation (PCFP), house construction material and assets (land and cultivation, domestic animal assets) and community variables. Dietary data was collected through a 24-hour diet recall.

Statistical analysis

Stunting and thinness were the main outcomes of interest, defined as height-for-age z-score (HAZ) <-2 and BMI-for-age z-score (BAZ) <-2 respectively. The z-scores were calculated using the WHO 2007 reference (for children $\geq$5 years) and the WHO Growth Standards (for children $<$5 years old), both computed by WHO Anthro Plus software.

The dietary data collected through the 24-hour diet recall were computed into 9 food groups (1. Basic staples, 2. Vitamin A rich fruits and vegetables, 3. Other fruits, 4. Other vegetables, 5. Legumes and pulses, 6. Meat or Fish, 7. Oil, 8. Dairy and 9. Eggs) based on the FAO/FANTA Household Dietary Diversity Questionnaire and Guidelines [21].

Frequencies and percentages were used to summarize data and to explore the differences between rural and urban communities. These differences were assessed by Student's t-test and χ^2 tests for continuous and categorical variables, respectively.

Bivariate analyses for thinness and stunting and their related factors were performed, with stratification by setting. Age and sex, considered biologically relevant, and all variables associated with each of the outcomes at the p<0.10 level were included in the multivariable analysis. Logistic regression models stratified by setting for stunting and thinness were obtained by using a manual backward stepwise procedure. P-values less than or equal to 0.05 were considered statistically significant.

Data analysis was performed using Anthro Plus v1.02 (WHO, Geneva, Switzerland) and SPSS version 18.0 (SPSS Inc., Chicago, Illinois, USA).

Ethical considerations

The study was approved by the ethical review boards of the *Instituto de Salud Carlos III* (ISCIII), the Armauer Hansen Research Institute, and the Ethiopian National Ethical Review Committee. Support letters were obtained from the Amhara Regional State and the *woreda* health bureaus. Parents/guardians gave written informed consent before enrollment of their children in the study.

Results

Description of the sample

The study included a total of 886 children aged 4 to 15 years, of which 462 (52.0%) were males. Around 80% lived in the rural setting and 50.6% presented malnutrition. The prevalence of malnutrition was significantly higher in rural than in urban communities (53% and 42.1% respectively; p = 0.006).

The mean HAZ and BAZ for the overall study population were below the WHO references [28], −1.62 (SD = 1.34, range −6.12–5.74, p≤0.05) and −1.28 (SD = 1.00, range −4.95–3.82, p≤0.05), respectively.

Individual characteristics, including demographic data, nutritional status and diet habits are summarized in Table 1, disaggregated by rural and urban strata.

There were several differences between children living in rural and urban settings regarding child health status, behavior and dietary habits. Children living in rural areas slept under a bed net less frequently than urban children (41.1% vs. 67.4% respectively, p<0.001). On the day before the survey, 18.1% of children in the rural setting had consumed food from animal sources vs. 64% of those in the urban setting.. The proportion of children who had consumed food from four or more food groups was 16.3% vs. 39.9%, respectively (p<0.001 for each comparison).

Household characteristics are summarized in Table 2. The proportion of rural households that owned land was 97.6% vs. 10.1% in urban households, while the corresponding figures for ownership of domestic animals or chickens were 96.3% vs. 36.5%, respectively (p<0.001 for each). The distribution of the rest of the socio-demographic and household variables but one (years of education of the HH) also differed significantly between urban and rural areas.

Chronic malnutrition

The prevalence of stunting was 42.7% in the rural setting and 29.2% in the urban setting (p = 0.001).

Chronic malnutrition in rural communities. In the bivariate analysis (Table S1), the prevalence of chronic malnutrition was similar in males and females, however it was significantly higher inchildren age 10 and over than in those under 10 years of age (OR: 2.28; 95% CI: 1.66–3.11) in the rural group. Stunting was significantly more frequent in children with a previous history of splenomegaly (OR: 2.26; 95% CI: 1.11–4.59) or fever (OR: 1.59; 95% CI: 1.15–2.18), and less common in those who slept under a bed net (OR: 0.68; 95% CI: 0.50–0.92) or herded the cattle (OR: 0.70; 95% CI: 0.52–0.95). Regarding dietary habits in rural communities, the consumption of vitamin A rich fruits and vegetables and the consumption of any meat or fish the day before the survey were associated with a lower prevalence of chronic malnutrition (OR: 0.34 (95% CI: 0.13–0.93) and OR: 0.59 (95% CI: 0.36–0.97), respectively).

Results from the multivariable logistic analysis are presented in Table 3. The difference between the two age groups remained significant in the final model (OR: 3.12; 95% CI: 2.15–4.51), showing that the prevalence of chronic malnutrition was higher in children age 10 and over. Children with fever in the two weeks prior to the survey were 1.62 times more likely to be stunted (95% CI: 1.23–2.32). Herding cattle (OR: 0.43; 95% CI: 0.30–0.63) and the consumption of any food from animal sources (OR: 0.51; 95% CI: 0.29–0.91) showed a significant negative association with stunting. With regard to household socio demographic characteristics, children from rural areas were 2.97 times more likely to have chronic malnutrition if the HH was female (95%CI: 1.47–5.98). The number of people living in the house was positively associated with the prevalence of stunting (p = 0.042), while millet production (OR: 0.50; 95% CI: 0.27–0.93) and consumption of products from the family's own cattle (OR: 0.67; 95% CI: 0.46–0.96) were negatively associated.

Chronic malnutrition in urban communities. In the urban setting, the significant age differences (OR: 3.73; 95% CI: 1.89–7.39) found in the bivariate analysis occurred in the same direction as in the rural area (Table S1). Furthermore, the prevalence of stunting was significantly higher among children living in a house where the HH (OR: 1.58; 95% CI: 1.00–2.53) or the PCFP (OR: 1.60; 95% CI: 0.99–2.66) had not attended school.

Table 3 summarizes the results adjusted by logistic regression. Older children were more prone to stunting than younger children (OR: 4.62; 95% CI: 2.09–10.21). Years of school attendance of the PCFP was negatively associated with chronic malnutrition among children living in urban communities (OR: 0.88; 95% CI: 0.79–0.97).

Acute malnutrition

The prevalence of thinness was 21.6% in the rural setting and 20.8% in the urban setting (p>0.05).

Acute malnutrition in rural communities. In the bivariate analysis (Table S2), the prevalence of acute malnutrition was higher in children age 10 and over (OR: 4.74; 95% CI: 3.24–6.94) and among boys (OR: 1.58; 95% CI: 1.18–2.12). Children from rural communities who herded the cattle were 2.43 times more likely to be thin (95%CI: 1.63–3.61) than those who did not. The number of children living in the house (p = 0.007) and teff cultivation (OR: 1.53; 95% CI: 1.02–2.30) were positively associated with higher prevalence of thinness, while living with a HH under 40 years old and rice farming showed an inverse association with thinness (OR: 0.75; 95% CI: 0.56–0.99 and 0.63; 95% CI: 0.42–0.95, respectively).

Table 1. Individual characteristics, behavioral determinants and dietary habits of school-aged children in rural and urban areas of at Libokemkem and Fogera districts, Ethiopia, May–June 2009.

CHARACTERISTICS	RURAL (n = 711)		URBAN (n = 178)		p value
	No.	(%)	No.	(%)	
Sex (female)	339	47,68	88	49,44	0,676
Age group (≥10 years)	259	36,43	58	32,58	0,193
Stunting	302	42,66	52	29,21	0,001
Wasting	153	21,61	37	20,79	0,450
Splenomegaly	34	4,79	1	0,56	0,004
Fever in the last 15 days	223	31,41	37	20,79	0,003
Sleeps under a bed net	292	41,13	120	67,42	<0.001
Herds the cattle	413	58,17	7	3,93	<0.001
Consumption on day before survey of:					
Food of animal source	129	18,14	114	64,04	<0.001
Basic staples	708	99,58	178	100	0,511
VitA rich fruits and vegetables	24	3,38	11	6,18	0,071
Other fruits	0	0	3	1,69	0,008
Other vegetables	53	7,45	22	12,36	0,029
Legumes and pulses	643	90,44	106	59,55	<0.001
Meat/fish	79	11,11	103	57,87	<0.001
Oil	644	90,58	166	93,26	0,164
Dairy	53	7,45	15	8,43	0,381
Eggs	5	0,7	5	2,81	0,032
5 or more food groups	28	3,94	16	8,99	0,007
4 or more food groups	116	16,32	71	39,89	<0.001
	Mean	**s.d.**	**Mean**	**s.d.**	**p value**
Sum of food groups	3,12	0,60	3,42	0,77	<0.001

After adjusting for socio demographic and household characteristics in the model, sex differences lost significance, and the relationship between thinness and age was slightly weakened (OR: 4.11; 95% CI: 2.74–6.16) (Table 4). Children from rural communities were significantly less likely to be thin if the HH was female (OR: 0.40; 95% CI: 0.16–0.70). The number of children living in the house showed a positive relationship with thinness in this setting ($p = 0.027$), while children from households that cultivate rice were less likely to be thin (OR: 0.64; 95% CI: 0.41–0.99).

Acute malnutrition in urban communities. In the bivariate analysis (Table S2), no significant associations with thinness were found apart from age group (OR: 2.76; 95% CI: 1.13–5.80).

After adjusting the analysis, age group remained significantly related to thinness (OR: 3.67; 95% CI: 1.63–8.30). Food consumption from animal sources on the day before the survey was inversely associated with acute malnutrition (OR: 0.26; 95% CI: 0.10–0.67) and thinness prevalence was lower among in households headed by literate persons (OR: 0.24; 95% CI: 0.09–0.65) (Table 4).

Discussion

Our study shows that there is a high prevalence of stunting (39.8%) and thinness (21.4%) among school-aged children in Libo Kemkem and Fogera regions of Ethiopia. The prevalence of stunting was significantly higher in rural areas (42.7% vs. 29.2%), but no significant differences were observed for thinness. These results are similar to those observed in other developing countries [29]. Various intermediate and distal factors like age, consumption of food from animal sources and family size were associated with both types of malnutrition in one or both settings. Other determinants such as years of school attendance of the PCFP and consumption of the family's own cattle products were related to only one kind of malnutrition. Although malnutrition among pre-school children has been well documented in Ethiopia [5,30,31], to our knowledge this is the first research to assess factors related to acute and chronic malnutrition stratified by setting in school aged children. These results may assist stakeholders in planning and undertaking contextual and evidence-based policy initiatives.

We found that the probability of a child being malnourished increases with age. Age-group differences were significant in both strata for stunting and thinness. No sex differences were found in either strata. As children mature, household socioeconomic characteristics may emerge in conjunction with behavioral and biological variables as important risk factors [32].

Chronic malnutrition

The prevalence of stunting in rural areas in our study was higher (42.7%) than that found in a study conducted in the same age group in rural settings of Fogera in 2012 (30.7%) [33]. Our study was carried out in 2009, which may partially explain this difference due to possible improvements in local conditions;

Table 2. Parental and household characteristics of school-aged children in rural and urban areas of Libo Kemkem and Fogera districts, Ethiopia, May–June 2009.

CHARACTERISTICS	RURAL (n = 711)		URBAN (n = 178)		p value
	No.	(%)	No.	(%)	
Sex head of household (HH)					
Female	52	7.31	75	42.13	<0.001
Age HH					
≥40 years	351	49.72	65	36.93	0.008
HH literacy (read and write)					
Yes	282	39.83	97	54.49	<0.001
Person in charge of food preparation (PCFP)					
Wife or HH(she)	690	97.05	144	80.9	<0.001
Other	21	2.95	34	19.1	
Years of HH education	**Mean**	**s.d.**	**Mean**	**s.d.**	**p value**
	2.70	12.6	4.27	4.92	0.106
Years of education of the PCFP					
	0.22	1	3.30	4.53	<0.001
Number of people living in the house					
	6.41	1.71	5.24	1.58	<0.001
Number children in the house					
	2.85	1.13	2.17	0.89	<0.001
Does the household own land?	**No.**	**(%)**	**No.**	**(%)**	**p value**
Yes	694	97.61	18	10.11	<0.001
Have domestic animals or chickens?					
Yes	685	96.34	65	36.52	<0.001
Does the household....					
cultivate teff?					
Yes	481	67.65	4	2.25	<0.001
cultivate rice?					
Yes	231	32.49	2	1.12	<0.001
cultivate millet?					
Yes	70	9.85	5	2.81	<0.001
cultivate beans?					
Yes	22	3.09	1	0.56	0.038
consume products from their own cattle?					
Do not consume own cattle products	224	31.68	0		
Consume own cattle products	419	59.26	11	6.29	<0.001
Do not have cattle	64	9.05	164	93.71	
consume products from their own goats?					
Do not consume own goat products	35	4.96	0		
Consume own goat products	34	4.82	7	3.93	0.008
Do not have goats	637	90.23	171	96.07	
consume products from their own sheep?					
Do not consume own sheep products	62	8.81	2	1.12	
Consume own sheep products	90	12.78	6	3.37	<0.001
Do not have sheep	552	78.41	170	95.51	
consume products from their own chickens?					
Do not consume own chicken products	80	11.28	2	1.12	
Consume own chicken products	343	48.38	47	26.40	<0.001
Do not have chickens	286	40.34	129	72.47	

Table 3. Multivariable logistic regression analysis of stunting in school-aged children stratified by setting in Libo Kemkem and Fogera districts, Ethiopia, May–July 2009.

VARIABLES		RURAL (N=711)				URBAN (N=178)			
		n (%)	AOR	95% CI	p value	n (%)	AOR	95% CI	p value
CHILD CHARACTERISTICS									
Sex	**male**	166 (44.86)	1			27 (30.00)	1		
	female	136 (40.24)	0.78	(0.55–1.10)	0.160	25 (28.41)	1.29	(0.56–2.96)	0.554
Age group	**<10 years**	159 (35.24)	1			24 (20.01)	1		
	≥10 years	143 (55.26)	3.12	(2.15–4.51)	0.000	28 (48.39)	4.62	(2.09–10.21)	0.000
Fever in the last 15 days?	**No**	112 (50.45)	1			13 (35.14)	1		
	Yes	190 (39.09)	1.62	(1.23–2.32)	0.009	39 (27.66)	1.80	(0.73–4.47)	0.204
Does the child herd the cattle?	**No**	141 (47.64)	1			39 (29.24)	1		
	Yes	160 (38.93)	0.43	(0.30–0.63)	0.000	13 (28.57)	0.75	(0.07–7.71)	0.811
DOES THE CHILD CONSUME...									
Any food from animal sources*	**No**	254 (43.87)	1			20 (31.25)	1		
	Yes	48 (37.21)	0.51	(0.29–0.91)	0.022	32 (28.07)	0.72	(0.31–1.71)	0.463
vit A rich fruits and vegetables*	**No**	297 (43.42)	1			48 (28.74)	1		
	Yes	5 (20.83)	0.29	(0.83–1.04)	0.057	4 (36.36)	1.32	(0.29–5.99)	0.717
Other vegetables*	**No**	284 (43.36)	1			42 (26.92)	1		
	Yes	18 (33.96)	1.08	(0.49–2.38)	0.855	10 (45.45)	3.00	(0.97–9.38)	0.058
HOUSEHOLD AND LAND PRODUCTION									
Sex of head of household	**Male**	267 (40.70)	1			29 (28.16)	1		
	Female	35 (67.31)	2.97	(1.47–5.98)	0.002	23 (30.67)	0.66	(0.27–1.64)	0.370
Age of head of household	**<40 years**	151 (42.66)	1			37 (28.16)	1		
	≥40 years	147 (42.14)	0.73	(0.50–1.06)	0.097	23 (30.67)	0.43	(0.17–1.06)	0.069
Years of school-person in charge of food preparation		**Mean (sd)**	**AOR**	**95% CI**	**p value**	**Mean (sd)**	**AOR**	**95% CI**	**p value**
		0.16 (0.86)	0.84	(0.70–1.01)	0.065	2.19 (4.0)	0.88	(0.79–0.97)	0.014
Number of people living in the house									
		6.43 (1.85)	1.12	(1.01–1.25)	0.042	5.08 (1.41)	0.84	(0.63–1.13)	0.260
		n (%)	**AOR**	**95% CI**	**p value**	**n (%)**	**AOR**	**95% CI**	**p value**
Does the family cultivate millet?	**No**	280 (43.82)	1			50 (28.90)	1		
	Yes	22 (31.88)	0.50	(0.27–0.93)	0.029	2 (40.00)	2.35	(0.27–20.19)	0.435
Does the family consume products from their own cattle?	**Do not consume own products**	39 (60.94)	1			47 (28.66)	1		
	Consume own products	107 (48.20)	0.67	(0.46–0.96)	0.030	0	-	-	N.A.
	Do not have cattle	154 (36.84)	1.36	(0.72–2.56)	0.348	3 (27.27)	1.07	(0.11–9.23)	0.989

Table 3. Cont.

VARIABLES		RURAL (N = 711)				URBAN (N = 178)			
		n (%)	AOR	95% CI	p value	n (%)	AOR	95% CI	p value
Does the family consume products from their own goats?	Do not consume own products	277 (43.69)	1			52 (30.41)	1		
	Consume own products	16 (45.71)	0.37	(0.12–1.16)	0.090	0	-	-	N.A.
	Do not have goats	8 (23.53)	0.92	(0.43–1.96)	0.833	0	-	-	N.A.

*day before the survey.

another reason may be that children in the Fogera study had to be enrolled in school in order to participate, which could result in selection bias. In addition, our sampling was done in sub-districts with a high incidence of VL, a characteristic that may be associated with fewer resources and worse health status in children. The prevalence of chronic malnutrition in the urban area (29.2%) could not be compared to previous data due to the lack of research targeting this particular age group in this setting.

In rural communities, the setting with the highest stunting prevalence, we found several factors associated with chronic malnutrition: age group, fever in the previous 15 days, herding the cattle, consumption of any food from animal sources, sex of the HH, family size, cultivation of millet and consumption of the family's own cattle products. These factors should be considered when targeting chronic malnutrition in this region.

Children who had fever in the previous 15 days were 62% more likely to be stunted than those who did not. Infection and malnutrition are intricately linked through extensive, synergistic, antagonistic, and cyclical interactions [34,35]. Although our study area is known to be a low endemic area for malaria and leishmaniasis [25,36], other specific infections associated with malnutrition (such as chronic parasitic infestations) are highly prevalent [37,38]. Infectious diseases manifested in the form of fever affect both dietary intake and utilization, which may affect child growth. Not having empirical data on specific infections is a limitation, but we considered fever in the previous 15 days could act as a proxy for non-specific infection. On the other hand, stunted growth and related immunosuppression may lead to intermittent fever [39].

In our research, children who herd the cattle were less likely to be stunted. This could be explained by better activity levels in non-stunted children, given that stunted children show behavioral differences in early childhood including apathy and reduced activity, play and exploration [40].

Finally, children from households with millet farming and from families who consume their own cattle products were less likely to be stunted in rural communities. Although most rural families own land and animals (97.6% and 96.3% respectively), we observed that they do not consume their own products as often. Only 11.1% of the children had eaten any meat or fish over the last 24 hours, while 99.6% and 90.4%, respectively, had consumed basic staples and legumes and/or pulses respectively. In Ethiopia, child diet is based mainly based on plant foods like the traditional Ethiopian staple food called "*injera*", a yeast-risen flatbread made of a blend of cereals, usually served with legumes or pulses. This may not provide all the nutritional requirements of children [41]. We are aware that market access in this livelihood zone is poor; moreover what little trade interaction exists is restricted to cash crops that are attractive for their high price (i.e. rice and teff), while other essential crops cultivated mainly for personal consumption face disincentives [16,42].

In urban communities, age group and years of school of the PCFP were significantly associated with chronic malnutrition in children. This educational factor may operate indirectly to affect children's nutritional status by determining the quality of the child's diet, care and physical environment [30]. The level of education of the PCFP may have a positive impact on his/her knowledge on food facilities, controlling contamination, time and temperature parameters for controlling pathogens, and advice on good dietary habits [43].

Acute malnutrition

The prevalence of acute malnutrition in the rural settings of Fogera and Libo Kemkem was 21.6%. The prevalence of

Table 4. Multivariable logistic regression analysis of thinness in school-aged children, stratified by setting in Libo Kemkem and Fogera districts, Ethiopia, May–July 2009.

VARIABLES		RURAL (N=711)				URBAN (N=178)			
		n (%)	Adjusted OR	95% CI	p value	n (%)	Adjusted OR	95% CI	p value
CHILD CHARACTERISTICS									
Sex	**male**	97 (26.22)	1			21 (23.33)	1		
	female	56 (16.57)	0.69	(0.46–1.03)	0.073	16 (18.18)	0.86	(0.39–1.92)	0.717
Age group	**<10 years**	53 (11.83)	1			18 (15.02)	1		
	≥10 years	100 (38.84)	4.11	(2.74–6.16)	0.000	19 (32.81)	3.67	(1.63–8.30)	0.002
Does the child herd the cattle?	**No**	40 (13.51)	1			36 (21.05)	1		
	Yes	113 (27.49)	1.50	(0.96–2.36)	0.076	1 (14.29)	0.55	(0.06–5.03)	0.598
DOES THE CHILD CONSUME...									
Any food from animal sources	**No**	129 (22.28)	1			18 (28.13)	1		
	Yes	24 (18.60)	0.83	(0.49–1.41)	0.493	19 (16.67)	0.26	(0.10–0.67)	0.005
HOUSEHOLD AND LAND PRODUCTION									
Sex of head of household	**Male**	146 (22.26)	1			23 (22.33)	1		
	Female	7 (13.46)	0.40	(0.16–0.70)	0.043	14 (18.67)	0.67	(0.26–1.72)	0.407
Literacy of head of household (can read and write)	**No**	93 (21.83)	1			25 (25.77)	1		
	Yes	60 (21.51)	1.39	(0.91–2.11)	0.127	12 (14.81)	0.24	(0.09–0.65)	0.005
Number of people living in the house		**Mean (sd)**	**AOR**	**95% CI**	**p value**	**Mean (sd)**	**AOR**	**95% CI**	**p value**
		6.45 (1.68)	0.87	(0.75–1.00)	0.054	5.14 (1.72)	0.87	(0.64–1.20)	0.403
Number of children in the house									
		3.06 (1.14)	1.28	(1.03–1.60)	0.027	2.19 (0.94)	1.02	(0.61–1.70)	0.955
		n (%)	**AOR**	**95% CI**	**p value**	**n (%)**	**AOR**	**95% CI**	**p value**
Does the family cultivate rice?	**No**	115 (24.01)	1			36 (20.45)	1		
	Yes	38 (16.59)	0.64	(0.41–0.99)	0.045	1 (50.00)	3.26	(0.15–72.94)	0.456

underweight found in the study conducted in Fogera was 37.2% [33]. These results cannot be directly compared as different anthropometric indices were used. And again, we did not find any data on thinness to compare with our results in the urban population.

In rural settings, age group, sex of the HH, number of children in the house and rice cultivation were factors associated with thinness. The number of children in a household and the prevalence of thinness were positively associated. Larger family size may put children at higher risk for acute malnutrition, which could be due to the imbalance between family size and resources [44].

Those whose families cultivate rice were less likely to be thin in rural communities. In this zone, rice production might be acting as a proxy for better socioeconomic status, as rice consumption is relatively recent but is one of the main cash crops in the area [16]. The low consumption of animal source foods and its association with acute malnutrition has been previously identified as a major contributing factor to delayed growth in children [45] and suboptimal dietary practices among adolescents in Ethiopia [17].

In urban areas, children with a literate HH were 4 times less likely to be thin than those living in houses headed by illiterate adults. Some studies have shown that parental education is associated with more efficient management of limited household resources, improved utilization of available health care services, and better health-promoting behaviors, all of which are associated with better child nutrition [46,47]. This result is similar to what we previously observed for stunting and PCFP years of education in the urban setting. A possible explanation could be the existence of an educational gap in urban but not in rural areas.

Stunting versus thinness: associated factors

Clear differences among risk factors for stunting (Table 3) and thinness (Table 4) emerged from this study. The literature on the causes of stunting is vast, and conventional thinking is summarized in the *Lancet* series on maternal and child under-nutrition [48]. Recognized causal factors include prenatal and postnatal periods. Stunting is seen as closely tied to poverty and access to services. Less knowledge is available on risk factors for thinness [1]. In our research, risk factors for chronic malnutrition encompass a wide range of variables.. The relatively consistent pattern of related factors for stunting suggests that continued exposure to adverse conditions retards children's linear growth. Conversely, the greater diversity observed in the factors associated with thinness is consistent with the fact that a relatively short period of risk exposure can precipitate its onset in children [32].

In rural communities, children from male-headed households were more likely to be thin than children from female-headed households ($p = 0.043$), while stunting was significantly more frequent in female-headed households ($p = 0.002$). The disparate sample size in rural and urban areas may have influenced these results. However, the result in the rural area is consistent with the study conducted in North Ethiopia by Haidar et al. [49]. This study found a significantly higher proportion of stunted and underweight pre-school children in female headed-households, whereas the prevalence of thinness was similar [48–50]. Women who are single HH may be removed from their support structures and may face constraints in accessing services, including food, as a result of insecurity, cultural discrimination and limited mobility [48,50]. This situation may have a long-term impact in child nutrition.

Rural versus urban: associated factors

Ethiopia remains one of the least urbanized countries in the world [42]. Globally, malnutrition is less common in urban areas [2,31]. We found that malnutrition in rural communities was associated with food habits and the lack of material resources whereas in the urban area, it was better predicted by socio demographic factors. Inequalities in child health outcomes are known to vary between rural and urban areas, and are often due to unequal allocation of resources [51].

Significant urban-rural differences remained in the multivariable model. This shows that even in the presence of important individual factors and socioeconomic variables, area of residence is still a predictor of children's nutritional status. Our results highlight the need to stratify data when rural and urban communities are targeted in nutritional research in this kind of context.

Limitations

The present study was conducted in two single districts in Ethiopia, thus, the findings may not be generalizable to a larger population. Additionally, the cross-sectional nature of this data does not allow us to examine causality in the relationship between malnutrition and diverse risk factors. Seasonality should be given special attention; the season of the year has a significant effect not only on food security and nutritional status, but also on patterns and trends of infectious disease incidence. Therefore, consecutive measurements are desirable..

This research is part of a project which aimed to characterize nutritional, immunological, and parasitological aspects in school-aged children from urban and rural villages with a high incidence of VL in 2005–07. However, the VL prevalence found in the study was very low [25], and no association was found between nutritional status and asymptomatic infection [24]. Therefore, we are confident that this limitation does not alter our general conclusions.

Conclusions

Our findings suggest that improving food availability is a necessary but not sufficient condition to improve the nutritional status of school-aged children in this region. Especially in rural areas, the challenge will be for health and development extension workers to build on this knowledge through educational campaigns when advising households about balanced diet, food production and consumption, and hygienic behavior. It is also important to emphasize that nutritional programs should not be biased towards rural areas at the cost of excluding the urban poor.

To effectively tackle malnutrition, nutritional programs should be oriented to the local needs. Our findings can be used to help policy makers plan and undertake regional initiatives to streamline recommendations.

Supporting Information

Table S1 Factors related to stunting in school-aged children by setting in Libokemkem and Fogera districts, Ethiopia, May–June 2009. Bivariate analysis.
(DOCX)

Table S2 Factors related to thinness in school-aged children by setting in Libokemkem and Fogera districts, Ethiopia, May–June 2009. Bivariate analysis.
(DOCX)

Acknowledgments

We thank the study participants for volunteering to participate in the study; the data collectors for performing field work; the Armauer Hansen Research Institute/All Africa Leprosy Rehabilitation and Training Center and the Fundación Española para la Cooperación Internacional, Salud y Política Social for providing logistic and technical support; the Amhara Regional State Laboratory for allowing us to use their laboratory facility and for creating a conducive environment during the field work.

Author Contributions

Conceived and designed the experiments: LS EG JM JN AA CC EC. Performed the experiments: ZH AB LS EG EC. Analyzed the data: ZH AB LS EC. Contributed reagents/materials/analysis tools: AB JM AA JN CC. Wrote the paper: ZH EC LS. Critically reviewed the manuscript: EG JM JN AB AA CC.

References

1. United Nations Children's Fund, World Health Organization, The World Bank (2012) UNICEF-WHO-World Bank Joint Child Malnutrition Estimates. UNICEF, New York; WHO, Geneva; The World Bank, Washington, DC; 2012. Available: http://www.who.int/nutgrowthdb/jme_unicef_who_wb.pdf. Accessed: 2013 Aug 19.
2. de Onis M, Blossner M, Borghi E (2012) Prevalence and trends of stunting among pre-school children, 1990–2020. Public Health Nutr 15: 142–148.
3. de Onis M, Onyango A, Borghi E, Siyam A, Blossner M, et al. (2012) Worldwide implementation of the WHO Child Growth Standards. Public Health Nutr 15: 1603–1610.
4. Ezzati M, Hoorn SV, Lopez AD, Danaei G, Rodgers A, et al. (2006) Comparative Quantification of Mortality and Burden of Disease Attributable to Selected Risk Factors. In: Lopez AD, Mathers CD, Ezzati M, et al., editors. Global Burden of Disease and Risk Factors. Washington (DC): World Bank; 2006. Chapter 4. Available: http://www.ncbi.nlm.nih.gov/books/NBK11813/. Accessed: 2013 Sep 1.
5. United Nations System Standing Committee on Nutrition (2010) Progress in Nutrition: 6th Report on the World Nutrition Situation (Geneva, Switzerland: UNSCN Secretariat, 2010), Available: www.unscn.org/files/Publications/RWNS6/report/SCN_report.pdf. Accessed: 2013 Aug 19.
6. United Nations Children's Fund (UNICEF) (1991) Strategy for improved nutrition of children and women in developing countries: a UNICEF policy review. New York, USA: 1991. Available: http://repository.forcedmigration.org/show_metadata.jsp?pid=fmo:3066. Accessed: 2013 Aug 19.
7. Owusu WB, Lartey A, de Onis M, Onyango AW, Frongillo EA (2004) Factors associated with unconstrained growth among affluent Ghanaian children. Acta Paediatr 93: 1115–1119.
8. Abubakar A, Uriyo J, Msuya SE, Swai M, Stray-Pedersen B (2012) Prevalence and risk factors for poor nutritional status among children in the Kilimanjaro region of Tanzania. Int J Environ Res Public Health 9: 3506–3518.
9. Engebretsen IM, Tylleskar T, Wamani H, Karamagi C, Tumwine JK (2008) Determinants of infant growth in Eastern Uganda: a community-based cross-sectional study. BMC Public Health 8: 418.
10. Van de Poel E, O'Donnell O, Van DE (2007) Are urban children really healthier? Evidence from 47 developing countries. Soc Sci Med 65: 1986–2003.
11. Central Statistical Agency [Ethiopia] and ICF International (2012) Ethiopia Demographic and Health Survey 2011. Addis Ababa, Ethiopia and Calverton, Maryland, USA: Central Statistical Agency and ICF International. Available: http://www.usaid.gov/sites/default/files/documents/1860/Demographic%20Health%20Survey%202011%20Ethiopia%20Final%20Report.pdf. Accessed: 2013 Aug 20.
12. Demissie T, Ali A, Mekonnen Y, Haider J, Umeta M (2009) Demographic and health-related risk factors of subclinical vitamin A deficiency in Ethiopia. J Health Popul Nutr 27: 666–673.
13. Woldehanna T, Mekonnen A, Alemu T (2008) Young Lives: Ethiopia Round 2 Survey Report. University of Oxford, UK; 2008. Available: http://www.younglives.org.uk/files/country-reports/country-report-ethiopia-2008. Accessed: 2013 Aug 23.
14. Fotso JC (2006) Child health inequities in developing countries: differences across urban and rural areas. Int J Equity Health 5: 9.
15. Frank E (1999) Gender, Agricultural Development and Food Security in Amhara, Ethiopia: The Contested Identity of Women Farmers in Ethiopia. Agency for International Development, Washington, DC. Available: http://pdf.usaid.gov/pdf_docs/pnacg552.pdf. Accessed: 2013 Aug 23.
16. Tools for Food Security and Nutrition Analysis, Household Economy Approach and Cost of the Diet (2007) Livelihood Profile Amhara Region, Ethiopia. Tana Zuria Livelihood Zone (TZA). Available: http://www.heawebsite.org/countries/ethiopia/reports/hea-lz-profile-tana-zuria-livelihood-zone-tza-amhara-region-ethiopia-2007. Accessed: 2013 Aug 23.
17. Belachew T, Lindstrom D, Gebremariam A, Hogan D, Lachat C, et al. (2013) Food insecurity, food based coping strategies and suboptimal dietary practices of adolescents in Jimma zone Southwest Ethiopia. PLoS One 8 [2]: e57643.
18. Food and Agriculture Organization of the United Nations (FAO) (2009) Declaration of the World Summit on Food Security. Rome, Italy; 16–18 November 2009. Available: http://www.fao.org/fileadmin/templates/wsfs/Summit/Docs/Final_Declaration/WSFS09_Declaration.pdf. Accessed: 2013 Aug 20.
19. USAID Collaborative Research Support Programs Team (2000) Amhara National Regional State Food Security- Research Assessment Report. Available: http://www.ctahr.hawaii.edu/sm-crsp/phase1/pdf/amhara.pdf. Accessed 2013 Sep 1.
20. International Food Policy Research Institute (2005) An assessment of the causes of malnutrition in Ethiopia. A contribution to the formulation of a National Nutrition Strategy for Ethiopia. Washington, DC, USA Available: http://www.ifpri.org/sites/default/files/publications/ethionutrition.pdf. Accessed: 2013 Sep 1.
21. Food and Agriculture Organization of the United Nations and Food and Nutrition Technical Assistance Project (2008) Guidelines for Measuring Household and Individual Dietary Diversity. FAO, Rome, Italy; Reprinted 2013..Available: http://www.fao.org/docrep/014/i1983e/i1983e00.pdf. Accessed 2013 Sep 2.
22. Lyons S, Veeken H, Long J (2003) Visceral leishmaniasis and HIV in Tigray, Ethiopia. Trop Med Int Health 8: 733–739.
23. Amati L, Cirimele D, Pugliese V, Covelli V, Resta F, et al. (2003) Nutrition and immunity: laboratory and clinical aspects. Curr Pharm Des 9: 1924–1931.
24. Custodio E, Gadisa E, Sordo L, Cruz I, Moreno J, et al. (2012) Factors associated with Leishmania asymptomatic infection: results from a cross-sectional survey in highland northern Ethiopia. PLoS Negl Trop Dis 6: e1813.
25. Sordo L, Gadisa E, Custodio E, Cruz I, Simon F, et al. (2012) Low prevalence of Leishmania infection in post-epidemic areas of Libo Kemkem, Ethiopia. Am J Trop Med Hyg 86: 955–958.
26. Gadisa E, Custodio E, Canavate C, Sordo L, Abebe Z, et al. (2012) Usefulness of the rK39-immunochromatographic test, direct agglutination test, and leishmanin skin test for detecting asymptomatic Leishmania infection in children in a new visceral leishmaniasis focus in Amhara State, Ethiopia. Am J Trop Med Hyg 86: 792–798.
27. World Health Organization Working Group (1986) Use and interpretation of anthropometric indicators of nutritional status. Bull World Health Organ 64: 929–941.
28. de Onis M, Garza C, Victora CG, Onyango AW, Frongillo EA, et al. (2004) The WHO Multicentre Growth Reference Study: planning, study design, and methodology. Food Nutr Bull 25: S15–S26.
29. Food and Agriculture Organization of the United Nations (FAO) (2010) Assessment of Nutritional Status in Urban Areas. Available: http://www.fao.org/ag/agn/nutrition/urban_assessment_en.stm. Accessed: 2013 Sep 2.
30. Girma W, Genebo T (2002) Determinants of Nutritional Status of Women and Children in Ethiopia. ORC Macro, Calverton, Maryland, USA. Available: http://dhsprogram.com/pubs/pdf/FA39/02-nutrition.pdf. Accessed: 2013 Sep 2.
31. World Health Organization (WHO) (2006) The African Regional Health Report. WHO, Geneva, Switzerland; 2007. Available: http://www.who.int/mediacentre/news/releases/2006/pr68/en/. Accessed: 2013 Sep 2.
32. Ricci JA, Becker S (1996) Risk factors for wasting and stunting among children in Metro Cebu, Philippines. Am J Clin Nutr 63: 966–975.
33. Mekonnen H, Tadesse T, Kisi T (2013) Malnutrition and its Correlates among Rural Primary School Children of Fogera District, Northwest Ethiopia. J NutrDisorders Ther S12: 002.
34. Custodio E, Descalzo MA, Villamor E, Molina L, Sanchez I, et al. (2009) Nutritional and socio-economic factors associated with Plasmodium falciparum infection in children from Equatorial Guinea: results from a nationally representative survey. Malar J 8: 225.
35. Katona P, Katona-Apte J (2008) The interaction between nutrition and infection. Clin Infect Dis 46: 1582–1588.
36. Ayele DG, Zewotir TT, Mwambi HG (2012) Prevalence and risk factors of malaria in Ethiopia. Malar J 11: 195.
37. Amare B, Ali J, Moges B, Yismaw G, Belyhun Y, et al. (2013) Nutritional status, intestinal parasite infection and allergy among school children in Northwest Ethiopia. BMC Pediatr 13: 7.
38. Mahmud MA, Spigt M, Mulugeta BA, Lopez P, Dinant GJ, et al. (2013) Risk factors for intestinal parasitosis, anaemia, and malnutrition among school children in Ethiopia. Pathog Glob Health 107: 58–65.
39. Ehrhardt S, Burchard GD, Mantel C, Cramer JP, Kaiser S, et al. (2006) Malaria, anemia, and malnutrition in african children–defining intervention priorities. J Infect Dis 194: 108–114.
40. Black RE, Victora CG, Walker SP, Bhutta ZA, Christian P, et al. (2013) Maternal and child undernutrition and overweight in low-income and middle-income countries. Lancet 382: 427–451.
41. Mekonnen A, Jones N, Tefera B (2005) Tackling child malnutrition in Ethiopia: do the Sustainable development poverty reduction programme's underlying policy assumptions reflect local realities? Young Lives-Save the Children Working Paper 19, London, UK. Available: http://www.younglives.org.uk/

files/working-papers/wp19-tackling-child-malnutrition-in-ethiopia-do-the-sustainable-development-poverty-reduction-programme2019s-underlying-policy-assumptions-reflect-local-realities. Accessed: 2013 Sept 7.
42. Dorosh P, Schmidt E (2010) The Rural-Urban Transformation in Ethiopia. Development Strategy and Governance Division, International Food Policy Research Institute.. Working Paper 13. Addis Ababa, Ethiopia; Washington, DC, USA; 2010. Available: http://www.ifpri.org/sites/default/files/publications/esspwp013.pdf. Accessed 2013 Sep 7.
43. Coates J, Swindale A, Bilinsky P (2007) Household Food Insecurity Access Scale (HFIAS) for Measurement of Food Access: Indicator Guide. Food and Nutrition Technical Assistance Project (FANTA). USAID, Washington, DC, USA; August 2007. Available: http://www.fao.org/fileadmin/user_upload/eufao-fsi4dm/doc-training/hfias.pdf. Accessed: 2013 Sep 7.
44. Filmer D, Friedman J, Schady N (2009) Development, Modernization, and Childbearing: The Role of Family Sex Composition. World Bank Econ Rev 23: 371–398.
45. Ayele Z, Peacock C (2003) Improving access to and consumption of animal source foods in rural households: the experiences of a women-focused goat development program in the highlands of Ethiopia. J Nutr 133: 3981S–3986S.
46. Glewwe P (2005) The impact of child health and nutrition on education in developing countries: theory, econometric issues, and recent empirical evidence. Food Nutr Bull 26: S235–S250.
47. Abuya BA, Onsomu EO, Kimani JK, Moore D (2011) Influence of maternal education on child immunization and stunting in Kenya. Matern Child Health J 15: 1389–1399.
48. Inter-agency Standing Committee (IASC) (2006) Women, Girls, Boys and Men. Different Needs. Equal Opportunities. Gender Handbook in Humanitarian Action. IASC, December 2006. Available: http://www.humanitarianinfo.org/iasc/gender. Accessed: 2013 Sep 8.
49. Haidar J, Kogi-Makau W (2009) Gender differences in the household-headship and nutritional status of pre-school children. East Afr Med J 86: 69–73.
50. Woldehann T, Tefera B, Jones N, Bayrau A (2005) Child labour, gender inequality and rural/urban disparities: how can Ethiopia national development strategies best address negative spill-over impacts on child education and well-being?. Young Lives-Save the Children Working Paper No 20; Addis Ababa, Ethiopia; London, UK. Available: http://r4d.dfid.gov.uk/PDF/Outputs/YoungLives/wp20-execsummary.pdf. Accessed: 2013 Oct 8.
51. Siddiqi A, Irwin LG, Hertzman C (2007) Early child development: a powerful equalizer. Final Report for the World Health Organization's Commission on the Social Determinants of Health. WHO, Geneva, Switzerland, June 2007. Available: http://www.who.int/social_determinants/resources/ecd_kn_report_07_2007.pdf. Accessed: 2013 OCt 8.

The Immune System in Children with Malnutrition

Maren Johanne Heilskov Rytter[1]*, Lilian Kolte[2], André Briend[1,3], Henrik Friis[1], Vibeke Brix Christensen[4]

1 Department of Nutrition, Exercise and Sports, Faculty of Science, University of Copenhagen, Frederiksberg, Denmark, **2** Department of Infectious Diseases, Copenhagen University Hospital, Hvidovre, Denmark, **3** Department for International Health, University of Tampere, School of Medicine, Tampere, Finland, **4** Department of Paediatrics, Copenhagen University Hospital Rigshospitalet, Copenhagen, Denmark

Abstract

Background: Malnourished children have increased risk of dying, with most deaths caused by infectious diseases. One mechanism behind this may be impaired immune function. However, this immune deficiency of malnutrition has not previously been systematically reviewed.

Objectives: To review the scientific literature about immune function in children with malnutrition.

Methods: A systematic literature search was done in PubMed, and additional articles identified in reference lists and by correspondence with experts in the field. The inclusion criteria were studies investigating immune parameters in children aged 1–60 months, in relation to malnutrition, defined as wasting, underweight, stunting, or oedematous malnutrition.

Results: The literature search yielded 3402 articles, of which 245 met the inclusion criteria. Most were published between 1970 and 1990, and only 33 after 2003. Malnutrition is associated with impaired gut-barrier function, reduced exocrine secretion of protective substances, and low levels of plasma complement. Lymphatic tissue, particularly the thymus, undergoes atrophy, and delayed-type hypersensitivity responses are reduced. Levels of antibodies produced after vaccination are reduced in severely malnourished children, but intact in moderate malnutrition. Cytokine patterns are skewed towards a Th2-response. Other immune parameters seem intact or elevated: leukocyte and lymphocyte counts are unaffected, and levels of immunoglobulins, particularly immunoglobulin A, are high. The acute phase response appears intact, and sometimes present in the absence of clinical infection. Limitations to the studies include their observational and often cross-sectional design and frequent confounding by infections in the children studied.

Conclusion: The immunological alterations associated with malnutrition in children may contribute to increased mortality. However, the underlying mechanisms are still inadequately understood, as well as why different types of malnutrition are associated with different immunological alterations. Better designed prospective studies are needed, based on current understanding of immunology and with state-of-the-art methods.

Editor: Taishin Akiyama, University of Tokyo, Japan

Funding: The work was supported by a PhD grant from University of Copenhagen. The funders had no role in study design, data collection and analysis, decision to publish, or preparation of the manuscript.

Competing Interests: The authors have declared that no competing interests exist.

* Email: marenrytter@hotmail.com

Introduction

Malnutrition in children is a global public health problem with wide implications. Malnourished children have increased risk of dying from infectious diseases, and it is estimated that malnutrition is the underlying cause of 45% of global deaths in children below 5 years of age [1–2]. The association between malnutrition and infections may in part be due to confounding by poverty, a determinant of both, but also possibly due to a two-way causal relationship (**Figure 1**): malnutrition increases susceptibility to infections while infections aggravate malnutrition by decreasing appetite, inducing catabolism, and increasing demand for nutrients [3]. Although it has been debated whether malnutrition increases incidence of infections, or whether it only increases severity of disease [3], solid data indicates that malnourished children are at higher risk of dying once infected [2–4]. The increased susceptibility to infections may in part be caused by impairment of immune function by malnutrition [5]. The objective of this study was to investigate the associations of different types of malnutrition with immune parameters in children, through a systematic review of the literature.

Since most infections and deaths in malnourished children occur in low-income settings, the organisms causing disease are rarely identified. Therefore, little is known about whether these differ from pathogens infecting well-nourished children, and whether malnourished children are susceptible to opportunistic

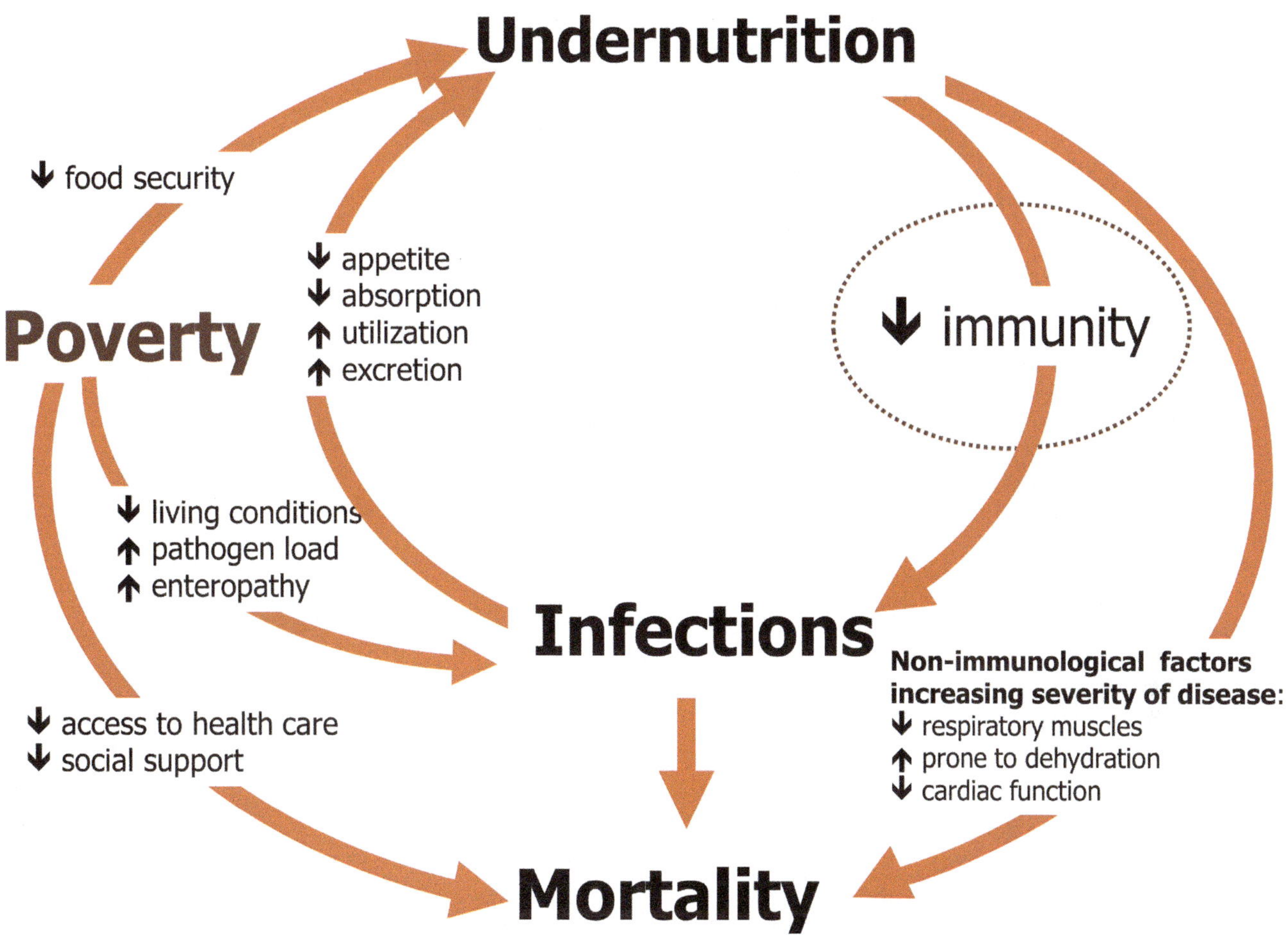

Figure 1. Conceptual framework on the relationship between malnutrition, infections and poverty.

infections. Although opportunistic infections like *Pneumocystis jirovecii* and severe varicella has been reported in malnourished children [6–7], these studies were carried out before the discovery of HIV, and may represent cases of un-diagnosed paediatric AIDS. More recent studies have found that *Pneumocystis jirovecii* pneumonia is not frequent in malnourished children not infected with HIV [8]. However, quasi-opportunistic pathogens like cryptosporidium and yeast are frequent causes of diarrhoea in malnourished children [9], and malnourished children have a higher risk of invasive bacterial infections, causing bacterial pneumonia [8], bacterial diarrhoea [10–11], and bacteraemia [12–14], with a predominance of gram negative bacteria. Due to the high prevalence of invasive bacterial infections, current guidelines recommend antibiotic treatment to all children with severe acute malnutrition, even though the evidence behind is not very strong [14].

Non-immunological factors may also contribute to increased mortality in malnourished children: reduced muscle mass may impair respiratory work with lung infections [15]; reduced electrolyte absorption from the gut [16] and impaired renal concentration capacity may increase susceptibility to dehydration from diarrhoea [5]; and diminished cardiac function may increase risk of cardiac failure [17]. Thus, immune function may only be one of several links between malnutrition, infections and increased mortality, but most likely an important one.

Definitions of malnutrition

This review considers childhood malnutrition in the sense of under-nutrition, causing growth failure or weight loss, or severe acute malnutrition, either oedematous, or non-oedematous.

Growth failure caused by malnutrition has commonly been defined by low weight-for-age (underweight), length-for-age (stunting), or weight-for-length (wasting) [5]. Generally, older studies diagnosed malnutrition using weight-for-age, while newer studies tend to use weight-for-length. Recently, mid-upper arm circumference (MUAC) has been promoted to diagnose severe acute malnutrition, because of its feasibility and because it predicts mortality risk better than other anthropometric indices [18]. Other definitions of malnutrition include specific micronutrient deficiencies, intra-uterine growth restriction, and obesity, but these conditions are outside the scope of this review.

Severe Acute Malnutrition

Two forms of severe acute malnutrition in children exist: non-oedematous malnutrition, also known as marasmus, characterized by severe wasting and currently defined by weight-for-length z-score <-3 of the WHO growth standard, or MUAC $<11{,}5$ cm; and oedematous malnutrition defined by bilateral pitting oedema (**Figure 2**) [19]. Kwashiorkor refers to a form of oedematous malnutrition, the fulminant syndrome including enlarged fatty liver, mental changes as well as skin and hair changes [20]. The term "marasmic kwashiorkor", has been used to describe children

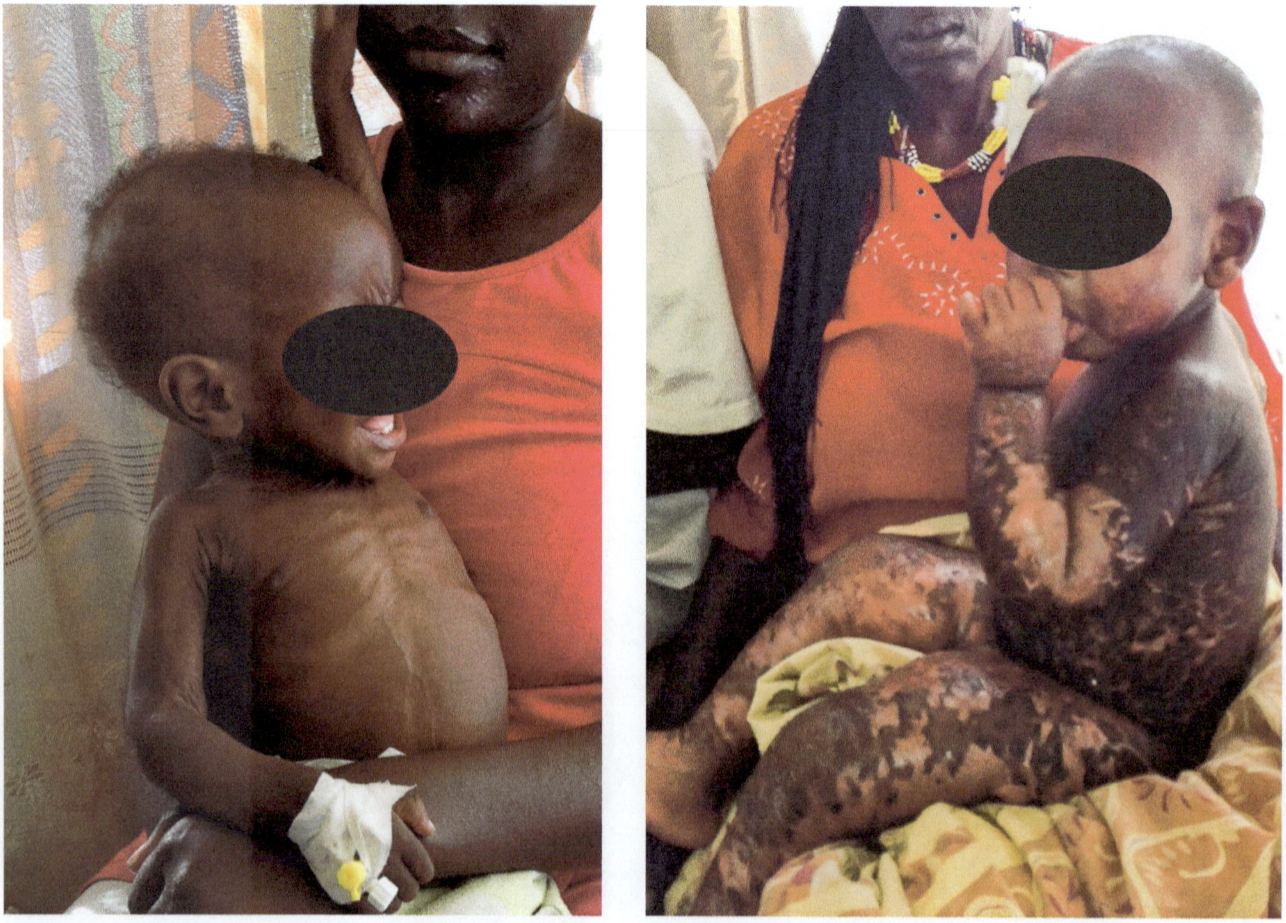

Figure 2. Clinical picture: two forms of severe acute malnutrition, oedematous and non-oedematous malnutrition.

with both wasting and oedema [21]. It is still unknown why some children develop oedematous malnutrition, and unclear whether this form of malnutrition is associated with a different degree of immune deficiency.

Materials and Methods

A systematic literature search was carried out in PubMed using combinations of the search terms related to malnutrition and immune parameters. The full search strategy and the search terms used are described in **Figure 3**.

Inclusion criteria were: studies presenting original clinical data regarding immune parameters in children, aged 1–60 months, where a comparison was made, either between malnourished and well-nourished children, or between malnourished children before and after nutritional rehabilitation. Exclusion criteria were studies of children with another primary diagnosis such as cancer, congenital heart disease or endocrine disease. Studies were accepted where children had co-morbid infections, since this is typically seen in malnourished children. Articles by RK Chandra were excluded, due to concerns about possible fraud [22]. Studies published in peer-reviewed scientific journals, as well as in books were included. Only articles in English were included.

The search was carried out in August 2013, and updated in December 2013. The search results were sorted by MJHR, based on titles, abstracts or full-text-articles. Additional literature was obtained from reference lists, text books and by personal communication with experts.

For data retrieval, studies were sorted according to whether they investigated barrier function (skin and gut), innate immunity or acquired immune system, and listed in tables based on the specific immune parameter studied. Some studies were included in more than one table. The following data was extracted from each article: year and country, number and age range of malnourished and well-nourished participants, type of malnutrition and whether included children fulfilled WHOs current diagnostic criteria for severe acute malnutrition, whether infections were present, immune parameter studied, methods used, how the parameter was associated with malnutrition, and whether children with oedematous and non-oedematous malnutrition were differentially affected.

The results of the included articles were summarized for each immune parameter. Due to the heterogeneous nature of study designs, participants and outcomes, it was not meaningful to synthesize the results in a meta-analysis. The main potential bias was presence of infection. For this reason, presence and effect of infection was considered for each study as well as for each outcome. The PRISMA (Preferred Reporting Items for Systematic Reviews and Meta-Analyses) guideline was followed, except for the items relating to meta-analysis (**Checklist S1**).

Search terms:

"malnutrition" OR "undernutrition" OR "marasmus" OR "kwashiorkor" OR "wasting" OR "stunting" OR "underweight"

AND

"immune" OR "antibodies" OR "thymus" OR "lymphatic" OR "delayed-type hypersensitivity" OR "leucocytes" OR "lymphocyte" OR "activation" OR "B-cell" OR "T-cell" OR "complement" OR "humoral" OR "cytokine" OR "chemotaxis"OR "acute phase response" OR "phagocytosis" OR "flow cytometry" OR "enteropathy" OR "barrier" OR "intestinal permeability" OR "microbiota" .

Filters: human studies, children from 0-18 years, and publications in English.

Figure 3. Full search strategy in PubMed, including search terms and filters.

Results

The search in PubMed yielded 3402 articles. By contacting experts in the field, an additional 631 papers were obtained. Reference list of all papers read were screened for relevant papers not included in the initial search. Of all the screened papers, 245 met the inclusion criteria (**Figure S1**). Another 49 articles were identified which, in addition to children 1–60 months old, also included older children. These studies were not included in the main analysis, but used in a sensitivity analysis in which all studies were included. The result of this additional analysis was essentially similar to the results obtained with studies only including children less than 60 month (results not shown). The studies were published between 1957–2014, mainly in the 1970s and 1980s. Only 33 studies were published after 2003 (**Figure 4**). The studies included 29 prospective studies that compared malnourished children to themselves after nutritional recovery, and 216 cross-sectional studies. Of the cross-sectional studies, 51 were community-based, comparing immune parameters in children according to nutritional status. The remaining 165 cross-sectional studies compared hospitalised malnourished children to well-nourished children, often recruited outside the hospital. In 53 studies, all children fulfilled WHOs diagnostic criteria for severe acute malnutrition [23]. The vast majority of these studies included children with oedematous malnutrition, while only two studies included children with non-oedematous malnutrition based on the new WHO growth standard.

The results of each immune parameter are summarized in **Table 1**, and the results of individual articles are summarized in **Tables S1–14**.

Epithelial barrier function

The barrier function of the skin and mucosal surfaces is considered the first-line defence of the immune system, upheld by the physical integrity of the epithelia, anti-microbial factors in secretions (e.g. lysozyme, secretory IgA and gastric acidity) and the commensal bacterial flora [24].

Of the articles describing barrier function in malnourished children, six described skin structure and function, 21 described structure and permeability of intestinal mucosa, 19 protective factors in secretions and 11 the microbial flora colonizing mucosal surfaces.

Skin. *Skin barrier* has mostly been studied in children with oedematous malnutrition, who may develop a characteristic dermatosis, characterized by hyper-pigmentation, cracking and scaling of the epidermis, resembling "peeling paint", providing a potential entry port for pathogens [25].

Six articles assessed barrier and immune function of the skin in malnourished children (**table S1**). Two articles describing histology reported atrophy of skin layers, but did not describe cutaneous immune cells [26–27]. Four articles described the "cutaneous inflammatory response": They made small abrasions in the skin, and placed microscopy slides over the sites. Similar or higher numbers of white blood cells migrated onto slides in malnourished children, predominantly granulocytes and a lower proportion of monocytes and macrophages [28–31]. This pattern was noted to resemble a neonatal immature immune response [30]. All four articles found this pattern in patients with oedematous malnutrition, while one study found that the response of non-oedematous children resembled that of well-nourished [30].

Structure and function of the intestinal mucosa. The intestinal mucosa of malnourished children was described in 21 articles (**table S2**). Autopsy-studies from as early as 1965 described a thin-walled intestine in malnourished children, and noted that "… the *tissue paper intestine* of kwashiorkor is well known to tropical pathologists." [32]. Small-intestinal biopsies showed thinning of the mucosa [33–36], decrease in villous height [37–43], altered villous morphology [32] [40] [44] and infiltration of lymphocytes [32] [34–38]. Electron-microscopy studies found sparse brush border with shortened microvilli and sparse endoplasmatic reticulum [42]. Others found increased intestinal permeability to lactulose [45–48]. Such an intestine may predispose to bacterial translocation, and likewise, one of the included articles described high levels of lipopolysaccharide in the blood of malnourished children, probably originating from gut bacteria translocating into the bloodstream [49]. However, the mucosal atrophy and functional changes did not only occur in malnourished children. Although sometimes found to be most severe in malnourished children [33] [35–36] [46–47], similar

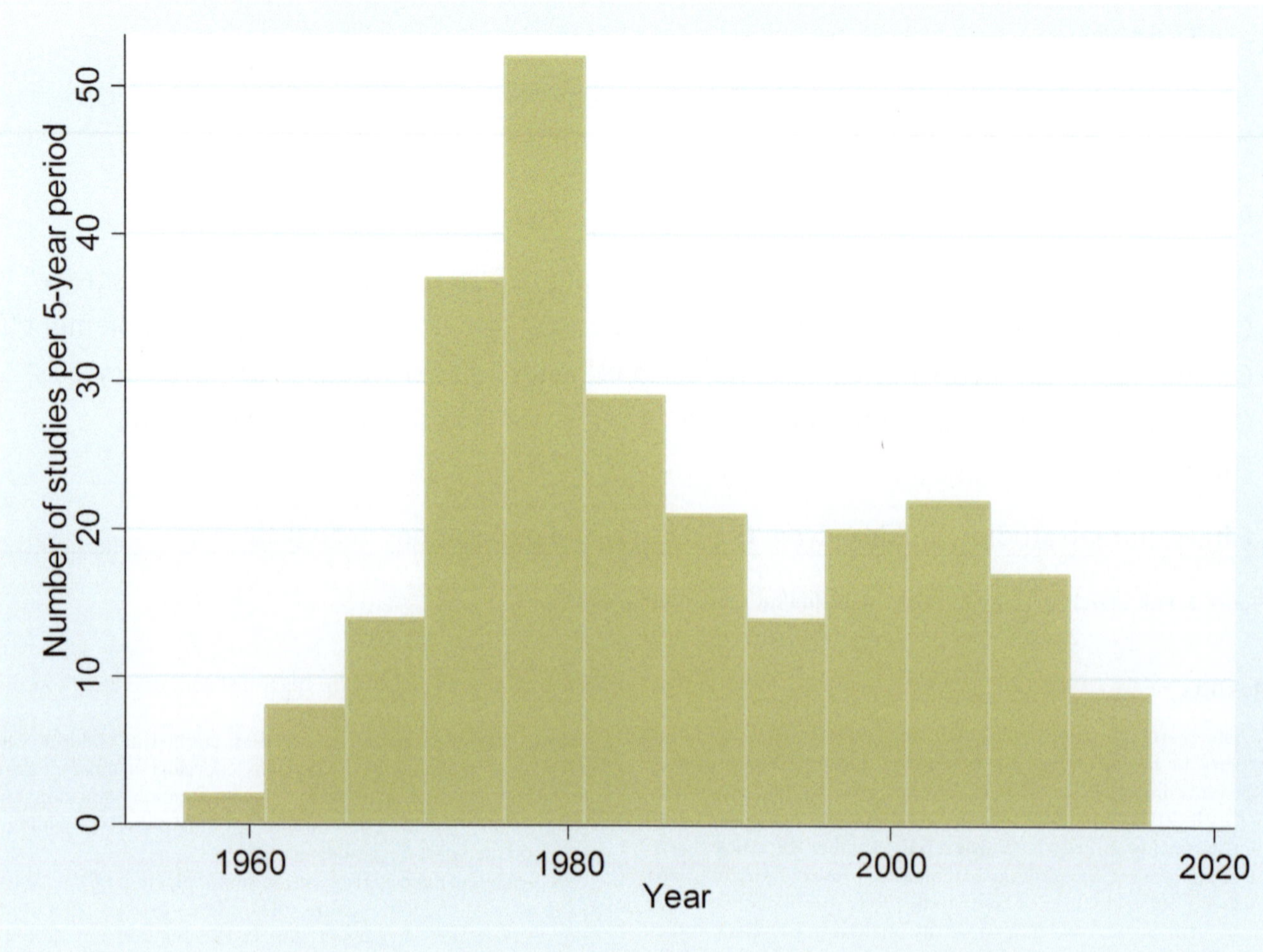

Figure 4. Number of studies published per 5-year period about immune function in malnourished children.

abnormalities were present in apparently well-nourished children from the same environment [38–40] [43] [50], and frequently persisted after nutritional recovery [34] [37] [51].

Two articles described immune cells in small intestinal biopsies from malnourished children in Gambia and Zambia: both reported increased lymphocyte infiltration, more T-cells, and cells expressing HLA-DR in malnourished children compared to English children [37–38]. However, it was similar to Gambian well-nourished children [38], and unaltered by nutritional recovery [37]. Both well-nourished and malnourished Gambian children had high levels of intestinal cytokine expression, but malnourished children had an increased ratio of cells expression pro-inflammatory to regulatory cytokines, compared to the well-nourished Gambian children [38].

The colon was only described in one article, reporting increased vascularity, atrophy of the mucosa and a tendency to rectal prolapse in children with oedematous malnutrition [52].

Four articles compared the intestine of children with oedematous and non-oedematous malnutrition: one study from South Africa found that the histological changes were most severe in those with oedema [40]. Two articles from Chile found that children with non-oedematous malnutrition had a thinner mucosa, whereas children with oedema had more villous atrophy and more cellular infiltration [35–36]. In contrast, a more recent study from Zambia found higher numbers of T-cells and cells expressing HLA-DR in the intestines of children with non-oedematous than oedematous malnutrition, while the intestines of oedematous children were deficient in sulphated glycosaminoglycan [37].

Antimicrobial factors in mucosal secretions. Nineteen articles were published on anti-microbial factors in secretions from malnourished children (**table S3**). Secretory IgA (sIgA) was investigated in 15 studies, of which 11 investigated saliva, urine, tears, nasal washings and duodenal fluid [53–63] and three investigated small intestinal biopsies [39–40] [64].

SIgA in saliva, tears and nasal washings was frequently reduced in severely malnourished children [54–55] [57–58]. One article from Egypt reported increased levels in children with oedematous malnutrition [56], but may have overestimated sIgA, since saliva flow was reduced in malnourished children, and sIgA was expressed as g/l, whereas other articles expressed it as sIgA as % of protein content. Studies of sIgA in duodenal fluid showed conflicting results [57] [59], as did studies quantifying sIgA in small intestinal biopsies [39–40] [64]. The sIgA content of urine was increased or normal in severely malnourished children [60–61]. In mild to moderately underweight children, inconsistent results were found for sIgA in tears [63] and saliva [53–54] [62–63].

Tear lysozyme content was found to be reduced in malnourished children [54] [63], while saliva lysozyme was unaffected [53–54]. Gastric acid secretion was consistently reduced in severely

Table 1. Summary of results in studies of each immune parameter.

Immune parameter	Number of studies	Period	In children with severe malnutrition?	In children with moderate malnutrition?	Different in OM compared to NOM?	Comments	Listed in table
Skin	6	1968–1989	- Atrophy - Cells in skin abrasions: ↑ GRAN, ↓ monocytes	Not assessed	Cells in abrasions only affected in OM		S1
Gut function	21	1965–2013	Thin mucosa, shorter villi, infiltration of immune cells. Increased intestinal permeability.	No linear relationship	↕	Also in well-nourished children	S2
Factors in secretions	19	1968–2012	sIgA in saliva, tears, nasal washings: ↓ in duodenal fluids: ↕, in urine: 0 Lysozyme: ↕. Gastric juice and acidity: ↓	↕	Saliva flow ↓ in OM; sIgA ↑ in OM		S3
Microbial flora	11	1972–2014	Different pattern of stool micro-biota; bacterial growth in small intestine; ↑ yeast and g. neg. bact.	↑ yeast in mouth	Not assessed		S4
White blood cells	38	1964–2009	Leukocytes in blood: 0; Microbicidal activity ↓, Chemotaxis ↓; Phagocytosis: ↕.	Leukocytes in blood: 0; NK cells: 0	Bactericidal activity ↓ in OM		S5
Acute phase	24	1970–2006	Positive APP ↑, negative APP ↓ with infection, sometimes also without clinical infection	Few studies	↕		S6
Complement	24	1973–2011	C3, C6, C1, C9, Factor B: ↓; C5, C activity: ↕; C4: 0	Not affected	All parameters ↓ in OM	Signs of in-vivo consumption in OM	S7
Lymphatic tissue	12	1956–2009	Thymic atrophy. Fewer lymphocytes in thymus cortex. Less atrophy of other lymphatic tissue.	Linear relationship of thymus size with nutritional status	↕	Also ↓ by infections and zinc deficiency	S8 and S9
DTHR	21	1965–2092	Mantoux after BCG vaccination: ↓; Reaction to other antigens: ↓	: ↕;	↕	Also ↓ by infections and zinc deficiency	S10
Lymphocytes	58	1971–2009	Total lymphocytes 0; T-cells: 0/↑; CD4 count: 0/↑; B-cells: ↓; Response to PHA: ↓	Not affected	CD4 count ↑ in OM	Conflicting result by flow cytometry older methods	S11
Antibody levels	32	1962–2008	IgG: 0; IgM: 0; IgA: ↑; IgE: ↕; IgD: ↑ in OM, ↕ in NOM	Not affected	IgA and IgD ↑ in OM		S12
Vaccination response	35	1957–2009	Antibody titre: ↓; Most acceptable sero-conversion; Possibly delay in antibody response	Antibody titre: 0; Sero-conversion: 0	Titres: ↓ in OM		S13
Cytokines	35	1975–2013	Th1-cytokines: IL1. Il2, IL12, IFN-γ: ↓; Th2 cytokines: IL10, IL14: ↑; Inflammatory cytokines (IL6, TNFα): ↕	Few studies: Same pattern as severe malnutrition	Th2-response ↑, IL6 ↑ in OM; Altered leukotrienes		S14

Legend: ↑ = higher in malnourished than well-nourished, ↓ = lower in malnourished than well-nourished, 0 = similar in malnourished and well-nourished; ↕ = inconsistent results; OM = Oedematous malnutrition, NOM = Non-oedematous malnutrition, GRAN = Granulocytes (Polymorph nuclear cells); sIgA = secretory immunoglobulin A; NK = Natural killer; APP = Acute phase protein; C = Complement component, BCG = Bacille Calmette-Guérin, PHA: phyto-hemaglutinin; Ig = immunoglobulin; IL = Interleukin; IFNγ = Interferon-gamma; TNFα = Tumour-necrosis-factor-alpha.

malnourished children [65–68], and higher pH was associated with bacterial colonization of the stomach [65].

Microbial colonization. Microbes colonizing skin and mucosa may protect against infections by competing with pathogens, by producing specific antimicrobial substances, and by stimulating host immune function [69]. Despite much recent interest in the subject, of 11 articles describing the micro-flora in malnourished children, only four were published during the last ten years (**table S4**). All found malnourished children to host a different flora from well-nourished children. Their mouths and throats contained more yeast [70–72], and their stomach and duodenum, which in healthy children is considered to be almost sterile, contained a large number of microorganisms [72–75]. Although one study found similar degree of small intestinal bacterial overgrowth in diarrhoeal patients with and without malnutrition [75], another found more small intestinal bacteria in malnourished than in well-nourished children with diarrhoea [72]. While gram positive cocci predominated in the small intestine of well-nourished children, malnourished children hosted more gram negative bacteria [65] and yeast [74].

The colonic flora, containing the vast majority of commensal bacteria, was described by sequencing bacterial DNA from stool samples in four recent articles, which consistently found that the pattern of bacteria was different in malnourished and well-nourished children [76–79]. More bacteria with pathogenic potential were found in the malnourished children [77–78], and their flora was less mature [79] and less diverse [76] [78]. A twin study from Malawi suggested that micro-flora pattern could also play a role in developing malnutrition [76]. No articles have so far reported whether the intestinal flora is different in children with oedematous and non-oedematous malnutrition.

Innate immune system

The innate immune system delivers an unspecific response relying on leukocytes (like granulocytes, monocytes and macrophages), as well as soluble factors in blood (like acute phase proteins and the complement system) [24]. Of the articles describing innate immune response, 38 described number and function of leucocytes, 25 acute phase proteins and 24 complement components and activity.

White blood cells of the innate immune system. Thirty-eight articles described number and function of leukocytes of the innate immune system (**table S5**). Most reported similar or higher numbers of total leukocytes in blood of malnourished children [49] [80–92], and three found that granulocytes were higher in malnourished children [81] [86] [93].

Two studies from Nigeria and one from Ghana found no difference in the mean percentage of natural-killer-cells among malnourished or well-nourished children [94–96], although two reported that more malnourished children had abnormally low numbers of natural-killer cells. In Zambia, levels of dendritic cells were lower in blood from malnourished children before nutritional rehabilitation than after, and elevated inflammation markers were associated with a paradoxical lower level of dendritic cell activation. This was associated with endotoxin levels in the blood, and was interpreted as a type of immune-paralysis, related to inflammation and bacterial translocation [49]. Unfortunately, it was not assessed whether this was different from well-nourished children with severe infections.

Chemotaxis of granulocytes was reduced in malnourished children in three of five studies [80] [83] [97–99], and one study found a diminished ability to adhere to foreign material [100]. Results for phagocytosis were mixed: five of 12 studies found that leukocytes of malnourished children had reduced ability to ingest particles or bacteria [81] [83] [88–89] [97–98] [101–106]. Microbicidal activity of granulocytes was reduced in malnourished children in five of seven studies [80] [83] [88] [97–98] [103] [107], while two of three studies found macrophages from malnourished children to have normal microbicidal activity [89] [108–109]. Neutrophils may kill microorganisms by producing reactive oxygen compounds; assessable by the Nitroblue Tetrazolenium (NBT) test, which, however, gave inconsistent results in malnourished children [83] [105] [110–114]. It has been hypothesized, that reactive oxygen production is involved in the pathogenesis of oedematous malnutrition [115]; however, the NBT test results did not show any clear pattern in children with oedematous compared to non-oedematous malnutrition.

One study found the levels of enzymes, like alkaline and acid phosphatase, to be increased in leukocytes from children with malnutrition [116]. More leukocytes of malnourished children were found to have markers of apoptosis (CD95) [92], and signs of DNA damage [117–118].

No articles have yet described the expression of pattern-recognition molecules, like Toll-like receptors in malnourished children, although these are fundamental to the function of the innate immune system.

Acute phase response. Acute phase responses is induced by infection or trauma, and mediated by cytokines like IL-6 and TNF-α. It involve temporal suppression of acquired, and amplification of innate immune responses, with secretion of positive acute phase proteins (APP) like C-reactive protein (CRP), serum-amyloid-A (SAA), complement factors, α-1-acid-glycoprotein or ferritin [119], while levels of other proteins are reduced, as albumin, pre-albumin, transferrin, α -2-HS-glycoprotein, and α -fetoprotein. These are sometimes called 'negative acute phase proteins', although it is not clear whether their reduced level are due to active down-regulation, or because of competition with production of positive acute phase proteins. Twenty-four articles described the levels of acute phase proteins in malnourished children with or without infection (**table S6**).

Acute phase response in children with infections. Most studies found elevated positive APP in malnourished children with infections. This included CRP [120–128], α-1 acid-glycoprotein [120–121] [129], haptoglobin [120–121] [125] [127] [129] while the results for ceruloplasmin [125] [130], and α-1-antitrysin were inconsistent [120–121] [125] [127–129]. Only one study found lower CRP levels in malnourished than well-nourished children with similar infections, despite higher levels of IL-6 [129]. So-called negative APP were uniformly low in children with malnutrition and infection, including transferrin [94] [127] [130–133], α-2-HS-glycoprotein [134–136], pre-albumin [122], fibronectin [132], and α-2-macroglobulin[127].

Acute phase response in children without infections. Three studies found elevated CRP in malnourished children without apparent infections [94] [124] [128], while two studies found similar CRP-levels in malnourished and well-nourished children [122] [137]. Results for α-1-antitrysin were inconsistent [128]. So-called negative acute phase proteins like transferrin [94] [130], α-2-HS-glycoprotein [135], fibronectin [133] [138] and pre-albumin [122] [138–139] were consistently reduced in malnourished children, even without infections.

Acute phase response to a controlled stressor. Four articles described the acute phase response induced by a vaccine. Two reported a normal [140] or increased [141] febrile response to measles vaccine in malnourished children. In another study, a similar rise in APP was seen in malnourished and well-nourished children [137], in response to a diphtheria-pertussis-tetanus-vaccination, but the increase in APP was greater when the vaccination was repeated after nutritional rehabilitation. The same was found for the febrile response to a repeated vaccine in malnourished children [142]. Since no repeated vaccine was given to well-nourished children, it is unknown whether they would also have had a stronger response to the second dose.

Complement. The complement system consists of plasma proteins secreted by the liver that, upon activation, react to recruit immune cells, opsonize and kill pathogens [24]. Three main pathways activate the complement system: the classical pathway, the alternative pathway and the lectin pathway [143], with the complement protein C3 playing a central role in all three pathways.

Twenty-four articles described levels or in-vitro activity of complement proteins (**table S7**). In 17 of 21 studies, levels of C3 were depressed in malnourished children [89] [94] [99] [106] [124–125] [127–130] [144–154]. Two studies found C3 to correlate with albumin [94] [148], and with one exception [94], C3 levels were lower in children with oedematous than non-oedematous malnutrition [89] [146] [149] [150–151] [153].

Few studies assessed C6, C9, and factor B, and most found reduced levels in malnourished children [145] [148–149] [151] [153], most so in oedematous malnutrition [148–149] [151] [153].

Levels of C1 and C4 were mostly normal in malnourished children [94] [99] [145] [148] [150–153], while two studies found reduced levels of C4 in patients with oedematous, but not non-oedematous malnutrition [89] [149]. Studies assessing C5 showed inconsistent results [145] [148–149] [151] [153].

Classical pathway activity was either unaffected [106] [145–146] [152], reduced [148] [155] [156], or reduced only in oedematous, but not in non-oedematous malnutrition [157]. Alternative pathway activity was reduced in two studies [145] [156] and unaffected in one [146]. General opsonic activity of serum was reduced in one study [156]. No articles reported the activity of the lectin pathway.

Both reduced production and increased consumption may explain the reduced levels of complement factors. Complement components are produced by the liver, and their levels correlated with albumin levels, the production of which is also impaired in malnutrition [158]. However, increased consumption is also supported by one study showing high levels of C3d, a by-product after activation of C3, in malnourished children, most pronounced in oedematous malnutrition [148].

Acquired immunity

Acquired immunity is characterized by specialized cellular and antibody-mediated immune responses, generated by T- and B-lymphocytes reacting with high specificity towards pathogens and creating long-lasting immunological memory. The acquired immune system also orchestrates tolerance to self and other non-pathogenic material like gut bacteria [24]. Of the articles describing acquired immunity, 12 described the thymo-lymphatic system, 21 delayed-type hypersensitivity responses (DTHR), 58 lymphocyte subsets in blood, 32 immunoglobulins in blood, 35 vaccination responses and 35 cytokines.

Thymus. The thymus gland is the central lymphatic organ in the acquired immune system, where maturation and proliferation of T-lymphocytes take place. The thymus is large at birth and undergoes gradual involution after childhood [159], with diminished output of T-lymphocytes [160].

Six articles reported autopsy studies of the thymo-lymphatic system in malnourished children, published between 1956 and 1988 [161–166] **table S8**). All reported thymus atrophy in malnourished children, to an extent termed "nutritional thymectomy" [164]. Histology revealed depleted thymocytes, replacement with connective tissue, and decreased cortico-medullar differentiation [163] [165–166].

Eight articles reported thymic size measured by ultrasound, in relation to nutritional status [91] [167–173] (**table S9**). Five of these studied children with severe malnutrition and found severe thymic atrophy [91] [167–170], reversible with nutritional rehabilitation, although thymic size did not reach normal levels as fast as anthropometric recovery [91] [170]. Thymic size was also measured by ultrasound in cohorts of children to determine patterns of thymic growth [159] [171], in a vaccination trial in Guinea Bissau [172] and in a pre-natal nutritional supplementation trial in Bangladesh [171]. These studies confirmed that thymus size was associated with nutritional status, even in mild malnutrition. Breastfed children often had a larger thymus than artificially fed children [174], possibly explained by IL-7 in breast milk [175], and children with a large thymus were found to have a higher chance of surviving than those with a small thymus [172] [176].

Other lymphatic tissue. Six articles reported investigations of other lymphatic tissue. Four autopsy studies found atrophy of lymph nodes, spleen, tonsils, appendix and Peyer's patches, although not as pronounced as in the thymus. Histology revealed a reduction in germinal centres and depletion of lymphocytes from para-cortical areas [161] [163–165]. Two studies in living children also found that the tonsils were smaller in malnourished than in well-nourished children [163] [177].

Delayed type hypersensitivity response (DTHR). Cellular immune function can be examined by dermal DTHR, the prototype of which is the Mantoux test. Intradermal application of substances like candida or phyto-hemaglutinin (PHA) are also used, as well as sensitizing skin with a local contact sensitizer such as 2-4-di-nitro-clorobenzene (DNCB). Twenty-one articles reported DTHR in relation to malnutrition (**table S10**).

The majority of studies found that malnourished children less frequently developed a positive Mantoux after BCG vaccination [154] [177–185]. Most also found diminished reactivity to *Candida*, PHA and other common antigens [29] [145] [179] [183] [186–190], and after sensitizing with DNCB [163] [177] [179] [183] [188] [191–192]. Conflicting results were found for DTHR in children with different types of severe malnutrition: Three studies found most impaired response in oedematous malnutrition [179] [181] [191], while one found that it was worst in non-oedematous malnutrition [184], and two studies found similar responses [186] [187].

The proportion of positive DTHR varied from study to study, both in well-nourished and malnourished children. Inconsistent results were found in moderately malnourished children [178] [180–181] [185–187] [193]. Other studies found that DTHR was improved with zinc supplementation [190] [194–195] diminished by infections [178] [181] [196], and in slightly older children, a strong interaction was seen between infections and nutritional status [197].

Lymphocytes in blood. Fifty-eight articles reported either total numbers of lymphocytes or lymphocyte subsets in blood (**table S11**). Of 16 articles, 13 reported similar or higher levels of lymphocytes in peripheral blood of malnourished children [80–83] [85–87] [90] [93] [101] [177] [179] [187] [191] [198] [199].

Three studies found that children with oedematous malnutrition had more atypical lymphocytes in blood, resembling plasma cells [81] [87] [93]. Other indicators of functional differences were higher density [200], different pattern of gene expression [201], and more markers of apoptosis in lymphocytes of malnourished children [92] [202].

T-lymphocytes in blood. Numbers of T-lymphocytes were described in 29 articles (**table S11**). Early studies identified T-lymphocytes as those forming rosettes with sheep red blood cells, while later studies used monoclonal antibodies to CD3. Using the rosette-method, 19 of 20 studies found lower levels of T-lymphocytes [28] [87] [93] [101] [128] [130] [144] [183] [186–187] [191] [199] [203–210]. Four studies using monoclonal CD3-antibodies and cell-counting by microscopy also found reduced levels of T-lymphocytes in malnourished children [144] [167–168] [207]. In contrast, only one flow cytometry study found lower levels of T-lymphocytes in malnourished children [211], while four did not [86] [94] [210] [212]. Accordingly, it seems like the rosette-based method identifies different T-lymphocytes than flow cytometry. Some studies found that the numbers of T-lymphocytes were reduced in acute infections [86] [90] [212].

Lymphocyte response to PHA stimulation. In healthy children, incubation of lymphocytes with PHA results in T-lymphocytes to proliferate. Seventeen out of 23 articles reported a reduced proliferative response to PHA in lymphocytes of malnourished children [93] [97–98] [101] [147] [154] [163] [177] [179] [186–187] [189–190] [192] [196] [203] [212–218]. Zinc supplementation improved the response in malnourished children [190].

CD4+ lymphocytes. With assessment of CD4 counts becoming widely available, it has been investigated whether the number of CD4+ lymphocytes was affected by malnutrition. In children without HIV, two of four studies using monoclonal antibodies and microscopy found reduced levels of CD4+ lymphocyte in malnourished children [144] [168] [219] [207], while all seven flow cytometry-studies except one [211] found similar or higher levels [86] [90] [91] [94] [198] [212]. Bacterial infections were noted to reduce the CD4-count [86]. For malnourished children infected with HIV, it was hoped that renutrition alone could increase their level of CD4+ lymphocytes. However, a study from Zambia found that CD4 counts declined during nutritional rehabilitation in HIV-infected malnourished children without anti-retroviral treatment [198]. Thus, a low level of CD4+ lymphocytes can probably not be attributed to malnutrition, regardless of whether the child has HIV or not.

Three studies noted that level of CD4+ lymphocytes were higher in children with oedematous than with non-oedematous malnutrition [91] [198] [220], and several studies have noted that children with HIV were less likely to develop oedematous malnutrition [198] [220] [221], suggesting that some level of CD4+ lymphocytes could be required to develop the syndrome.

Activation markers on T-lymphocytes. Most flow cytometry studies assessing surface markers on T-lymphocytes have been carried out in Mexico, all comparing malnourished infected children with similarly infected well-nourished children. Malnourished children were found to have fewer effector T-lymphocytes, identified as cells lacking the "naïve" markers CD62L and CD28 [90], fewer activated T-lymphocytes, with the markers CD69 and/or CD25 [212] [222] [223], and fewer memory T-lymphocytes identified by the marker CD45RO+ [86]. In contrast, a study from Ghana found similar numbers of activated T-lymphocytes, identified by HLA-DR, in malnourished and well-nourished children [94].

B-lymphocytes. Articles published before 1990 measured B-lymphocytes as those forming rosettes when incubated with sheep erythrocytes and C3, while more recent studies used monoclonal antibodies to CD20 and flow cytometry. All seven rosette-based studies found unaffected or higher B-lymphocyte counts in malnourished children [130] [186] [200] [204] [206] [213] [224], as did one study using anti-CD20 and microscopy [167]. In contrast, all four studies using flow cytometry found reduced numbers of B-lymphocytes in malnourished children [86] [94] [211] [212].

Antibody levels. Thirty-two articles described immunoglobulins in blood of malnourished children (**table S12**). Nineteen of 27 studies found no difference in IgG antibodies or total γ-globulin between malnourished and well-nourished children [94] [53] [63–64] [82] [130] [144] [147] [150] [154] [179] [186] [224–238]. Likewise, IgM levels were most frequently similar, or higher in malnourished than well-nourished children [94] [53] [63–64] [82] [130] [144] [147] [154] [179] [186] [224–225] [227–238].

IgA was elevated in malnourished children in 19 of 27 studies [94] [53] [55–56] [63–64] [82] [130] [144] [147] [150] [154] [179] [224–225] [227–238]. With a few exceptions [150] [232], all studies found elevated levels of IgA in oedematous malnutrition, while 11 of 19 studies found that IgA in non-oedematous or underweight children was normal [94] [53] [55–56] [63] [82] [130] [144] [150] [154] [179] [224] [227] [230] [233–238]. One study noted that levels of IgA correlated with the degree of dermatosis in children with Kwashiorkor [231].

IgE showed no clear pattern, but was elevated in malnourished children in three of six studies [82] [147] [211] [233] [238–239]. IgD, present in low amounts in healthy children, was elevated in children with malnutrition in two studies[130] [233], or elevated in oedematous but not non-oedematous malnutrition [179], while one study found that it was similar to well-nourished children [82].

Antibody vaccination responses. Thirty-five articles described vaccination responses to a specific antigen (**table S13**). The articles either reported *sero-conversion rates*, or *antibody titre* response. Studies assessing sero-conversion rates in children with severe malnutrition found mixed results: Six of 10 studies found reduced sero-conversion rates in children with severe malnutrition to typhoid [101] [240], diphtheria [101], tetanus[101] [206], tetanus-diphtheria-pertussis (DTP) [234], hepatitis B [241], measles [141] [149] [242] and yellow fever [243–244], and two studies found that sero-conversion was delayed in malnourished children [245] [238]. Ten of 11 studies found that severely malnourished children responded with reduced antibody titres [101] [141] [149] [206] [233–234] [238] [240–242] [246], despite some of the studies finding acceptable sero-conversion rates. No study found that children with oedematous malnutrition had a normal antibody response to vaccination. One study from 1964 found improved antibody response to DTP in children with oedematous malnutrition randomized to a high-protein diet [247]. There did not seem to be any specific vaccines whose antibody response was more affected than others by malnutrition, nor was there any pattern in terms of responses to live or dead vaccines.

In contrast, mild and moderately malnourished children were most often found to seroconvert normally when vaccinated against smallpox [248], diphtheria [101] [178] [249] [284] , DTP [178] [234], measles [139] [140] [178] [245] [250–255], polio [178] [256], meningococcus[178] [257], and hepatitis B [258], and 9 of 11 articles reported similar level of antibody titres response in moderately malnourished, as well-nourished children [101] [140] [154] [178] [234] [248–249] [252–253] [258–259].

Three of five articles reported similar adverse reactions to vaccination in malnourished as in well-nourished [140–141] [242] [245–255]. In contrast, one study found that malnourished children given measles vaccine frequently developed diarrhoea, pneumonia and fever, compared to well-nourished children, who, in turn, more often developed a rash [141].

Results were inconsistent for studies assessing levels of specific antibodies to non-vaccine antigens, like blood type antigens [260] malaria [261], H. *influenza*, E. *Coli* [235] [262], *Ascaris* [211],

Rotavirus and Lipopolysaccharide [262]. Most of these studies were done in children with moderate malnutrition.

Cytokines. Cytokines are signal molecules acting locally between immune cells, and sometimes with systemic effects. Thirty-five articles described cytokines in malnourished children (**table S14**).

Early works identified cytokines as factors in serum influencing various in-vitro functions of immune cells. Thus, three of five studies found that "Leucocyte Migration Inhibiting factor" was lower in malnourished children [84] [263–264], that serum from malnourished children contained an "E-rosette inhibiting substance" [128] [265], "lympho-cytotoxin" [266], and a substance inhibiting lymphocyte response to PHA [218] [147] [267–268], sometimes called IL-1 [269]. Similarly, Interferon (IFN) was quantified by the antiviral effect of plasma on a cell culture [95] [196]. In neither of these bioassays, the substance responsible for the effect was known. More recent studies assessed levels of cytokines by immunoassays, looking for structurally known cytokines in plasma [123] [270–272] or in cultured leucocytes [89], with flow cytometry staining for intracellular cytokines [222–223], or by identifying mRNA coding for the protein [273–274], with remarkably consistent results.

Cytokines commonly found to be low in malnourished children included IL- 1 and IL-2 [222–223] [269–270] [273–274], although one study found both cytokines to be normal in non-oedematous malnutrition and lower in oedematous malnutrition [89]. IFN-γ was low in malnourished children in six studies [49] [222–223] [273–275], unaltered in malnourished children in one [276], and elevated in one [272]. IL-12 [49] [274], IL-18 and IL-21 [274], and Granulocyte Macrophage Colony Stimulating Factor [270] were also found to be lower in malnourished children. Blunted cytokine response after in-vitro stimulation with LPS was found in malnourished children [276–278], while incubation with leptin normalized their pattern of intracellular cytokines [223].

Other cytokines were mostly found to be elevated in malnutrition: IL10 was elevated in four of five studies [49] [222–223] [272–273], so was IL-4 [211] [273] [276] and soluble receptors to Tumour Necrosis Factor-α [123]. IL-8 was elevated [277] or unaltered [272].

Tumour Necrosis Factor-α (TNFα) [49] [129] [271–273] [276] [279–280] and IL-6 [120] [122–123] [129] [271–273] [276–278] were mostly similar or higher compared to well-nourished, most often in studies of infected children.

Comparing cytokine pattern between children with oedematous and non-oedematous malnutrition, most found that the difference from well-nourished was greatest in children with oedematous malnutrition [84] [89] [123] [265] [269–270] [277], while two studies found no difference between oedematous and non-oedematous malnutrition [218] [271].

Leukotrienes (LT) are not strictly cytokines, but immune modulating molecules derived from long chain polyunsaturated fatty acids. Levels of LTC4 and LTE4 were higher, and LTB4 lower, in children with oedematous than with non-oedematous malnutrition, whose levels were similar to well-nourished [281], and prostaglandin E2 [282] was higher in children with oedematous malnutrition than in well-nourished.

Discussion

We identified and reviewed 245 articles about immune function in malnourished children. Some general problems apply to many of the studies, mostly related to their observational design. For this reason they can only describe associations, not causalities.

First, many studies were done in severely malnourished children from hospital settings, who were ill with infections, making it difficult to disentangle the immunological effect of malnutrition from the effect of infection. This problem has caused some to propose that there really is no immune impairment by malnutrition, and that all alterations seen are due to infections or underlying unknown immune deficiencies, which are also responsible for the poor growth [283]. Enteropathy could be an example of such an "invisible" condition, causing both immune deficiency and malnutrition. This hypothesis is difficult to test. However, some studies did try to account for this problem by selecting malnourished children without clinical infections, or by comparing them to well-nourished infected children. In studies from central Africa in the 1970s and 1980s, some malnourished children may have suffered from unrecognized paediatric HIV [284], giving obvious problems for interpretation.

Second, publication bias is a well-known problem, and may have occurred, particularly in older studies, where some small studies showed a dramatic effect.

Third, studies used different diagnostic criteria for malnutrition, making it difficult to determine the children's degree of malnutrition as defined by present-day criteria. While children in 52 of the studies fulfilled WHOs present criteria for severe acute malnutrition, only two diagnosed children based on the new WHO growth reference. Those defined as severely malnourished based on old growth references would most likely also be classified as severely malnourished today, since the new WHO standard tend to classify more children as severely malnourished, while some children then defined as moderately malnourished would be classified as severely malnourished today. The studies including children based on weight-for-age probably included children with stunting and wasting, without differentiating between the two.

Fourth, even using uniform criteria, malnourished children are a heterogeneous group. Anthropometric measurements are only crude markers of body composition, which - among other things - reflect nutrient deficiencies. It is unknown what specific nutrients were deficient, and to what extent infection contributed. Deficits in lean tissue and fat tissue are plausibly different physiologic conditions, and children appearing similarly malnourished may be so for entirely different reasons, with different immunological consequences. No articles have so far reported reliable measures of body composition, simultaneously with markers of immune function. Probably, the consequence of malnutrition on immune function may also depend on the pattern and load of infections. Although most studies were carried out in low-income settings with high infectious loads, a few were from middle- or high-income countries. This may also contribute to inconsistencies in the results.

In spite of these limitations, common patterns emerge from the studies, summarized below (**Figure 5**).

Immune parameters apparently not affected by malnutrition

Total white blood cell and lymphocyte counts in peripheral blood are not decreased in malnourished children, and granulocytes are frequently elevated. Likewise, T-lymphocytes and CD4 counts appear normal in malnourished children, when measured by flow cytometry, the gold standard for characterizing cell subsets. Their levels seem to be determined more by infections than by nutritional state, and do not reflect the degree of malnutrition-related immune deficiency, as high infectious mortality is seen in malnourished children, despite unaffected white blood cell counts [49].

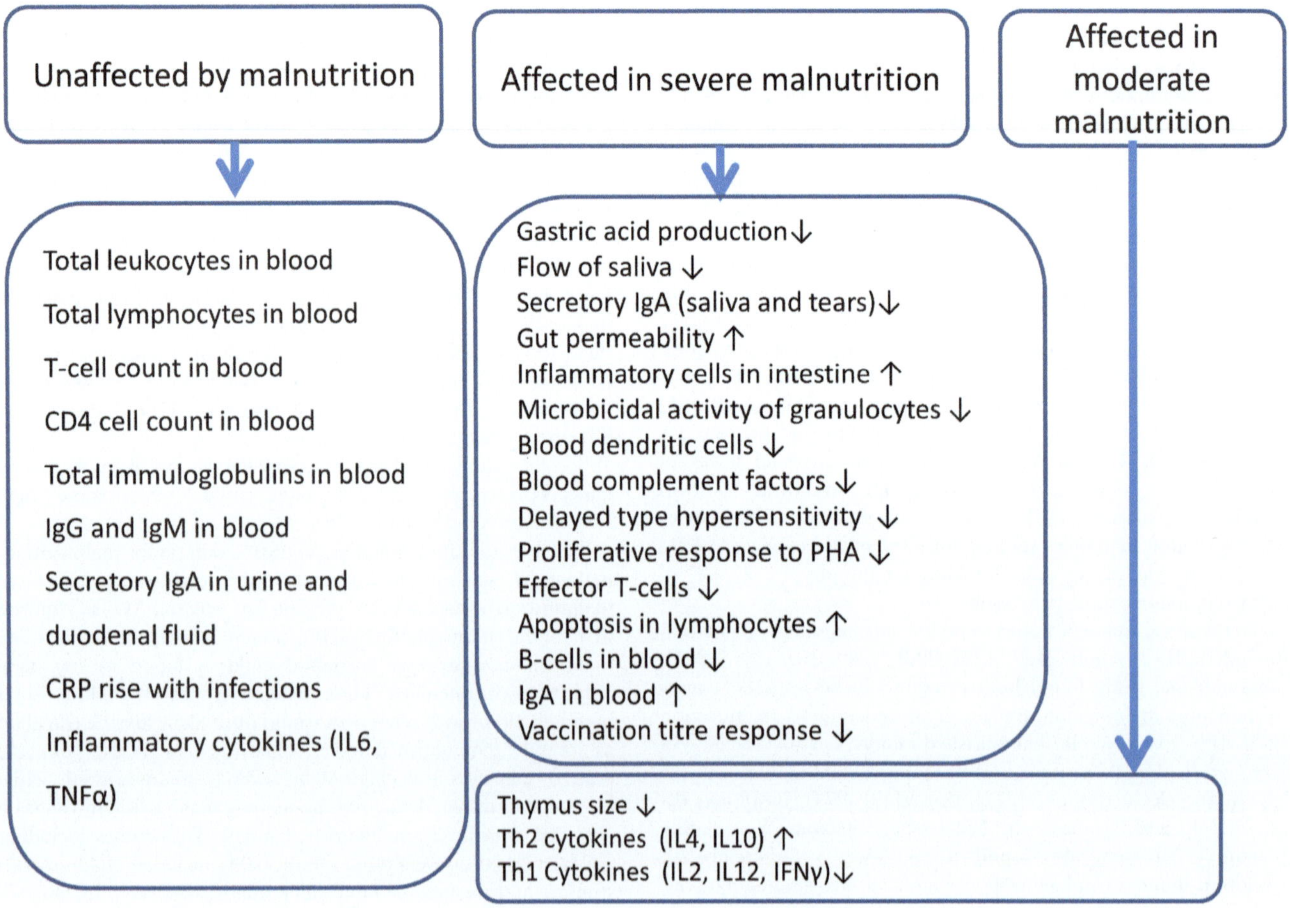

Figure 5. Summary of immune parameters affected and not affected by malnutrition.

Malnourished children can mount an acute phase response to infections, with elevated CRP and low negative acute phase reactants, and this can also be seen in absence of clinical infection. Thus, based on available evidence, the acute phase response, if anything, seems exaggerated rather than diminished. Levels of IgM and IgG are normal or elevated in malnourished children. Secretory IgA is not consistently lower in duodenal fluid, and frequently elevated in urine.

Immune parameters affected by malnutrition

The gut mucosa is atrophied and permeable in malnourished children. This enteropathy also affects well-nourished children in poor communities, but probably most severely in malnourished children. The condition appears similar to *tropical sprue* described in adults, and the term *enteropathy of malnutrition* has been replaced by the broader term *environmental enteropathy* [285]. At present, this condition is thought to result from high pathogen load rather than nutrient deficiencies, and thus primarily a cause of malnutrition, particularly of stunting [286] [287].

Production of gastric acid and flow of saliva is reduced in malnourished children. Secretory IgA is also reduced in saliva, tears and nasal washings from children with severe, but not moderate malnutrition. The small bowel of malnourished children is often colonized with abundant bacteria, and their pattern of commensal flora is altered. Granulocytes kill ingested microorganisms less effectively. Levels of complement proteins are low in blood from malnourished children, particularly in children with oedematous malnutrition, and less in children with moderate malnutrition.

Lymphatic tissue, particularly the thymus, undergoes atrophy in malnutrition in a dose-response fashion: thymic size depends on nutritional status even in milder degrees of malnutrition, and thymus size is a predictor of survival in children.

DTHR is diminished in malnourished children. Lymphocytes of malnourished children are less responsive to stimulation with PHA, fewer are activated and more cells have markers of apoptosis. Plasma IgA is mostly elevated in malnourished children, particular in those with oedema. Children with severe, but not moderate, malnutrition mount a lower specific antibody response to vaccination, although for most children sufficient to obtain protection. The lower titres seen in malnourished may be due to a delay in vaccination response.

Cytokines can be classified as those promoting a Th1 response of predominantly cellular immunity, and those promoting a Th2-response of humoral immunity [24]. Although this approach has somewhat been replaced by other classifications [288], it seems useful to describe the profile of malnourished children, whose immune system seems tuned towards a Th2 response, with high IL4 and IL10, and low levels of IL-2, IL-12 and IFN-γ. Elevated levels of IL-6 and TNFα may primarily be related to infections, and support the observation that induction of an acute phase response is intact in malnutrition. A more recent classification focuses on whether cytokines are predominantly inflammatory or anti-inflammatory [289]. Malnourished children appear to have high levels of anti-inflammatory cytokines and less clearly affected levels of pro-inflammatory cytokines in blood, in contrast to the predominantly pro-inflammatory cytokine expression in the gut of malnourished children.

Mechanisms

The mechanisms behind these immunological alterations are still not adequately understood. Some explain it by lack of energy and building blocks to synthesize the proteins required [290]. However, lack of building blocks does not explain why some immune parameters seem intact, or paradoxically elevated in malnutrition, such as plasma IgA, acute-phase proteins, leucocytes in blood, and production of Th2 cytokines. If it was simply a matter of lack of building blocks, all parameters of the immune system should be equally affected. The fact that the pattern of cytokines in malnourished children is tuned towards at Th2-response fits with their high levels of immunoglobulins, reduction in thymus size and diminished DTHR. Still, the pathophysiology behind this Th2 skewedness remains unexplained.

Infections could obviously contribute to the changes seen, and interactions have been noted between infection and malnutrition in their respective effects on immune parameters [197]. However, although many of the immunological changes appear to be synergistically affected by malnutrition and infections, malnutrition also seems to be independently associated with altered immune function.

Animal studies suggest hormonal factors to be involved in the immune profile of malnutrition. Leptin [291], prolactin [292] and growth hormone [293] all stimulate thymic growth and function, and their levels are low in malnourished children. In support of this, a recent study found that a low leptin level was associated with a higher risk of death in malnourished children [272]. Growth hormone therapy increased thymic size and output in adult HIV patients [294]. In contrast, cortisol and adrenalin induce thymic atrophy in mice [295–296], and cortisol is high in children with malnutrition and other forms of stress. It is plausible that this hormonal interplay is implicated in the immune deficiency in malnourished children.

This hormonal profile is similar to that of an acute phase response, where thymus atrophy also occurs, acquired immunity is temporarily suppressed and innate immunity takes over [296]. This could explain why some malnourished children have elevated positive APP and most have depressed negative APP in absence of clinical infections. Zinc deficiency causes thymic atrophy [297–298], and acute phase responses lower plasma zinc, so zinc status may contribute to the immune deficiency of both malnutrition and acute phase responses.

In HIV infection, persisting subclinical inflammation and immune activation is frequently present, and may be partly responsible for immune deficiency and disease manifestations [299]. Given the frequent finding of elevated acute phase proteins in malnourished children, it seems plausible that a similar state of subclinical inflammation could be involved in both the impairment of immune function, and in the vicious circle of catabolism and deterioration of the nutritional status. However, in spite of elevated acute phase proteins, most studies have reported unaffected or even paradoxically lowered levels of activated T-cell and dendritic cells in malnourished children.

The intracellular receptor, *mammalian target of Raptomycin* (mTOR), is present in most cells. It responds to concentrations of nutrients in the cell's surroundings, and to other signs of stress, such as hypoxia, enabling the cell to adapt its metabolism to locally available nutrients. Immune cells also use mTOR to regulate their state of activation. Nutrient availability may thereby determine whether an immune cell is activated [300], and whether T-cells differentiate towards a pro-inflammatory or a tolerance-inducing phenotype [301]. Some immune cells may even deplete the micro-environment of certain nutrients, to manipulate the activation of mTOR. Accordingly, the significance of nutrients in the micro-environment expands from simple building blocks to signal molecules. Obviously, this mechanism could be involved in the immunological profile in malnutrition. However, no articles have yet described the activity of mTOR in malnourished children.

A research group working with animal models of malnutrition has proposed a theory called the "tolerance hypothesis" [302]. This suggests that the depression of cellular immunity in malnutrition is an adaptive response to prevent autoimmune reactions, which would otherwise occur as a result of catabolism and release of self-antigens. Although adaptive in this sense, it happens at the price of increased susceptibility to infections [303]. However, if this tolerance hypothesis holds true, one would expect to see occasional break-through of auto-immune reactions in malnourished children. Such phenomena have apparently not been studied.

The pathogenesis of oedematous malnutrition is still unknown. Many immune parameters seem affected to a different degree in children with oedematous malnutrition, with higher levels of IgA, higher levels of abnormal antibodies like IgD, poorer vaccination responses and cytokines more skewed towards a Th2-response; their complement levels are lower, which may partly be caused by increased consumption of complement in-vivo. The pattern of leukotrienes is different in children with oedematous compared to non-oedematous malnutrition. This immunological profile resembles that seen in autoimmune diseases such as lupus erythematosus [304–305]. Moreover, elevated immunoglobulins in children with oedematous malnutrition seem to correlate with its unexplainable manifestations, like dermatosis and oedema [231] [233]. It could be speculated whether this syndrome could indeed represent some kind of autoimmune reaction to malnutrition, perhaps resulting from a failure to induce efficient tolerance.

Conclusion

In spite of the prevalence of malnutrition, and its fatal consequences, scientific interest in the immune deficiency of malnutrition seems dwindling, and little research has been carried out on the topic during the last ten years. For this reason, most evidence on the subject relies on immunological methods used 30 to 40 years ago, many of which are no longer in use, and little research has been done with modern methods, and with the present understanding of immunology. Moreover, most studies have looked at isolated aspects of immune function, despite the fact that the parameters are interdependent, and the division into innate and adaptive immune function seems to be a simplification. Thus, our understanding of immune function in malnutrition is still very limited.

This review illuminates the little that we know about the immunological alterations associated with malnutrition, and also points to significant gaps in our knowledge. Future well designed prospective cohort studies should examine how immune parameters are related to morbidity and mortality in malnourished children, with detailed characteristic of nutritional status, preferably body composition, of infections, enteropathy and of low-grade inflammation. When testing nutritional and medical interventions for malnutrition, immune parameters should be included as outcomes. Studies should investigate newer immunological parameters in malnutrition, like expression of innate pattern recognition receptors (as the Toll-like receptor), the lectin pathway of the complement system and mTOR expression and activity. It should be investigated whether a small thymus is associated with lower output of recent thymic-derived T-cells, and how it correlates with hormones like leptin, cortisol, insulin and Insulin Growth Factor-1. Innate and adaptive immune parameters should be assessed simultaneously, taking into account their dynamic interdependency. To understand whether malnutrition is indeed associated with active down-regulation of immune reactivity (as formulated in the "tolerance hypothesis"), the balance between regulatory T-lymphocytes and their counterparts, Th17 lymphocytes should be measured. Finally, prospective studies among children at risk should assess whether immune profiles differ in those who subsequently develop oedematous and non-oedematous malnutrition, and it should be investigated whether children with oedematous malnutrition have markers suggestive of auto-immune or inflammatory diseases. Such studies would reduce our current ignorance on the interplay between malnutrition and infectious diseases.

Supporting Information

Figure S1 PRISMA Flow diagram showing study retrieval and selection.
(DOCX)

Table S1 Articles describing barrier and immune function of skin in malnourished children.
(DOCX)

Table S2 Articles describing intestinal function and mucosal structure in children with malnutrition.
(DOCX)

Table S3 Articles describing anti-microbial factors in mucosal secretions of malnourished children.
(DOCX)

Table S4 Articles describing commensal flora in children with malnutrition.
(DOCX)

Table S5 Articles describing function of innate immune cells: polymorph-nuclear cells and monocytes/macrophages in children with malnutrition.
(DOCX)

Table S6 Articles describing acute phase response in malnourished children.
(DOCX)

Table S7 Articles describing complement in malnourished children.
(DOCX)

Table S8 Articles describing thymus and other lymphatic tissue in autopsies of malnourished children.
(DOCX)

Table S9 Articles describing ultrasound scans of thymus in malnourished children.
(DOCX)

Table S10 Articles describing delayed type hypersensitivity response in children with malnutrition.
(DOCX)

Table S11 Articles describing lymphocyte subsets in children with malnutrition.
(DOCX)

Table S12 Articles describing antibody levels in children with malnutrition.
(DOCX)

Table S13 Articles describing humoral vaccination responses in children with malnutrition.
(DOCX)

Table S14 Articles describing cytokines in malnourished children.
(DOCX)

Checklist S1 PRISMA Checklist.
(DOCX)

Acknowledgments

We are grateful to Dr Michael Golden for providing an extensive list of literature on the subject, and to Professor Kim Fleischer Michaelsen and Charlotte Gylling Mortensen for critically reviewing the manuscript.

Author Contributions

Conceived and designed the experiments: MJHR VBC. Performed the experiments: MJHR. Analyzed the data: MJHR. Contributed to the writing of the manuscript: MJHR LK AB HF VBC.

References

1. Black RE, Victora CG, Walker SP, Bhutta ZA, Christian P, et al. (2013) Maternal and child undernutrition and overweight in low-income and middle-income countries. Lancet 382: 427–451. doi:10.1016/S0140-6736(13)60937-X.
2. Pelletier DL, Frongillo EA Jr, Schroeder DG, Habicht JP (1995) The effects of malnutrition on child mortality in developing countries. Bull World Health Organ 73: 443–448.
3. Tomkins A, Watson F (1989) Malnutrition and Infection - A Review - Nutrition Policy Discussion Paper No. 5. United Nations - Administrative Commitee on Coordination - Subcommitee on Nutrition.
4. Chisti MJ, Tebruegge M, La Vincente S, Graham SM, Duke T (2009) Pneumonia in severely malnourished children in developing countries - mortality risk, aetiology and validity of WHO clinical signs: a systematic review. Trop Med Int Health TM IH 14: 1173–1189. doi:10.1111/j.1365-3156.2009.02364.x.
5. Waterlow JC (1992) Protein Energy malnutrition, 2nd ed. London: Hodder&Stouton.
6. Dutz W, Jennings-Khodadad E, Post C, Kohout E, Nazarian I, et al. (1974) Marasmus and Pneumocystis carinii pneumonia in institutionalised infants. Observations during an endemic. Z Für Kinderheilkd 117: 241–258.
7. Purtilo DT, Connor DH (1975) Fatal infections in protein-calorie malnourished children with thymolymphatic atrophy. Arch Dis Child 50: 149–152.
8. Ikeogu MO, Wolf B, Mathe S (1997) Pulmonary manifestations in HIV seropositivity and malnutrition in Zimbabwe. Arch Dis Child 76: 124–128.
9. Amadi B, Kelly P, Mwiya M, Mulwazi E, Sianongo S, et al. (2001) Intestinal and systemic infection, HIV, and mortality in Zambian children with persistent diarrhea and malnutrition. J Pediatr Gastroenterol Nutr 32: 550–554.
10. Mondal D, Haque R, Sack RB, Kirkpatrick BD, Petri WA Jr (2009) Attribution of malnutrition to cause-specific diarrheal illness: evidence from a prospective study of preschool children in Mirpur, Dhaka, Bangladesh. Am J Trop Med Hyg 80: 824–826.
11. Khatun F, Faruque ASG, Koeck JL, Olliaro P, Millet P, et al. (2011) Changing species distribution and antimicrobial susceptibility pattern of Shigella over a 29-year period (1980–2008). Epidemiol Infect 139: 446–452. doi:10.1017/S0950268810001093.
12. Berkley JA, Lowe BS, Mwangi I, Williams T, Bauni E, et al. (2005) Bacteremia among children admitted to a rural hospital in Kenya. N Engl J Med 352: 39–47. doi:10.1056/NEJMoa040275.
13. Aiken AM, Mturi N, Njuguna P, Mohammed S, Berkley JA, et al. (2011) Risk and causes of paediatric hospital-acquired bacteraemia in Kilifi District Hospital, Kenya: a prospective cohort study. Lancet 378: 2021–2027. doi:10.1016/S0140-6736(11)61622-X.
14. Alcoba G, Kerac M, Breysse S, Salpeteur C, Galetto-Lacour A, et al. (2013) Do children with uncomplicated severe acute malnutrition need antibiotics? A systematic review and meta-analysis. PloS One 8: e53184. doi:10.1371/journal.pone.0053184.

15. Soler-Cataluña JJ, Sánchez-Sánchez L, Martínez-García MA, Sánchez PR, Salcedo E, et al. (2005) Mid-arm muscle area is a better predictor of mortality than body mass index in COPD. Chest 128: 2108–2115. doi:10.1378/chest.128.4.2108.
16. Roediger WE (1990) The starved colon–diminished mucosal nutrition, diminished absorption, and colitis. Dis Colon Rectum 33: 858–862.
17. Faddan NHA, Sayh KIE, Shams H, Badrawy H (2010) Myocardial dysfunction in malnourished children. Ann Pediatr Cardiol 3: 113–118. doi:10.4103/0974-2069.74036.
18. Myatt M, Khara T, Collins S (2006) A review of methods to detect cases of severely malnourished children in the community for their admission into community-based therapeutic care programs. Food Nutr Bull 27: S7–23.
19. World Health Organization, United Nations Children's Fund (2009) WHO child growth standards and the identification of severe acute malnutrition in infants and children A Joint Statement. Available: http://www.who.int/maternal_child_adolescent/documents/9789241598163/en/. Accessed 2014 Aug 5.
20. Williams C (1935) Kwashiorkor - a nutritional disease in children associated with a maize diet. The Lancet nov 16, 1935: 1151–1152.
21. Wellcome Trust Working Party (1970) Classification of infantile malnutrition. The Lancet aug 8: 302–303.
22. Smith R (2005) Investigating the previous studies of a fraudulent author. BMJ 331: 288–291. doi:10.1136/bmj.331.7511.288.
23. WHO (2009) WHO child growth standards and the identification of severe acute malnutrition in infants and children. Geneva: WHO. Available: http://www.who.int/nutrition/publications/severemalnutrition/9789241598163_eng.pdf. Accessed 7 July 2013.
24. Murphy K (2012) Janeways's Immunobiology. 2012th ed. Garland Science, Taylor & Francis Group.
25. Heilskov S, Rytter MJH, Vestergaard C, Briend A, Babirekere E, et al. (2014) Dermatosis in children with oedematous malnutrition (Kwashiorkor): a review of the literature. J Eur Acad Dermatol Venereol JEADV. doi:10.1111/jdv.12452.
26. Sims RT (1968) The ultrastructure of depigmented skin in kwashiorkor. Br J Dermatol 80: 822–832.
27. Thavaraj V, Sesikeran B (1989) Histopathological changes in skin of children with clinical protein energy malnutrition before and after recovery. J Trop Pediatr 35: 105–108.
28. Kulapongs P, Edelman R, Suskind R, Olson RE (1977) Defective local leukocyte mobilization in children with kwashiorkor. Am J Clin Nutr 30: 367–370.
29. Bhaskaram P, Reddy V (1982) Cutaneous inflammatory response in kwashiorkor. Indian J Med Res 76: 849–853.
30. Freyre EA, Chabes A, Poémape O, Chabes A (1973) Abnormal Rebuck skin window response in kwashiorkor. J Pediatr 82: 523–526.
31. Edelman R, Suskind R, Olson RE, Sirisinha S (1973) Mechanisms of defective delayed cutaneous hypersensitivity in children with protein-calorie malnutrition. Lancet 1: 506–508.
32. Burman D (1965) The jejunal mucosa in kwashiorkor. Arch Dis Child 40: 526–531.
33. Brunser O, Castillo C, Araya M (1976) Fine structure of the small intestinal mucosa in infantile marasmic malnutrition. Gastroenterology 70: 495–507.
34. Schneider RE, Viteri FE (1972) Morphological aspects of the duodenojejunal mucosa in protein-calorie malnourished children and during recovery. Am J Clin Nutr 25: 1092–1102.
35. Brunser O, Reid A, Monckeberg F, Maccioni A, Contreras I (1968) Jejunal mucosa in infant malnutrition. Am J Clin Nutr 21: 976–983.
36. Brunser O, Reid A, Mönckeberg F, Maccioni A, Contreras I (1966) Jejunal biopsies in infant malnutrition: with special reference to mitotic index. Pediatrics 38: 605–612.
37. Amadi B, Fagbemi AO, Kelly P, Mwiya M, Torrente F, et al. (2009) Reduced production of sulfated glycosaminoglycans occurs in Zambian children with kwashiorkor but not marasmus. Am J Clin Nutr 89: 592–600. doi:10.3945/ajcn.2008.27092.
38. Campbell DI, Murch SH, Elia M, Sullivan PB, Sanyang MS, et al. (2003) Chronic T cell-mediated enteropathy in rural west African children: relationship with nutritional status and small bowel function. Pediatr Res 54: 306–311. doi:10.1203/01.PDR.0000076666.16021.5E.
39. Green F, Heyworth B (1980) Immunoglobulin-containing cells in jejunal mucosa of children with protein-energy malnutrition and gastroenteritis. Arch Dis Child 55: 380–383.
40. Kaschula RO, Gajjar PD, Mann M, Hill I, Purvis J, et al. (1979) Infantile jejunal mucosa in infection and malnutrition. Isr J Med Sci 15: 356–361.
41. Theron JJ, Wittmann W, Prinsloo JG (1971) The fine structure of the jejunum in kwashiorkor. Exp Mol Pathol 14: 184–199.
42. Shiner M, Redmond AO, Hansen JD (1973) The jejunal mucosa in protein-energy malnutrition. A clinical, histological, and ultrastructural study. Exp Mol Pathol 19: 61–78.
43. Römer H, Urbach R, Gomez MA, Lopez A, Perozo-Ruggeri G, et al. (1983) Moderate and severe protein energy malnutrition in childhood: effects on jejunal mucosal morphology and disaccharidase activities. J Pediatr Gastroenterol Nutr 2: 459–464.
44. Stanfield JP, Hutt MS, Tunnicliffe R (1965) Intestinal biopsy in kwashiorkor. Lancet 2: 519–523.
45. Behrens RH, Lunn PG, Northrop CA, Hanlon PW, Neale G (1987) Factors affecting the integrity of the intestinal mucosa of Gambian children. Am J Clin Nutr 45: 1433–1441.
46. Brewster DR, Manary MJ, Menzies IS, O'Loughlin EV, Henry RL (1997) Intestinal permeability in kwashiorkor. Arch Dis Child 76: 236–241.
47. Hossain MI, Nahar B, Hamadani JD, Ahmed T, Roy AK, et al. (2010) Intestinal mucosal permeability of severely underweight and nonmalnourished Bangladeshi children and effects of nutritional rehabilitation. J Pediatr Gastroenterol Nutr 51: 638–644. doi:10.1097/MPG.0b013e3181eb3128.
48. Boaz RT, Joseph AJ, Kang G, Bose A (2013) Intestinal permeability in normally nourished and malnourished children with and without diarrhea. Indian Pediatr 50: 152–153.
49. Hughes SM, Amadi B, Mwiya M, Nkamba H, Tomkins A, et al. (2009) Dendritic cell anergy results from endotoxemia in severe malnutrition. J Immunol Baltim Md 1950 183: 2818–2826. doi:10.4049/jimmunol.0803518.
50. Mishra OP, Dhawan T, Singla PN, Dixit VK, Arya NC, et al. (2001) Endoscopic and histopathological evaluation of preschool children with chronic diarrhoea. J Trop Pediatr 47: 77–80.
51. Sullivan PB, Lunn PG, Northrop-Clewes C, Crowe PT, Marsh MN, et al. (1992) Persistent diarrhea and malnutrition–the impact of treatment on small bowel structure and permeability. J Pediatr Gastroenterol Nutr 14: 208–215.
52. Redmond AO, Kaschula RO, Freeseman C, Hansen JD (1971) The colon in kwashiorkor. Arch Dis Child 46: 470–473.
53. McMurray DN, Rey H, Casazza LJ, Watson RR (1977) Effect of moderate malnutrition on concentrations of immunoglobulins and enzymes in tears and saliva of young Colombian children. Am J Clin Nutr 30: 1944–1948.
54. Watson RR, McMurray DN, Martin P, Reyes MA (1985) Effect of age, malnutrition and renutrition on free secretory component and IgA in secretions. Am J Clin Nutr 42: 281–288.
55. Sirisinha S, Suskind R, Edelman R, Asvapaka C, Olson RE (1975) Secretory and serum IgA in children with protein-calorie malnutrition. Pediatrics 55: 166–170.
56. Ibrahim AM, el-Hawary MF, Sakr R (1978) Protein-calorie malnutrition (PCM) in Egypt immunological changes of salivary protein in PCM. Z Für Ernährungswissenschaft 17: 145–152.
57. Reddy V, Raghuramulu N, Bhaskaram C (1976) Secretory IgA in protein-calorie malnutrition. Arch Dis Child 51: 871–874.
58. Yakubu AM (1982) Secretory IgA in nasal secretions of children with acute gastroenteritis and kwashiorkor. Ann Trop Paediatr 2: 139–142.
59. Bell RG, Turner KJ, Gracey M, Suharjono Sunoto (1976) Serum and small intestinal immunoglobulin levels in undernourished children. Am J Clin Nutr 29: 392–397.
60. Buchanan N, Fairburn JA, Schmaman A (1973) Urinary tract infection and secretory urinary IgA in malnutrition. South Afr Med J Suid-Afr Tydskr Vir Geneeskd 47: 1179–1181.
61. Marei MA, al-Hamshary AM, Abdalla KF, Abdel-Maaboud AI (1998) A study on secretory IgA in malnourished children with chronic diarrhoea associated with parasitic infections. J Egypt Soc Parasitol 28: 907–913.
62. Miller EM, McConnell DS (2012) Brief communication: chronic undernutrition is associated with higher mucosal antibody levels among Ariaal infants of northern Kenya. Am J Phys Anthropol 149: 136–141. doi:10.1002/ajpa.22108.
63. Watson RR, Reyes MA, McMurray DN (1978) Influence of malnutrition on the concentration of IgA, lysozyme, amylase and aminopeptidase in children's tears. Proc Soc Exp Biol Med Soc Exp Biol Med N Y N 157: 215–219.
64. Beatty DW, Napier B, Sinclair-Smith CC, McCabe K, Hughes EJ (1983) Secretory IgA synthesis in Kwashiorkor. J Clin Lab Immunol 12: 31–36.
65. Gilman RH, Partanen R, Brown KH, Spira WM, Khanam S, et al. (1988) Decreased gastric acid secretion and bacterial colonization of the stomach in severely malnourished Bangladeshi children. Gastroenterology 94: 1308–1314.
66. Shashidhar S, Shah SB, Acharya PT (1976) Gastric acid, pH and pepsin in healthy and protein calorie malnourished children. Indian J Pediatr 43: 145–151.
67. Gracey M, Cullity GJ, Suharjono S (1977) The stomach in malnutrition. Arch Dis Child 52: 325–327.
68. Adesola AO (1968) The influence of severe protein deficiency (kwashiorkor) on gastric acid secretion in Nigerian children. Br J Surg 55: 866.
69. Vael C, Desager K (2009) The importance of the development of the intestinal microbiota in infancy. Curr Opin Pediatr 21: 794–800. doi:10.1097/MOP.0b013e328332351b.
70. Scheutz F, Matee MI, Simon E, Mwinula JH, Lyamuya EF, et al. (1997) Association between carriage of oral yeasts, malnutrition and HIV-1 infection among Tanzanian children aged 18 months to 5 years. Community Dent Oral Epidemiol 25: 193–198.
71. Matee MI, Simon E, Christensen MF, Kirk K, Andersen L, et al. (1995) Association between carriage of oral yeasts and malnutrition among Tanzanian infants aged 6–24 months. Oral Dis 1: 37–42.
72. Omoike IU, Abiodun PO (1989) Upper small intestinal microflora in diarrhea and malnutrition in Nigerian children. J Pediatr Gastroenterol Nutr 9: 314–321.
73. Mata LJ, Jiménez F, Cordón M, Rosales R, Prera E, et al. (1972) Gastrointestinal flora of children with protein–calorie malnutrition. Am J Clin Nutr 25: 118–126.

74. Gracey M, Stone DE, Suharjono Sunoto (1974) Isolation of Candida species from the gastrointestinal tract in malnourished children. Am J Clin Nutr 27: 345–349.
75. Neto UF, Toccalino H, Dujovney F (1976) Stool bacterial aerobic overgrowth in the small intestine of children with acute diarrhoea. Acta Paediatr Scand 65: 609–615.
76. Smith MI, Yatsunenko T, Manary MJ, Trehan I, Mkakosya R, et al. (2013) Gut microbiomes of Malawian twin pairs discordant for kwashiorkor. Science 339: 548–554. doi:10.1126/science.1229000.
77. Monira S, Nakamura S, Gotoh K, Izutsu K, Watanabe H, et al. (2011) Gut microbiota of healthy and malnourished children in bangladesh. Front Microbiol 2: 228. doi:10.3389/fmicb.2011.00228.
78. Gupta SS, Mohammed MH, Ghosh TS, Kanungo S, Nair GB, et al. (2011) Metagenome of the gut of a malnourished child. Gut Pathog 3: 7. doi:10.1186/1757-4749-3-7.
79. Subramanian S, Huq S, Yatsunenko T, Haque R, Mahfuz M, et al. (2014) Persistent gut microbiota immaturity in malnourished Bangladeshi children. Nature. doi:10.1038/nature13421.
80. Rosen EU, Geefhuysen J, Anderson R, Joffe M, Rabson AR (1975) Leucocyte function in children with kwashiorkor. Arch Dis Child 50: 220–224.
81. Schopfer K, Douglas SD (1976) Fine structural studies of peripheral blood leucocytes from children with kwashiorkor: morphological and functional properties. Br J Haematol 32: 573–577.
82. Purtilo DT, Riggs RS, Evans R, Neafie RC (1976) Humoral immunity of parasitized, malnourished children. Am J Trop Med Hyg 25: 229–232.
83. Schopfer K, Douglas SD (1976) Neutrophil function in children with kwashiorkor. J Lab Clin Med 88: 450–461.
84. Fongwo NP, Arinola OG, Salimonu LS (1999) Leucocyte migration inhibition factor (L-MIF) in malnourished Nigerian children. Afr J Med Med Sci 28: 17–20.
85. Nájera O, González C, Toledo G, López L, Cortés E, et al. (2001) CD45RA and CD45RO isoforms in infected malnourished and infected well-nourished children. Clin Exp Immunol 126: 461–465.
86. Nájera O, González C, Toledo G, López L, Ortiz R (2004) Flow cytometry study of lymphocyte subsets in malnourished and well-nourished children with bacterial infections. Clin Diagn Lab Immunol 11: 577–580. doi:10.1128/CDLI.11.3.577-580.2004.
87. Keusch G, Urritia J, Guerrero O, Castenada G, Douglas S (1977) Rosette-Forming Lymphocytes in Guatemalan Children with Protein-Calorie Malnutrition. Malnutrition and the Immune Response, Edited by Robert M Suskind. New York: Raven Press, Vol. 1977.pp. 117–124.
88. Keusch G, Urrutia JJ, Fernandez R, Guerrero O, Casteneda G (1977) Humoral and Cellular Aspects of Intracellular Bactericidal killing in Guatemalan Children with Protein-Energy Malnutrition. Malnutrition and the Immune Response, Edited by Robert M Suskind. New York: Raven Press.pp. 245–251.
89. Lotfy OA, Saleh WA, el-Barbari M (1998) A study of some changes of cell-mediated immunity in protein energy malnutrition. J Egypt Soc Parasitol 28: 413–428.
90. Nájera O, González C, Cortés E, Toledo G, Ortiz R (2007) Effector T lymphocytes in well-nourished and malnourished infected children. Clin Exp Immunol 148: 501–506. doi:10.1111/j.1365-2249.2007.03369.x.
91. Nassar MF, Younis NT, Tohamy AG, Dalam DM, El Badawy MA (2007) T-lymphocyte subsets and thymic size in malnourished infants in Egypt: a hospital-based study. East Mediterr Health J Rev Santé Méditerranée Orient Al-Majallah Al-Ṣiḥḥīyah Li-Sharq Al-Mutawassiṭ 13: 1031–1042.
92. Nassar MF, El-Batrawy SR, Nagy NM (2009) CD95 expression in white blood cells of malnourished infants during hospitalization and catch-up growth. East Mediterr Health J Rev Santé Méditerranée Orient Al-Majallah Al-Ṣiḥḥīyah Li-Sharq Al-Mutawassiṭ 15: 574–583.
93. Schopfer K, Douglas SD (1976) In vitro studies of lymphocytes from children with kwashiorkor. Clin Immunol Immunopathol 5: 21–30.
94. Rikimaru T, Taniquchi K, Yartey J, Kennedy D, Nkrumah F (1998) Humoral and cell-mediated immunity in malnourished children in Ghana. Eur J Clin Nutr 1998 May; 52: 344–350.
95. Salimonu LS, Ojo-Amaize E, Williams AI, Johnson AO, Cooke AR, et al. (1982) Depressed natural killer cell activity in children with protein-calorie malnutrition. Clin Immunol Immunopathol 24: 1–7.
96. Salimonu LS, Ojo-Amaize E, Johnson AO, Laditan AA, Akinwolere OA, et al. (1983) Depressed natural killer cell activity in children with protein–calorie malnutrition. II. Correction of the impaired activity after nutritional recovery. Cell Immunol 82: 210–215.
97. Vásquez-Garibay E, Campollo-Rivas O, Romero-Velarde E, Méndez-Estrada C, García-Iglesias T, et al. (2002) Effect of renutrition on natural and cell-mediated immune response in infants with severe malnutrition. J Pediatr Gastroenterol Nutr 34: 296–301.
98. Vásquez-Garibay E, Méndez-Estrada C, Romero-Velarde E, García-Iglesias MT, Campollo-Rivas O (2004) Nutritional support with nucleotide addition favors immune response in severely malnourished infants. Arch Med Res 35: 284–288. doi:10.1016/j.arcmed.2004.03.002.
99. Rich K, Neumann C, Stiehm R (1977) Neutrophil Chemotaxis in Malnourished Ghaninan Children. In: Suskind RM, editor.Malnutrition and the Immune Response.New York: Raven Press. pp. 271–275.
100. Goyal HK, Kaushik SK, Dhamieja JP, Suman RK, Kumar KK (1981) A study of granulocyte adherence in protein calorie malnutrition. Indian Pediatr 18: 287–292.
101. Reddy V, Jagadeesan V, Ragharamulu N, Bhaskaram C, Srikantia SG (1976) Functional significance of growth retardation in malnutrition. Am J Clin Nutr 29: 3–7.
102. Tejada C, Argueta V, Sanchez M, Albertazzi C (1964) Phagocytic and alkaline phosphatase activity of leucocytes in kwashiorkor. J Pediatr 64: 753–761.
103. Douglas SD, Schopfer K (1974) Phagocyte function in protein-calorie malnutrition. Clin Exp Immunol 17: 121–128.
104. Leitzmann C, Vithayasai V, Windecker P, Suskind R, Olson R (1977) Phagocytosis and Killing Function of Polymorphnuclear Leukocytes in Thai Children with Protein-Energy Malnutrition. In: Suskind RM, editor.Malnutri-Malnutrition and the Immune Response.New York: Raven Press. pp. 253–257.
105. Shousha S, Kamel K (1972) Nitro blue tetrazolium test in children with kwashiorkor with a comment on the use of latex particles in the test. J Clin Pathol 25: 494–497.
106. Forte WCN, Martins Campos JV, Leao RC (1984) Non specific immunological response in moderate malnutrition. Allergol Immunopathol (Madr) 12: 489–496.
107. Chhangani L, Sharma ML, Sharma UB, Joshi N (1985) In vitro study of phagocytic and bactericidal activity of neutrophils in cases of protein energy malnutrition. Indian J Pathol Microbiol 28: 199–203.
108. Bhaskaram P (1980) Macrophage function in severe protein energy malnutrition. Indian J Med Res 71: 247–250.
109. Bhaskaram P, Reddy V (1982) Macrophage function in kwashiorkor. Indian J Pediatr 49: 497–499.
110. Shilotri PG (1976) Hydrogen peroxide production by leukocytes in protein-calorie malnutrition. Clin Chim Acta Int J Clin Chem 71: 511–514.
111. Raman TS (1992) Nitroblue tetrazolium test in protein energy malnutrition. Indian Pediatr 29: 355–356.
112. Altay C, Dogramaci N, Bingol A, Say B (1972) Nitroblue tetrazolium test in children with malnutrition. J Pediatr 81: 392–393.
113. Machado RM, da Costa JC, de Lima Filho EC, Brasil MR, da Rocha GM (1985) Longitudinal study of the nitroblue tetrazolium test in children with protein-calorie malnutrition. J Trop Pediatr 31: 74–77.
114. Wolfsdorf J, Nolan R (1974) Leucocyte function in protein deficiency states. South Afr Med J Suid-Afr Tydskr Vir Geneeskd 48: 528–530.
115. Golden MH, Ramdath D (1987) Free radicals in the pathogenesis of kwashiorkor. Proc Nutr Soc 46: 53–68.
116. Shousha S, Kamel K, Ahmad KK (1974) Cytochemistry of polymorphonuclear neutrophil leukocytes in kwashiorkor. J Egypt Med Assoc 57: 298–308.
117. González C, Nájera O, Cortés E, Toledo G, López L, et al. (2002) Hydrogen peroxide-induced DNA damage and DNA repair in lymphocytes from malnourished children. Environ Mol Mutagen 39: 33–42.
118. González C, Nájera O, Cortés E, Toledo G, López L, et al. (2002) Susceptibility to DNA damage induced by antibiotics in lymphocytes from malnourished children. Teratog Carcinog Mutagen 22: 147–158.
119. Berczi I, Quintanar-Stephano A, Kovacs K (2009) Neuroimmune regulation in immunocompetence, acute illness, and healing. Ann N Y Acad Sci 1153: 220–239. doi:10.1111/j.1749-6632.2008.03975.x.
120. Reid M, Badaloo A, Forrester T, Morlese JF, Heird WC, et al. (2002) The acute-phase protein response to infection in edematous and nonedematous protein-energy malnutrition. Am J Clin Nutr 76: 1409–1415.
121. Morlese JF, Forrester T, Jahoor F (1998) Acute-phase protein response to infection in severe malnutrition. Am J Physiol 275: E112–117.
122. Malavé I, Vethencourt MA, Pirela M, Cordero R (1998) Serum levels of thyroxine-binding prealbumin, C-reactive protein and interleukin-6 in protein-energy undernourished children and normal controls without or with associated clinical infections. J Trop Pediatr 44: 256–262.
123. Sauerwein RW, Mulder JA, Mulder L, Lowe B, Peshu N, et al. (1997) Inflammatory mediators in children with protein-energy malnutrition. Am J Clin Nutr 65: 1534–1539.
124. Ekanem E, Umotong A, Raykundalia C, Catty D (1997) Serum C-reactive protein and C3 complement protein levels in severely malnourished Nigerian children with and without bacterial infections. Acta Pædiatrica 86: 1317–1320. doi:10.1111/j.1651-2227.1997.tb14905.x.
125. Razban SZ, Olusi SO, Ade-Serrano MA, Osunkoya BO, Adeshina HA, et al. (1975) Acute phase proteins in children with protein-calorie malnutrition. J Trop Med Hyg 78: 264–266.
126. El-Sayed HL, Nassar MF, Habib NM, Elmasry OA, Gomaa SM (2006) Structural and functional affection of the heart in protein energy malnutrition patients on admission and after nutritional recovery. Eur J Clin Nutr 60: 502–510. doi:10.1038/sj.ejcn.1602344.
127. McFarlane H (1977) Acute-Phase Proteins in Malnutrition. In: Suskind RM, editor.Malnutrition and the Immune Response.New York: Raven Press. pp. 403–405.
128. Salimonu LS (1985) Soluble immune complexes, acute phase proteins and E-rosette inhibitory substance in sera of malnourished children. Ann Trop Paediatr 5: 137–141.
129. Manary MJ, Yarasheski KE, Berger R, Abrams ET, Hart CA, et al. (2004) Whole-body leucine kinetics and the acute phase response during acute infection in marasmic Malawian children. Pediatr Res 55: 940–946. doi:10.1203/01.pdr.0000127017.44938.6d.

130. Nahani J, Nik-Aeen A, Rafii M, Mohagheghpour N (1976) Effect of malnutrition on several parameters of the immune system of children. Nutr Metab 20: 302–306.
131. Parent MA, Loening WE, Coovadia HM, Smythe PM (1974) Pattern of biochemical and immune recovery in protein calorie malnutrition. South Afr Med J Suid-Afr Tydskr Vir Geneeskd 48: 1375–1378.
132. Akenami FO, Koskiniemi M, Siimes MA, Ekanem EE, Bolarin DM, et al. (1997) Assessment of plasma fibronectin in malnourished Nigerian children. J Pediatr Gastroenterol Nutr 24: 183–188.
133. Hassanein el-S A, Assem HM, Rezk MM, el-Maghraby RM (1998) Study of plasma albumin, transferrin, and fibronectin in children with mild to moderate protein-energy malnutrition. J Trop Pediatr 44: 362–365.
134. Schelp FP, Thanangkul O, Supawan V, Pongpaew P (1980) α2HS-glycoprotein serum levels in protein–energy malnutrition. Br J Nutr 43: 381–383. doi:10.1079/BJN19800101.
135. Abiodun PO, Ihongbe JC, Dati F (1985) Decreased levels of alpha 2 HS-glycoprotein in children with protein-energy-malnutrition. Eur J Pediatr 144: 368–369.
136. Abiodun PO, Olomu IN (1987) Alpha 2 HS-glycoprotein levels in children with protein-energy malnutrition and infections. J Pediatr Gastroenterol Nutr 6: 271–275.
137. Doherty JF, Golden MH, Raynes JG, Griffin GE, McAdam KP (1993) Acute-phase protein response is impaired in severely malnourished children. Clin Sci Lond Engl 1979 84: 169–175.
138. Yoder MC, Anderson DC, Gopalakrishna GS, Douglas SD, Polin RA (1987) Comparison of serum fibronectin, prealbumin, and albumin concentrations during nutritional repletion in protein-calorie malnourished infants. J Pediatr Gastroenterol Nutr 6: 84–88.
139. Dao H, Delisle H, Fournier P (1992) Anthropometric status, serum prealbumin level and immune response to measles vaccination in Mali children. J Trop Pediatr 38: 179–184.
140. McMurray DN, Loomis SA, Casazza LJ, Rey H (1979) Influence of moderate malnutrition on morbidity and antibody response following vaccination with live, attenuated measles virus vaccine. Bull Pan Am Health Organ 13: 52–57.
141. Idris S, El Seed AM (1983) Measles vaccination in severely malnourished Sudanese children. Ann Trop Paediatr 3: 63–67.
142. Doherty JF, Golden MH, Griffin GE, McAdam KP (1989) Febrile response in malnutrition. West Indian Med J 38: 209–212.
143. Degn SE, Thiel S, Jensenius JC (2007) New perspectives on mannan-binding lectin-mediated complement activation. Immunobiology 212: 301–311. doi:10.1016/j.imbio.2006.12.004.
144. Ozkan H, Olgun N, Saşmaz E, Abacioğlu H, Okuyan M, et al. (1993) Nutrition, immunity and infections: T lymphocyte subpopulations in protein–energy malnutrition. J Trop Pediatr 39: 257–260.
145. Sakamoto M, Nishioka K (1992) Complement system in nutritional deficiency. World Rev Nutr Diet 67: 114–139.
146. Kumar R, Kumar A, Sethi RS, Gupta RK, Kaushik AK, et al. (1984) A study of complement activity in malnutrition. Indian Pediatr 21: 541–547.
147. Beatty DW, Dowdle EB (1978) The effects of kwashiorkor serum on lymphocyte transformation in vitro. Clin Exp Immunol 32: 134–143.
148. Haller L, Zubler RH, Lambert PH (1978) Plasma levels of complement components and complement haemolytic activity in protein-energy malnutrition. Clin Exp Immunol 34: 248–252.
149. Hafez M, Aref GH, Mehareb SW, Kassem AS, El-Tahhan H, et al. (1977) Antibody production and complement system in protein energy malnutrition. J Trop Med Hyg 80: 36–39.
150. Olusi SO, McFarlane H, Osunkoya BO, Adesina H (1975) Specific protein assays in protein-calorie malnutrition. Clin Chim Acta Int J Clin Chem 62: 107–116.
151. Olusi SO, McFarlane H, Ade-Serrano M, Osunkoya BO, Adesina H (1976) Complement components in children with protein-calorie malnutrition. Trop Geogr Med 28: 323–328.
152. Forte WC, Forte AC, Leão RC (1992) Complement system in malnutrition. Allergol Immunopathol (Madr) 20: 157–160.
153. Sirisinha S, Edelman R, Suskind R, Charupatana C, Olson RE (1973) Complement and C3-proactivator levels in children with protein-calorie malnutrition and effect of dietary treatment. Lancet 1: 1016–1020.
154. Kielman A (1977) Nutritional and Immune Responses of Subclinically Malnourished Indian Children. In: Suskind RM, editor.Malnutrition and the Immune Response.New York: Raven Press. pp. 429–440.
155. Abdulrhman MA, Nassar MF, Mostafa HW, El-Khayat ZA, Abu El Naga MW (2011) Effect of honey on 50% complement hemolytic activity in infants with protein energy malnutrition: a randomized controlled pilot study. J Med Food 14: 551–555. doi:10.1089/jmf.2010.0082.
156. Keusch GT, Torun B, Johnston RB Jr, Urrutia JJ (1984) Impairment of hemolytic complement activation by both classical and alternative pathways in serum from patients with kwashiorkor. J Pediatr 105: 434–436.
157. Suskind R, Edelman R, Kulapongs P, Pariyanonda A, Sirisinha S (1976) Complement activity in children with protein-calorie malnutrition. Am J Clin Nutr 29: 1089–1092.
158. Jahoor F, Badaloo A, Reid M, Forrester T (2008) Protein metabolism in severe childhood malnutrition. Ann Trop Paediatr 28: 87–101. doi:10.1179/146532808X302107.
159. Hasselbalch H, Ersbøll AK, Jeppesen DL, Nielsen MB (1999) Thymus size in infants from birth until 24 months of age evaluated by ultrasound. A longitudinal prediction model for the thymic index. Acta Radiol Stockh Swed 1987 40: 41–44.
160. Gui J, Mustachio LM, Su D-M, Craig RW (2012) Thymus Size and Age-related Thymic Involution: Early Programming, Sexual Dimorphism, Progenitors and Stroma. Aging Dis 3: 280–290.
161. Naeye RL (1965) Organ and cellular development in congenital heart disease and in alimentary malnutrition. J Pediatr 67: 447–458.
162. Watts T (1969) Thymus weights in malnourished children. J Trop Pediatr 15: 155–158.
163. Smythe PM, Brereton-Stiles GG, Grace HJ, Mafoyane A, Schonland M, et al. (1971) Thymolymphatic deficiency and depression of cell-mediated immunity in protein-calorie malnutrition. Lancet 2: 939–943.
164. Schonland M (1972) Depression of immunity in protein-calorie malnutrition: a post-mortem study. J Trop Pediatr Environ Child Health 18: 217–224.
165. Aref GH, Abdel-Aziz A, Elaraby II, Abdel-Moneim MA, Hebeishy NA, et al. (1982) A post-mortem study of the thymolymphatic system in protein energy malnutrition. J Trop Med Hyg 85: 109–114.
166. Jambon B, Ziegler O, Maire B, Hutin MF, Parent G, et al. (1988) Thymulin (facteur thymique serique) and zinc contents of the thymus glands of malnourished children. Am J Clin Nutr 48: 335–342.
167. Parent G, Chevalier P, Zalles L, Sevilla R, Bustos M, et al. (1994) In vitro lymphocyte-differentiating effects of thymulin (Zn-FTS) on lymphocyte subpopulations of severely malnourished children. Am J Clin Nutr 60: 274–278.
168. Chevalier P, Sevilla R, Zalles L, Sejas E, Belmonte G, et al. (1994) Study of thymus and thymocytes in Bolivian preschool children during recovery from severe acute malnutrition. J Nutr Immunol Vol 3, 1994: 27–39.
169. Chevalier P (1997) Thymic ultrasonography in children, a non-invasive assessment of nutritional immune deficiency. Nutr Res 17: 1271–1276. doi:10.1016/S0271-5317(97)00110-3.
170. Chevalier P, Sevilla R, Sejas E, Zalles L, Belmonte G, et al. (1998) Immune recovery of malnourished children takes longer than nutritional recovery: implications for treatment and discharge. J Trop Pediatr 44: 304–307.
171. Collinson AC, Moore SE, Cole TJ, Prentice AM (2003) Birth season and environmental influences on patterns of thymic growth in rural Gambian infants. Acta Paediatr Oslo Nor 1992 92: 1014–1020.
172. Garly M-L, Trautner SL, Marx C, Danebod K, Nielsen J, et al. (2008) Thymus size at 6 months of age and subsequent child mortality. J Pediatr 153: 683–688, 688.e1–3. doi:10.1016/j.jpeds.2008.04.069.
173. Moore SE, Prentice AM, Wagatsuma Y, Fulford AJC, Collinson AC, et al. (2009) Early-life nutritional and environmental determinants of thymic size in infants born in rural Bangladesh. Acta Paediatr Oslo Nor 1992 98: 1168–1175. doi:10.1111/j.1651-2227.2009.01292.x.
174. Hasselbalch H, Jeppesen DL, Engelmann MD, Michaelsen KF, Nielsen MB (1996) Decreased thymus size in formula-fed infants compared with breastfed infants. Acta Paediatr Oslo Nor 1992 85: 1029–1032.
175. Ngom PT, Collinson AC, Pido-Lopez J, Henson SM, Prentice AM, et al. (2004) Improved thymic function in exclusively breastfed infants is associated with higher interleukin 7 concentrations in their mothers' breast milk. Am J Clin Nutr 80: 722–728.
176. Moore SE, Fulford AJ, Wagatsuma Y, Persson LÅ, Arifeen SE, et al. (2013) Thymus development and infant and child mortality in rural Bangladesh. Int J Epidemiol. doi:10.1093/ije/dyt232.
177. McMurray DN, Loomis SA, Casazza LJ, Rey H, Miranda R (1981) Development of impaired cell-mediated immunity in mild and moderate malnutrition. Am J Clin Nutr 34: 68–77.
178. Greenwood BM, Bradley-Moore AM, Bradley AK, Kirkwood BR, Gilles HM (1986) The immune response to vaccination in undernourished and well-nourished Nigerian children. Ann Trop Med Parasitol 80: 537–544.
179. McMurray DN, Watson RR, Reyes MA (1981) Effect of renutrition on humoral and cell-mediated immunity in severely malnourished children. Am J Clin Nutr 34: 2117–2126.
180. Seth V, Kukreja N, Sundaram KR, Malaviya AN (1981) Delayed hypersensitivity after BCG in preschool children in relation to their nutritional status. Indian J Med Res 74: 392–398.
181. Satyanarayana K, Bhaskaram P, Seshu VC, Reddy V (1980) Influence of nutrition on postvaccinial tuberculin sensitivity. Am J Clin Nutr 33: 2334–2337.
182. Heyworth B (1977) Delayed hypersensitivity to PPD-S following BCG vaccination in African children–an 18-month field study. Trans R Soc Trop Med Hyg 71: 251–253.
183. Smith N, Khadroui S, Lopez V, Hamza B (1977) Cellular Immune Response in Tunisian Children with Severe Infantile Malnutrition. Malnutrition and the Immune Response, Edited by Robert Suskind. New York: Raven Press, Vol. 1977.
184. Abbassy AS, el-Din MK, Hassan AI, Aref GH, Hammad SA, et al. (1974) Studies of cell-mediated immunity and allergy in protein energy malnutrition. I. Cell-mediated delayed hypersensitivity. J Trop Med Hyg 77: 13–17.
185. Harland PS (1965) Tuberculin reactions in malnourished children. Lancet 2: 719–721.
186. Puri V, Misra PK, Saxena KC, Saxsena PN, Saxena RP, et al. (1980) Immune status in malnutrition. Indian Pediatr 17: 127–133.

187. Bhaskaram C, Reddy V (1974) Cell mediated immunity in protein-calorie malnutrition. J Trop Pediatr Environ Child Health 20: 284–286.
188. Edelman R (1973) Cutaneous hypersensitivity in protein-calorie malnutrition. Lancet 1: 1244–1245.
189. Geefhuysen J, Rosen EU, Katz J, Ipp T, Metz J (1971) Impaired cellular immunity in kwashiorkor with improvement after therapy. Br Med J 4: 527–529.
190. Castillo-Duran C, Heresi G, Fisberg M, Uauy R (1987) Controlled trial of zinc supplementation during recovery from malnutrition: effects on growth and immune function. Am J Clin Nutr 45: 602–608.
191. Fakhir S, Ahmad P, Faridi MA, Rattan A (1989) Cell-mediated immune responses in malnourished host. J Trop Pediatr 35: 175–178.
192. Schlesinger L, Stekel A (1974) Impaired cellular Immunity in marasmic infants. Am J Clin Nutr 27: 615–620.
193. Ziegler HD, Ziegler PB (1975) Depression of tuberculin reaction in mild and moderate protein-calorie malnourished children following BCG vaccination. Johns Hopkins Med J 137: 59–64.
194. Golden MH, Harland PS, Golden BE, Jackson AA (1978) Zinc and immunocompetence in protein-energy malnutrition. Lancet 1: 1226–1228.
195. Schlesinger L, Arevalo M, Arredondo S, Diaz M, Lönnerdal B, et al. (1992) Effect of a zinc-fortified formula on immunocompetence and growth of malnourished infants. Am J Clin Nutr 56: 491–498.
196. Schlesinger L, Ohlbaum A, Grez L, Stekel A (1977) Cell-mediated Immune studies in Marasmic Children from Chile: Delayed Hypersensitivity, Lymphocyte transformation, and Interferon Production. Suskind RM, editor. Malnutrition and the Immune Response. New York: Raven Press, Vol. 1977.
197. Wander K, Shell-Duncan B, Brindle E, O'Connor K (2013) Predictors of delayed-type hypersensitivity to Candida albicans and anti-Epstein-Barr virus antibody among children in Kilimanjaro, Tanzania. Am J Phys Anthropol 151: 183–190. doi:10.1002/ajpa.22250.
198. Hughes SM, Amadi B, Mwiya M, Nkamba H, Mulundu G, et al. (2009) CD4 counts decline despite nutritional recovery in HIV-infected Zambian children with severe malnutrition. Pediatrics 123: e347–351. doi:10.1542/peds.2008-1316.
199. Olusi SO, Thurman GB, Goldstein AL (1980) Effect of thymosin on T-lymphocyte rosette formation in children with kwashiorkor. Clin Immunol Immunopathol 15: 687–691.
200. Mahalanabis D, Jalan KN, Chatterjee A, Maitra TK, Agarwal SK, et al. (1979) Evidence for altered density characteristics of the peripheral blood lymphocytes in kwashiorkor. Am J Clin Nutr 32: 992–996.
201. González C, González H, Rodríguez L, Cortés L, Nájera O, et al. (2006) Differential gene expression in lymphocytes from malnourished children. Cell Biol Int 30: 610–614. doi:10.1016/j.cellbi.2006.02.011.
202. El-Hodhod MAA, Nassar MF, Zaki MM, Moustafa A (2005) Apoptotic changes in lymphocytes of protein energy malnutrition patients. Nutr Res 25: 21–29. doi:10.1016/j.nutres.2004.10.005.
203. Ferguson AC, Lawlor GJ Jr, Neumann CG, Oh W, Stiehm ER (1974) Decreased rosette-forming lymphocytes in malnutrition and intrauterine growth retardation. J Pediatr 85: 717–723.
204. Bang BG, Mahalanabis D, Mukherjee KL, Bang FB (1975) T and B lymphocyte rosetting in undernourished children. Proc Soc Exp Biol Med Soc Exp Biol Med N Y N 149: 199–202.
205. Rabson AR, Geefhuyzen J, Rosen EU, Joffe M (1975) Letter: Rosette-forming T-lymphocytes in malnutrition. Br Med J 1: 40.
206. Salimonu LS, Johnson AO, Williams AI, Adeleye GI, Osunkoya BO (1982) Lymphocyte subpopulations and antibody levels in immunized malnourished children. Br J Nutr 48: 7–14.
207. Joffe MI, Kew M, Rabson AR (1983) Lymphocyte subtypes in patients with atopic eczema, protein calorie malnutrition, SLE and liver disease. J Clin Lab Immunol 10: 97–101.
208. Cruz JR, Chew F, Fernandez RA, Torun B, Goldstein AL, et al. (1987) Effects of nutritional recuperation on E-rosetting lymphocytes and in vitro response to thymosin in malnourished children. J Pediatr Gastroenterol Nutr 6: 387–391.
209. Keusch GT, Cruz JR, Torun B, Urrutia JJ, Smith H Jr, et al. (1987) Immature circulating lymphocytes in severely malnourished Guatemalan children. J Pediatr Gastroenterol Nutr 6: 265–270.
210. Fakhir S, Ahmed P, Faridi MM, Rattan A (1988) Early rosette forming T cell–a marker of cellular immunodeficiency in PEM. Indian Pediatr 25: 1017–1018.
211. Hagel I, Lynch NR, Puccio F, Rodriguez O, Luzondo R, et al. (2003) Defective regulation of the protective IgE response against intestinal helminth Ascaris lumbricoides in malnourished children. J Trop Pediatr 49: 136–142.
212. Nájera O, González C, Cortés E, Betancourt M, Ortiz R, et al. (2002) Early Activation of T, B and NK Lymphocytes in Infected Malnourished and Infected Well-Nourished Children. J Nutr Immunol 5: 85–97. doi:10.1300/J053v05n03_07.
213. Kulapongs P, Suskind R, Vithayasai V, Olson R (1977) In Vitro Cell-Mediated Immune Response in Thai Children with Protein-Calorie Malnutrition. Malnutrition and the Immune Response, Edited by Robert M Suskind. New York: Raven Press, Vol. 1977.
214. Grace HJ, Armstrong D, Smythe PM (1972) Reduced lymphocyte transformation in protein calorie malnutrition. South Afr Med J Suid-Afr Tydskr Vir Geneeskd 46: 402–403.
215. Murthy PB, Rahiman MA, Tulpule PG (1982) Lymphocyte proliferation kinetics in malnourished children measured by differential chromatid staining. Br J Nutr 47: 445–450.
216. Ortiz R, Campos C, Gómez JL, Espinoza M, Ramos-Motilla M, et al. (1995) Effect of renutrition on the proliferation kinetics of PHA stimulated lymphocytes from malnourished children. Mutat Res 334: 235–241.
217. Moore DL, Heyworth B, Brown J (1974) PHA-induced lymphocyte transformations in leucocyte cultures from malarious, malnourished and control Gambian children. Clin Exp Immunol 17: 647–656.
218. Moore DL, Heyworth B, Brown J (1977) Effects of autologous plasma on lymphocyte transformation in malaria and in acute protein-energy malnutrition. Comparison of purified lymphocyte and whole blood cultures. Immunology 33: 777–785.
219. Noureldin MS, Shaltout AA, El Hamshary EM, Ali ME (1999) Opportunistic intestinal protozoal infections in immunocompromised children. J Egypt Soc Parasitol 29: 951–961.
220. Bachou H, Tylleskär T, Downing R, Tumwine JK (2006) Severe malnutrition with and without HIV-1 infection in hospitalised children in Kampala, Uganda: differences in clinical features, haematological findings and CD4+ cell counts. Nutr J 5: 27–27. doi:10.1186/1475-2891-5-27.
221. Ndagije F, Baribwira C, Coulter JBS (2007) Micronutrients and T-cell subsets: a comparison between HIV-infected and uninfected, severely malnourished Rwandan children. Ann Trop Paediatr 27: 269–275. doi:10.1179/146532807X245652.
222. Rodríguez L, González C, Flores L, Jiménez-Zamudio L, Graniel J, et al. (2005) Assessment by flow cytometry of cytokine production in malnourished children. Clin Diagn Lab Immunol 12: 502–507. doi:10.1128/CDLI.12.4.502-507.2005.
223. Rodríguez L, Graniel J, Ortiz R (2007) Effect of leptin on activation and cytokine synthesis in peripheral blood lymphocytes of malnourished infected children. Clin Exp Immunol 148: 478–485. doi:10.1111/j.1365-2249.2007.03361.x.
224. Fakhir S, Ahmad P, Faridi MM, Rattan A (1988) Serum immunoglobulins and B cell count in protein energy malnutrition. Indian Pediatr 25: 960–965.
225. Rosen EU, Geefhuysen J, Ipp T (1971) Immunoglobulin levels in protein calorie malnutrition. South Afr Med J Suid-Afr Tydskr Vir Geneeskd 45: 980–982.
226. Cohen S, Hansen JD (1962) Metabolism of albumin and gamma-globulin in kwashiorkor. Clin Sci 23: 351–359.
227. Najjar SS, Stephan M, Asfour RY (1969) Serum levels of immunoglobulins in marasmic infants. Arch Dis Child 44: 120–123.
228. Keet MP, Thom H (1969) Serum immunoglobulins in kwashiorkor. Arch Dis Child 44: 600–603.
229. Watson CE, Freesemann C (1970) Immunoglobulins in protein-calorie malnutrition. Arch Dis Child 45: 282–284.
230. el-Gholmy A, Helmy O, Hashish S, Ragan HA, el-Gamal Y (1970) Immunoglobulins in marasmus. J Trop Med Hyg 73: 196–199.
231. el-Gholmy A, Hashish S, Helmy O, Aly RH, el-Gamal Y (1970) A study of immunoglobulins in kwashiorkor. J Trop Med Hyg 73: 192–195.
232. Aref GH, el-Din MK, Hassan AI, Araby II (1970) Immunoglobulins in kwashiorkor. J Trop Med Hyg 73: 186–191.
233. Suskind R, Sirishinha S, Vithayasai V, Edelman R, Damrongsak D, et al. (1976) Immunoglobulins and antibody response in children with protein-calorie malnutrition. Am J Clin Nutr 29: 836–841.
234. Awdeh ZL, Kanawati AK, Alami SY (1977) Antibody response in marasmic children during recovery. Acta Paediatr Scand 66: 689–692.
235. Cripps AW, Otczyk DC, Barker J, Lehmann D, Alpers MP (2008) The relationship between undernutrition and humoral immune status in children with pneumonia in Papua New Guinea. P N G Med J 51: 120–130.
236. Casazza LJ, Sunoto S, Sugiono M (1972) Immunoglobulin levels in malnourished children. Paediatr Indones 12: 263–270.
237. Taddesse WW (1988) Immunoglobulins in kwashiorkor. East Afr Med J 65: 393–396.
238. Suskind R, Sirisinha S, Edelman R, Vithayasai V, Damrongsak D, et al. (1977) Immunoglobulins and Antibody Response in Thai Children with Protein-Calirie Malnutrition. Suskind RM, editor. Malnutrition and the Immune Response. New York: Raven Press, Vol. 1977.
239. Forte WCN, Santos de Menezes MC, Horta C, Carneiro Leão Bach R (2003) Serum IgE level in malnutrition. Allergol Immunopathol (Madr) 31: 83–86.
240. Pretorius PJ, De Villiers LS (1962) Antibody response in children with protein malnutrition. Am J Clin Nutr 10: 379–383.
241. el-Gamal Y, Aly RH, Hossny E, Afify E, el-Taliawy D (1996) Response of Egyptian infants with protein calorie malnutrition to hepatitis B vaccination. J Trop Pediatr 42: 144–145.
242. Powell GM (1982) Response to live attenuated measles vaccine in children with severe kwashiorkor. Ann Trop Paediatr 2: 143–145.
243. Brown RE, Katz M (1966) Failure of antibody production to yellow fever vaccine in children with kwashiorkor. Trop Geogr Med 18: 125–128.
244. Brown RE, Katz M (1965) Antigenic Stimulation in Undernourished Children. East Afr Med J 42: 221–232.
245. Wesley A, Coovadia HM, Watson AR (1979) Immunization against measles in children at risk for severe disease. Trans R Soc Trop Med Hyg 73: 710–715.

246. el-Molla A, el-Ghoroury A, Hussein M, Badr-el-Din MK, Hassen AH, et al. (1973) Antibody production in protein calorie malnutrition. J Trop Med Hyg 76: 248–250.
247. Reddy V, Srikantia SG (1964) Antibody Response in Kwashiorkor. Indian J Med Res 52: 1154–1158.
248. Brown RE, Katz M (1966) Smallpox vaccination in malnourished children. Trop Geogr Med 18: 129–132.
249. Paul S, Saini L, Grover S, Ray K, Ray SN, et al. (1979) Immune response in malnutrition–study following routine DPT immunization! Indian Pediatr 16: 3–10.
250. Ekunwe EO (1985) Malnutrition and seroconversion following measles immunization. J Trop Pediatr 31: 290–291.
251. Halsey NA, Boulos R, Mode F, Andre J, Bowman L, et al. (1985) Response to measles vaccine in Haitian infants 6 to 12 months old. Influence of maternal antibodies, malnutrition, and concurrent illnesses. N Engl J Med 313: 544–549. doi:10.1056/NEJM198508293130904.
252. Baer CL, Bratt DE, Edwards R, McFarlane H, Utermohlen V (1986) Response of mildly to moderately malnourished children to measles vaccination. West Indian Med J 35: 106–111.
253. Smedman L, Silva MC, Gunnlaugsson G, Norrby E, Zetterstrom R (1986) Augmented antibody response to live attenuated measles vaccine in children with Plasmodium falciparum parasitaemia. Ann Trop Paediatr 6: 149–153.
254. Smedman L, Gunnlaugsson G, Norrby E, Silva MC, Zetterström R (1988) Follow-up of the antibody response to measles vaccine in a rural area of Guinea-Bissau. Acta Paediatr Scand 77: 885–889.
255. Bhaskaram P, Madhusudan J, Radhrakrishna KV, Raj S (1986) Immunological response to measles vaccination in poor communities. Hum Nutr Clin Nutr 40: 295–299.
256. Chopra K, Kundu S, Chowdhury DS (1989) Antibody response of infants in tropics to five doses of oral polio vaccine. J Trop Pediatr 35: 19–23.
257. Greenwood BM, Bradley AK, Blakebrough IS, Whittle HC, Marshall TF, et al. (1980) The immune response to a meningococcal polysaccharide vaccine in an African village. Trans R Soc Trop Med Hyg 74: 340–346.
258. Asturias EJ, Mayorga C, Caffaro C, Ramirez P, Ram M, et al. (2009) Differences in the immune response to hepatitis B and Haemophilus influenzae type b vaccines in Guatemalan infants by ethnic group and nutritional status. Vaccine 27: 3650–3654. doi:10.1016/j.vaccine.2009.03.035.
259. Waibale P, Bowlin SJ, Mortimer EA Jr, Whalen C (1999) The effect of human immunodeficiency virus-1 infection and stunting on measles immunoglobulin-G levels in children vaccinated against measles in Uganda. Int J Epidemiol 28: 341–346.
260. Kahn E, Stein H, Zoutendyk A (1957) Isohemagglutinins and immunity in malnutrition. Am J Clin Nutr 5: 70–71.
261. Fillol F, Sarr JB, Boulanger D, Cisse B, Sokhna C, et al. (2009) Impact of child malnutrition on the specific anti-Plasmodium falciparum antibody response. Malar J 8: 116. doi:10.1186/1475-2875-8-116.
262. Brüssow H, Sidoti J, Dirren H, Freire WB (1995) Effect of malnutrition in Ecuadorian children on titers of serum antibodies to various microbial antigens. Clin Diagn Lab Immunol 2: 62–68.
263. Lomnitzer R, Rosen EU, Geefhuysen J, Rabson AR (1976) Defective leucocyte inhibitory factor (LIF) production by lymphocytes in children with kwashiorkor. South Afr Med J Suid-Afr Tydskr Vir Geneeskd 50: 1820–1822.
264. Heresi GP, Saitúa MT, Schlesinger L (1981) Leukocyte migration inhibition factor production in marasmic infants. Am J Clin Nutr 34: 909–913.
265. Salimonu LS, Johnson AO, Williams AI, Adeleye GI, Osunkoya BO (1982) The occurrence and properties of E rosette inhibitory substance in the sera of malnourished children. Clin Exp Immunol 47: 626–634.
266. Kobielowa Z, Turowski G, Szumera B, Lankosz-Lauterbach J (1979) Direct lymphocytotoxic test in protein-calorie malnutrition in infants. Acta Med Pol 20: 265–272.
267. Beatty DW, Dowdle EB (1979) Deficiency in kwashiorkor serum of factors required for optimal lymphocyte transformation in vitro. Clin Exp Immunol 35: 433–442.
268. Heyworth B, Moore DL, Brown J (1975) Depression of lymphocyte response to phytohaemagglutinin in the presence of plasma from children with acute protein energy malnutrition. Clin Exp Immunol 22: 72–77.
269. Bhaskaram P, Sivakumar B (1986) Interleukin-1 in malnutrition. Arch Dis Child 61: 182–185.
270. Aslan Y, Erduran E, Gedik Y, Mocan H, Okten A, et al. (1996) Serum interleukin-1 and granulocyte-macrophage colony-stimulating factor levels in protein malnourished patients during acute infection. Cent Afr J Med 42: 179–184.
271. Dülger H, Arik M, Sekeroğlu MR, Tarakçioğlu M, Noyan T, et al. (2002) Pro-inflammatory cytokines in Turkish children with protein-energy malnutrition. Mediators Inflamm 11: 363–365. doi:10.1080/09629350210000051566.
272. Bartz S, Mody A, Hornik C, Bain J, Muehlbauer M, et al. (2014) Severe acute malnutrition in childhood: hormonal and metabolic status at presentation, response to treatment, and predictors of mortality. J Clin Endocrinol Metab 99: 2128–2137. doi:10.1210/jc.2013-4018.
273. González-Martínez H, Rodríguez L, Nájera O, Cruz D, Miliar A, et al. (2008) Expression of cytokine mRNA in lymphocytes of malnourished children. J Clin Immunol 28: 593–599. doi:10.1007/s10875-008-9204-5.
274. González-Torres C, González-Martínez H, Miliar A, Nájera O, Graniel J, et al. (2013) Effect of malnutrition on the expression of cytokines involved in Th1 cell differentiation. Nutrients 5: 579–593. doi:10.3390/nu5020579.
275. Solis B, Samartín S, Gómez S, Nova E, de la Rosa B, et al. (2002) Probiotics as a help in children suffering from malnutrition and diarrhoea. Eur J Clin Nutr 56 Suppl 3: S57–59. doi:10.1038/sj.ejcn.1601488.
276. Palacio A, Lopez M, Perez-Bravo F, Monkeberg F, Schlesinger L (2002) Leptin levels are associated with immune response in malnourished infants. J Clin Endocrinol Metab 87: 3040–3046.
277. Abo-Shousha SA, Hussein MZ, Rashwan IA, Salama M (2005) Production of proinflammatory cytokines: granulocyte-macrophage colony stimulating factor, interleukin-8 and interleukin-6 by peripheral blood mononuclear cells of protein energy malnourished children. Egypt J Immunol Egypt Assoc Immunol 12: 125–131.
278. Doherty JF, Golden MH, Remick DG, Griffin GE (1994) Production of interleukin-6 and tumour necrosis factor-alpha in vitro is reduced in whole blood of severely malnourished children. Clin Sci Lond Engl 1979 86: 347–351.
279. Giovambattista A, Spinedi E, Sanjurjo A, Chisari A, Rodrigo M, et al. (2000) Circulating and mitogen-induced tumor necrosis factor (TNF) in malnourished children. Medicina (Mex) 60: 339–342.
280. Hemalatha R, Bhaskaram P, Balakrishna N, Saraswathi I (2002) Association of tumour necrosis factor alpha & malnutrition with outcome in children with acute bacterial meningitis. Indian J Med Res 115: 55–58.
281. Mayatepek E, Becker K, Hoffmann G, Leichsenring M, Gana L (1993) Leukotrienes in the pathophysiology of kwashiorkor. The Lancet 342: 958–960. doi:10.1016/0140-6736(93)92003-C.
282. Iputo JE, Sammon AM, Tindimwebwa G (2002) Prostaglandin E2 is raised in kwashiorkor. South Afr Med J Suid-Afr Tydskr Vir Geneeskd 92: 310–312.
283. Morgan G (1997) What, if any, is the effect of malnutrition on immunological competence? Lancet 349: 1693–1695. doi:10.1016/S0140-6736(96)12038-9.
284. Saxinger WC, Levine PH, Dean AG, de Thé G, Lange-Wantzin G, et al. (1985) Evidence for exposure to HTLV-III in Uganda before 1973. Science 227: 1036–1038.
285. Prendergast A, Kelly P (2012) Enteropathies in the developing world: neglected effects on global health. Am J Trop Med Hyg 86: 756–763. doi:10.4269/ajtmh.2012.11-0743.
286. Keusch GT, Rosenberg IH, Denno DM, Duggan C, Guerrant RL, et al. (2013) Implications of acquired environmental enteric dysfunction for growth and stunting in infants and children living in low- and middle-income countries. Food Nutr Bull 34: 357–364.
287. Campbell DI, Elia M, Lunn PG (2003) Growth faltering in rural Gambian infants is associated with impaired small intestinal barrier function, leading to endotoxemia and systemic inflammation. J Nutr 133: 1332–1338.
288. Basso AS, Cheroutre H, Mucida D (2009) More stories on Th17 cells. Cell Res 19: 399–411. doi:10.1038/cr.2009.26.
289. Opal SM, DePalo VA (2000) Anti-inflammatory cytokines. Chest 117: 1162–1172.
290. Manary MJ, Yarasheski KE, Smith S, Abrams ET, Hart CA (2004) Protein quantity, not protein quality, accelerates whole-body leucine kinetics and the acute-phase response during acute infection in marasmic Malawian children. Br J Nutr 92: 589–595.
291. Howard JK, Lord GM, Matarese G, Vendetti S, Ghatei MA, et al. (1999) Leptin protects mice from starvation-induced lymphoid atrophy and increases thymic cellularity in ob/ob mice. J Clin Invest 104: 1051–1059. doi:10.1172/JCI6762.
292. De Mello-Coelho V, Savino W, Postel-Vinay MC, Dardenne M (1998) Role of prolactin and growth hormone on thymus physiology. Dev Immunol 6: 317–323.
293. Savino W, Postel-Vinay MC, Smaniotto S, Dardenne M (2002) The thymus gland: a target organ for growth hormone. Scand J Immunol 55: 442–452.
294. Hansen BR, Kolte L, Haugaard SB, Dirksen C, Jensen FK, et al. (2009) Improved thymic index, density and output in HIV-infected patients following low-dose growth hormone therapy: a placebo controlled study. AIDS Lond Engl 23: 2123–2131. doi:10.1097/QAD.0b013e3283303307.
295. Barone KS, O'Brien PC, Stevenson JR (1993) Characterization and mechanisms of thymic atrophy in protein-malnourished mice: role of corticosterone. Cell Immunol 148: 226–233. doi:10.1006/cimm.1993.1105.
296. Haeryfar SM, Berczi I (2001) The thymus and the acute phase response. Cell Mol Biol Noisy-Gd Fr 47: 145–156.
297. Golden MH, Jackson AA, Golden BE (1977) Effect of zinc on thymus of recently malnourished children. Lancet 2: 1057–1059.
298. Chevalier P (1995) Zinc and duration of treatment of severe malnutrition. Lancet 345: 1046–1047.
299. Miedema F, Hazenberg MD, Tesselaar K, van Baarle D, de Boer RJ, et al. (2013) Immune Activation and Collateral Damage in AIDS Pathogenesis. Front Immunol 4: 298. doi:10.3389/fimmu.2013.00298.
300. Cobbold SP (2013) The mTOR pathway and integrating immune regulation. Immunology. doi:10.1111/imm.12162.
301. Peter C, Waldmann H, Cobbold SP (2010) mTOR signalling and metabolic regulation of T cell differentiation. Curr Opin Immunol 22: 655–661. doi:10.1016/j.coi.2010.08.010.
302. Monk JM, Steevels TAM, Hillyer LM, Woodward B (2011) Constitutive, but not challenge-induced, interleukin-10 production is robust in acute pre-

pubescent protein and energy deficits: new support for the tolerance hypothesis of malnutrition-associated immune depression based on cytokine production in vivo. Int J Environ Res Public Health 8: 117–135. doi:10.3390/ijerph8010117.
303. Monk JM, Richard CL, Woodward B (2011) A non-inflammatory form of immune competence prevails in acute pre-pubescent malnutrition: new evidence based on critical mRNA transcripts in the mouse. Br J Nutr: 1–5. doi:10.1017/S0007114511004399.
304. Lo MS, Zurakowski D, Son MB, Sundel RP (2013) Hypergammaglobulinemia in the pediatric population as a marker for underlying autoimmune disease: a retrospective cohort study. Pediatr Rheumatol Online J 11: 42. doi:10.1186/1546-0096-11-42.
305. Chen M, Daha MR, Kallenberg CGM (2010) The complement system in systemic autoimmune disease. J Autoimmun 34: J276–J286. doi:10.1016/j.jaut.2009.11.014.

PERMISSIONS

All chapters in this book were first published in PLOS ONE, by The Public Library of Science; hereby published with permission under the Creative Commons Attribution License or equivalent. Every chapter published in this book has been scrutinized by our experts. Their significance has been extensively debated. The topics covered herein carry significant findings which will fuel the growth of the discipline. They may even be implemented as practical applications or may be referred to as a beginning point for another development.

The contributors of this book come from diverse backgrounds, making this book a truly international effort. This book will bring forth new frontiers with its revolutionizing research information and detailed analysis of the nascent developments around the world.

We would like to thank all the contributing authors for lending their expertise to make the book truly unique. They have played a crucial role in the development of this book. Without their invaluable contributions this book wouldn't have been possible. They have made vital efforts to compile up to date information on the varied aspects of this subject to make this book a valuable addition to the collection of many professionals and students.

This book was conceptualized with the vision of imparting up-to-date information and advanced data in this field. To ensure the same, a matchless editorial board was set up. Every individual on the board went through rigorous rounds of assessment to prove their worth. After which they invested a large part of their time researching and compiling the most relevant data for our readers.

The editorial board has been involved in producing this book since its inception. They have spent rigorous hours researching and exploring the diverse topics which have resulted in the successful publishing of this book. They have passed on their knowledge of decades through this book. To expedite this challenging task, the publisher supported the team at every step. A small team of assistant editors was also appointed to further simplify the editing procedure and attain best results for the readers.

Apart from the editorial board, the designing team has also invested a significant amount of their time in understanding the subject and creating the most relevant covers. They scrutinized every image to scout for the most suitable representation of the subject and create an appropriate cover for the book.

The publishing team has been an ardent support to the editorial, designing and production team. Their endless efforts to recruit the best for this project, has resulted in the accomplishment of this book. They are a veteran in the field of academics and their pool of knowledge is as vast as their experience in printing. Their expertise and guidance has proved useful at every step. Their uncompromising quality standards have made this book an exceptional effort. Their encouragement from time to time has been an inspiration for everyone.

The publisher and the editorial board hope that this book will prove to be a valuable piece of knowledge for researchers, students, practitioners and scholars across the globe.

LIST OF CONTRIBUTORS

Steve Collins
Valid International, Oxford, United Kingdom

Marko Kerac
Valid International, Oxford, United Kingdom
Department of Paediatrics and Child Health, College of Medicine, Blantyre, Malawi
Institute for Global Health, University College London, London, United Kingdom
Leonard Cheshire Disability and Inclusive Development Centre, University College London, London, United Kingdom

Paluku Bahwere
Valid International, Oxford, United Kingdom
Centre of Research in Epidemiology, Biostatistics and Clinical Research, Free University of Brussels, Brussels, Belgium

James Bunn
Department of Paediatrics and Child Health, College of Medicine, Blantyre, Malawi
Liverpool School of Tropical Medicine, Liverpool, United Kingdom

George Chagaluka
Department of Paediatrics and Child Health, College of Medicine, Blantyre, Malawi

Andrew Tomkins and Andrew Seal
Institute for Global Health, University College London, London, United Kingdom

Hwajiun Chen and Chun-Yao Chen
Department of Life Science, Tzu-Chi University, Hualien, Taiwan
Institute of Medical Sciences, Tzu-Chi University, Hualien, Taiwan
David T. Bolick, James K. Roche, Relana F. Pinkerton and Cirle A. Warren
Division of Infectious Diseases and International Medicine, Center for Global Health, School of Medicine, University of Virginia, Charlottesville, Virginia, United States of America

Aldo A. M. Lima and Richard L. Guerrant
Division of Infectious Diseases and International Medicine, Center for Global Health, School of Medicine, University of Virginia, Charlottesville, Virginia, United States of America
Laboratory of Infectious Diseases, Clinical Research Unit, Institute of the Brazilian Semi-Arid, School of Medicine, Federal University of Ceara, Fortaleza, Ceará, Brazil

Orleâncio G. R. Azevedo and Reinaldo B. Oriá
Division of Infectious Diseases and International Medicine, Center for Global Health, School of Medicine, University of Virginia, Charlottesville, Virginia, United States of America
Laboratory of the Biology of Tissue Healing, Ontogeny and Nutrition, Institute of the Brazilian Semi-arid, School of Medicine, Federal University of Ceara, Fortaleza, Ceará, Brazil

Michael P. Vitek
Duke University Medical Center, Department of Medicine, Durham, North Carolina, United States of America

Milinda Lakkam
Institute for Computational and Mathematical Engineering, Stanford University, Stanford, California, United States of America

Stefan Wager
Statistics Department, Stanford University, Stanford, California, United States of America

Paul H. Wise
School of Medicine, Stanford University, Stanford California, United States of America

Lawrence M. Wein
Graduate School of Business, Stanford University, Stanford, California, United States of America

Catarina Cardoso, Tatsiana Charnikhova, Muhammad Jamila and Maryam Aminic
Laboratory of Plant Physiology, Wageningen University, Wageningen, the Netherlands

Francel Verstappen and Harro Bouwmeester
Laboratory of Plant Physiology, Wageningen University, Wageningen, the Netherlands
Centre for Biosystems Genomics, Wageningen, the Netherlands

Carolien Ruyter-Spira
Laboratory of Plant Physiology, Wageningen University, Wageningen, the Netherlands France

Bioscience, Plant Research International, Wageningen, the Netherlands

Pierre-Marc Delauxb and Dominique Lauressergue
Laboratoire de Recherche en Sciences Végétales, Unité Mixte de Recherche
(UMR) 5546, Université de Toulouse, Castanet-Tolosan, France
Laboratoire de Recherche en Sciences Végétales, Unité Mixte de Recherche (UMR) 5546, Centre National de la Recherche Scientifique (CNRS), Castanet-Tolosan

Seyed-Mohammad Fereshtehnejad
Division of Clinical Geriatrics, Department of Neurobiology, Care Sciences, and Society (NVS), Karolinska Institutet, Stockholm, Sweden
Firoozgar Clinical Research vDevelopment Center (FCRDC), Firoozgar Hospital, Iran University of Medical Sciences, Tehran, Iran

Ahmad Delbari
Division of Clinical Geriatrics, Department of Neurobiology, Care Sciences, and Society (NVS), Karolinska Institutet, Stockholm, Sweden
Aging Research Center, Sabzevar University of Medical Sciences, Sabzevar, Khorasan, Iran

Johan Lökk
Division of Clinical Geriatrics, Department of Neurobiology, Care Sciences, and Society (NVS), Karolinska Institutet, Stockholm, Sweden
Department of Geriatric Medicine, Karolinska University Hospital, Stockholm, Sweden

Ladan Ghazi
Department of Biosciences and Nutrition, Karolinska Institutet, Stockholm, Sweden

Mahdiyeh Shafieesabet
Medical Students Research Committee (MSRC), Faculty of Medicine, Iran University of Medical Sciences, Tehran, Iran

Gholam Ali Shahidi
Movement Disorders Clinic, Department of Neurology, Faculty of Medicine, Iran University of Medical Sciences, Tehran, Iran

Kirsten R. Poore, Lisa J. Hollis, Robert J. S. Murray, Anna Warlow, Andrew Brewin, Laurence Fulford, Jane K. Cleal, Karen A. Lillycrop, Graham C. Burdge, Mark A. Hanson and Lucy R. Green
Academic Unit of Human Development and Health, Faculty of Medicine, University of Southampton, Southampton, United Kingdom

Eva Nouri, Florence Breuillin-Sessoms and Didier Reinhardt
Dept. of Biology, University of Fribourg, Fribourg, Switzerland

Urs Feller
Institute of Plant Science, University of Bern, Bern, Switzerland

Giancarlo A. Valle and Julio A. Poterico
CRONICAS Center of Excellence in Chronic Diseases, Universidad Peruana Cayetano Heredia, Lima, Peru

Christian Loret de Mola
CRONICAS Center of Excellence in Chronic Diseases, Universidad Peruana Cayetano Heredia, Lima, Peru
Post-Graduate Program in Epidemiology, Federal University of Pelotas, Pelotas, Rio Grande do Sul, Brazil

Renato Quispe
CRONICAS Center of Excellence in Chronic Diseases, Universidad Peruana Cayetano Heredia, Lima, Peru
CONEVID Unidad de Conocimiento y Evidencia, Universidad Peruana Cayetano Heredia, Lima, Peru

Jason M. Nagata
School of Medicine, University of California, San Francisco, San Francisco, California, United States of America

Craig R. Cohen
Department of Obstetrics, Gynecology and Reproductive Sciences, University of California, San Francisco, San Francisco, California, United States of America

Sera L. Young
Division of Nutritional Sciences, Cornell University, Ithaca, New York, United States of America

Catherine Wamuyu, Mary N. Armes, Elizabeth A. Bukusi and Benard O. Otieno
Family AIDS Care and Education Services, Center for Microbiology Research, Kenya Medical Research Institute, Nairobi, Kenya

Hannah H. Leslie
Division of Epidemiology, University of California, Berkeley, Berkeley, California, United States of America

Madhavi Dandu
Division of Hospital Medicine, University of California, San Francisco, San Francisco, California, United States of America

Christopher C. Stewart
Department of Pediatrics, University of California, San Francisco, San Francisco, California, United States of America

Sheri D. Weiser
Division of HIV/AIDS, University of California, San Francisco, San Francisco, California, United States of America

Eugenia Carrillo, Carmen Sanchez and Javier Moreno
WHO Collaborating Centre for Leishmaniasis, Centro Nacional de Microbiología, Instituto de Salud Carlos III, Madrid, Spain

MaAngeles Jimenez
Departamento Medicina y Cirugía Animal, Facultad de Veterinaria, Universidad Complutense de Madrid, Madrid, Spain

Joana Cunha
Instituto de Biología Molecular e Celular, Instituto de Ciências Biomédicas Abel Salazare Faculdade de Medicina, Universidade do Porto, Porto, Portugal

Camila Marinelli Martins and Anaiá da Paixão Sevá
Departamento Medicina Veterinária Preventiva e Saúde Animal, Faculdade de Medicina Veterináriae Zootecnia da Universidade de São Paulo, São Paulo, Brazil

Masoud Vaezghasemi and Ann Öhman
Department of Public Health and Clinical Medicine, Division of Epidemiology and Global Health, Umeå University, Umeå Sweden
UmeåCentre for Global Health Research, Umeå University, Umeå, Sweden, Umeå Centre for Gender Studies, Umeå University, Umeå, Sweden

Malin Eriksson, Lars Weinehall and Nawi Ng
Department of Public Health and Clinical Medicine, Division of Epidemiology and Global Health, Umeå University, Umeå, Sweden
Umeå Centre for Global Health Research, Umeå University, Umeå, Sweden

Mohammad Hakimi
Centre for Health and Nutrition Research Laboratory, Faculty of Medicine, Gadjah Mada University, Yogyakarta, Indonesia

Hari Kusnanto
Centre for Environmental Studies, Faculty of Medicine, Gadjah Mada University, Yogyakarta, Indonesia

Tarini Shankar Ghosh, Tanudeep Bhattacharya, Deepak Yadav and Sharmila S. Mande
Bio Sciences R&D, TCS Innovation Labs, Pune, India

Sourav Sen Gupta, Bhabatosh Das and G. Balakrish Nair
Center for Human Microbial Ecology, Translational Health Science and Technology Institute, Gurgaon, India

Anamitra Barik
Society for Health and Demographic Surveillance, West Bengal, India

Abhijit Chowdhury
Society for Health and Demographic Surveillance, West Bengal, India
Department of Hepatology, School of Digestive and Liver Diseases, Institute of Post Graduate Medical Education and Research, Kolkata, India

Els Willems, Johan Buyse and Eddy Decuypere
Laboratory of Livestock Physiology, Department of Biosystems, KU Leuven, Leuven, Belgium

Nadia Everaert
Laboratory of Livestock Physiology, Department of Biosystems, KU Leuven, Leuven, Belgium
Animal Science Unit, Gembloux Agro-Bio Tech, University of Liége, Gembloux, Belgium

Tjing-Tjing Hu and Lutgarde Arckens
Laboratory of Neuroplasticity and Neuroproteomics, KU Leuven, Leuven, Belgium

Laura Soler Vasco
Division of Livestock-Nutrition-Quality, Department of Biosystems, KU Leuven, Leuven, Belgium

Aaloke Mody and Sarah Bartz
Division of Pediatric Endocrinology and Diabetes, Pediatric Division of Quantitative Sciences, Duke University Medical Center, Durham, North Carolina, United States of America

Michael Freemark
Division of Pediatric Endocrinology and Diabetes, Pediatric Division of Quantitative Sciences, Duke University Medical Center, Durham, North Carolina, United States of America
Sarah W. Stedman Nutrition and Metabolism Center, Duke University Medical Center, Durham, North Carolina, United States of America
Duke Global Health Institute, Duke University Medical Center, Durham, North Carolina, United States of America

Christoph P. Hornik
Duke Clinical Research Institute, Duke University Medical Center, Durham, North Carolina, United States of America

James Bain, Michael Muehlbauer, Robert Stevens and Christopher B. Newgard
Sarah W. Stedman Nutrition and Metabolism Center, Duke University Medical Center, Durham, North Carolina, United States of America

John Bartlett
Duke Global Health Institute, Duke University Medical Center, Durham, North Carolina, United States of America

John V. St. Peter
Global Research & Development, Long Term Research, PepsiCo, Inc., Purchase, New York, United States of America

Elizabeth Kiboneka and Tonny Kiyimba
Mwanamugimu Nutrition Unit, Mulago Hospital Complex, Kampala, Uganda
Bruno F. Sunguya, Linda B. Mlunde, Junko Yasuoka and Masamine Jimba
Department of Community and Global Health, Graduate School of Medicine, The University of Tokyo, Tokyo, Japan

Krishna C. Poudel
Department of Public Health, School of Public Health and Health Sciences, University of Massachusetts Amherst, Amherst, Massachusetts, United States of America

David P. Urassa
School of Public Health and Social Sciences, Muhimbili University of Health and Allied Sciences, Dares Salaam, Tanzania

Linda Ambrosio, Stephanie Morriss, Ryan Bailey and Gustavo C. MacIntosh
Roy J. Carver Department of Biochemistry, Biophysics and Molecular Biology, Iowa State University, Ames, Iowa, United States of America

Ayesha Riaz
Interdepartmental Genetics Graduate Program, Iowa State University, Ames, Iowa, United States of America

Jian Ding
Children's Hospital Boston, Harvard Medical School, Boston, Massachusetts, United States of America

Shari E. Smith, Sarah A. Figley and Phyllis G. Paterson
College of Pharmacy and Nutrition, University of Saskatchewan, Saskatoon, Saskatchewan, Canada
Cameco MS Neuroscience Research Center, Saskatoon City Hospital, Saskatoon, Saskatchewan, Canada

David J. Schreyer
Department of Anatomy and Cell Biology, University of Saskatchewan, Saskatoon, Saskatchewan, Canada
Cameco MS Neuroscience Research Center, Saskatoon City Hospital, Saskatoon, Saskatchewan, Canada

Bharati J. Bhadbhade
Department of Microbiology, Abasaheb Garware College, Pune, Maharashtra, India

Ulfat I. Baig
Department of Microbiology, Abasaheb Garware College, Pune, Maharashtra, India
Department of Biology, Indian Institute of Science Education and Research, Pune, Maharashtra, India

Dincy Mariyam and Milind G. Watve
Department of Biology, Indian Institute of Science Education and Research, Pune, Maharashtra, India

Zaida Herrador, Agustín Benito and Estefania Custodio
National Centre of Tropical Medicine, Instituto de Salud Carlos III (ISCIII), Madrid, Spain
Tropical Diseases Research Network (RICET in Spanish), Madrid, Spain

Luis Sordo
National Centre of Epidemiology, ISCIII, Madrid, Spain
Department of Preventive Medicine and Public Health, Faculty of Medicine, Complutense University, Madrid, Spain
Network Biomedical Research Centers, Epidemiology and Public Health (CIBERESP in Spanish), Madrid, Spain

Endalamaw Gadisa and Abraham Aseffa
Armauer Hansen Research Institute, Addis Ababa, Ethiopia

Javier Moreno, Javier Nieto and Carmen Cañavate
National Centre of Microbiology, ISCIII, Madrid, Spain

Maren Johanne Heilskov Rytter and Henrik Friis
Department of Nutrition, Exercise and Sports, Faculty of Science, University of Copenhagen, Frederiksberg, Denmark

André Briend
Department of Nutrition, Exercise and Sports, Faculty of Science, University of Copenhagen, Frederiksberg, Denmark
Department for International Health, University of Tampere, School of Medicine, Tampere, Finland

Lilian Kolte
Department of Infectious Diseases, Copenhagen University Hospital, Hvidovre, Denmark

Vibeke Brix Christensen
Department of Paediatrics, Copenhagen University Hospital Rigshospitalet, Copenhagen, Denmark

Index